AN INTEGRATED VIEW OF THE MOLECULAR RECOGNITION AND TOXINOLOGY - FROM ANALYTICAL PROCEDURES TO BIOMEDICAL APPLICATIONS

Edited by **Gandhi Rádis Baptista**

An Integrated View of the Molecular Recognition and Toxinology - From Analytical Procedures to Biomedical Applications

http://dx.doi.org/10.5772/3429
Edited by Gandhi Rádis Baptista

Contributors

Miguel Reyes-Parada, Jerzy Radecki, Lida Khalafi, Mohammad Rafiee, Takashiro Akitsu, Luba Tchertanov, Rohit Arora, Yasushi Sako, Yoshiko Miura, Noriyuki Koizumi, Koji Mikami, Camila Yonamine, Ricardo Cunha, Jose M. Manuel Perez De La Lastra, Lourdes Mateos-Hernández, José De La Fuente, Elena Crespo, Silvana Giuliatti, Pawel Brzuzan, Maciej Woźny, Lidia Wolińska, Michał K. Łuczyński, Márcia Mortari, Alexandra Olimpio Siqueira Cunha, Matheus Freitas Fernandes-Pedrosa, Juliana Félix-Silva, Yamara Arruda Silva De Menezes Menezes, Ana Marisa Chudzinski-Tavassi, Linda Christian Carrijo-Carvalho, Maria Esther Ricci-Silva, Miryam Paola Alvarez-Flores, Leonardo Puerta, José Cantillo, Mirian A.F. Hayashi, Claudiana Lameu, Márcia Neiva, Yasser Ezzat Shahein, Amira Abouelella, Ragaa Hamed, Alba Torres, Yves Quinet, Alexandre Havt, Gandhi Rádis-Baptista, Alice Martins

Published by InTech

Janeza Trdine 9, 51000 Rijeka, Croatia

Publishing Process Manager Sandra Bakic
Typesetting InTech DTP Team
Cover InTech Design Team

Additional hard copies can be obtained from orders@intechopen.com

An Integrated View of the Molecular Recognition and Toxinology - From Analytical Procedures to Biomedical Applications, Edited by Gandhi Rádis Baptista
p. cm.
ISBN 978-953-51-1151-1

For EU product safety concerns:
IN TECH d.o.o., Prolaz Marije Krucifikse Kozulić 3, 51000 Rijeka, Croatia,
info@intechopen.com or visit our website at intechopen.com.

Meet the editor

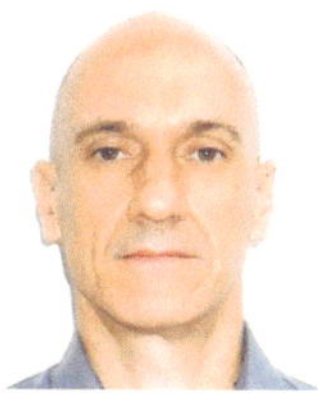

Gandhi Radis-Baptista obtained his BS degree in Pharmacy and Biochemistry from University of São Paulo (USP) in 1993; his MSc in Technology of Fermentation in 1996, and his PhD in Life Sciences (Biochemistry) in 2002, both from USP. He was associate researcher in the Butantan Institute, SP (2002-2003). Dr. Radis-Baptista participated in several scientific missions to the National Institute of Advanced Industrial Science and Technology (AIST/MITI), Japan and to the Biomedical Research Park in Barcelona, Spain. He served as an Associate Professor in the Department of Biochemistry at Federal University of Pernambuco (2005-2008). Presently, he is Associate Professor at the Institute of Marine Sciences (UFCE). His main scientific interests are polypeptides from marine and terrestrial organisms, cell receptors, molecular interaction, recombinant DNA technology, and drug discovery from nature.

Contents

Preface

Molecular Toxinology has been consolidated as a scientific field focused on the intertwined description of ecological, biochemical, clinical, pharmacological and structural aspects of animal toxins. In an inquiring biological world, where the practical scientific responses are given ultimately to improve the human health, animal toxins have arisen as an invaluable source for the discovery of therapeutic peptides and proteins. Both basic and applied research in academy and pharmaceutical industries are granted and benefited from million of years of natural history by which families of toxins in animal venoms have evolved and were improved in terms of selectivity and target specificity. Another advantage is that nature has selected several toxin structures and scaffolds to act effectively as poison but indeed have similar counterparts in the human body. No matter if organic or polypeptide, animal toxins rely on specific chemical interactions with their partner molecule to exert their biological actions.

Obviously, better the comprehension of how molecules interact and discriminate (recognize) their target, better the benefits we can achieve for rational exploration of the bioactive peptides and polypeptides as therapeutics. In this respect, a deep investigation of the molecular mechanism of interaction and recognition by which a given polypeptide acts as ligand or target molecule offers a window of opportunities for the pharmaceutical industry and clinical medicine.

This book is dedicated to present to the reader selected elegant examples of two interconnected themes - molecular recognition and toxinology–concerning to the integration between analytical procedures and biomedical applications. With this aim, the book is divided in three sections, where the first combines chapters on molecular toxinology, the second deals on molecular cloning and genetics, and the third brings into focus basic and applied works on molecular recognition.

Thus, by means of proteomic and pharmacological concepts, Cunha's group (Chapter 1) and Fernandes-Pedrosa (Chapter 2) describe several examples of venom toxins from the main poisonous animal groups and illustrate the potential application of isolated venom components to modulate physiological and pathological processes, particularly, in mammals. In Chapter 3, Mortari and Siqueira Cunha present a comprehensive review concerning to the arthropod neurotoxic polypeptides useful for target-driven drug discovery, and in Chapter 4 Giuliatti shows in detail how to apply distinct computational methods to elaborate three-dimensional protein models and search for binders and ligands. Lameu and collaborators, in Chapter 5, review the multiple biological roles of venom bradikinin potetiating peptides–a component of kallikrein-kinin system–and the importance of these molecules in programs of drug development for the treatment of cardiovascular diseases. In Chapter 6, Yanomine and co-workers discuss about serine proteases from snake venom, taking into account the cloning, expression and use of this class of thrombin-like enzymes in controlling coagulopathies. In Chapter 7, Chudzinski-Tavassi's group paradigmatically covers robust analytical procedures to understand the Lonomia obliqua (caterpillar) envenomation, compositional determination of bristle secretion, and biomedical application of its components on blood coagulation system. In a moment that several species of hymenoptera have their genome sequenced and annotated, Torres and co-authors bring to view, in Chapter 8, the current status and recent progress on the venom from ants, dedicating particular attention to the giant ant Dinoponera quadriceps. Connecting the molecular mechanism by which toxins induce tissue damage, Bruzan and collaborators (Chapter 9) elegantly discuss the role of miRNA in the mechanism of intoxication caused by microcystin - a hepatotoxin produced by cyanobacteria.

Section two is opened with a work written by Perez de la Lastra et al. (Chapter 10) devoted to the identification of key components from vulture immune system involved in the neutralization of noxious microorganisms taking during carcass feeding. Related to host mechanisms of detoxification and control of disease-causing plague's vector, the article authored by Shahein et al. (Chapter 11) introduces the genetic, structural and functional characteristics of GST from ticks and its amenability to serve as an antigen for parasite killing using anti-tick vaccines. In connection, Castillo & Porta (Chapter 12) focus on presenting concepts and practice of preparing structurally modified recombinant allergens for diagnosis and allergen-specific immunotherapy to treat allergy syndrome. In biotechnology, different biological platforms are used for genome modification and developed for recombinant protein expression. The review article (Chapter 13) by Murakami brings into focus the recent advances in genetic transformation of macroalgae–a photosynthetic biological system of high economic, industrial and medical importance. Closing the section two, Noriyuki and collaborators report, in Chapter 14, the genetic diversity and population balance of Hotoke loach in rivers from rural area of Japan, bringing to discussion an actual ecological case that can be applicable as model for the evaluation of population status and genetic background of other endangered species of animals.

Section three starts (Chapter 15) with the examination of the mechanistic and structural characteristics of molecular recognition between HIV-1 integrase and its inhibitor raltegravir, by Tchertanov and Arora. This survey sets the basis for target-based drug discovery and clinical application of highly specific allosteric inhibitor in HIV therapy. In Chapter 16, Fierro and collaborators present theoretical and original data from protein crystal structure and computational molecular modelling to evaluate ligand-binding sites of monoamine oxidases and experimentally test several selective inhibitors. Hibino and co-authors (Chapter 17) treat sharply on a powerful and sophisticated technology to investigate and quantify the ligand association/dissociation with their respective receptors based on single-molecule imaging (SMI). The authors offer some examples of the actual use of SMI in Life Sciences and its applicability in the field of Toxinology. The molecular interaction and recognition between saccharides and polypeptides play a crucial role in biological process and signaling. In Chapter 18, Miura and collaborators exemplify several aspects of sugar-protein discrimination and interaction, discussing the fabrication of glycopolymeric biomaterials for analytical and nanotechnological purposes. In Chapter 19, Khalafi and Rafiee present fundaments of how spectral changes of cyclodextrin are observed and illustrate practical uses of this system in molecular recognition of distinct compounds, including toxins. Another technique of evaluating recognition of molecules involves the application of potentiometry, as discussed by Radecki and Radecka, in Chapter 20. Closing the section three, Akitsu and Kominato bring into view the backgrounds of conformational changes occurring in consequence of molecular recognition based on Schiff-base interaction. This principle can be applicable for spectroscopic analysis and docking studies of metal-Schiff base complexes in proteins.

I hope the readers will enjoy the selected and interconnected themes compiled here and that the chapters in this book will serve as useful reference for productive research and technological application.

I am very thankful to all authors for their contribution and sharing their knowledge, what surely is the result from constant and dedicated works. I manifest my gratitude to InTech editorial office for making possible the concretization of this book project.

Dr. Gandhi Radis-Baptista
Universidade Federal do Ceara, Instituto de Ciencias do Mar - Labomar,
Brazil

Section 1

Molecular Toxinology

Chapter 1

Peptidomic Analysis of Animal Venoms

Ricardo Bastos Cunha

Additional information is available at the end of the chapter

http://dx.doi.org/10.5772/53773

1. Introduction

The last two decades have witnessed a growing interest in the discovery of new chemical and pharmacological substances of animal origin. Pharmacological tests of toxins obtained from animal venoms revealed its effects on central nervous system, mainly acting on ion channels in heart, intestine, in vascular permeability, etc. Potential applications of these substances have been proposed ranging from human disease treatment to plague control of agricultural interest. In this scenario, the peptidomic analysis has played an increasingly important role.

Venomous organisms are widespread throughout the animal kingdom, comprising more than 100,000 species distributed in all major phyla. Virtually all ecosystems on Earth have venomous or poisonous organisms. Venoms represent an adaptive trait, and an example of convergent evolution. They are truly mortal cocktails, comprising unique mixtures of peptides and proteins naturally tailored by natural selection to operate in defense or attack systems, for the prey or the victim. Venoms represent an enormous reservoir of bioactive compounds able to cure diseases that do not respond to conventional therapies. Darwinian evolution of animal venoms has accumulated in nature a wide variety of biological fluids which resulted in a true combinatorial libraries of hundreds of thousands of molecules potentially active and pharmacologically useful.

Venom is a general term which refers to a variety of toxins used by certain animals that inoculate its victims through a bite, a sting or other sharp body feature. Venoms of vertebrates and invertebrates contain a molecular diversity of proteins and peptides, and other classes of substances, which together form an arsenal of highly effective agents, paralyzing and lethal, mainly used for predation and defense. We must distinguish venom from poison, which is ingested or inhaled by the victim, being absorbed by its digestive system or respiratory system. Animal venoms, in contrast, are administered directly into the lymphatic system, where it acts faster. Only those organisms possessing injection devices (stingers, fangs, spines, hypostomes, spurs or harpoons) which allow the active use of venom for predation can be correctly characterized as venomous. Many other animals secrete lethal substances (insects, centipedes, frogs, fish, etc.), but, as these substances are used primarily for defense purposes, these animals are termed poisonous and cannot be accurately characterized as venomous.

Venomous and poisonous invertebrates include cnidarians [1, 2] (sea anemones, jellyfish and corals), some families of mollusks [3] (mainly Conidae) and arthropods [4] (scorpions, pseudoscorpions, spiders, centipedes, ticks and hymenoptera insects, like bees, ants and wasps). Arthropods inject their venom through fangs (spiders and centipedes) or stingers (scorpions and pungent insects). The sting, in some insects, such as bees and wasps, is a modified egg-laying device, called ovipositor. Some caterpillars have venom defense glands associated to specialized bristles in the body known as urticating hairs, which can be lethal to humans (such as the moth *Lonomia*) [5]. Bees use an acidic poison (apitoxin), which causes pain in those bitten, to defend their hives and food stocks [6]. Wasps, on the other hand, use its venom to only paralyze the prey [7]. In this way, the pray can be stored alive in food chambers for the young. The ant *Polyrhachis dives* produces a poison that is applied topically on the victim for pathogen sterilization [8]. There are many other venomous and poisonous invertebrates, including jellyfish [9], bugs [10] and snails [11-13]. The sea wasp (*Chironex fleckeri*), also called box jellyfish, has about 500,000 cnidocytes in each tentacle, containing nematocysts, a harpoon-shaped mechanism that injects an extremely potent venom into the victim, which causes severe physical and psychological symptoms known as Irukandji syndrome. In many cases, this inoculation leads to death of the victim, that is why sea wasp is popularly known as "the world's most venomous creature" [14].

Loxoscelism is a condition produced by the bite of spiders from the genus *Loxosceles*, and is the only proven cause of necrosis in humans of arachnological origin [15]. *Loxosceles* spiders can be found worldwide. However, their distribution is heavily concentrated at the Western Hemisphere, particularly at the Americas, with more evidence in the tropics. In urban areas of South America, the presence of this type of spider is so evident that loxoscelism is considered a public health problem. Although *Loxosceles* bite is usually mild, it may ulcerate or cause more serious dermonecrotic injurie and even systemic reactions. This injurie is mainly due to the presence of the enzyme sphingomyelinase D in spider venom. Because the great number of diseases which mimic the loxoscelism symptoms, it is frequently misdiagnosed by physicians [16]. Although there is no known fully effective therapy for loxoscelism, research about potential antivenoms and vaccines has been exhaustive, presently also using the peptidomic approach [17], and many palliative therapies are reported in literature [15, 18].

Among vertebrates, only few reptiles (snakes and lizards) have developed the machinery for venom production [9], although some fish [9, 19], amphibians [20] and mammals (platypus for example) [21] have venom glands. The best known venomous reptiles are the snakes, which normally inject venom into their prey through hollow fangs. The snake venom is produced by mandibular glands located below the eyes and is inoculated into the victim through tubular or channeled fangs. Snakes use their venom mainly for hunting, although they can also use it for defense. A snakebite can cause a variety of symptoms including pain, swelling, tissue damage, decreased blood pressure, seizures, bleeding, respiratory paralysis, kidney failure and coma, and may, in severe cases, cause the patient death. These symptoms will vary depending on snake specie. Snakebite is an important medical emergency in many parts of the world, particularly in tropical and subtropical regions. According to World Health Organization (WHO), the incidence of snakebite reaches 5 million per year, causing 2.5 million envenomations and 125,000 deaths [22]. About 80% of envenomation deaths worldwide are caused by snakebite, followed by scorpion bite, which causes 15% [23]. Most affected are healthy people, such as children and agricultural populations, usually in poor resources areas, away from health centers in low-income countries in Africa, Asia and Latin America. As a result, WHO declared snakebite as a health crisis and a neglected tropical disease.

In addition to snakes, there are other venomous reptiles, such as the beaded lizard (*Heloderma horridum*), the Gila monster (*Heloderma suspectum*) and other species of lizards [9]. The composition of the Komodo dragon (*Varanus komodoensis*) venom is as complex as snake venoms [24]. Because of recent studies of venom glands in squamata and analysis of nuclear protein-coding genes, a new hypothetical clade, Toxicofera, is being proposed [25]. This clade would include all poisonous Squamata: suborders Serpentes (snakes) and Iguania (iguanas, agamid lizards, chameleons, etc.) and the infraorder Anguimorpha, represented by the families Varanidae (monitor lizards), Anguidae (alligator lizards, glass lizards, etc.) and Helodermatidae (Gila monster and beaded lizard).

Venoms can also be found in some fish, such as cartilaginous (rays, sharks and chimaeras) and teleostean, including monognathus eel-like fishes, catfishes, rockfishes, waspfishes, scorpionfishes, lionfishes, goatfishes, rabbitfishes, spiderfishes, surgeonfishes, gurnards, scats, stargazers, weever, swarmfish, etc. [9, 19]. Another venomous fish, the doctor fish, also know as "reddish log sucker", is used by some spas to feed the affected and dead areas of the skin of psoriasis patients, leaving the healthy skin to grow. There are venomous mammals, including solenodons, shrews, slow loris and the male platypus [21]. There are few poisonous amphibian species [20]. Some salamanders can expel venom through a rib of a sharp edge. There are even reports of venomous dinosaurs [26]. *Sinornithosaurus*, a genus of Dromaeosauridae dinosaur with feathers, may have had a venomous bite. But this theory is still controversial. The coelophysoid dinosaur *Dilophosaurus* is commonly portrayed in popular culture as being poisonous, but this superstition is not considered likely by the scientific community.

Until recently, the work in toxinology involved prospecting highly toxic or lethal toxins in animal venoms that could explain the symptoms observed clinically. Typically, such an approach involved the isolation and structural characterization of the molecule which causes an specific adverse effect observed when a person is envenomed. However, small molecules with micro-effects that were not easily observed were neglected or poorly studied. This situation changed in recent years with the improvement in sensitivity, resolution and accuracy of mass spectrometry and other techniques used in proteomic toxinology. With the advent of these new technologies, small peptides from animal venoms with unexplored biological activities started to be studied systematically, emerging, then, this new area of knowledge and scientific research called peptidomics. These molecules are potential candidates for new drugs or compounds with significant therapeutic actions.

2. Chemical composition and strategic importance of venoms

Over 5000 years ago, the Mesopotamians used a cane with a serpent as an emblem of Ningizzida, the god of fertility, marriage and pests. In Christianity, the serpent has always been associated with evil because of the biblical allegory of Adam and Eve. There is also a biblical story in which Moses erected a post with a brazen serpent to release his people from the plague of snakes. Throughout the development of Christianity, this symbol was transformed and the post became a tau.

But not always and not in all cultures, serpents were associated with evil. Many people believed in the cure power of serpents, often associated with its venom. Indeed, the medicinal value of animal venoms has been known since Antiquity. The medicinal use of bee venom, apitoxin, is reported in ancient Egypt and in Europe and Asia history. Charlemagne and Ivan *the Terrible*, for example, would have used apitoxin to treat common diseases. The medical uses of scorpion and snake venoms are well documented in Chinese pharmacopoeia. In an Islamic traditional tale, Muhammed is sick and, in the face of no known cure, it allows the use of snake venom as a last resource.

To Greeks and Romans, the serpent was a symbol of cure because periodically abandons its old skin and seemingly reborn, in the same way that doctors remove the disease of the body and rejuvenate the men, and also because the serpent was a symbol of concentrated attention, which was required to the curers. However, the association of serpents with cure may also be related to its venom, represented symbolically by herbs in the Greek-Roman mythology of Aesculapius, the god of medicine and cure. Called to assist Glaucus, who had been killed by lightning, Aesculapius saw a snake enter the room where he was, and killed it with his staff. Soon, a second serpent entered the room carrying herbs in its mouth, which deposited at the mouth of another dead serpent, making it back to life. Watching this scene, Aesculapius decided to put the herbs into the Glaucus mouth, who also raised from dead. Since then, Aesculapius turned the serpent your pet guardianship. His staff with a coiled serpent became the symbol of modern medicine in a large number of countries and is present even in the banner of the World Health Organization (WHO).

However, despite the healing power of animal venoms be known for a long time, the systematic investigation of venom components as natural sources for the generation of pharmaceuticals was only performed over the past decades, after a peptide that potencialize bradykinin action was isolated from the venom of the Brazilian snake *Bothrops jararaca* [27]. This led to the development, in the 1950s, of the first commercial drug based on angiotensin I converting enzyme (ACE)-inhibitor (trade name captopril®), for the treatment of arterial hypertension and heart failure [28]. Prialt® (ziconotide) is another example of synthetic drug successfully isolated from an animal venom [11]. This is a synthetic non-opioid peptide, non-NSAID, non-local anesthetic calcium channel blocker, isolated from the secretions of the cone snail *Conus magus*. Prialt® is used for the alleviation of chronic intractable pain and is administered directly into the spinal cord, due to deep side effects or lack of efficacy when it is administered by the more common routes such as orally or intravenously.

The evolution of the venom secretion apparatus in animals is indeed an impressive biological achievement at the evolutionary point of view. Since venoms components result of biochemical and pharmacological refinement over a long period in evolutionary scale, they have been tuned for optimum activity by the natural evolution. Thus, nature has already prospected huge combinatorial libraries of potential therapeutic drugs. The biochemical evolution of proteins from salivary fluids or venom exocrine glands is remarkable, especially when one considers the highly specialized functions of these proteins and its high specificity with respect to the target molecule.

Several classes of organic molecules have been described in venoms, such as alkaloids and acylpolyamines. However, the main constituents are indeed polypeptides. Venoms of cone snail and arthropods, such as spiders, scorpions and insects, to a lesser extent, seem to be mainly peptidic, while snakes produce protein rich venoms. Snake venoms contain a variety of proteases, which hydrolyze peptide bonds of proteins, nucleases, which hydrolyze phosphodiester bonds of DNA, and neurotoxins, which disable signaling in the nervous system. The brown spider venom contains a variety of toxins, the most important of which is the tissue destruction agent sphingomyelinase D, present in the venom of all species of *Loxosceles* in different concentrations [29]. Only another spider genus (*Sicarius*) and several pathogenic bacteria are known to produce this enzyme.

Some venoms comprise several hundreds of components, which further expands its potential as a source of new medicines. Many components of venoms affect the nervous system and modulate the generation and propagation of action potentials, acting on multiple molecular sites, which include central and peripheral neurons, axons, synapses and neuromuscular junctions [30]. Many of these target receptors play important physiological roles or are associated with specific diseases. Therefore, the components of animal venoms are important biological tools for studying these receptors, and the discovery of molecules in venoms with selective activity for these receptors represents a very attractive approach to the search for new drugs. The venom components may therefore be probed for the development of new therapies for pain management [31], new anti-arrhythmic [32], anticonvulsant [33] or anxiolytic drugs [34], new antimicrobial agents [35-37] or pesticides [38, 39], etc. Even a substance that causes priapism has been isolated from the venom of a Brazilian spider [40], becoming a potential drug candidate to attend erectile dysfunction.

Another reason to study the composition of animal venoms is trying to seek more effective prophylaxis for envenomings. Doctors treat victims of venomous sting with serum, which is produced by injecting into an animal, such as sheep, horse, goat or rabbit, a small amount of specific venom. The animal's immune system responds to the target dose, producing antibodies to active molecules of the venom. These antibodies can then be isolated from the animal's blood and used in envenoming treatment in other animals, including humans.

However, this treatment can be effectively used only a limited number of times for a particular person, since that person will develop antibodies to neutralize the exogenous animal's antibodies used to produce the antiserum (antibodies antiantibodies). Even if that person does not suffer a severe allergic reaction to the antiserum, his own immune system can destroy the antiserum even before the antiserum destroys the venom toxins. Most people will never need an antiserum treatment throughout their lives. However, others, who work or live in risk areas habited by snakes or other venomous animals, such as agricultural areas for example, need that this treatment is available in public health network.

Some treatments are done not with antiserum, but herbal. *Aristolochia rugosa* and *Aristolochia trilobata*, or angelic, are medicinal plants used in Western India and in Central and South America against snake and scorpion bites [41]. Aristolochic acid, produced by those plants, inhibits inflammation induced by immune complexes and non-immunological agents (carrageenan or croton oil). It also inhibits the activity of phospholipases present in snake venoms (PLA2], forming a 1:1 complex with the enzyme. Phospholipases play an important role in the reactions cascade that lead to inflammatory response and pain. Therefore, its inhibition may reduce problems of scorpionism, snakebite and loxoscelism.

3. Proteomic and peptidomic analysis: A new approach to study venoms

Proteins are very large molecules formed by amino acids chains linked together as a polymer. Although biological systems uses only 20 amino acids to build their proteins, the different possible combinations among them is virtually infinite, resulting in tens of thousands different proteins, each one with a unique sequence, genetically defined, which determines its specific form and biological function. Furthermore, each protein may undergo a variety of post-translational modifications, which diversifies even more its form and function. Proteins are the main constituents of protoplasm of all cells. As the major components of cells metabolic pathways, proteins have vital functions in organism, such as: catalyze biochemical reactions (eg. enzymes), transmit messages (eg. neurotransmitters), regulate cellular reproduction, influence growth and development of various tissues (eg. trophic factors), carry oxygen in the blood (eg. hemoglobin), defend the body against diseases (eg. antibodies), among countless other achievements. There is no metabolic reaction in which the participation of at least one protein is dispensable.

The term "proteome" is derived from the junction of the word "PROTEin" with the word "genOME" and refers to the set of proteins expressed starting from a genome, i.e., all the proteins produced by an organism. Indeed, the word proteome is often be more related to the set of proteins expressed in a specific organ, or biological fluid, or cell, in a given state (eg. diseased cell). The proteome is therefore the complete complement of a genome, including the "makeup" that proteins receives after being synthesized, i.e., the post-translational modifications, all of them absolutely relevant for that proteins perform their biological function. The proteome of a cell or fluid varies with time and conditions under which the organism is subjected. The human body, for example, can contain more than 2 million different proteins, each one exerting a distinct role. Unlike the genome, which is relatively static, the proteome is constantly changing in response to tens of thousands of intra and extracellular environmental signals. The proteome varies with the nature of each tissue or organ, the cell development stage, the stress conditions to which the organism is subjected, the organism health state, the effects of drug treatment, etc. As such, the proteome is often defined as the proteins present in a sample (tissue, organism, cell culture, biological fluid, etc.) at a given point in time.

The term proteomics consists of comprehensive and systematic study of all proteins present in a given cell state, which was made possible by the huge development of mass spectrometry techniques over the past two decades. Proteomics and genomics run parallel and are interdependent. Genomics without proteomics is only an "alphabet soup", because it can only make inferences about their products (proteins). Moreover, proteomics requires genomics to identify the proteins expressed in a particular cell state. Briefly, genomics provides a static information of the various ways in which a cell may use its proteins, while proteomics gives a dynamic panorama of molecular diversity, showing not only which proteins are more or less expressed (or is not even expressed), but also how these proteins were modified and how these modifications affect its role in the cell theater.

Proteomic technologies can play an important role in new drugs discovery, new diagnostics and molecular medicine, because it is the connection between genes, proteins and diseases. For example, the discovery of defective proteins that cause specific diseases can help develop new drugs that either alter the shape of a defective protein or mimic its action. Most of the most popular drugs today either have proteinaceous nature or have a protein target. Through proteomics, one can create "custom" drugs, i.e., drugs specially designed for specific individuals. Such drugs are supposed to be more effective and cause fewer side effects. Another field to which proteomic studies can contribute is the biomarkers discovery for specific diseases, whose overexpression (or depletion) would indicate, quite early, the disease development. For example, serum levels of prostate specific antigen (PSA) is commonly used in the diagnosis of prostate cancer in men, which makes PSA a biomarker for cancer. Unfortunately, however, the diagnosis based on a single protein biomarker is not very reliable. Proteomics may help scientists to develop diagnostic tests that simultaneously analyze the expression of multiple proteins in order to improve the specificity and sensitivity of these tests.

Over time, new study areas with the suffix "omics" have emerged, such as metabolomics, lipidomics, carbohydratomics, degradomics etc. The term venomics did not slow to appear, and today it is defined as the study of all components (protean or not protean) of a venom. The word peptidomics has also been proposed to set the study of the peptides (instead of proteins) of a cell type or a biological fluid, such as venom. According to Ivanov and Yatskin [42]: "structure and biologic function of the entire multitude of peptides circulating in living organisms, their organs, tissues, cells and fluids comprises the scope of peptidomics". For these authors, "these two multitudes of polypeptides (proteins and peptides) play a dominant role in the functioning of any cellular system, tissue or organ. They are intimately connected with each other and exist in equilibrium as an essential part of homeostasis (i.e., the normal state of any living organism and the basis of life itself)".

Peptidomic analysis has been proposed by several authors [43-55] as a way to access information relevant to clinical diagnosis and/or to monitor the patient biochemical profile during the therapy. The growing interest in peptidomic analysis led some scientists to develop new analytical technologies to improve peptidomic analysis, such as: use of capillary electrophoresis to separate the peptides [46]; use of size exclusion chromatography as a pre-fractionation step [53, 56]; new technologies and methods for sample pretreatment [57], such as methods for isolation rare amino acid-containing peptides, terminal peptides, PTM peptides and endogenous peptides, automated sample pretreatment technologies (automated sample injection and on-line digestion) [58]; development of a new target plate for MALDI-MS for one step electric transfer of analytes from a 1-dimensional electrophoresis gel directly to the target plate [59, 60]; etc. In recent years, in the face of the remarkable development on nanotechnology, many researchers have produced different kind of nanoparticles, such as mesoporous silica nanoparticles [50, 51, 61, 62] and carbon nanotubes [52, 63], for selective peptide extraction (and, hence, its enrichment) from biological fluids for therapeutic purposes (clinical diagnosis and/or novel biomarker discovery).

In the case of animal venoms, however, peptidomics is a highly interesting area for different reasons, since most of the biologically active components of pharmacological interest are of peptidic nature [64]. For example, Biass and co-workers [12] studied the venom peptidomic profile of the cone snail-hunting fish, *Conus consors*, through approaches involving different sample preparation protocols and analysis by mass spectrometry. The cone snail was quoted in the television series *Animal Planet: The Most Extreme*, because it can quickly shoot a harpoon filled with deadly toxins. The conidia (Conidae) constitute a family of several shells divided into subfamilies. It is estimated that this genus produce more than 70,000 different pharmacologically active components, most of peptidic nature, whereas interspecies variations. It is a rich library of neuropharmacology and combinatorial chemistry. Precisely for this reason, the 6th Framework Programme of the European Union funded with € 10.7 million the international project CONCO involving 20 partners and 13 countries [65], whose objective is to explore new molecules therapeutically relevant produced by venomous marine cone snails.

4. The tools to peptidomic analysis

Mass spectrometry is an analytical tool that has evolved dramatically over the past 20 years in terms of sensitivity, resolving power and versatility, and is currently one of the main tools for studying the molecular components of biological systems, including venoms. The development of techniques such as electrospray ionization (ESI) and matrix-assisted laser desorption ionization (MALDI) was essential for allowing polypeptides be analyzed by mass spectrometry. Hyphenation of separation techniques such as high performance liquid chromatography (HPLC) with mass spectrometry was also decisive for this progress. As a consequence, the highly combinatorial nature of venom components and their underlying pharmacologic complexity have been progressively revealed by mass spectrometry. Currently, major challenges remain on samples complexity, lack of biological material and databases absence to peptide and protein identification based on sequence information.

Peptidomic analysis of a sample will consist of essentially four steps: (I) peptides extraction from the sample; (II) separation of these peptides – including their prior separation from other polypetidic components of the sample, i.e., proteins, defined as the protean components with molecular weight above 10 kDa –; (III) peptides detection – which is commonly performed by mass spectrometry –, (IV) and finally identification of the peptides – which usually involves fragmentation of those peptides in a tandem mass spectrometer (MS/MS).

With respect to peptide sequencing for identification purposes, the technique traditionally used is Edman degradation-based sequencing [66, 67]. But nowadays this kind of sequencing is increasingly being replaced by sequencing techniques based on mass spectrometry [68, 69]. This is due to the fact that mass spectrometry is much more rapid and sensitive than Edman sequencing and prenscinde of prior separation of the peptides, which means that peptides can be sucessfully analyzed and sequenced by mass spectrometry from a complex peptide matrix, which is impossible by Edman sequencing. This is only possible because the peptide of interest is selected (i.e., separated from others) in the first mass spectrometer. Then, this parent ion is fragmented in a collision chamber and the daughter ions are analyzed in a second mass spectrometer (MS/MS). Figure 3 gives an example of peptide *de novo* sequencing by tandem mass spectrometry. For more details about this kind of polypeptide sequencing, see reference [69].

In proteomics, the most widely used technique to separate protean components of a sample is the two-dimensional polyacrylamide gel electrophoresis (2D-PAGE). In peptidomics, however, techniques based on liquid chromatography coupled to mass spectrometry (LC-MS) appear to be more popular, since peptides are not well resolved by electrophoresis [70]. Despite this, capillary electrophoresis has also been used successfully in peptidomic analysis, mainly to analyze biological fluids for clinical applications, such as disease diagnosis and response to therapy [46].

As an example, Valente and co-workers [71] ran a two-dimensional gel from the venom of *Bothrops insularis*, an endemic snake specie in Queimada Grande Island, Brazil. The result is shown in Figure 1. This is an example of venomics, i.e., the study of all protean components of a venom. Using the proteomic approach, the authors detected 494 spots in the gel using an image analysis software, from which 69 proteins were identified by current identification techniques, using mass spectrometry and heavy bioinformatics to interpret the mass spectra and also to make a comparative search of protein sequences deposited in databases. The identified proteins include metalloproteinases, serine proteinases, phospholipases A2, lectins, growth factors, L-amino acid oxidases, the developmental protein G10, a disintegrin, a nuclear protein of the BUD31 family, and putative novel bradykinin-potentiating peptides. In the same study, the authors also performed a peptidomic analysis of the venom, by direct analysis of the crude venom by MALDI-TOF-TOF and LC-ESI-Q-TOF. Many new peptides were partially or completely sequenced by both MALDI-MS/MS and LC-ESI-MS/MS. Using the proteomic approach associated with peptidomic analysis, the authors could speculate about the existence of posttranslational modifications and a proteolytic processing of precursor molecules which could lead to diverse multifunctional proteins.

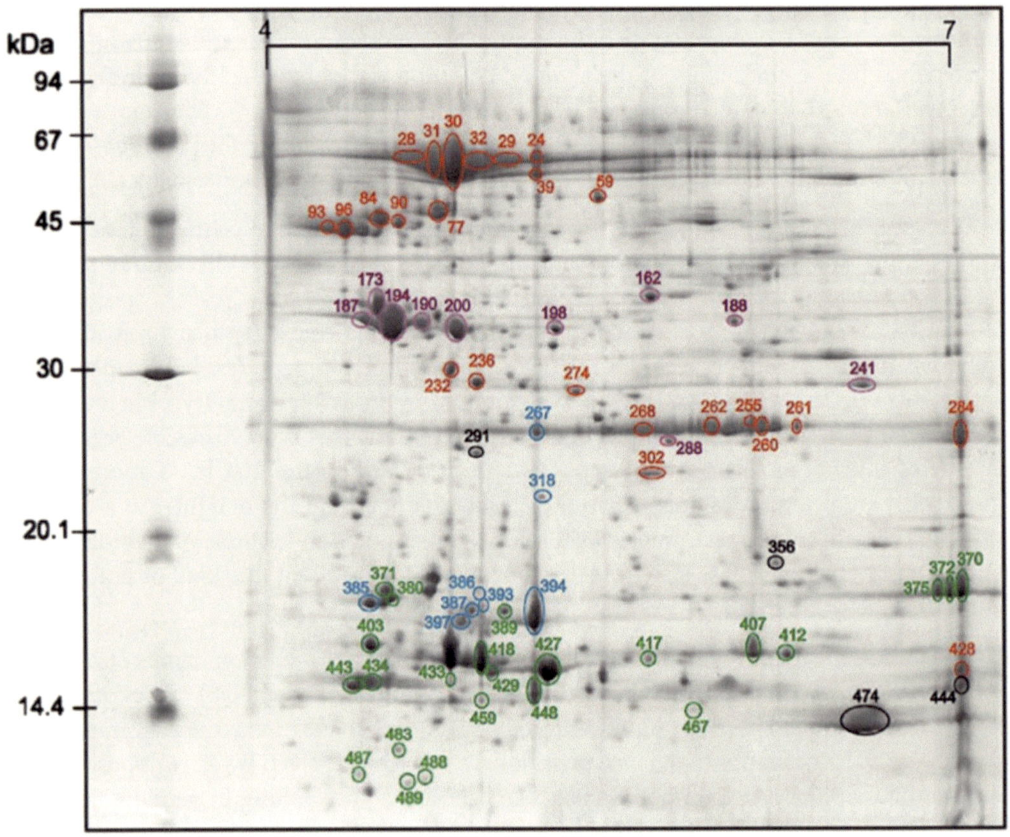

Figure 1. Proteomic profile of *Bothrops insularis* venom: 2D-PAGE reference map (copyed from reference [71]).

Liao and co-workers [72] also applied proteomic and peptidomic approaches together to analyze the venom of *Chilobrachys jingzhao* (a type of tarantula; one of the most venomous spiders in southern China). They developed a protocol which consists in run a gel filtration of the crude venom and then divide the fractions in two parts. The fraction containing protean components with molecular mass above 10 kDa they underwent proteomic analysis, which consisted of 2-DE, in gel trypsin digestion, MALDI-TOF-TOF and ESI-Q-TOF analysis of the spots, protein identification by PMF, *de novo* sequencing of the peptides, and protein identification by MS BLAST sequence similarity search. The fraction containing protein components with molecular weight below 10 kDa was used for peptidomic analysis, consisting in separation of the peptides by ion-exchange HPLC followed by reverse phase HPLC, MALDI-TOF analysis of the chromatographic fractions, Edman peptide sequencing, and peptide identification by MS BLAST. The authors reported that peptides were the predominant components [69%) of the dry crude venom, while proteins accounted only for 6%. Nonprotean components (low MW inorganic and organic molecules, such as polyamines, salts, free acids, glucose, etc.) complete the remaining 25% of the crude venom.

Another good example of peptidomic analysis was presented by Rates and co-workers [73], who studied the *Tityus serrulatus* (a specie of scorpion whose venom has been most extensively studied) venom peptide diversity. In this work, the authors fracionated the venom by gel filtration followed by reverse phase chromatography of each fraction obtained in the first separation. The results are shown in Figure 2. Then, the chromatographic fractions were analyzed by MALDI-TOF-TOF. The peptides were sequenced using *de novo* methodology (Figure 3) and the sequences obtained were compared with protein databases in sequence similarity searches. The authors also reported the finding of novel peptides without sequence similarities to other known molecules.

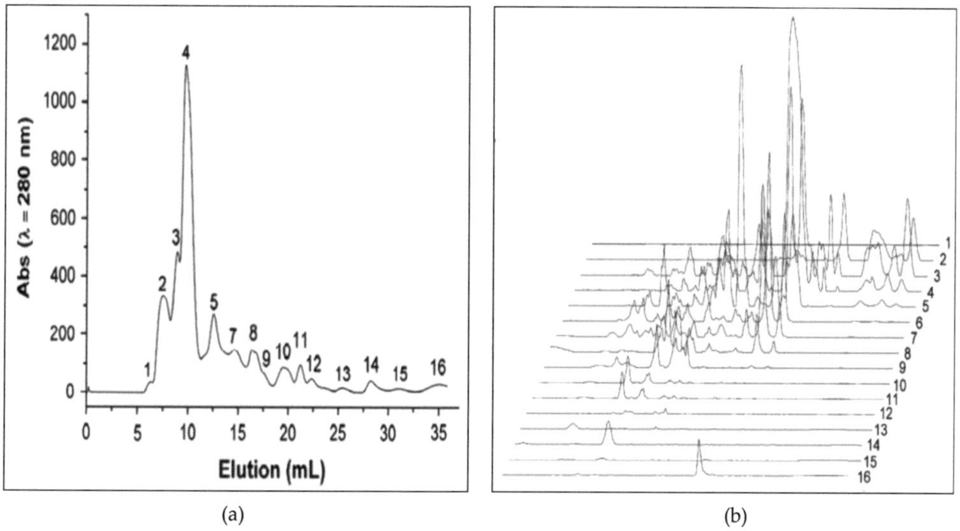

Figure 2. *Tityus serrulatus* venom fractionation through gel filtration (A) and re-chromatography of each fraction by reverse phase chromatography (B) (copyed from reference [73]).

One of the biggest difficulties currently encountered by researchers working with peptidomic analysis of animal venoms is that organisms with unsequenced genomes, including venomous animals, still represent the overwhelming majority of species in the biosphere. Fortunately, Andrej Shevchenko, from Max Planck Institute of Molecular Cell Biology and Genetics, at Dresden, Germany, paved the way for homology-driven proteomic approaches to explore proteomes of organisms with unsequenced genomes [74-76]. Through this new methodology, the search against sequences databases is made not by the exact sequence, but by sequence similarity to other protein sequences deposited in the database. This new approach does not fully solve the problem, but allows peptides to be positively identified in peptidomic experiments through cross-species identification. Wang and colleagues [77] developed an alternative strategy to circumvent the problem of absence of systematic online database information, and used this technique to analyze the peptidome of amphibian skin secretions. Although amphibian skin secretion is not exactly a venom, it is still a biological model also very promising for the search of new pharmacologically active substances. First, the authors deduced all of putative bioactive peptide sequences by shotgun cloning the cDNAs encoding peptide precursors. Then, they separated the entire peptidome by UPLC/MS/MS, and confirmed those sequences deduced before by *de novo* MS/MS sequencing.

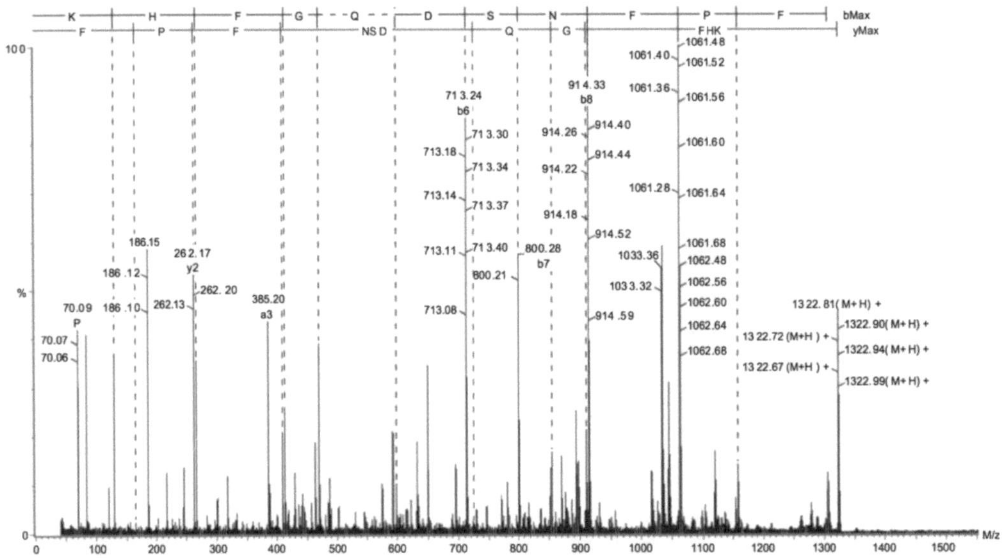

Figure 3. MS/MS spectra interpretation (*de novo* sequencing) for peptide NH_2-FPFNSD(K/Q)GFH(K/Q)-CO_2H (copyed from reference [73]). The K/Q denotes a doubt about the possibility of being lysine or glutamine, as these two amino acids are isobaric. However, as trypsin cleaves on C-terminal sides of arginines and lysines, it is likely that the middle amino acid is glutamine and the last one is lysine.

5. Concluding remarks

Animal venoms are true "cocktails" of substances normally harmful, but that can be explored with intelligence for medical use. Many authors even use the word "cornucopia" to define a venom. The cornucopia — junction of the Latin "*cornu*" (horn) with "*copiae*" (strength) -, also called "horn of plenty", is a symbol of nourishment and abundance in classical mythology, usually represented by a large horn-shaped container overflowing with products such as flowers, dried fruit, other foodstuffs, and other types of wealthiness. Nowadays it is particularly associated with the Thanksgiving holiday. In toxinology, cornucopia represents the chemical wealth of animal venoms, where one can find thousands of such substances with interesting biological effects that can be explored as candidates for future pharmaceutical products.

Much (perhaps the largest) of this pool of substances is of peptidic nature, i.e., polypeptides with molecular weight below 10 kDa. These are biologically active peptides with diverse functions, ranging from heart hypotensors to erectile dysfunction controllers. Thus, the peptidomic analysis of animal venoms is an emerging and promising area of science, and can be considered a frontier area as it includes researchers from toxinology, proteomics, pharmacology, therapeutics, drug discovery, peptide chemistry, analytical chemistry, etc.

In this chapter we tried to show the importance of animal venoms for molecular toxinology and its potential use for biomedical applications. We also sought to demonstrate the recent advent and rapid growth of peptidomic analysis as the main tool to explore the molecular features of these venoms, not only to produce more efficient antisera against venomous bites but also and mainly to characterize the components of peptide nature in search for new products of pharmacological interest. Although this new science is still in its early stages of development, it is already very mature. This is a science field that has enough potential to grow and provide creative solutions to problems that affect human health. Hopefully more and more researchers become interested on this topic. Medicine has much to gain from it.

Author details

Ricardo Bastos Cunha

Bioanalytical Chemistry Laboratory, Division of Analytical Chemistry, Institute of Chemistry, University of Brasília, Brazil

References

[1] Russell FE. Venomous animal injuries. Current problems in pediatrics. 1973;3(9):1-47. Epub 1973/07/01.

[2] Bedry R, de Haro L. [Venomous and poisonous animals. V. Envenomations by venomous marine invertebrates]. Medecine tropicale : revue du Corps de sante colonial. 2007;67(3):223-31. Epub 2007/09/06. Envenimations ou intoxications par les animaux venimeux ou veneneux. V--invertebres marins venimeux.

[3] Hermitte LC. Venomous marine molluscs of the genus Conus. Transactions of the Royal Society of Tropical Medicine and Hygiene. 1946;39:485-512. Epub 1946/06/01.

[4] Ghosh SM. Injuries by Venomous Arthropods. Bulletin of the Calcutta School of Tropical Medicine. 1965;13:30-3. Epub 1965/01/01.

[5] Veiga AB, Blochtein B, Guimaraes JA. Structures involved in production, secretion and injection of the venom produced by the caterpillar Lonomia obliqua (Lepidoptera, Saturniidae). Toxicon : official journal of the International Society on Toxinology. 2001;39(9):1343-51. Epub 2001/06/01.

[6] Tannenberg J, Kosseff A. Fatal anaphylactic shock due to a bee sting in the finger. Proceedings of the New York State Association of Public Health Laboratories. 1945;25(2):33. Epub 1945/01/01.

[7] Seward EH. Wasp venoms and anaesthesia. Proceedings of the Royal Society of Medicine. 1954;47(12):1032-4. Epub 1954/12/01.

[8] Blum MS, Walker JR, Callahan PS, Novak AF. Chemical, insecticidal and antibiotic properties of fire ant venom. Science. 1958;128(3319):306-7. Epub 1958/08/08.

[9] Warrell DA. Venomous bites, stings, and poisoning. Infectious disease clinics of North America. 2012;26(2):207-23. Epub 2012/05/29.

[10] Viswanathan M, Srinivasan K. Poisoning by bug poison. A preliminary study. Journal of the Indian Medical Association. 1962;39:345-9. Epub 1962/10/01.

[11] McIntosh M, Cruz LJ, Hunkapiller MW, Gray WR, Olivera BM. Isolation and structure of a peptide toxin from the marine snail Conus magus. Archives of biochemistry and biophysics. 1982;218(1):329-34. Epub 1982/10/01.

[12] Biass D, Dutertre S, Gerbault A, Menou JL, Offord R, Favreau P, et al. Comparative proteomic study of the venom of the piscivorous cone snail Conus consors. Journal of proteomics. 2009;72(2):210-8. Epub 2009/05/22.

[13] Eugster PJ, Biass D, Guillarme D, Favreau P, Stocklin R, Wolfender JL. Peak capacity optimisation for high resolution peptide profiling in complex mixtures by liquid chromatography coupled to time-of-flight mass spectrometry: Application to the Conus consors cone snail venom. Journal of chromatography A. 2012. Epub 2012/06/05.

[14] Pearn J, Fenner P. The Jellyfish hunter--Jack Barnes: a pioneer medical toxinologist in Australia. Toxicon : official journal of the International Society on Toxinology. 2006;48(7):762-7. Epub 2006/10/31.

[15] Swanson DL, Vetter RS. Loxoscelism. Clinics in dermatology. 2006;24(3):213-21. Epub 2006/05/23.

[16] Bennett RG, Vetter RS. An approach to spider bites. Erroneous attribution of dermonecrotic lesions to brown recluse or hobo spider bites in Canada. Canadian family physician Medecin de famille canadien. 2004;50:1098-101. Epub 2004/10/01.

[17] Guimarães AB. Análise peptidômica comparativa das peçonhas de duas espécies de aranhas marrom: Loxosceles laeta e Loxosceles intermedia [dissertation]. http://capesdw.capes.gov.br/capesdw/resumo.html?idtese=20092753001010005P5: University of Brasilia; 2009.

[18] da Silva PH, da Silveira RB, Appel MH, Mangili OC, Gremski W, Veiga SS. Brown spiders and loxoscelism. Toxicon : official journal of the International Society on Toxinology. 2004;44(7):693-709. Epub 2004/10/27.

[19] Maretic Z. [Experience with venomous fish bites]. Acta tropica. 1957;14(2):157-61. Epub 1957/01/01. Erfahrungen mit Stichen von Giftfischen.

[20] Chippaux JP, Goyffon M. [Venomous and poisonous animals--I. Overview]. Medecine tropicale : revue du Corps de sante colonial. 2006;66(3):215-20. Epub 2006/08/24. Envenimations et intoxications par les animaux venimeux ou veneneux--I. Generalits.

[21] Whittington CM, Koh JM, Warren WC, Papenfuss AT, Torres AM, Kuchel PW, et al. Understanding and utilising mammalian venom via a platypus venom transcriptome. Journal of proteomics. 2009;72(2):155-64. Epub 2009/01/21.

[22] Girish KS, Kemparaju K. Overlooked issues of snakebite management: time for strategic approach. Current topics in medicinal chemistry. 2011;11(20):2494-508. Epub 2011/06/28.

[23] Calvete JJ, Sanz L, Angulo Y, Lomonte B, Gutierrez JM. Venoms, venomics, antivenomics. FEBS Lett. 2009;583(11):1736-43. Epub 2009/03/24.

[24] Fry BG, Wroe S, Teeuwisse W, van Osch MJ, Moreno K, Ingle J, et al. A central role for venom in predation by Varanus komodoensis (Komodo Dragon) and the extinct giant Varanus (Megalania) priscus. Proceedings of the National Academy of Sciences of the United States of America. 2009;106(22):8969-74. Epub 2009/05/20.

[25] Vidal N, Hedges SB. The phylogeny of squamate reptiles (lizards, snakes, and amphisbaenians) inferred from nine nuclear protein-coding genes. Comptes rendus biologies. 2005;328(10-11):1000-8. Epub 2005/11/16.

[26] Gong E, Martin LD, Burnham DA, Falk AR. The birdlike raptor Sinornithosaurus was venomous. Proceedings of the National Academy of Sciences of the United States of America. 2010;107(2):766-8. Epub 2010/01/19.

[27] Rocha ESM, Beraldo WT, Rosenfeld G. Bradykinin, a hypotensive and smooth muscle stimulating factor released from plasma globulin by snake venoms and by trypsin. The American journal of physiology. 1949;156(2):261-73. Epub 1949/02/01.

[28] Fernandez JH, Neshich G, Camargo AC. Using bradykinin-potentiating peptide structures to develop new antihypertensive drugs. Genetics and molecular research : GMR. 2004;3(4):554-63. Epub 2005/02/03.

[29] Merchant ML, Hinton JF, Geren CR. Sphingomyelinase D activity of brown recluse spider (Loxosceles reclusa) venom as studied by 31P-NMR: effects on the time-course of sphingomyelin hydrolysis. Toxicon : official journal of the International Society on Toxinology. 1998;36(3):537-45. Epub 1998/06/24.

[30] Pungercar J, Krizaj I. Understanding the molecular mechanism underlying the presynaptic toxicity of secreted phospholipases A2. Toxicon : official journal of the International Society on Toxinology. 2007;50(7):871-92. Epub 2007/10/02.

[31] Reid PF. Cobra venom: A review of the old alternative to opiate analgesics. Alternative therapies in health and medicine. 2011;17(1):58-71. Epub 2011/05/28.

[32] Ma H, Zhou J, Jiang J, Duan J, Xu H, Tang Y, et al. The novel antidote Bezoar Bovis prevents the cardiotoxicity of Toad (Bufo bufo gargarizans Canto) Venom in mice. Experimental and toxicologic pathology : official journal of the Gesellschaft fur Toxikologische Pathologie. 2012;64(5):417-23. Epub 2010/11/19.

[33] Fachim HA, Cunha AO, Pereira AC, Beleboni RO, Gobbo-Neto L, Lopes NP, et al. Neurobiological activity of Parawixin 10, a novel anticonvulsant compound isolated from Parawixia bistriata spider venom (Araneidae: Araneae). Epilepsy & behavior : E&B. 2011;22(2):158-64. Epub 2011/07/19.

[34] Cesar-Tognoli LM, Salamoni SD, Tavares AA, Elias CF, Costa JC, Bittencourt JC, et al. Effects of Spider Venom Toxin PWTX-I (6-Hydroxytrypargine) on the Central Nervous System of Rats. Toxins. 2011;3(2):142-62. Epub 2011/11/10.

[35] Samy RP, Stiles BG, Gopalakrishnakone P, Chow VT. Antimicrobial proteins from snake venoms: direct bacterial damage and activation of innate immunity against Staphylococcus aureus skin infection. Current medicinal chemistry. 2011;18(33): 5104-13. Epub 2011/11/05.

[36] Azevedo Calderon L, Silva Ade A, Ciancaglini P, Stabeli RG. Antimicrobial peptides from Phyllomedusa frogs: from biomolecular diversity to potential nanotechnologic medical applications. Amino acids. 2011;40(1):29-49. Epub 2010/06/08.

[37] Remijsen Q, Verdonck F, Willems J. Parabutoporin, a cationic amphipathic peptide from scorpion venom: much more than an antibiotic. Toxicon : official journal of the International Society on Toxinology. 2010;55(2-3):180-5. Epub 2009/10/31.

[38] Bosmans F, Tytgat J. Sea anemone venom as a source of insecticidal peptides acting on voltage-gated Na+ channels. Toxicon : official journal of the International Society on Toxinology. 2007;49(4):550-60. Epub 2007/01/17.

[39] Rohou A, Nield J, Ushkaryov YA. Insecticidal toxins from black widow spider venom. Toxicon : official journal of the International Society on Toxinology. 2007;49(4): 531-49. Epub 2007/01/11.

[40] Nunes KP, Costa-Goncalves A, Lanza LF, Cortes SF, Cordeiro MN, Richardson M, et al. Tx2-6 toxin of the Phoneutria nigriventer spider potentiates rat erectile function. Toxicon : official journal of the International Society on Toxinology. 2008;51(7): 1197-206. Epub 2008/04/10.

[41] Martz W. Plants with a reputation against snakebite. Toxicon : official journal of the International Society on Toxinology. 1992;30(10):1131-42. Epub 1992/10/01.

[42] Ivanov VT, Yatskin ON. Peptidomics: a logical sequel to proteomics. Expert review of proteomics. 2005;2(4):463-73. Epub 2005/08/16.

[43] Tammen H, Schulte I, Hess R, Menzel C, Kellmann M, Mohring T, et al. Peptidomic analysis of human blood specimens: comparison between plasma specimens and serum by differential peptide display. Proteomics. 2005;5(13):3414-22. Epub 2005/07/23.

[44] Tammen H, Hess R, Schulte I, Kellmann M, Appel A, Budde P, et al. Prerequisites for peptidomic analysis of blood samples: II. Analysis of human plasma after oral glucose challenge -- a proof of concept. Combinatorial chemistry & high throughput screening. 2005;8(8):735-41. Epub 2006/02/09.

[45] Tammen H, Schulte I, Hess R, Menzel C, Kellmann M, Schulz-Knappe P. Prerequisites for peptidomic analysis of blood samples: I. Evaluation of blood specimen qualities and determination of technical performance characteristics. Combinatorial chemistry & high throughput screening. 2005;8(8):725-33. Epub 2006/02/09.

[46] Schiffer E, Mischak H, Novak J. High resolution proteome/peptidome analysis of body fluids by capillary electrophoresis coupled with MS. Proteomics. 2006;6(20): 5615-27. Epub 2006/09/23.

[47] Geho DH, Liotta LA, Petricoin EF, Zhao W, Araujo RP. The amplified peptidome: the new treasure chest of candidate biomarkers. Current opinion in chemical biology. 2006;10(1):50-5. Epub 2006/01/19.

[48] Traub F, Jost M, Hess R, Schorn K, Menzel C, Budde P, et al. Peptidomic analysis of breast cancer reveals a putative surrogate marker for estrogen receptor-negative carcinomas. Laboratory investigation; a journal of technical methods and pathology. 2006;86(3):246-53. Epub 2006/02/18.

[49] Mischak H, Julian BA, Novak J. High-resolution proteome/peptidome analysis of peptides and low-molecular-weight proteins in urine. Proteomics Clinical applications. 2007;1(8):792. Epub 2007/07/10.

[50] Tian R, Zhang H, Ye M, Jiang X, Hu L, Li X, et al. Selective extraction of peptides from human plasma by highly ordered mesoporous silica particles for peptidome analysis. Angew Chem Int Ed Engl. 2007;46(6):962-5. Epub 2006/12/14.

[51] Tian R, Ye M, Hu L, Li X, Zou H. Selective extraction of peptides in acidic human plasma by porous silica nanoparticles for peptidome analysis with 2-D LC-MS/MS. Journal of separation science. 2007;30(14):2204-9. Epub 2007/08/09.

[52] Li X, Xu S, Pan C, Zhou H, Jiang X, Zhang Y, et al. Enrichment of peptides from plasma for peptidome analysis using multiwalled carbon nanotubes. Journal of separation science. 2007;30(6):930-43. Epub 2007/06/01.

[53] Hu L, Li X, Jiang X, Zhou H, Jiang X, Kong L, et al. Comprehensive peptidome analysis of mouse livers by size exclusion chromatography prefractionation and nanoLC-MS/MS identification. Journal of proteome research. 2007;6(2):801-8. Epub 2007/02/03.

[54] Tammen H, Hess R, Rose H, Wienen W, Jost M. Peptidomic analysis of blood plasma after in vivo treatment with protease inhibitors--a proof of concept study. Peptides. 2008;29(12):2188-95. Epub 2008/09/23.

[55] Gelman JS, Sironi J, Castro LM, Ferro ES, Fricker LD. Peptidomic analysis of human cell lines. Journal of proteome research. 2011;10(4):1583-92. Epub 2011/01/06.

[56] Hu L, Ye M, Zou H. Peptidome analysis of mouse liver tissue by size exclusion chromatography prefractionation. Methods Mol Biol. 2010;615:207-16. Epub 2009/12/17.

[57] Beaudry F. Stability comparison between sample preparation procedures for mass spectrometry-based targeted or shotgun peptidomic analysis. Analytical biochemistry. 2010;407(2):290-2. Epub 2010/08/24.

[58] Jiang X, Ye M, Zou H. Technologies and methods for sample pretreatment in efficient proteome and peptidome analysis. Proteomics. 2008;8(4):686-705. Epub 2008/01/23.

[59] Tanaka K, Tsugawa N, Kim YO, Sanuki N, Takeda U, Lee LJ. A new rapid and comprehensive peptidome analysis by one-step direct transfer technology for 1-D electrophoresis/MALDI mass spectrometry. Biochemical and biophysical research communications. 2009;379(1):110-4. Epub 2008/12/17.

[60] Araki Y, Nonaka D, Tajima A, Maruyama M, Nitto T, Ishikawa H, et al. Quantitative peptidomic analysis by a newly developed one-step direct transfer technology without depletion of major blood proteins: its potential utility for monitoring of pathophysiological status in pregnancy-induced hypertension. Proteomics. 2011;11(13):2727-37. Epub 2011/06/02.

[61] Tian R, Ren L, Ma H, Li X, Hu L, Ye M, et al. Selective enrichment of endogenous peptides by chemically modified porous nanoparticles for peptidome analysis. Journal of chromatography A. 2009;1216(8):1270-8. Epub 2008/10/22.

[62] Hu L, Ye M, Zou H. Recent advances in mass spectrometry-based peptidome analysis. Expert review of proteomics. 2009;6(4):433-47. Epub 2009/08/18.

[63] Li F, Dever B, Zhang H, Li XF, Le XC. Mesoporous materials in peptidome analysis. Angew Chem Int Ed Engl. 2012;51(15):3518-9. Epub 2012/02/07.

[64] Pimenta AM, De Lima ME. Small peptides, big world: biotechnological potential in neglected bioactive peptides from arthropod venoms. Journal of peptide science : an official publication of the European Peptide Society. 2005;11(11):670-6. Epub 2005/08/17.

[65] ; Available from: http://www.toxinomics.org/conco_project.html.

[66] Edman P. A method for the determination of amino acid sequence in peptides. Archives of biochemistry. 1949;22(3):475. Epub 1949/07/01.

[67] Niall HD. Automated Edman degradation: the protein sequenator. Methods in enzymology. 1973;27:942-1010. Epub 1973/01/01.

[68] Roepstorff P, Fohlman J. Proposal for a common nomenclature for sequence ions in mass spectra of peptides. Biomedical mass spectrometry. 1984;11(11):601. Epub 1984/11/01.

[69] Steen H, Mann M. The ABC's (and XYZ's) of peptide sequencing. Nature reviews Molecular cell biology. 2004;5(9):699-711. Epub 2004/09/02.

[70] Songping L. Protocols for peptidomic analysis of spider venoms. Methods Mol Biol. 2010;615:75-85. Epub 2009/12/17.

[71] Valente RH, Guimaraes PR, Junqueira M, Neves-Ferreira AG, Soares MR, Chapeaurouge A, et al. Bothrops insularis venomics: a proteomic analysis supported by transcriptomic-generated sequence data. Journal of proteomics. 2009;72(2):241-55. Epub 2009/02/13.

[72] Liao Z, Cao J, Li S, Yan X, Hu W, He Q, et al. Proteomic and peptidomic analysis of the venom from Chinese tarantula Chilobrachys jingzhao. Proteomics. 2007;7(11): 1892-907. Epub 2007/05/04.

[73] Rates B, Ferraz KK, Borges MH, Richardson M, De Lima ME, Pimenta AM. Tityus serrulatus venom peptidomics: assessing venom peptide diversity. Toxicon : official journal of the International Society on Toxinology. 2008;52(5):611-8. Epub 2008/08/23.

[74] Shevchenko A, Sunyaev S, Liska A, Bork P, Shevchenko A. Nanoelectrospray tandem mass spectrometry and sequence similarity searching for identification of proteins from organisms with unknown genomes. Methods Mol Biol. 2003;211:221-34. Epub 2002/12/20.

[75] Liska AJ, Shevchenko A. Expanding the organismal scope of proteomics: cross-species protein identification by mass spectrometry and its implications. Proteomics. 2003;3(1):19-28. Epub 2003/01/28.

[76] Sunyaev S, Liska AJ, Golod A, Shevchenko A, Shevchenko A. MultiTag: multiple error-tolerant sequence tag search for the sequence-similarity identification of proteins by mass spectrometry. Analytical chemistry. 2003;75(6):1307-15. Epub 2003/03/28.

[77] Wang L, Evaristo G, Zhou M, Pinkse M, Wang M, Xu Y, et al. Nigrocin-2 peptides from Chinese Odorrana frogs--integration of UPLC/MS/MS with molecular cloning in amphibian skin peptidome analysis. The FEBS journal. 2010;277(6):1519-31. Epub 2010/02/18.

Chapter 2

Toxins from Venomous Animals: Gene Cloning, Protein Expression and Biotechnological Applications

Matheus F. Fernandes-Pedrosa,
Juliana Félix-Silva and Yamara A. S. Menezes

Additional information is available at the end of the chapter

http://dx.doi.org/10.5772/52380

1. Introduction

Venoms are the secretion of venomous animals, which are synthesized and stored in specific areas of their body i.e., venom glands. The animals use venoms for defense and/or to immobilize their prey. Most of the venoms are complex mixture of biologically active compounds of different chemical nature such as multidomain proteins, peptides, enzymes, nucleotides, lipids, biogenic amines and other unknown substances. Venomous animals as snakes, spiders, scorpions, caterpillars, bees, insects, wasps, centipedes, ants, toads and frogs have largely shown biotechnological or pharmacological applications. During long-term evolution, venom composition underwent continuous improvement and adjustment for efficient functioning in the killing or paralyzing of prey and/or as a defense against aggressors or predators. Different venom components act synergistically, thus providing efficiency of action of the components. Venom composition is highly species-specific and depends on many factors including age, sex, nutrition and different geographic regions. Toxins, occurring in venoms and poisons of venomous animals, are chemically pure toxic molecules with more or less specific actions on biological systems [1-3]. A large number of toxins have been isolated and characterized from snake venoms and snake venoms repertoire typically contain from 30 to over 100 protein toxins. Some of these molecules present enzymatic activities, whereas several others are non-enzymatic proteins and polypeptides. The most frequent enzymes in snake venoms are phospholipases A_2, serine proteinases, metalloproteinases, acetylcholinesterases, L-amino acid oxidases, nucleotidases and hyaluronidases. Higher catalytic efficiency, heat stability and resistance to proteolysis as well as abundance of snake venom enzymes provide them attractive models for biotechnologists, pharmacologists and biochemists [3-4]. Scorpion toxins are classified according to their structure, mode of action, and binding site on different channels or channel subtypes. The venom is constituted by mucopolysaccharides, hyaluronidases, phospholipases, serotonins, histamines, enzyme inhibitors, antimicrobials and proteins namely neurotoxic peptides. Scorpion peptides presents specificity and high affinity and have been used as pharmacological tools to characterize various receptor proteins involved in normal ion channel functionating, as abnormal channel functionating in cases of diseases. The venoms can be characterized by identification of peptide toxins analysis of the structure of the toxins and also have proven to be among the most and selective antagonists available for voltage-gated channels permeable to K^+, Na^+, and Ca^{2+}. The neurotoxic peptides and small proteins lead to dysfunction and provoke pathophysiological actions, such as membrane destabilization, blocking of the central, and peripheral nervous systems or alteration of smooth or skeletal muscle activity [5-8]. Spider venoms are complex mixtures of biologically active compounds of different chemical nature, from salts to peptides and proteins. Specificity of action of some spider toxins is unique along with high toxicity for insects, they can be absolutely harmless for members of other taxons, and this could be essential for investigation of insecticides. Several spider toxins have been identified and characterized biochemically. These include mainly ribonucleotide phosphohydrolase, hyaluronidases, serine proteases, metalloproteases, insecticidal peptides and phospholipases D [9-10]. Venoms from toads and frogs have been extensively isolated and characterized showing molecules endowed with antimicrobial and/or cytotoxic activities [11]. Studies involving the molecular repertoire of the venom of bees and wasps have revealed the partial isolation, characterization and biological activity assays of histamines, dopamines, kinins, phospholipases and hyaluronidases. The venom of caterpillars has been partially characterized and contains mainly ester hydrolases, phospholipases and proteases [12]. The purpose of this chapter is to present the main toxins isolated and characterized from the venom of venomous animals, focusing on their biotechnological and pharmacological applications.

2. Biotechnological and pharmacological applications of snake venom toxins

While the initial interest in snake venom research was to understand how to combat effects of snakebites in humans and to elucidate toxins mechanisms, snake venoms have become a fertile area for the discovery of novel products with biotechnological and/or pharmacological applications [13-14]. Since then, many different products have been developed based on purified toxins from snake venoms, as well recent studies have been showing new potential molecules for a variety of applications [15].

2.1. Toxins acting on cardiovascular system

Increase in blood pressure is often a transient physiological response to stressful stimuli, which allows the body to react to dangers or to promptly increase activity. However, when the blood pressure is maintained at high levels for an extended period, its long term effects

http://dx.doi.org/10.5772/52380

are highly undesirable. Persistently high blood pressure could cause or accelerate multiple pathological conditions such as organ (heart and kidney) failure and thrombosis events (heart attack and stroke) [14]. So, it is important to lower the blood pressure of high-rick patients through use of specific anti-hypertensive agents, and in this scenario, snake venom toxins has been shown to be promising sources [14-15]. This is because it has long been noted that some snake venoms drastically lower the blood pressure in human victims and experimental animals [15]. The first successful example of developing a drug from an isolated toxin was the anti-hypertensive agent Capoten® (captopril), an angiotensin-converting enzyme (ACE) inhibitor modeled from a venom peptide isolated from *Bothrops jararaca* venom [16]. These bradykinin-potentiating peptides (BPPs) are venom components which inhibits the breakdown of the endogenous vasodilator bradykinin while also inhibiting the synthesis of the endogenous vasoconstrictor angiotensin II, leading to a reduction in blood pressure [15]. BPPs have also been identified in *Crotalus durissus terrificus* venom [17]. Snake venom represents one of the major sources of exogenous natriuretic peptides (NPs) [18]. The first venom NP was identified from *Dendroaspis angusticeps* snake venom and was named *Dendroaspis* natriuretic peptide (DNP) [19]. Other venom NPs were also reported in various snake species, such as *Micrurus corallinus* [20], *B. jararaca* [4], *Trimeresurus flavoviridis*, *Trimeresurus gramineus*, *Agkistrodon halys blomhoffii* [21], *Pseudocerastes persicus* [22], *Crotalus durissus cascavella* [23], *Bungarus flaviceps* [24], among others. L-type Ca^{2+}-channels blockers identified in snake venoms include calciseptine [25] and FS2 toxins [26] from *Dendroaspis polylepis polylepis*, C10S2C2 from *D. angusticeps* [27], S4C8 from *Dendroaspis jamesoni kaimosae* [28] and stejnihagin, a metalloproteinase from *Trimeresurus stejnegeri* [29].

2.2. Toxins acting on hemostasis

Desintegrins are a family of cysteine-rich low molecular weight proteins that inhibits various integrins and that usually contain the integrin-binding RGD motif, that binds the GPIIa/IIIb receptor in platelets, thus prevents the binding of fibrinogen to the receptor and consequently platelet aggregation [13]. Two drugs, tirofiban (Aggrastat®) and eptifibatide (Integrillin®) were designed based on snake venom disintegrins and are avaliable in the market as antiplatelet agents, approved for preventing and treating thrombotic complications in patients undergoing percutaneous coronay intervention and in patients with acute cornonary sydrome [30-31]. Tirofiban has a non-peptide structure mimicking the RDG motif of the disintegrin echistatin from *Echis carinatus* [30]. Eptifibatide is a cyclic peptide based on the KGD motif of barbourin from *Sisturus miliaris barbouri* snake [31]. Recently, leucurogin, a new recombinant disintegrin was cloned from *Bothrops leucurus*, being a potent agent upon platelet aggregation [32]. Thrombin-like enzymes (TLEs) are proteases reported from many different crotalid, viperid and colubrid snakes that share some functional similarity with thrombin [13]. TLEs are not inactivated by heparin-antithrombin III complex (the physiological inhibitor of thrombin), and, differently to thrombin, they are not able to activate FXIII (the enzyme that covalently cross-links fibrin monomer to form insoluble clots). These are interesting properties, because although being procoagulants *in vitro*, TLEs have the clinical results of being anti-coagulants, by the depletion of plasma level of fibrinogen, and the clots formed are easily soluble and removed from the body. At same time, thrombolysis is enhanced by stimulation of endogenous plasminogen activators binding to the noncrosslinked fibrin [13]. Batroxobin (Defibrase®) was isolated and purified from *Bothrops atrox* venom [33] and ancrod (Viprinex®) from *Agkistrodon rhodostoma* [34]. Haemocoagulase® is a mixture of two proteinases isolated from *B. atrox* venom, acting on blood coagulation by two mechanisms: the first having a thrombin-like activity and the second having a thromboplastin-like activity, activating FX which in turn converts prothrombin into thrombin. It is indicated for the prevention and treatment of hemorrhages of a variety of origins [13]. Other toxins acting on hemostasis with potential biotechnological/pharmacological applications has been purified and characterized from several snake venoms, such as bhalternin from *Bothrops alternatus* [35], bleucMP from *B. leucurus* [36], VLH2 from *Vipera lebetina* [37], trimarin from *Trimeresurus malabaricus* [38], BE-I-PLA_2 from *Bothrops erythromelas* [39], among others.

2.3. Toxins with antibiotic activity

Antibiotics are a heterogeneous group of molecules produced by several organisms, including bacteria and fungi, presenting an antimicrobial profile, inducing the death of the agent or inhibiting microbial growth [40]. L-amino acid oxidases (LAAOs) are enantioselective flavoenzymes catalyzing the stereospecific oxidative deamination of a wide range of L-amino acids to form α-keto acids, ammonia and hydrogen peroxide (H_2O_2). Antimicrobial activities are reported to various LAAOs, such as TJ-LAO from *Trimeresurus jerdonii* [41], Balt-LAAO-I from *Bothrops alternatus* [42], TM-LAO *Trimeresurus mucrosquamatus* [43], BpirLAAO-I from *Bothrops pirajai* [44], casca LAO from *Crotalus durissus cascavella* [45], a LAAO from *Naja naja oxiana* [46], BmarLAAO from *Bothrops marajoensis* [47], among others. Recently, studies revealed that *B. jararaca* venom induced programmed cell death in epimastigotes of *Trypanossoma cruzi*, being this anti-*T. cruzi* activity associated with fractions of venoms with LAAO activity [48]. Secreted phospholipases A_2 ($sPLA_2s$) constitute a diverse group of enzymes that are widespread in nature, being particularly abundant in snake venoms. In addition to their catalytic activity, hydrolyzing the sn-2 ester bond of glycerophospholipids, $sPLA_2s$ display a range of biological actions, which may be either dependent or independent of catalytic action [49]. Eight $sPLA_2$ myotoxins purified from crotalid snake venoms, including both Lys49 and Asp49-type isoforms, were all found to express bactericidal activity [50]. EcTx-I from *Echis carinatus* [51], $PnPLA_2$ from *Porthidium nasutum* [52] and BFPA [53] from *Bungarus fasciatus* also presented antimicrobial activity. Vgf-1, a small peptide from *Naja atra* venom had *in vitro* activity against clinically isolated multidrug-resistant strains of *Mycobacterium tuberculosis* [54]. Neuwiedase, a metalloproteinase from *Bothrops neuwiedi* snake venom, showed considerable effects of *Toxoplasma gondii* infection inhibition *in vitro* [55]. Recently, a study revealed that whole venom, crotoxin and $sPLA_2s$ (PLA_2-CB and PLA_2-IC) isolated from *Crotalus durissus terrificus* venom showed antiviral activity against dengue and yellow fever viruses, which are two of the most important arboviruses in public health [56].

2.4. Toxins acting on inflammatory and nociceptive responses

Various snake venoms are rich in secretory phospholipases A_2 ($sPLA_2$), which are potent pro-inflammatory enzymes producing different families of inflammatory lipid mediators such as arachidonic acid derived eicosanoids, various lysophospholipids and platelet activating factors through cyclooxygenase and lipoxygenase pathways [57]. In a recent study, was described the first complete nucleotide sequence of a βPLI from venom glands of *Lachesis muta* by a transcriptomic analysis [58]. Recently, was purified from the venom of *Crotalus durissus terrificus* a hyaluronidase (named Hyal) that was able to provide a highly antiedematogenic acitivity [59]. Crotapotin, a subunit of crotoxin, from *C. d. terrificus*, has been reported to possess immunossupressive activity, associated to an increase in the production of prostaglandin E_2 by macrophages, consequently reducing the proliferative response of lymphocytes [60]. Various elapid and viperid venoms have been reported to induce antinociception through their neurotoxins and myotoxins [61]. *C. d. terrificus* venom induces neurological symptoms in their victims, but, contrary to most venoms from other species, it does not induce pain or severe tissue destruction at the site of inoculation, being usual the sensation of paresthesia in the affected area [62]. Based on this, several studies have been carried out with this venom, being reported in the literature several molecules with antinociceptive activity from *C. d. terrificus* venom, such as crotamine [63] and crotoxin [64]. Has been demonstrated that the anti-nociceptive effect of crotamine involve both central and peripheral mechanisms, being 30-fold higher than the produced by morphine [63]. Studies suggest that crotoxin has antinociceptive effect mediated by an action on the central nervous system, without involvement of muscarinic and opioid receptors [64]. Other antinociceptive peptides isolated from snake venoms are cobrotoxin, a neurotoxin isolated from *Naja atra* [65] and hannalgesin, a neurotoxin isolated from *Ophiophagus hannah* [66].

2.5. Toxins acting on immunological system

Venom-derived peptides are being evaluated as immunosuppressants for the treatment of autoimmune diseases and the prevention of graft rejection [67]. Studies have shown that anti-crotalic serum possesses an antibody content usually inferior to the antibody content of other anti-venom serum suggesting that the crotalic venom is a poor immunogen or that it has components with immunosuppressor activity [68]. Indeed, the immunosuppressive effect of venom and crotoxin (a toxin isolated from *Crotalus durissus terrificus*) was reported [68]. Crotapotin, an acidic and non-toxic subunit of crotoxin, administrated by intraperitoneal route, significantly reduces the severity of experimental autoimmune neuritis, an experimental model for Guillain-Barré syndrome, which indicate a novel path for neuronal protection in this autoimmune disease and other inflammatory demyelinating neuropathies [69]. Inappropriate activation of complement system occurs in a large number of inflammatory, ischaemic and other diseases. Cobra venom factor (CVF) is an unusual venom component which exists in the venoms of different snake species, such as *Naja* sp., *Ophiophagus* sp. and *Hemachatus* sp. that activate complement system [70]. Due its similarity with C3 complement system component, after binding to mammalian fB in plasma and cleavage of fB by fD, produces a C3 convertase, that is more stable than the other C3 convertases, and resistant to the fluid phase regulators. The CVF-Bb convertase consumes all plasma C3 obliterating the functionality of complement system [70]. Recently, a CVF named OVF was purified from the crude venom of *Ophiophagus hannah* and cloned by cDNA transcriptomic analysis of the snake venom glands [71].

2.6. Toxins with anticancer and cytotoxic activities

Anticancer therapy is an important area for the application of proteins and peptides from venomous animals. Integrins play multiple important roles in cancer pathology including tumor cell proliferation, angiogenesis, invasion and metastasis [72]. Inhibition of angiogenesis is one of the heavily explored treatment options for cancer, and in this scenario snake venom disintegrins represent a library of molecules with different structure, potency and specificity [1]. RGD-containing disintegrins was identified in several snake venoms, inhibiting tumor angiogenesis and metastasis, such as accutin (from *Agkistrodon acutus*) [73], salmosin (from *Agkistrodon halys brevicaudus*) [74], contortrostatin (from *Agkistrodon contortrix*) [75], jerdonin (from *Trimeresurus jerdonii*) [76], crotatroxin (from *Crotalus atrox*) [77], rhodostomin (from *Calloselasma rhodostoma*) [78] and a novel desintegrin from *Naja naja* [79]. The cytostatic effect of L-amino acid oxidases (LAAOs) have been demonstrated using various models of human and animal tumors. Studies show that LAAOs induces apoptosis in vascular endothelial cells and inhibits angiogenesis [80]. Examples of LAAOs isolated from snake venoms with anticancer potential are a LAAO isolated from *Ophiophagus hannah* [81], ACTX-6 from *A. acutus* [82], OHAP-1 from *Trimeresurus flavoviridis* [83] and Bl-LAAO from *Bothrops leucurus* [84]. Secretory phospholipases A_2 (sPLA_2) also figures the snake toxins with anticancer potential [1]. sPLA_2 with cytotoxic activity to tumor cells was described in *Bothrops neuwiedii* [85], *Bothrops brazili* [86], *Naja naja naja* [87], among others. Crotoxin, the main polypeptide isolated from *C. d. terrificus* has shown potent antitumor activity as well the whole venom, highlighting thereby the potential of venom as a source of pharmaceutical templates for cancer therapy [88]. BJcuL, a lectin purified from *Bothrops jararacussu* venom [89] and a metalloproteinase [90] and a lectin from *B. leucurus* [91] are other examples of toxins from snake venoms with anticancer potential.

3. Biotechnological and pharmacological applications of scorpion venom toxins

Scorpions are venomous arthropods, members of Arachnida class and order Scorpiones. These animals are found in all continents except Antarctica, and are known to cause problems in tropical and subtropical regions. Actually these animals are represented by 16 families and approximately 1500 different species and subspecies which conserved their morphology almost unaltered [92-93]. The scorpion species that present medically importance belonging to the family Buthidae are represented by the genera *Androctonus, Buthus, Mesobuthus, Buthotus, Parabuthus,* and *Leirus* located in North Africa, Asia, the Middle East, and India. *Centruroides* spp. are located in Southwest of United States, Mexico, and Central America, while *Tityus* spp. are found in Central and South America and Caribbean. In these different regions of the world the scorpionism is considered a public health problem, with frequent statements that scorpion stings are dangerous [8]. It is generally known that scorpion venom is a complex mixture composed of a wide array of substances. It contains mucopolysaccharides, hyaluronidase, phopholipase, low relative molecular mass molecules like

http://dx.doi.org/10.5772/52380

serotonin and histamine, protease inhibitors, histamine releasers and polypeptidyl compounds. Scorpion venoms are a particularly rich source of small, mainly neurotoxic proteins or peptides interacting specifically with various ionic channels in excitable membranes [94].

3.1. Toxins acting on cardiovascular system

The first peptide from scorpion endowed effects of bradykinin and on arterial blood pressure was isolated from the Brazilian scorpion *Tityus serrulatus* [95]. These peptides named *Tityus serrulatus* Hypotensins have molecular masses ranging approximately from 1190 to 2700 Da [96]. Other scorpion bradykinin-potentiating peptides (BPPs) were reported to be found in the venom of the scorpions *Buthus martensii* Karsch [97] and *Leiurus quinquestriatus* [98]. These molecules can display potential as new drugs and could be of interest for biotechnological purposes.

3.2. Toxins with antibiotic activity

In order to defend themselves against the hostile environment, scorpions have developed potent defensive mechanisms that are part of innate and adaptive immunity [99]. Cysteine-free antimicrobial peptides have been identified and characterized from the venom of six scorpion species [100]. Antimicrobial peptides isolated from scorpion venom are important in the discovery of novel antibiotic molecules [101]. The first antimicrobial peptide isolated from scorpions were of the defensin type from *Leiurus quinquestriatus hebraeus* [102]. Later cytolitic and/or antibacterial peptides were isolated from scorpions belonging to the Buthidae, Scorpionidae, Ischnuridae, and Iuridae superfamilies hemo-lymph and venom [103-108]. The discovery of these peptides in venoms from Eurasian scorpions, Africa and the Americas, confirmed their widespread occurrence and significant biological function. Scorpine, a peptide from *Pandinus imperator* with 75 amino acids, three disulfide bridges, and molecular mass of 8350 Da has anti-bacterial and anti-malaria effects [104]. A cationic amphipatic peptide consisting of 45 amino acids has been purified from the venom of the southern African scorpion, *Parabuthus schlechteri.* At higher concentrations it forms non-selective pores into membranes causing depolarization of the cells [109]. Opistoporin1 and 2 (OP 1 and 2) was isolated from the venom of *Opistophthalmus carinatus.* These are amphipathic, cationic peptides which differ only in one amino acid residue. OP1 and PP were active against Gram-negative bacteria and both had hemolytic activity and antifungal activity. These effects are related to membrane permeabilization [106]. A new antimicrobial peptide, hadrurin, was isolated from *Hadrurus aztecus.* It is a basic peptide composed of 41 amino-acid residues with a molecular mass of 4436 Da, and contains no cysteines. It is a unique peptide among all known antimicrobial peptides described, only partially similar to the N-terminal segment of gaegurin 4 and brevinin 2e, isolated from frog skin. It would certainly be a model molecule for studying new antibiotic activities and peptide-lipid interactions [110]. Pandinin 1 and 2 are antimicrobial peptides have been identified and characterized from venom of the African scorpion *Pandinus imperator* [101]. Recently six novel peptides, named bactridines, were isolated from *Tityus discrepans* scorpion venom by mass spectrometry. The antimicrobial effects on membrane Na^+ permeability induced by bactridines were observed on *Yersinia enterocolitica* [111]. The profile of gene in the venom glands of *Tityus stigmurus* scorpions was studied by transcriptome. Data revealed that 41 % of ESTs belong to recognized toxin-coding sequences, with transcripts encoding antimicrobial toxins (AMP-like) being the most abundant, followed by alfa KTx-like, beta KTx-like, beta NaTx-like and alfa NaTx-like. Parallel, 34% of the transcripts encode "other possible venom molecules", which correspond to anionic peptides, hypothetical secreted peptides, metalloproteinases, cystein-rich peptides and lectins [7].

3.3. Toxins acting on acting on inflammatory and nociceptive response

The use of toxins as novel molecular probes to study the structure-function relationship of ion-channels and receptors as well as potential therapeutics in the treatment of wide variety of diseases is well documented. The high specificity and selectivity of these toxins have attracted a great deal of interest as candidates for drug development [8]. At least five peptides have been identified from *Buthus martensii* (Chinese scorpion) venom that have anti-inflammatory and antinociceptive properties [61]. One peptide, J123, blocks potassium channels that activate memory T-cells [112]. The venom also contains a 61-amino acid peptide that has demonstrated antiseizure properties in an animal model [113] as well as other constituents that act as analgesics in mice, rats, and rabbits [114]. The polypeptide BmK IT2 from scorpion *Buthus martensi* Karsh stops rats from reacting to experimentally-induced pain [115]. A protein from the Indian black scorpion, *Heterometrus bengalensis*, bengalin caused human leukemic cells to undergo apoptosis *in vitro* [116]. The peptide chlorotoxin, found in the venom of the scorpion *Leiurus quinquestriatus*, retarded the activity of human glioma cells *in vitro* [117]. An investigation about the role of kinins, prostaglandins and nitric oxide in mechanical hypernociception, spontaneous nociception and paw oedema after intraplantar have been done with *Tityus serrulatus* venom in male wistar rats, proving the potential of use of the venom to alleviate pain and oedema formation [118].

3.4. Toxins acting on acting on immunological system

OSK1 (alpha-KTx3.7) is a 38-residue toxin cross-linked by three disulphide bridges initially purified from the venom of the central Asian scorpion *Orthochirus scrobiculosus* [119]. OSK1 and several structural analogues were produced by solid-phase chemical synthesis, and were tested for lethality in mice and for their efficacy in blocking a series of 14 voltage-gated and Ca^{2+} activated K^+ channels *in vitro*. The literature report that OSK1 could serve as leads for the design and production of new immunosuppressive drugs [119]. Margatoxin, a peptidyl inhibitor of K^+ channels has been purified to homogeneity from venom of the new world scorpion *Centruroides margaritatus* showed that could be used as immunosuppressive agent [120]. Kaliotoxin, a peptidyl inhibitor of the high conductance Ca^{2+}-activated K^+ channels (KCa) has been purified to homogeneity from the venom of the scorpion *Androctonus mauretanicus mauretanicus*. This peptide appears to be a useful tool for elucidating the molecular pharmacology of the high conductance Ca^{2+}-activated K^+ channel [121]. Agitoxin 1, 2, and 3, from the venom of the scorpion *Leiurus quinquestriatus* var. hebraeus have been identified on the basis of their ability to block the shaker K^+ channel [122]. Hongotoxin, a pep-

http://dx.doi.org/10.5772/52380

tide inhibitor of shaker-type (K(v)1) K^+ channels have been purified to homogeneity from venom of the scorpion *Centruroides limbatus* [123]. Noxiustoxin, component II-11 from the venom of scorpion *Centruroides noxius* Hoffmann, was obtained in pure form after fractionation by Sephadex G-50 chromatography followed by ion exchange separation on carboxymethylcellulose columns. This peptide is the first short toxin directed against mammals and the first K^+ channel blocking polypeptide-toxin found in scorpion venoms [124]. Pi1 is a peptide purified and characterized from the venom of the scorpion *Pandinus imperato,* showing ability to block the shaker K^+ channel [125]. All of these peptides obtained from scorpions venoms are potential toxins acting on immunological system as immunosuppressant for autoimmune diseases.

3.5. Toxins with anticancer and cytotoxic activities

One of the most notable active principles found in scorpion venom is chlorotoxin (Cltx), a peptide isolated from the species *Leiurus quinquestriatus.* Cltx has 36 amino acids with four disulfide bonds, and inhibits chloride influx in the membrane of glioma cells [126]. This peptide binds only to glioma cells, displaying little or no activity at all in normal cells. The toxin appears to bind matrix metalloproteinase II [117]. A synthetic version of this peptide (TM601) is being produced by the pharmaceutical industry coupled to iodine 131 (131I-TM601), to carry radiation to tumor cells [127]. A recent study shows that TM601 inhibited angiogenesis stimulated by pro-angiogenic factors in cancer cells, and when TM601 was co-administered with bevacizumab, the combination was significantly more potent than a ten-fold increase in bevacizumab dose [128]. A chlorotoxin-like peptide has also been isolated, cloned and sequenced from the venom of another scorpion species, *Buthus martensii* Karsch [129]. In reference [130] was expressed the recombinant chlorotoxin like peptide from *Leiurus quinquestriatus* and named rBmK CTa. Two novel peptides named neopladine 1 and neopladine 2 were purified from *Tityus discrepans* scorpion venom and found to be active on human breast carcinoma SKBR3 cells. Inmunohistochemistry assays revealed that neopladines bind to SKBR3 cell surface inducing FasL and BcL-2 expression [131]. Results indicate the venom from this scorpion represents a great candidate for the development of new clinical treatments against tumors.

3.6. Toxins with insecticides applications

Evidence for the potential application of scorpions toxins as insecticides has emerged in recent years. The precise action mechanism of several of these molecules remains unknown; many have their effects via interactions with specific ion channels and receptors of neuromuscular systems of insects and mammals. These highly potent and specific interactions make venom constituents attractive candidates for the development of novel therapeutics, pesticides and as molecular probes of target molecules [132].

Toxin Lqhα IT from the scorpion *Leiurus quinquestriatus hebraeus* venom is the best representative of anti-insect alpha toxins [133-134]. A similar effect was observed after applying the insect-selective toxin Bot IT1 from *Buthus occitanus tunetanus* venom [135]. Selective inhibition of the inactivation process of the insect para/tipNav expressed in *Xenopus oocyteswas*

was observed in the presence of Bjα IT [136] and OD1 [137], which are toxins from *Buthotus judaicus* and *Odonthobuthus doriae* scorpion venom, respectively. A second group of scorpion toxins slowing insect sodium channel inactivation was called alpha-like toxins. The first precisely described toxins from this group were the Lqh III/Lqh3 (from *L. q. hebraeus*), Bom III/ Bom 3 and Bom IV/ Bom 4 (from *B. o. mardochei*). They were all tested on cockroach axonal preparation [138-139]. BmKM1 toxin from *B. martensi* Karsch was the first alpha-like toxin available in recombinant form that was tested also on cockroach axonal preparation [140]. Toxins Lqh6 and Lqh7 from *L. q. hebraeus* scorpion venom show high structural similarity with Lqh3 toxin. Their toxicity to cockroach is in the range found for other alpha-like toxins [141]. Alpha-like toxins from scorpion venoms show lower efficiency when applied to insects, as compared to α anti-insect toxins. Therefore they seem to be less interesting from the point of view of future insecticide development [132]. Scorpion contractive and depressant toxins are highly selective for insect sodium channels. Several of these toxins were tested on cockroach axonal preparations; toxin AaH IT1 from the *A. australis* scorpion venom was the first one [142-143]. All other contractive toxins tested on cockroach axon produced very similar effects, as for example Lqq IT1 from *L. q. quinquestriatus* [133]; Bj IT1 from *B. judaicus* [143], Bm 32-1 and Bm 33-1 from *B. martensi* [144].

4. Biotechnological and pharmacological applications of spider venom toxins

Spider venoms contain a complex mixture of proteins, polypeptides, neurotoxins, nucleic acids, free amino acids, inorganic salts and monoamines that cause diverse effects in vertebrates and invertebrates [145]. Regarding the pharmacology and biochemistry of spider venoms, they present a variety of ion channel toxins, novel non-neurotoxins, enzymes and low molecular weight compounds [146].

4.1. Toxins acting on cardiovascular system

Venom from the South American tarantula *Grammostola spatulata* presents GsMtx-4, a small peptide belonging to the "cysteine-knot" family that blocks cardiac stretch-activated ion channels and suppresses atrial fibrillation in rabbits [147]. Studies are being conducted to develop therapeutics for atrial fibrillation based on GsMtx-4.

4.2. Toxins acting on hemostasis

ARACHnase (Hemostasis Diagnostics International Co., Denver, CO) is a normal plasma that contains a venom extract from the brown recluse spider, *Loxosceles reclusa*, which mimics the presence of a lupus anticoagulant (LA). ARACHnase is a biotechnological product usefulness like a positive control for lupus anticoagulant testing [148]. Native dermonecrotic toxins (phospholipase-D) from *Loxosceles* sp. are agents that stimulate platelet aggregation [149].

4.3. Toxins with antibiotic activity

Two peptide toxins with antimicrobial activity, lycotoxins I and II, were identified from venom of the wolf spider *Lycosa carolinensis* (Araneae: Lycosidae). The lycotoxins may play a dual role in spider-prey interaction, functioning both in the prey capture strategy as well as to protect the spider from potentially infectious organisms arising from prey ingestion. Spider venoms may represent a potentially new source of novel antimicrobial agents with important medical implications [150].

4.4. Toxins acting on inflammatory and nociceptive response

Psalmotoxin 1, a peptide extracted from the South American tarantula *Psalmopoeus cambridgei*, has very potent analgesic properties against thermal, mechanical, chemical, inflammatory and neuropathic pain in rodents. It exerts its action by blocking acid-sensing ion channel 1a, and this blockade results in an activation of the endogenous enkephalin pathway [151]. Phospholipases from both *Loxosceles laeta* and *Loxosceles reclusa* cleaved LPC (lysophosphatidylcholine) to LPA (lysophosphatidic acid) and choline. LPA receptors are potential targets for *Loxosceles* sp. envenomation treatment [152]. The possibilities for biotechnological applications in this area are enormous. Recombinant dermonecrotic toxins could be used as reagents to establish a new model to study the inflammatory response, as positive inducers of the inflammatory response and edema [9, 153-154]. The phospholipase-D from *Loxosceles* venom could be used in phospholipid studies, specially studies on cell membrane constituents with emphasis upon sphingophospholipids, lysophospholipids, lysophosphatidic acid and ceramide-1-phosphate, as models for elucidating lipid product receptors, signaling pathways and biological activities; this new wide field of *Loxosceles* research could also reveal new targets for the treatment of envenomation [10].

4.5. Toxins acting on immunological system

The antiserum most commonly used for treatment of loxoscelism in Brazil is anti-arachnidic serum. This serum is produced by the Instituto Butantan (São Paulo, Brazil) by hyperimmunization of horses with venoms of the spiders *Loxosceles gaucho* and *Phoneutria nigriventer* and the scorpion *Tityus serrulatus*. Several studies have indicated that sphingomyelinase D (SMase D) in venom of *Loxosceles* sp. spiders is the main component responsible for local and systemic effects observed in loxoscelism [153, 155]. Neutralization tests showed that anti-SMase D serum has a higher activity against toxic effects of *L. intermedia* and *L. laeta* venoms and similar or slightly weaker activity against toxic biological effects of *L. gaucho* than that of Arachnidic serum. These results demonstrate that recombinant SMase D can replace venom for anti-venom production and therapy [155].

4.6. Toxins with anticancer and cytotoxic activities

Psalmotoxin 1 was evaluated on inhibited Na^+ currents in high-grade human astrocytoma cells (glioblastoma multiforme, or GBM). These observations suggest this toxin may prove useful in determining whether GBM cells express a specific ASIC-containing ion channel type that can serve as a target for both diagnostic and therapeutic treatments of aggressive malignant gliomas [156]. The antitumor activity of a potent antimicrobial peptide isolated from hemocytes of the spider *Acanthoscurria gomesiana*, named gomesin, was tested *in vitro* and *in vivo*. Gomesin showed cytotoxic and antitumor activities in cell lines, such as melanoma, breast cancer and colon carcinoma [157].

4.7. Toxins with insecticides applications

Several spider toxins have been studied as potential insecticidal bioactive with great biotechnological possible applications [10]. A component of the venom of the Australian funnel web spider *Hadronyche versuta* that is a calcium channel antagonist retains its biological activity when expressed in a heterologous system. Transgenic expression of this toxin in tobacco effectively protected the plants from *Helicoverpa armigera* and *Spodoptera littoralis* larvae, with 100% mortality within 48h [158]. LiTxx1, LiTxx2 and LiTxx3 from *Loxosceles intermedia* venom were identified containing peptides that were active against *Spodoptera frugiperda*. These venom-derived products open a source of insecticide toxins that could be used as substitutes for chemical defensives and lead to a decrease in environmental problems [159]. An insecticidal peptide referred to as Tx4(6-1) was purified from the venom of the spider *Phoneutria nigriventer* by a combination of gel filtration, reverse-phase fast liquid chromatography on Pep-RPC, reverse-phase high performance liquid chromatography (HPLC) on Vydac C18 and ion-exchange HPLC. The protein contains 48 amino acids including 10 Cys and 6 Lys. The results showed that Tx4(6-1) has no toxicity for mice, and suggest that it is a specific anti-insect toxin [160]. SMase D and homologs in the SicTox gene family are the most abundantly expressed toxic protein in venoms of *Loxosceles* and *Sicarius* spiders (Sicariidae). A recombinant SMase D from *Loxosceles arizonica* was obtained and compared its enzymatic and insecticidal activity to that of crude venom. SMase D and crude venom have comparable and high potency in immobilization assays on crickets. These data indicate that SMase D is a potent insecticidal toxin, the role for which it presumably evolved [161]. δ-PaluIT1 and δ-paluIT2 are toxins purified from the venom of the spider *Paracoelotes luctuosus*. Similar in sequence to μ-agatoxins from *Agelenopsis aperta*, their pharmacological target is the voltage-gated insect sodium channel, of which they alter the inactivation properties in a way similar to α-scorpion toxins. Electrophysiological experiments on the cloned insect voltage-gated sodium channel heterologously co-expressed with the tipE subunit in *Xenopus laevis* oocytes, that δ-paluIT1 and δ-paluIT2 procure an increase of Na^+ current [162]. Recently, several toxins have been isolated from spiders with potential biotechnological application as insecticide.

5. Biotechnological and pharmacological applications of toad and frog toxins

Amphibians (toads, frogs, salamanders etc.) during their evolution have developed skin glands covering most parts of their body surface. From these glands small amounts of a mucous slime are secreted permanently, containing substances with different pharmacologic activities such as cardiotoxins, neurotoxins, hypotensive as well as hypertensive agents, hemolysins, and many others. Chemically they belong to a wide variety of substance classes such as steroids, alkaloids, indolalkylamines, catecholamines and low molecular peptides [11, 163]. Several studies have been showing new potential molecules for a variety of pharmacological applications from toads and frogs venoms.

5.1. Toxins acting on cardiovascular system

Neurotensin-like peptides has been identified from frog skin, such as margaratensin, isolated from *Rana margaratae* [164], a potential antihypertensive drug. Similar to the cardiac glycosides, bufadienolides from *Bufo bufo gargarizans* toad skin are able of inhibiting Na^+/K^+-ATPase, having an important role on treatment of congestive heart failure and arterial hypertension [165]. Examples of these bufadienolides are arenobufagin [166], cinobufagin, bufalin, resibufogenin, among others [165]. In the skin of *Rana temporaria* and *Rana igromaculata* frogs, bradykinin, a hypotensive and smooth muscle exciting substance, has been found [11]. Atelopidtoxin, a water-soluble toxin from skin of *Atelopus zeteki* frog, when injected into mammals, produces hypotension and ventricular fibrillation [167]. Semi-purified skin extracts from *Pseudophryne coriacea* frog displayed effects on systemic blood pressure, reducing it by a probably cholinergic mechanism [168].

5.2. Toxins acting on hemostasis

Annexins are a well-known multigene family of Ca^{2+}-regulated membrane-binding and phospholipid-binding proteins. A novel annexin A2 (Bm-ANXA2) was isolated and purified from *Bombina maxima* skin homogenate, being the first annexin A2 protein reported to possess platelet aggregation-inhibiting activity [169].

5.3. Toxins with antibiotic activity

Toxins with antibiotic activity are the most well studied toxins in toads and frogs. Two antimicrobial bufadienolides, telocinobufagin and marinobufagin, were isolated from skin secretions of the Brazilian toad *Bufo rubescens* [170]. Antimicrobial peptides, named syphaxins (SPXs), were isolated from skin secretions of *Leptodactylus syphax* frog [171]. The alkaloids apinaceamine, 6-methyl-spinaceamine isolated from the skin gland secretions of *Leptodactylus pentadactylus* showed in screening tests bactericidal activity [172]. The cinobufacini and its active components bufalin and cinobufagin, from *Bufo bufo gargarizans* Cantor skin, presented anti-hepatitis B virus (HBV) activity [173]. Telocinobufagin from *Rhinella jimi* toad were demonstrated to be active against *Leishmania chagasi* promastigotes and *Trypanosoma cruzi* trypomastigotes, while hellebrigenin, from same source, was active against only *T. cruzi* trypomastigotes [174].

5.4. Toxins acting on inflammatory and nociceptive responses

Epibatidine, an azabicycloheptane alkaloid isolated from the skin of frog *Epipedobates tricolor,* was found to be a potent antinociceptive compound. Although its toxicity, this toxin could be a lead compound in the development of therapeutic agents for pain relief as well for treatment of disorders whose pathogenesis involves nicotinic receptors [175]. A variety of toxins acting on opioid receptors have been isolated from amphibians. Dermorphin (Tyr-D-Ala-Phe-Gly-Tyr-Pro-Ser-NH_2) and related heptapeptide [Hyp^6]-dermorphin isolated from the frog skin of *Phyllomedusa* sp., show higher affinity for μ-opioid receptors. Several peptides belonging to the dermorphin family have been isolated from frog skin [61]. Deltorphins (also referred as dermenkephalin) and related peptides isolated from the frog skin have been found to exhibit high selectivity for δ-opiate receptors [176].

5.5. Toxins with anticancer and cytotoxic activities

Venenum Bufonis is a traditional Chinese medicine obtained from the dried white secretion of auricular and skin glands of Chinese toads (*Bufo melanostictus* Schneider or *Bufo bufo gargarzinas* Cantor). Cinobufagin (CBG), isolated from *Venenum Bufonis,* had potential immune system regulatory effects and is suggested that this compound could be developed as a novel immunotherapeutic agent to treat immune-mediated diseases such as cancer [177]. Bufadienolides from toxic glands of toads are used as anticancer agents, mainly on leukemia cells. Bufalin and cinobufagin from *Bufo bufo gargarizans* Cantor were tested and studies shown that these toxins suppress cell proliferation and cause apoptosis in prostate cancer cells via a sequence of apoptotic modulators [178]. Bufotalin, one of the bufadienolides isolated from Formosan Ch'an Su, which is made of the skin and parotid glands of toads, induce apoptosis in human hepatocellular carcinoma, probably involving caspases and apopotosis-inducing factor [179]. Cutaneous venom of *Bombina variegata pachypus* toad presented a cytolitic effect on the growth of the human HL 60 cell line [180]. Brevinin-2R, a non-hemolytic defensin has been isolated from the skin of the frog *Rana ridibunda,* showing pronounced cytotoxicity towards malignant cells [181].

5.6. Toxins with insulin releasing activity

Diabetes mellitus is a disease in which the body is unable to sufficiently produce or properly use insulin. Newer therapeutic modalities for this disease are extremely needed. Peptides with insulin-releasing activity have been isolated from the skin secretions of the frog *Agalychnis litodryas* and may serve as templates for a novel class of insulin secretagogues [182].

6. Biotechnological and pharmacological applications of bee and wasp toxins

Stinging accidents caused by wasps and bees generally produce severe pain, local damage and even death in various vertebrates including man, caused by action of their venoms. Bee venom contains a variety of compounds peptides including melittin, apamin, adolapin, and mast cell degranulating (MCD) peptide, in addition of hyaluronidase and phospholipase A enzymes, that plays a variety of biological activities. The chemical constituents of venoms from wasps species include acetylcholine, serotonin, norepinephrine, hyaluronidase, histidine decarboxylase, phospholipase A_2 and several polycationic peptides and proteins [12].

6.1. Toxins acting on cardiovascular system

Honey bee venom and its main constituents have a marked effect on the cardiovascular system, most notably a fall in arterial blood pressure [183]. From the hemodynamic point of view, the venom, in higher doses, is extremely toxic to the circulatory system and in smaller doses, however, produce a stimulatory effect upon the heart [184]. Melittin, a strongly basic 26 amino-acid polypeptide which constitutes 40–60% of the whole dry honeybee venom, induces contractures and depolarization in skeletal muscle [12]. Melittin is cardiotoxic *in vitro*, causing arrest of the rat heart, but only induces a slight hypertension *in vivo* [183]. Apamin, without direct effect on contraction or relaxation, could attenuate the relaxation evoked by melittin at lower concentrations, and thus contribute to the conversion of melittin's relaxing activity into the contractile activity of the venom. Another peptide found in bee venom that outlines effects on the cardiovascular system is the Cardiopep. Cardiopep is a relatively nonlethal component, compared to phospholipase A, melittin, or whole bee venom itself. It is a potent nontoxic beta-adrenergio-like stimulant that possesses definite anti-arrhythmic properties [185]. Studies on the cardiovascular effects of mastoparan B, isolated from the venom of the hornet *Vespa basalis*, has shown that the peptide caused a dose-dependent inhibition of blood pressure and cardiac function in the rat. Research has shown that the cardiovascular effects of mastoparan B are mainly due to the actions of serotonin, and by a lesser extent to other autacoids, released from mast cells as well from other biocompartments [186].

6.2. Toxins acting on hemostasis

The mechanism by which bee venom affects the hemostatic system remains poorly understood [187]. Among the serine proteases isolated from bees, which acts as a fibrin(ogen)olytic enzyme, activator prothrombin and directly degrades fibrinogen into fibrin degradation products, are the Bi-VSP (*Bombus ignitus*) [188], Bt-VSP (*Bombus terrestris*) [189] and Bs-VSP (*Bombus hypocrita sapporoensis*) [190]. According reference [188], the activation of prothrombin and fibrin(ogen)olytic activity may cooperate to effectively remove fibrinogen, and thus reduce the viscosity of blood. The injection fibrin(ogen)olytic enzyme can be used to facilitate the propagation of components of bee venom throughout the bloodstream of mammals. Bumblebee venom also affects the hemostatic system through by Bi-KTI (*B. ignitus*), a Kunitz-type inhibitor, that strongly inhibited plasmin during fibrinolysis, indicating that Bi-KTI specifically targets plasmin [187]. A toxin protein named magnvesin was purified of *Vespa magnifica*. This protein contains serine protease-like activity inhibits blood coagulation, and was found to act on factors TF, VII, VIII, IX and X [191]. Other anticoagulant protein (protease I) with proteolytic activity was purified from *Vespa orientalis* venom, involving mainly coagulation factors VIII and IX [192]. Magnifin, a phospholipase A_1 (PLA_1) purified from wasp venoms of *V. magnifica*, is very similar to other (PLA_1), especially to other wasp allergen PLA_1. Magnifin can activate platelet aggregation and induce thrombosis *in vivo*. It was the first report of PLA_1 from wasp venoms that can induce platelet aggregation [193].

6.3. Toxins with antibiotic activity

Antimicrobial peptides have attracted much attention as a novel class of antibiotics, especially for antibiotic-resistant pathogens. They provide more opportunities for designing novel and effective antimicrobial agents [194]. Melittin has various biological, pharmacological and toxicological actions including antibacterial and antifungal activities [195]. Bombolitin (structural and biological properties similar to those of melittin), isolated from the venom of *B. ignitus* worker bees, possesses antimicrobial activity and show inhibitory effects on bacterial growth for Gram-positive, Gram-negative bacteria and fungi, suggesting that bombolitin is a potential antimicrobial agent [196]. Osmin, isolated of solitary bee *Osmia rufa*, shows some similarities with the mast cell degranulation (MCD) peptide family. Free acid and C-terminally amidated osmins were chemically synthesized and tested for antimicrobial and haemolytic activities. Antimicrobial and antifungal tests indicated that both peptides were able to inhibit bacterial and fungal growth [197]. Two families of bioactive peptides which belongs to mastoparans (12a and 12b) and chemotactic peptides (5e, 5g and 5f) were purified and characterized from the venom of *Vespa magnifica*. MP-VBs (vespa mastoparan) and VESP-VBs (vespa chemotactic peptide) were purified from the venom of the wasp *Vespa bicolor* Fabricius and demonstrated antimicrobial action [198]. The amphipathic α-helical structure and net positive charge (which permits electrostatic interaction with the negatively charged microbial cell membrane) of mastoparan appear to be critical for MCD activity and because of these structural properties, mastoparans are often highly active against the cell membranes of bacteria, fungi, and erythrocytes, as well as mast cells [199].

6.4. Toxins acting on inflammatory and nociceptive responses

Bee venom has been used in Oriental medicine and evidence from the literature indicates that bee venom plays an anti-inflammatory or anti-nociceptive role against inflammatory reactions associated with arthritis and other inflammatory diseases [200]. Bee venom demonstrated neuroprotective effect against motor neuron cell death and suppresses neuroinflammation-induced disease progression in symptomatic amyotrophic lateral sclerosis (ALS) mice model [200]. Melittin has effects on the secretion of phospholipase A_2 and inhibits its enzymatic activity, which is important because phospholipases may release arachidonic acid which is converted into prostaglandins [201]. Have also been reported that melittin decreased the high rate of lethality, attenuated hepatic inflammatory responses, alleviated hepatic pathological injury and inhibited hepatocyte apoptosis. Protective effects were probably carried out through the suppression of NF-jB activation, which inhibited TNF-α liberation. Therefore, melittin may be useful as a potential therapeutic agent for attenuating acute liver injury [202]. In addition of melittin, others agents has shown anti-inflammatory activity. Among them are adolapin and MCDP. Adolapin showed marked anti-inflammatory and anti-nociceptive properties due to inhibition of prostaglandin synthase

http://dx.doi.org/10.5772/52380

system [203]. MCDP, isolated of *Apis mellifera* venom, is a strong mediator of mast cell degranulation and releases histamine at low concentrations [204].

6.5. Toxins acting on immunological system

Characterization of the primary structure of allergens is a prerequisite for the design of new diagnostic and therapeutic tools for allergic diseases. Major allergens in bee venom (recognized by IgE in more than 50% of patients) include phospholipase A_2 (PLA_2), acid phosphatase, hyaluronidase and allergen C, as well as several proteins of high molecular weights (MWs) [205]. Besides these, Api m 6, was frequently (42%) recognized by IgE from bee venom hypersensitive patients [206]; from wasp venom were purified Vesp c 1 (phospholipase A1) and Vesp c 5 (antigen-5) from *Polistes gallicus*, and Vesp ma 2 and Vesp ma 5 from *Vespa magnifica*, [207-208]. Formulations of poly(lactic-co-glycolic acid) (PLGA) microspheres represent a strategy for replacing immunotherapy in multiple injections of venom. The results obtained with bee venom proteins encapsulated showed that the allergens may still be effective in the induction of an immune response and so may be a new formulation for VIT [209]. Recombinant proteins with immunosuppressive properties have been reported in the literature, such as rVPr1 and rVRr3, identified, cloned and expressed from isolated VPR1 and VPr2 from *Pimpla hypochondriaca* [210]. Chemotactic peptide protonectin 1-6 (ILGTIL-NH2) was detected in the venom of the social wasp *Agelaia pallipes pallipes* [211]. Polybia-MPI and Polybia-CP were isolated from the venom of the social wasp *Polybia paulista* and characterized as chemotactic peptides for PMNL cells [212]. Under the diagnosis, the microarray was reported. Protein chips can be spotted with thousands of proteins or peptides, permitting to analyses the IgE responses against a tremendous variety of allergens. First attempts to microarray with Hymenoptera venom allergens included Api m 1, Api m 2, Ves v 5, Ves g 5 and Pol a 5 in a set-up with 96 recombinant or natural allergen molecules representative of most important allergen sources. The venom allergens from different bee, wasp and ant species can be offered on a single chip, allowing to differentiate the species that has stung based on species-specific markers. The allergen microarray allows the determination and monitoring of allergic patients' IgE reactivity profiles to large numbers of disease-causing allergens by using single measurements and minute amounts of serum [213].

6.6. Toxins with anticancer and cytotoxic activities

Bee venom is the most studied among the arthropods covered in this chapter regarding its anti-cancer activities, due mainly to two substances that have been isolated and characterized: melittin and phospholipase A_2 (PLA_2). Melittin and PLA_2 are the two major components in the venom of the species *Apis mellifera* [214]. Melittin is inhibitor of calmodulin activity and is an inhibitor of cell growth and clonogenicity of human and murine leukemic cells [215]. Study indicated that key regulators in bee venom-induced apoptosis are Bcl-2 and caspase-3 in human leukemic U937 cells through down-regulation of the ERK and Akt signal pathway [216]. Furthermore recent reports indicate that BV is also able to inhibit tumor growth and exhibit anti-tumor activity *in vitro* and *in vivo* and can be used as a chemotherapeutic agent against malignancy [217]. The adjuvant treatment with PLA_2 and phosphatidylinositol-(3,4)-bisphosphate was more effective in the blocking of tumor cell growth [218]. New peptides have been isolated from bee venom and tested in tumor cells, exhibiting promising activities in the treatment of cancer. Lasioglossins isolated from the venom of the bee *Lasioglossum laticeps* exhibited potency to kill various cancer cells *in vitro* [219]. Briefly the bee venom acts inhibiting cell proliferation and promoting cell death by different means: increasing Ca^{2+} influx; inducing cytochrome C release; binding calmodulin; decreasing or increasing the expression of proteins that control cell cycle or activating PLA_2, causing damage to cell membranes interfering in the apoptotic pathway [220]. Among potential anticancer compounds, one of the most studied is mastoparan, peptide isolated from wasp venom that has been reported to induce a potent facilitation of the mitochondrial permeability transition. It should be noted that this recognized action of mastoparan is marked at concentrations <1 μM [221]. Two novel mastoparan peptides, Polybia-MP-II e Polybia-MP-III isolated from venom of the social wasp *Polybia paulista*, exhibited hemolytic activity on erythrocytes [222]. Polybia-MPI, also was purified from the venom of the social wasp *P. paulista*, synthesized and studied its antitumor efficacy and cell selectivity. Results revealed that polybia-MPI exerts cytotoxic and antiproliferative efficacy by pore formation and have relatively lower cytotoxicity to normal cells [223].

6.7. Toxins with insulin releasing activity

Bee venom inhibits insulitis and development of diabetes in non-obese diabetic (NOD) mice. The cumulative incidence of diabetes at 25 weeks of age in control was 58% and NOD mice bee venom treated was 21% [224]. Mastoparan, component of wasp venom, is known to affect phosphoinositide breakdown, calcium influx, exocytosis of hormones and neurotransmitters and stimulate the GTPase activity of guanine nucleotide-binding regulatory proteins [225]. Thus, it is reported in the literature that mastoparan stimulates insulin secretion in human, as well as in rodent. Furthermore, glucose and alpha-ketoisocaproate (alfa-KIC) increase the mastoparan-stimulated insulin secretion [226].

7. Biotechnological and pharmacological applications of ant, centipede and caterpillar venom toxins

Ant, centipede and caterpillar venoms have not been studied so extensively as the venoms of snakes, scorpions and spiders. Ant venoms are rich in the phospholipase A_2 and B, hyaluronidase, and acid and alkaline phosphatase as well as in histamine itself [227]. Centipede venoms have been poorly characterized in the literature. Studies have reported in centipede venoms the presence of esterases, proteinases, alkaline and acid phosphatases, cardiotoxins, histamine, and neurotransmitter releasing compounds in *Scolopendra* genus venoms [228]. Among the most studied caterpillar venoms are *Lonomia obliqua* and *Lonomia achelous* venoms, which cause similar clinical effects [229]. Based on cDNA libraries, was possible to identify several proteins from *L. obliqua,* such as cysteine proteases, group III phospholipase A_2, C-type lectins, lipocalins, in addition to protease inhibitors including serpins, Kazal-type inhibitors, cystatins and trypsin inhibitor-like molecules [230].

7.1. Toxins acting on cardiovascular system

A study showed that the *Lonomia obliqua* caterpillar bristles extract (LOCBE) directly releases kinin from low-molecular weight kininogen, being suggested that kallikrein-kinin system plays a role in the edematogenic and hypotensive effects during *L. obliqua* envenomation [231].

7.2. Toxins acting on hemostasis

There are numerous studies in literature reporting the effects on the hemostatic system of toxins from caterpillars. The effect of a crude extract of spicules from *Lonomia obliqua* caterpillar on hemostasis was found to activate both prothrombin and factor X [232]. Lopap is a prothrombin activator isolated from the bristles of *L. obliqua* caterpillar. Lopap demonstrated ability to induce activation, expression of adhesion molecules and to exert an anti-apoptotic effect on human umbilical vein endothelial cells [233]. Lonofibrase, an α-fibrinogenase from *L. obliqua* was isolated from venomous secretion [234]. Losac, a protein with procoagulant activity, which acts as a growth stimulator and an inhibitor of cellular death for endothelial cells, was purified of the bristle extract of *L. obliqua*. Losac may have biotechnological applications, including the reduction of cell death and consequently increased productivity of animal cell cultures [235]. Lonomin V, serine protease isolated from *Lonomia achelous* caterpillar, inhibited platelet aggregation, probably caused by the degradation of collagen. It is emphasized that Lonomin V shows to be a potentially useful tool for investigating cell-matrix and cell-cell interactions and for the development of antithrombotic agents in terms of their anti-adhesive activities [236]. The venom from the tropical ant, *Pseudomyrmex triplarinus,* inhibited arachidonic acid and induced platelet aggregation, suggesting that venom prevented the action of prostaglandins. The venom was fractionated and factor F (adenosine) with antiplatelet activity were detected [237].

7.3. Toxins with antibiotic activity

Venom alkaloids from *Solenopsis invicta,* fire ant, inhibit the growth of Gram-positive and Gram-negative bacteria and presumably act as a brood antibiotic. Peptides named ponericins were identified from the venom of ant *Pachycondyla goeldii*. Fifteen peptides were classified into three different families according to their primary structure similarities: ponericins G, W, and L. Ponericin G1, G3, G4 and G6 demonstrated antimicrobial activity. Ponericins G share about 60% sequence similarity with cecropins and these have a broad spectrum of activity against bacteria. Peptides family W shares about 70% sequence similarity with Gaegurin 5 (*Rana rugosa*) and melittin (discussed in previous topics). Gaegurin 5 exhibits a broad spectrum of antimicrobial action against bacteria, fungi, and protozoa and has very little hemolytic action. The ponericin L2 from the third family has only an antibacterial action, and shares important sequence similarities with dermaseptin 5, which has strong antimicrobial action against bacteria, yeast, fungi, and protozoa [238]. A cytotoxic peptide from the venom of the ant *Myrmecia pilosula*, Pilosulin 1, was identified as a potential novel antimicrobial peptide sequence. It outlined a potent and broad spectrum antimicrobial activity including standard and multi-drug resistant gram-positive and gram-negative bacteria and

Candida albicans [239]. Two antimicrobial peptides from centipede venoms, scolopin 1 and 2 were identified from venoms of *Scolopendra subspinipes mutilan* [240].

7.4. Toxins acting on inflammatory and nociceptive responses

Venom from the tropical ant *Pseudomyrex triplarinus* relieves pain and inflammation in rheumatoid arthritis [241]. Venom from the *P. triplarinus* contains peptides called myrmexins that relieve pain and inflammation in patients with rheumatoid arthritis and inhibit inflammatory carragenin-induced edema in mice [242].

7.5. Toxins acting on immunological system

The most frequent cause of insect venom allergy in the Southeastern USA is the imported fire ant and the allergens are among the most potent known. Fire ant venom is a potent allergy-inducing agent containing four major allergens, Sol i I, Sol i II, Sol i III and Sol i IV [243-244].

7.6. Toxins with anticancer and cytotoxic activities

Solenopsin A, a primary alkaloid from the fire ant *Solenopsis invicta,* exhibits antiangiogenic activity. Among the results obtained in this study, one of the most interesting was the selective inhibition of Akt by solenopsin *in vitro,* that is of great interest since few Akt inhibitors have been developed, and Akt is a key molecular target in the pharmacological treatment of cancer [245]. Glycosphingolipid 7, identified in the millipede *Parafontaria laminata armigera,* suppressed cell proliferation and this effect was associated with suppression of the activation of FAK (focal adhesion kinase), Erk (extracellular signal-regulated kinase), and Akt in melanoma B16F10 cells. Cells treated with glycosphingolipid 7 reduced the expression of the proteins responsible for the progression of cell cycle, cyclin D1 and CDK4 [246].

7.7. Toxins with insecticides applications

Peptides named ponericins from ant *Pachycondyla goeldii* have a marked action as insecticides. Among the peptides showed insecticidal activity are the ponericins G1, G2 and ponericins belonging to the family W [238].

In Table 1, is presented a summary of the main biotechnological/pharmacological applications of toxins from venomous animals covered in this chapter.

Source		**Toxin**	**Application**	**Ref.**
		Toxins acting on cardiovascular system		
Snakes	*Agkistrodon halys blomhoffii*	NP	Anti-hypertensive agent	[21]
	Bothrops jararaca	BPP	Anti-hypertensive agent (development of captopril and derivatives)	[16]

		NP	Anti-hypertensive agent	[4]
	Bungarus flaviceps	NP	Anti-hypertensive agent	[24]
	Crotalus durissus cascavella	NP	Anti-hypertensive agent	[23]
	Crotalus durissus terrificus	BPP	Anti-hypertensive agent	[17]
	Dendroaspis angusticeps	DNP	Anti-hypertensive agent: natriuretic peptide	[19]
		C10S2C2	Anti-hypertensive drug: L-type Ca^2+channels blocker	[27]
	Dendroaspis jamesoni kaimosae	S4C8	Anti-hypertensive agent: L-type Ca^2+channels blocker	[27]
	Dendroaspis polylepis polylepis	Calciseptine	Anti-hypertensive agent: L-type Ca^2+channels blocker	[25]
		FS2 toxins	Anti-hypertensive agent: L-type Ca^2+channels blocker	[26]
	Micrurus corallinus	NP	Anti-hypertensive agent	[20]
	Pseudocerastes persicus	NP	Anti-hypertensive agent	[22]
	Trimeresurus flavoviridis	NP	Anti-hypertensive agent	[21]
	Trimeresurus stejnegeri	Stejnihagin	Anti-hypertensive agent: L-type Ca^2+channels blocker	[29]
Scorpions	*Buthus martensii*	BPP	Anti-hypertensive agent	[97]
	Leiurus quinquestriatus	BPP	Anti-hypertensive agent	[98]
	Tityus serrulatus	BPP	Anti-hypertensive agent	[96]
Spiders	*Grammostola spatulata*	GsMtx-4	Blocks cardiac stretch-activated ion channels and suppresses atrial fibrillation in rabbits	[147]
Toads and Frogs	*Atelopus zeteki*	Atelopidtoxin	Hypotensive agent and ventricular fibrillation inductor	[167]
	Bufo bufo gargarizans	Bufalin	Na^K+-ATPase inhibitor	[165]
	Pseudophryne coriacea	Semi-purified skin extracts	Hypotensive agent	[168]
	Rana igromaculata	Bradykinin	Hypotensive agent and smooth muscle exciting substance	[11]
	Rana margaratae	Margaratensin	Neurotensin-like peptide	[164]
		Cinobufagin	Na^K+ATPase inhibitor	[165]
	Rana temporaria	Bradykinin	Hypotensive agent and smooth muscle exciting substance	[11]
Bees and Wasps	*Apis mellifera*	Cardiopep	Beta-adrenergio-like stimulant and anti-arrhythmic agent	[185]

	Vespa basalis	Mastoparan B	Anti-hypertensive agent	[186]
		Toxins acting on hemostasis		
Snakes	*Agkistrodon rhodostoma*	Ancrod	Anticoagulant and defibrinogenating agent (Viprinex®)	[34]
	Bothrops alternatus	Bhalternin	Treatment and prevention of thrombotic disorders	[35]
	Bothrops atrox	Batroxobin	Anticoagulant and defibrinogenating agent (Defibrase®)	[33]
		Mixture of a TLE with a thromboplastin-like enzyme	Treatment of hemorrhages (Haemocoagulase®)	[13]
	Bothrops erythromelas	BE-I-PLA2	Antiplatelet agent	[39]
	Bothrops leucurus	BleucMP	Treatment and prevention of cardiovascular disorders and strokes	[36]
		Leucurogin	Antiplatelet agent	[32]
	Echis carinatus	Echistatin	Antiplatelet agent	[30]
	Sisturus miliaris barbouri	Barbourin	Antiplatelet agent	[31]
	Trimeresurus malabaricus	Trimarin	Treatment and prevention of thrombotic disorders	[38]
	Vipera lebetina	VLH2	Treatment and prevention of thrombotic disorders	[37]
Spiders	*Loxosceles.*	Phospholipase-D	Platelet aggregation inductor	[149]
Toads and Frogs	*Bombina maxima*	Bm-ANXA2	Antiplatelet agent	[169]
Bees and Wasps	*Bombus hypocrita sapporoensis*	Bs-VSP	Prothrombin activator, thrombin-like protease and a plasmin-like protease agent	[190]
	Bombus ignites	Bi-VSP	Prothrombin activator, thrombin-like protease and a plasmin-like protease agent	[188]
		Bi-KTI	Plasmin inhibitor agent	[187]
	Bombus terrestris	Bt-VSP	Prothrombin activator, thrombin-like protease and a plasmin-like protease agent	[189]
	Vespa orientalis	Protease I	Anticoagulant agent	[192]
	Vespa magnifica	Magnifin	Inductor platelet aggregation agent	[193]
		Magnvesin	Anticoagulant agent	[191]
Ants, Centipedes and Caterpillars	*Lonomia achelous*	Lonomin V	Inhibitor platelet aggregation agent	[236]
	Lonomia obliqua	Lopap	Prothrombin activator agent	[233]
		Lonofibrase	Fibrinogenolytic and fibrinolytic agent Agent	[234]
		Losac	Procoagulant agent	[235]
		Toxins with antibiotic activity		
Snakes	*Bothrops alternatus*	Balt-LAAO-I	Anti-bacterial agent	[42]

	Bothrops asper	Myotoxin II	Anti-bacterial agent	[50]
	Bothrops jararaca	LAAO	Antiparasitic agent	[48]
	Bothrops marajoensis	BmarLAAO	Anti-bacterial, antifungal and antiparasitic agent	[47]
	Bothrops neuwiedi	Neuwiedase	Antiparasitic agent	[55]
	Bothrops pirajai	BpirLAAO-I	Anti-bacterial and antiparasitic agent	[44]
	Bungarus fasciatus	BFPA	Anti-bacterial agent	[53]
	Crotalus durissus cascavella	Casca LAO	Anti-bacterial agent	[45]
	Crotalus durissus terrificus	Crotoxin	Antiviral agent	[56]
		PLA_2-CB	Antiviral agent	[56]
		PLA_2-IC	Antiviral agent	[56]]
	Echis carinatus	EcTx-I	Anti-bacterial agent	[51]
	Naja atra	Vgf-1	Anti-bacterial agent	[54]
	Naja naja oxiana	LAAO	Anti-bacterial agent	[46]
	Porthidium nasutum	$PnPLA_2$	Anti-bacterial agent	[52]
	Trimeresurus jerdonii	TJ-LAO	Anti-bacterial agent	[41]
	Trimeresurus mucrosquamatus	TM-LAO	Anti-bacterial agent	[43]
Scorpions	*Hadrurus aztecus*	Hadrurin	Anti-bacterial agent	[110]
	Leiurus quinquestriatus	Defensin	Anti-bacterial agent	[102]
	Opistophthalmus carinatus	Opistoporin I/II	Anti-bacterial and antifungal agent	[106]
	Pandinus imperator	Pandinin I/II	Antimicrobial agent	[101]
		Scorpine	Anti-bacterial and antiparasitic agent	[104]
	Parabuthus schlechteri	Cationic amphipatic peptide	Antimicrobial agent	[109]
	Tityus discrepans	Bactridines	Anti-bacterial agent	[111]
Spiders	*Lycosa carolinensis*	Lycotoxins I/II	Antimicrobial agent	[150]
Toads and Frogs	*Bufo bufo gargarizans*	6-methyl-spinaceamine	Anti-bacterial agent	[172]
		Bufalin	Antiviral agent	[173]
		Cinobufagin	Antiviral agent	[173]
	Bufo rubescens	Telocinobufagin	Anti-bacterial agent	[170]
		Marinobufagin	Anti-bacterial agent	[170]
	Leptodactylus pentadactylus	Apinaceamine	Anti-bacterial agent	[172]
	Leptodactylus syphax	SPXs	Anti-bacterial agent	[171]
	Rhinella jimi	Telocinobufagin	Antiparasitic agent	[174]

		Hellebrigenin	Antiparasitic agent	[174]
Bees and Wasps	*Apis mellifera*	Melittin	Anti-bacterial agent	[195]
	Bombus ignites	Bi-Bombolitin	Anti-bacterial and antifungal agent	[196]
	Osmia rufa	Osmin	Anti-bacterial and antifungal agent	[197]
	Vespa bicolor	MP-VB1	Anti-bacterial and antifungal agent	[198]
		VESP-VB1	Anti-bacterial and antifungal agent	[198]
Ants, Centipedes and Caterpillars	*Myrmecia pilosula*	Pilosulin 1	Anti-bacterial and antifungal agent	[239]
	Scolopendra subspinipes mutilan	Scolopin 1	Anti-bacterial and antifungal agent	[240]
		Scolopin 2	Anti-bacterial and antifungal agent	[240]
Toxins acting on inflammatory and nociceptive responses				
Snakes	*Crotalus durissus terrificus*	Crotamine	Antinociceptive agent	[63]
		Crotoxin	Antinociceptive agent	[64]
		Hyal	Anti-edematogenic agent	[59]
	Lachesis muta	βPLI	Phospholipase inhibitor	[58]
	Naja atra	Cobrotoxin	Antinociceptive agent	[65]
	Ophiophagus hannah	Hannalgesin	Antinociceptive agent	[66]
Scorpions	*Buthus martensii*	BmKIT2	Antinociceptive agent	[115]
		J123 peptide	K^+ channel blocker	[112]
Spiders	*Loxosceles laeta*	SMase D	Pro-inflammatory agent	[152]
	Loxosceles reclusa	Phospholipase D	Pro-inflammatory agent	[152]
	Psalmopoeus cambridgei	Psalmotoxin 1	Antinociceptive and anti-inflammatory agent	[151]
Toads and Frogs	*Epipedobates tricolor*	Epibatidine	Antinociceptive agent	[175]
	Phyllomedusa sp	Deltorphins	Opioid analgesic agents	[176]
		Dermorphins	Opioid analgesic agents	[61]
Bees and Wasps	*Apis mellifera*	Melittin	Anti-inflammatory agent	[202]
		MCDP	Anti-inflammatory agent	[204]
Ants, Centipedes and Caterpillars	*Pseudomyrex triplarinus*	Myrmexins	Anti-inflammatory agent	[242]
Toxins acting on immunological system				
Snakes	*Crotalus durissus terrificus*	Crotapotin	Immunossupressive agent	[69]
		Crotoxin	Immunossupressive agent	[68]
	Ophiophagus hannah	OVF	Complement system activator agent	[71]
Scorpions	*Androctonus mauretanicus*	Kaliotoxin	Ca^{2+} activated K^+ channel	[121]
	Centruroides limbatus	Hongotoxin	K^+ channel blocker	[123]
	Centruroides margaritatus	Margatoxin	Immunosuppressive agent	[120]
	Centruroides noxius	Noxiustoxin	K^+ channel blocker	[124]

	Leiurus quinquestriatus	Agitoxin I/II/III	K^+ channel blocker	[122]
	Orthochirus scrobiculosus	OSK1	Immunosuppressive agent	[119]
	Pandinus imperator	Pi1	K^+ channel blocker	[125]
Spiders	*Loxosceles laeta*	SMase D	Antiserum	[155]
	Loxosceles reclusa	SMase D	Antiserum	[155]
Bees and Wasps	*Agelaia pallipes pallipes*	Protonectin 1-6	Chemotactic agent	[211]
	Apis mellifera	Api m 1	Allergen	[213]
		Api m 2	Allergen	[213]
		Api m 6	Allergen	[206]
	Pimpla hypochondriaca	rVPr1	Immunosuppressive agent	[210]
		rVPr3	Immunosuppressive agent	[210]
	Polistes annularis	Pol a 5	Allergen	[213]
	Polistes gallicus	Vesp c 1 (phospholipase A1)	Allergen	[207-208]
		Vesp c 5 (antigen-5)	Allergen	[207-208]
	Polybia paulista	Polybia-MPI	Chemotactic agent	[212]
		Polybia-CP	Chemotactic agent	[212]
	Vespa magnifica	Vesp ma 2	Allergen agent	[207-208]
		Vesp ma 5	Allergen	[207-208]
	Vespula germanica	Ves g 5	Allergen	[213]
	Vespula vulgaris	Ves v 5	Allergen	[213]
Ants, Centipedes and Caterpillars	*Solenopsis invicta*	Sol i I	Allergen	[244]
		Sol i II	Allergen	[243]
		Sol i III	Allergen	[243]
		Sol i IV	Allergen	[243]
Toxins with anticancer and cytotoxic activity				
Snakes	*Agkistrodon acutus*	Accutin	Anticancer agent: disintegrin	[73]
		ACTX-6	Anticancer agent: L-amino acid oxidase	[82]
	Agkistrodon contortrix	Contortrostatin	Anticancer agent: disintegrin	[75]
	Agkistrodon halys brevicaudus	Salmosin	Anticancer agent: disintegrin	[74]
	Bothrops brazili	$sPLA_2$	Anticancer agent	[86]
	Bothrops jararacussu	BJcuL	Anticancer agent	[89]
	Bothrops leucurus	Bl-LAAO	Anticancer agent	[84]

		Metalloproteinase	Anticancer agent	[90]
		Lectin	Anticancer agent	[91]
	Bothrops neuwiedii	$sPLA_2$	Anticancer agent	[85]
	Calloselasma rhodostoma	Rhodostomin	Anticancer agent: disintegrin	[78]
	Crotalus atrox	Crotatroxin	Anticancer agent: disintegrin	[77]
	Naja naja	Disintegrin	Anticancer agent	[79]
	Naja naja naja	$sPLA_2$	Anticancer agent	[87]
	Ophiophagus hannah	LAAO	Anticancer agent	[81]
	Trimeresurus flavoviridis	OHAP-1	Anticancer agent: L-amino acid oxidase	[83]
	Trimeresurus jerdonii	Jerdonin	Anticancer agent: disintegrin	[76]
Scorpions	*Heterometrus bengalensis*	Bengalin	Anticancer agent	[116]
	Leiurus quinquestriatus	Chlorotoxin	Anticancer agent	[126]
		rBmK CTa	Anticancer agent	[130]
	Tityus discrepans	Neopladine 1 and 2	Anticancer agent	[131]
Spiders	*Acanthoscurria gomesiana*	Gomesin	Cytotoxic and anticancer agent	[157]
	Psalmopoeus cambridgei	Psalmotoxin 1	Anticancer agent	[156]
Toads and Frogs	*Bombina variegata pachypus*	Cutaneous venom	Anticancer agent	[180]
	Bufo bufo gargarizans	Bufalin	Anticancer agent	[178]
		Cinobufagin	Anticancer agent	[178]
	Formosan Ch'an Su	Bufotalin	Anticancer agent	[179]
	Rana ridibunda	Brevinin-2R	Anticancer agent	[181]
	Venenum Bufonis	CBG	Anticancer and immunotherapeutic agent to treat immune-mediated diseases	[177]
Bees and Wasps	*Lasioglossum laticeps*	Lasioglossins	Anticancer agent	[219]
	Polybia paulista	Polybia-MPI	Cytotoxic and antiproliferative agent	[223]
		Polybia-MP-II	Cytotoxic agent (hemolytic activity on erythrocytes)	[222]
		Polybia-MP-III	Cytotoxic agent (hemolytic activity on erythrocytes)	[222]
Ants, Centipedes and Caterpillars	*Parafontaria laminata armigera*	Glycosphingolipid 7	Anticancer agent	[246]
	Solenopsis invicta	Solenopsin A	Anticancer agent	[245]
Toxins with insulin releasing activity				

Toads and Frogs	*Agalychnis litodryas*	Peptides from skin secretion	Insulin-releasing activity	[182]
Bees and Wasps	Wasp venom	Mastoparan	Stimulator of insulin secretion agent	[226]
		Toxins with insecticides applications		
Scorpions	*Androctonus australis*	AaH IT1	Anti-insect agent	[142]
	Buthotus judaicu	Bjα IT	Anti-insect agent	[137]
	Buthus martensii	BmKM1	Anti-insect agent	[140]
	Buthus martensii	Bm 32/33	Anti-insect agent	[144]
	Buthus occitanus	Bot IT1	Anti-insect agent	[135]
	Buthus occitanus mardochei	Bom III/IV	Anti-insect agent	[139]
	Leiurus quinquestriatus	Lqhα IT	Anti-insect agent	[134]
	Leiurus quinquestriatus hebraeus	Lqh III/ VI/ VII	Anti-insect agent	[141]
	Odonthobuthus doriae	OD1	Anti-insect agent	[137]
Spiders	*Loxosceles arizonica*	SMase D	Anti-insect agent	[161]
	Loxosceles intermedia	LiTxx1/ LiTxx2/ LiTxx3	Anti-insect agent	[158]
	Paracoelotes luctuosus	δ-PaluIT1/ δ-PaluIT2	Anti-insect agent	[162]
	Phoneutria nigriventer	Tx4(6-1)	Anti-insect agent	[160]
Ants, Centipedes and Caterpillars	*Pachycondyla goeldii*	Ponericins G1	Insecticide Agent	[238]
		Ponericins G2	Insecticide Agent	[238]
		Ponericins family W	Insecticide Agent	[238]

Table 1. Summary of the main biotechnological/pharmacological applications of toxins from venomous animals.

8. Conclusion

The biodiversity of venoms and toxins made it a unique source of leads and structural templates from which new therapeutic agents may be developed. Such richness can be useful to biotechnology and/or pharmacology in many ways, with the prospection of new toxins in this field. Venoms of several animal species such as snakes, scorpions, toads, frogs and their active components have shown potential biotechnological applications. Recently, using molecular biology techniques and advanced methods of fractionation, researchers have obtained different native and/or recombinant toxins and enough material to afford deeper insight into the molecular action of these toxins. The mechanistic elucidation of toxins as well as their use as drugs will depend on insight into toxin biochemical classification, structure/conformation determination and elucidation of toxin biological activities based on their molecular organization, in addition to their mechanism of action upon different cell models as well as their cellular receptors. Furthermore, expansions in the fields of chemistry and biology have guided new drug discovery strategies to maximize the identification of biotechnological relevant toxins. In fact, with so much diversity in the terrestrial fauna to be explored in the future, is extremely important providing a further stimulus to the preservation of the precious ecosystem in order to develop the researches focusing on identify and isolate new molecules with importance in biotechnology or pharmacology.

Acknowledgements

Our research on this field is supported by Fundação de Amparo à Pesquisa do Estado do Rio Grande do Norte (FAPERN), Coordenação de Aperfeiçoamento de Pessoal de Nível Superior (CAPES) and Conselho Nacional de Desenvolvimento Científico e Tecnológico (CNPq).

Author details

Matheus F. Fernandes-Pedrosa*, Juliana Félix-Silva and Yamara A. S. Menezes

*Address all correspondence to: mpedrosa@ufrnet.br

Universidade Federal do Rio Grande do Norte, Brazil

References

[1] Gomes, A., Bhattacharjee, P., Mishra, R., Biswas, A. K., Dasgupta, S. C., Giri, B., Debnath, A., Gupta, S. D., & Das, T. (2010). Anticancer potential of animal venoms and toxins. *Indian Journal of Experimental Biology*, 48(2), 93-103.

[2] Braud, S., Bon, C., & Wisner, A. (2000). Snake venom proteins acting on hemostasis. *Biochimie*, 82(9-10), 851-9.

[3] Kang, T. S., Georgieva, D., Genov, N., Murakami, M. T., Sinha, M., Kumar, R. P., Kaur, P., Kumar, S., Dey, S., Sharma, S., Vrielink, A., Betzel, C., Takeda, S., Arni, R. K., Singh, T. P., & Kini, R. M. (2011). Enzymatic toxins from snake venom: Structural characterization and mechanism of catalysis. *FEBS Journal*, 278(23), 4544-4576.

[4] Murayama, N., Hayashi, M. A. F., Ohi, H., Ferreira, L. A. F., Hermann, V. V., Saito, H., Fujita, Y., Higuchi, S., Fernandes, B. L., Yamane, T., & Camargo, A. C. M. (1997). Cloning and sequence analysis of a Bothrops jararaca cDNA encoding a precursor of seven bradykinin-potentiating peptides and a C-type natriuretic peptide. *Proceedings of the National Academy of Sciences of the United States of America*, 94(4), 1189-1193.

[5] Quintero-Hernández, V., Ortiz, E., Rendón-Anaya, M., Schwartz, E. F., Becerril, B., Corzo, G., & Possani, L. D. (2011). Scorpion and spider venom peptides: Gene cloning and peptide expression. *Toxicon*, 58(8), 644-663.

[6] Verano-Braga, T., Rocha-Resende, C., Silva, D. M., Ianzer, D., Martin-Eauclaire, M. F., Bougis, P. E., De Lima, ME, Santos, R. A. S., & Pimenta, A. M. C. (2008). Tityus serrulatus Hypotensins: A new family of peptides from scorpion venom. *Biochemical and Biophysical Research Communications*, 371(3), 515-520.

[7] Almeida, D. D., Scortecci, K. C., Kobashi, L. S., Agnez-Lima, L. F., Medeiros, S. R. B., Silva-Junior, A. A., Junqueira-de-Azevedo, I. L. M., & Fernandes-Pedrosa, M. F. (2012). Profiling the resting venom gland of the scorpion Tityus stigmurus through a transcriptomic survey. *BMC Genomics*, 13, 362.

[8] Petricevich, V. L. (2010). Scorpion venom and the inflammatory response. *Mediators of Inflammation*, 903295.

[9] Tambourgi, D. V., Pedrosa, M. F. F., Van Den, Berg. C. W., Gonçalves-de-Andrade, R. M., Ferracini, M., Paixão-Cavalcante, D., Morgan, B. P., & Rushmere, N. K. (2004). Molecular cloning, expression, function and immunoreactivities of members of a gene family of sphingomyelinases from Loxosceles venom glands. *Molecular Immunology*, 41(8), 831-840.

[10] Senff-Ribeiro, A., Henrique, da., Silva, P., Chaim, O. M., Gremski, L. H., Paludo, K. S., Bertoni da. Silveira, R., Gremski, W., Mangili, O. C., & Veiga, S. S. (2008). Biotechnological applications of brown spider (Loxosceles genus) venom toxins. *Biotechnology Advances*, 26(3), 210-218.

[11] Habermehl, GG. (1995). Antimicrobial activity of amphibian venoms. *Studies in Natural Products Chemistry, Part C*, 327-339.

[12] Habermann, E. (1972). Bee and wasp venoms. *Science*, 177(4046), 314-322.

[13] Sajevic, T., Leonardi, A., & Križaj, I. (2011). Haemostatically active proteins in snake venoms. *Toxicon*, 57(5), 627-645.

[14] Koh, C. Y., & Kini, R. M. (2012). From snake venom toxins to therapeutics- cardiovascular examples. *Toxicon*, 59(4), 497-506.

[15] Hodgson, W. C., & Isbister, G. K. (2009). The application of toxins and venoms to cardiovascular drug discovery. *Current Opinion in Pharmacology*, 9(2), 173-176.

[16] Ferreira, S. H. (1965). A bradykinin-potentiating factor (BPF) present in the venom of Bothrops jararaca. *British Journal of Pharmacology and Chemotherapy*, 24(1), 163-169.

[17] Barreto, S. A., Chaguri, L. C. A. G., Prezoto, B. C., & Lebrun, I. (2012). Characterization of two vasoactive peptides isolated from the plasma of the snake Crotalus durissus terrificus. Biomedicine and Pharmacotherapy , 66(4), 256-265.

[18] Vink, S., Jin, A. H., Poth, K. J., Head, G. A., & Alewood, P. F. (2012). Natriuretic peptide drug leads from snake venom. *Toxicon*, 59(4), 434-445.

[19] Schweitz, H., Vigne, P., Moinier, D., Frelin, C., & Lazdunski, M. (1992). A new member of the natriuretic peptide family is present in the venom of the green mamba (Dendroaspis angusticeps). Journal of Biological Chemistry Jul 15; , 267(20), 13928-13932.

[20] Ho, P. L., Soares, M. B., Maack, T., Gimenez, I., Puorto, G., Furtado, M. D. F. D., & Raw, I. (1997). Cloning of an unusual natriuretic peptide from the South American coral snake Micrurus corallinus. *European Journal of Biochemistry*, 250(1), 144-149.

[21] Higuchi, S., Murayama, N., Saguchi, K., Ohi, H., Fujita, Y., Camargo, A. C. M., Ogawa, T., Deshimaru, M., & Ohno, M. (1999). Bradykinin-potentiating peptides and C-type natriuretic peptides from snake venom. *Immunopharmacology*, 44(1-2), 129-135.

[22] Amininasab, M., Elmi, M. M., Endlich, N., Endlich, K., Parekh, N., Naderi-Manesh, H., Schaller, J., Mostafavi, H., Sattler, M., Sarbolouki, M. N., & Muhle-Goll, C. (2004). Functional and structural characterization of a novel member of the natriuretic family of peptides from the venom of Pseudocerastes persicus. *FEBS Letters*, 557(1-3), 104-108.

[23] Evangelista, J. S. A. M., Martins, A. M. C., Nascimento, N. R. F., Sousa, C. M., Alves, R. S., Toyama, D. O., Toyama, M. H., Evangelista, J. J. F., Menezes, D. B., Fonteles, M. C., Moraes, M. E. A., & Monteiro, H. S. A. (2008). Renal and vascular effects of the natriuretic peptide isolated from Crotalus durissus cascavella venom. *Toxicon*, 52(7), 737-744.

[24] Siang, AS, Doley, R., Vonk, F. J., & Kini, R. M. (2010). Transcriptomic analysis of the venom gland of the red-headed krait (Bungarus flaviceps) using expressed sequence tags. *BMC Molecular Biology*, 11.

[25] De Weille, J. R., Schweitz, H., Maes, P., Tartar, A., & Lazdunski, M. (1991). Calciseptine, a peptide isolated from black mamba venom, is a specific blocker of the L-type calcium channel. *Proceedings of the National Academy of Sciences of the United States of America*, 88(6), 2437-2440.

[26] Yasuda, O., Morimoto, S., Jiang, B., Kuroda, H., Kimura, T., Sakakibara, S., Fukuo, K., Chen, S., Tamatani, M., & Ogihara, T. (1994). FS2. A mamba venom toxin, is a specific blocker of the L-type calcium channels. *Artery DCOM- 19961204*, 21(5), 287-302.

[27] Joubert, F. J., & Taljaard, N. (1980). The complete primary structures of two reduced and S-carboxymethylated Angusticeps-type toxins from Dendroaspis angusticeps (green mamba) venom. *BBA- Protein Structure*, 623(2), 449-456.

[28] Joubert, F. J., & Taljaard, N. (1980). The primary structure of a short neurotoxin homologue (S4C8) from Dendroaspis jamesoni kaimosae (Jameson's mamba) venom. *International Journal of Biochemistry*, 12(4), 567-574.

[29] Zhang, P., Shi, J., Shen, B., Li, X., Gao, Y., Zhu, Z., Zhu, Z., Ji, Y., Teng, M., & Niu, L. (2009). Stejnihagin, a novel snake metalloproteinase from Trimeresurus stejnegeri venom, inhibited L-type Ca^{2+} channels. *Toxicon*, 53(2), 309-315.

[30] Bilgrami, S., Tomar, S., Yadav, S., Kaur, P., Kumar, J., Jabeen, T., Sharma, S., & Singh, T. P. (2004). Crystal structure of Schistatin, a disintegrin homodimer from Saw-scaled Viper (Echis carinatus) at 2.5 Å Resolution. *Journal of Molecular Biology*, 341(3), 829-837.

[31] Scarborough, R. M., Rose, J. W., Hsu, MA, Phillips, D. R., Fried, V. A., Campbell, A. M., Nannizzi, L., & Charo, I. F. (1991). Barbourin: a GPIIb-IIIa-specific integrin antagonist from the venom of Sistrurus m. barbouri. *Journal of Biological Chemistry*, 266(15), 9359-9362.

[32] Higuchi, D. A., Almeida, M. C., Barros, C. C., Sanchez, E. F., Pesquero, P. R., Lang, E. A. S., Samaan, M., Araujo, R. C., Pesquero, J. B., & Pesquero, J. L. (2011). Leucurogin, a new recombinant disintegrin cloned from Bothrops leucurus (white-tailed-jararaca) with potent activity upon platelet aggregation and tumor growth. *Toxicon*, 58(1), 123-129.

[33] Stocker, K., & Barlow, G. H. (1976). The coagulant enzyme from Bothrops atrox venom (batroxobin). *Methods in Enzymology*, 45-214.

[34] Nolan, C., Hall, L. S., & Barlow, G. H. (1976). Ancrod, the coagulating enzyme from Malayan pit viper (Agkistrodon rhodostoma) venom. *Methods in Enzymology*, 45-205.

[35] Costa, J. O., Fonseca, K. C., Mamede, C. C. N., Beletti, M. E., Santos-Filho, N. A., Soares, A. M., Arantes, E. C., Hirayama, S. N. S., Selistre-de-Araújo, H. S., Fonseca, F., Henrique-Silva, F., Penha-Silva, N., & Oliveira, F. (2010). Bhalternin: functional and structural characterization of a new thrombin-like enzyme from Bothrops alternatus snake venom. *Toxicon*, 55(7), 1365-1377.

[36] Gomes, M. S. R., Queiroz, M. R., Mamede, C. C. N., Mendes, MM, Hamaguchi, A., Homsi-Brandeburgo, M. I., Sousa, M. V., Aquino, E. N., Castro, Oliveira. F., & Rodrigues, V. M. (2011). Purification and functional characterization of a new metalloproteinase (BleucMP) from Bothrops leucurus snake venom. *Comparative Biochemistry and Physiology, Part C: Toxicology and Pharmacology*, 153(3), 290-300.

[37] Hamza, L., Gargioli, C., Castelli, S., Rufini, S., & Laraba-Djebari, F. (2010). Purification and characterization of a fibrinogenolytic and hemorrhagic metalloproteinase isolated from Vipera lebetina venom. *Biochimie*, 92(7), 797-805.

[38] Kumar, R. V., Gowda, C. D. R., Shivaprasad, H. V., Siddesha, J. M., Sharath, B. K., & Vishwanath, B. S. (2010). Purification and characterization of 'Trimarin' a hemorrhagic metalloprotease with factor Xa-like activity, from Trimeresurus malabaricus snake venom. *Thrombosis Research*, 126(5), e356-e364.

[39] Modesto, J. C. A., Spencer, P. J., Fritzen, M., Valença, R. C., Oliva, M. L. V., Silva, M. B., Chudzinski-Tavassi, A. M., & Guarnieri, M. C. (2006). BE-I-PLA_2, a novel acidic phospholipase A_2 from Bothrops erythromelas venom: isolation, cloning and characterization as potent anti-platelet and inductor of prostaglandin I_2 release by endothelial cells. *Biochemical Pharmacology*, 72(3), 377-384.

[40] Chopra, I., Hesse, L., & O'Neill, A. J. (2002). Exploiting current understanding of antibiotic action for discovery of new drugs. Symposium Series Society for Applied Microbiology;, 31, 4S-15S.

[41] Lu, Q. M., Wei, Q., Jin, Y., Wei, J. F., Wang, W. Y., & Xiong, Y. L. (2002). L-amino acid oxidase from Trimeresurus jerdonii snake venom: purification, characterization, platelet aggregation-inducing and antibacterial effects. *Journal of Natural Toxins*, 11(4), 345-352.

[42] Stábeli, R. G., Marcussi, S., Carlos, G. B., Pietro, R. C. L. R., Selistre-de-Araújo, H. S., Giglio, J. R., Oliveira, E. B., & Soares, A. M. (2004). Platelet aggregation and antibacterial effects of an L-amino acid oxidase purified from Bothrops alternatus snake venom. *Bioorganic and Medicinal Chemistry*, 12(11), 2881-2886.

[43] Wei, J. F., Wei, Q., Lu, Q. M., Tai, H., Jin, Y., Wang, W. Y., & Xiong, Y. L. (2003). Purification, characterization and biological activity of an L-amino acid oxidase from Trimeresurus mucrosquamatus venom. *Acta Biochimica et Biophysica Sinica*, 35(3), 219-224.

[44] Izidoro, L. F. M., Ribeiro, M. C., Souza, G. R. L., Sant'Ana, C. D., Hamaguchi, A., Homsi-Brandeburgo, M. I., Goulart, L. R., Beleboni, R. O., Nomizo, A., Sampaio, S. V., Soares, A. M., & Rodrigues, V. M. (2006). Biochemical and functional characterization of an L-amino acid oxidase isolated from Bothrops pirajai snake venom. *Bioorganic and Medicinal Chemistry*, 14(20), 7034-7043.

[45] Toyama, M. H., Toyama, D. D. O., Passero, L. F. D., Laurenti, M. D., Corbett, C. E., Tomokane, T. Y., Fonseca, F. V., Antunes, E., Joazeiro, P. P., Beriam, L. O. S., Martins, M. A. C., Monteiro, H. S. A., & Fonteles, M. C. (2006). Isolation of a new L-amino acid oxidase from Crotalus durissus cascavella venom. *Toxicon*, 47(1), 47-57.

[46] Samel, M., Tõnismägi, K., Rönnholm, G., Vija, H., Siigur, J., Kalkkinen, N., & Siigur, E. (2008). L-amino acid oxidase from Naja naja oxiana venom. *Comparative Biochemistry and Physiology Part B: Biochemistry and Molecular Biology*, 149(4), 572-580.

[47] Torres, A. F. C., Dantas, R. T., Toyama, M. H., Diz-Filho, E., Zara, F. J., Queiroz, M. G. R., Nogueira, N. A. P., Oliveira, M. R., Toyama, D. O., Monteiro, H. S. A., & Martins, A. M. C. (2010). Antibacterial and antiparasitic effects of Bothrops marajoensis venom and its fractions: phospholipase A2 and L-amino acid oxidase. *Toxicon*, 55(4), 795-804.

[48] Deolindo, P., Teixeira-Ferreira, A. S., Da Matta, R. A., & Alves, E. W. (2010). L-Amino acid oxidase activity present in fractions of Bothrops jararaca venom is responsible for the induction of programmed cell death in Trypanosoma cruzi. *Toxicon*, 56(6), 944-955.

[49] Arni, R. K., & Ward, R. J. (1996). Phospholipase A2- a structural review. *Toxicon*, 34(8), 827-841.

[50] Santamaría, C., Larios, S., Angulo, Y., Pizarro-Cerda, J., Gorvel-P, J., Moreno, E., & Lomonte, B. (2005). Antimicrobial activity of myotoxic phospholipases A_2 from crotalid snake venoms and synthetic peptide variants derived from their C-terminal region. *Toxicon*, 45(7), 807-815.

[51] Samy, R. P., Gopalakrishnakone, P., Bow, H., Puspharaj, P. N., & Chow, V. T. K. (2010). Identification and characterization of a phospholipase A2 from the venom of the Saw-scaled viper: novel bactericidal and membrane damaging activities. *Biochimie*, 92(12), 1854-1866.

[52] Vargas, L. J., Londoño, M., Quintana, J. C., Rua, C., Segura, C., Lomonte, B., & Núñez, V. (2012). An acidic phospholipase A_2 with antibacterial activity from Porthidium nasutum snake venom. *Comparative Biochemistry and Physiology Part B: Biochemistry and Molecular Biology*, 161(4), 341-347.

[53] Xu, C., Ma, D., Yu, H., Li, Z., Liang, J., Lin, G., Zhang, Y., & Lai, R. (2007). A bactericidal homodimeric phospholipases A_2 from Bungarus fasciatus venom. *Peptides*, 28(5), 969-973.

[54] Xie, J. P., Yue, J., Xiong, Y. L., Wang, W. Y., Yu, S. Q., & Wang, H. H. (2003). In vitro activities of small peptides from snake venom against clinical isolates of drug-resistant Mycobacterium tuberculosis. *International Journal of Antimicrobial Agents*, 22(2), 172-174.

[55] Bastos, L. M., Júnior, R. J. O., Silva, D. A. O., Mineo, J. R., Vieira, C. U., Teixeira, D. N. S., Homsi-Brandeburgo, M. I., Rodrigues, V. M., & Hamaguchi, A. (2008). Toxoplasma gondii: Effects of neuwiedase, a metalloproteinase from Bothrops neuwiedi snake venom, on the invasion and replication of human fibroblasts in vitro. *Experimental Parasitology*, 120(4), 391-396.

[56] Muller, V. D. M., Russo, R. R., Oliveira, Cintra. A. C., Sartim, M. A., Alves-Paiva, R.d. M., Figueiredo, L. T. M., Sampaio, S. V., & Aquino, V. H. (2012). Crotoxin and phospholipases A2 from Crotalus durissus terrificus showed antiviral activity against dengue and yellow fever viruses. *Toxicon*, 59(4), 507-515.

[57] Kini, R. M. (2003). Excitement ahead: structure, function and mechanism of snake venom phospholipase A2 enzymes. *Toxicon*, 42(8), 827-840.

[58] Lima, R. M., Estevão-Costa, M. I., Junqueira-de-Azevedo, I. L. M., Lee, Ho. P., Vasconcelos, Diniz. M. R., & Fortes-Dias, C. L. (2011). Phospholipase A_2 inhibitors (βPLIs) are encoded in the venom glands of Lachesis muta (Crotalinae, Viperidae) snakes. *Toxicon*, 57(1), 172-175.

[59] Bordon, K. C. F., Perino, M. G., Giglio, J. R., & Arantes, E. C. (2012). 198. Isolation, enzymatic characterization and action as spreading factor of a hyaluronidase from Crotalus durissus terrificus snake venom. *Toxicon*, 60(2), 197.

[60] Garcia, F., Toyama, M. H., Castro, F. R., Proença, P. L., Marangoni, S., & Santos, L. M. B. (2003). Crotapotin induced modification of T lymphocyte proliferative response through interference with PGE_2 synthesis. *Toxicon*, 42(4), 433-437.

[61] Rajendra, W., Armugam, A., & Jeyaseelan, K. (2004). Toxins in anti-nociception and anti-inflammation. *Toxicon*, 44(1), 1-17.

[62] Giorgi, R., Bernardi, MM, & Cury, Y. (1993). Analgesic effect evoked by low molecular weight substances extracted from Crotalus durissus terrificus venom. *Toxicon*, 31(10), 1257-1265.

[63] Mancin, A. C., Soares, A. M., Andrião-Escarso, S. H., Faça, V. M., Greene, L. J., Zuccolotto, S., Pelá, I. R., & Giglio, J. R. (1998). The analgesic activity of crotamine, a neurotoxin from Crotalus durissus terrificus (South American rattlesnake) venom: A biochemical and pharmacological study. *Toxicon*, 36(12), 1927-1937.

[64] Zhang, H. L., Han, R., Chen, Z. X., Chen, B. W., Gu, Z. L., Reid, P. F., Raymond, L. N., & Qin, Z. H. (2006). Opiate and acetylcholine-independent analgesic actions of crotoxin isolated from Crotalus durissus terrificus venom. *Toxicon*, 48(2), 175-182.

[65] Chen, R., & Robinson, S. E. (1992). The effect of cobrotoxin on cholinergic neurons in the mouse. *Life Sciences*, 51(13), 1013-1019.

[66] Pu, X. C., Wong, P. T. H., & Gopalakrishnakone, P. (1995). A novel analgesic toxin (Hannalgesin) from the venom of king cobra (Ophiophagus hannah). *Toxicon*, 33(11), 1425-1431.

[67] Mirshafiey, A. (2007). Venom therapy in multiple sclerosis. *Neuropharmacology*, 53(3), 353-361.

[68] Rangel-Santos, A., Lima, C., Lopes-Ferreira, M., & Cardoso, D. F. (2004). Immunosuppresive role of principal toxin (crotoxin) of Crotalus durissus terrificus venom. *Toxicon*, 44(6), 609-616.

[69] Castro, F. R., Farias, AS, Proença, P. L. F., De La Hoz, C., Langone, F., Oliveira, E. C., Toyama, M. H., Marangoni, S., & Santos, L. M. B. (2007). The effect of treatment with crotapotin on the evolution of experimental autoimmune neuritis induced in Lewis rats. *Toxicon*, 49(3), 299-305.

[70] Vogel, C. W., & Fritzinger, D. C. (2010). Cobra venom factor: structure, function, and humanization for therapeutic complement depletion. *Toxicon*, 56(7), 1198-1222.

[71] Zeng, L., Sun, Q. Y., Jin, Y., Zhang, Y., Lee, W. H., & Zhang, Y. (2012). Molecular cloning and characterization of a complement-depleting factor from king cobra, Ophiophagus hannah. *Toxicon*, 60(3), 290-301.

[72] Goodman, S. L., & Picard, M. (2012). Integrins as therapeutic targets. *Trends in Pharmacological Sciences*, 33(7), 405-412.

[73] Yeh, C. H., Peng, H. C., & Huang, T. F. (1998). Accutin, a new disintegrin, inhibits angiogenesis in vitro and in vivo by acting as integrin α(v)β3 antagonist and inducing apoptosis. *Blood*, 92(9), 3268-3276.

[74] Kang, I. C., Kim, DS, Jang, Y., & Chung, K. H. (2000). Suppressive mechanism of salmosin, a novel disintegrin in B16 melanoma cell metastasis. *Biochemical and Biophysical Research Communications*, 275(1), 169-173.

[75] Minea, R., Swenson, S., Costa, F., Chen, T. C., & Markland, F. S. (2006). Development of a novel recombinant disintegrin, contortrostatin, as an effective anti-tumor and anti-angiogenic agent. *Pathophysiology of Haemostasis and Thrombosis*, 34(4-5), 177-183.

[76] Zhou, X. D., Jin, Y., Chen, R. Q., Lu, Q. M., Wu, J. B., Wang, W. Y., & Xiong, Y. L. (2004). Purification, cloning and biological characterization of a novel disintegrin from Trime resurus jerdonii venom. Toxicon , 43(1), 69-75.

[77] Galán, J. A., Sánchez, E. E., Rodríguez-Acosta, A., Soto, J. G., Bashir, S., Mc Lane, M. A., Paquette-Straub, C., & Pérez, J. C. (2008). Inhibition of lung tumor colonization and cell migration with the disintegrin crotatroxin 2 isolated from the venom of Crotalus atrox. *Toxicon*, 51(7), 1186-1196.

[78] Yeh, C. H., Peng, H. C., Yang, R. S., & Huang, T. F. (2001). Rhodostomin, a snake venom disintegrin, inhibits angiogenesis elicited by basic fibroblast growth factor and suppresses tumor growth by a selective αv/β3 blockade of endothelial cells. *Molecular Pharmacology*, 59(5), 133-1342.

[79] Thangam, R., Gunasekaran, P., Kaveri, K., Sridevi, G., Sundarraj, S., Paulpandi, M., & Kannan, S. (2012). A novel disintegrin protein from Naja naja venom induces cytotoxicity and apoptosis in human cancer cell lines in vitro. *Process Biochemistry*, 47(8), 1243-1249.

[80] Guo, C., Liu, S., Yao, Y., Zhang, Q., & Sun, M. Z. (2012). Past decade study of snake venom L-amino acid oxidase. *Toxicon*, 60(3), 302-311.

[81] Ahn, M. Y., Lee, B. M., & Kim, Y. S. (1997). Characterization and cytotoxicity of L-amino acid oxidase from the venom of king cobra (Ophiophagus hannah). *International Journal of Biochemistry and Cell Biology*, 29(6), 911-919.

[82] Zhang, L., & Wu, W. T. (2008). Isolation and characterization of ACTX-6: a cytotoxic L-amino acid oxidase from Agkistrodon acutus snake venom. *Natural Product Research*, 22(6), 554-563.

[83] Sun, L. K., Yoshii, Y., Hyodo, A., Tsurushima, H., Saito, A., Harakuni, T., Li, Y. P., Kariya, K., Nozaki, M., & Morine, N. (2003). Apoptotic effect in the glioma cells induced by specific protein extracted from Okinawa Habu (Trimeresurus flavoviridis) venom in relation to oxidative stress. *Toxicology in Vitro*, 17(2), 169-177.

[84] Naumann, G. B., Silva, L. F., Silva, L., Faria, G., Richardson, M., Evangelista, K., Kohlhoff, M., Gontijo, C. M. F., Navdaev, A., Rezende, F. F., Eble, J. A., & Sanchez, E.

F. (2011). Cytotoxicity and inhibition of platelet aggregation caused by an L-amino acid oxidase from Bothrops leucurus venom. *Biochimica et Biophysica Acta (BBA)- General Subjects*, 1810(7), 683-694.

[85] Daniele, J. J., Bianco, I. D., Delgado, C., Carrillo, D. B., & Fidelio, G. D. (1997). A new phospholipase A_2 isoform isolated from Bothrops neuwiedii (Yarara chica) venom with novel kinetic and chromatographic properties. *Toxicon*, 35(8), 1205-1215.

[86] Costa, T. R., Menaldo, D. L., Oliveira, C. Z., Santos-Filho, N. A., Teixeira, S. S., Nomizo, A., Fuly, A. L., Monteiro, M. C., De Souza, B. M., Palma, M. S., Stábeli, R. G., Sampaio, S. V., & Soares, A. M. (2008). Myotoxic phospholipases A2 isolated from Bothrops brazili snake venom and synthetic peptides derived from their C-terminal region: cytotoxic effect on microorganism and tumor cells. *Peptides*, 29(10), 1645-1656.

[87] Rudrammaji, L. M. S., & Gowda, T. V. (1998). Purification and characterization of three acidic, cytotoxic phospholipases A2 from Indian cobra (Naja naja naja) venom. *Toxicon*, 36(6), 921-932.

[88] Soares, M. A., Pujatti, P. B., Fortes-Dias, C. L., Antonelli, L., & Santos, R. G. (2010). Crotalus durissus terrificus venom as a source of antitumoral agents. *Journal of Venomous Animals and Toxins Including Tropical Diseases*, 16(3), 480-492.

[89] Nolte, S., Damasio, D. C., Baréa, A. C., Gomes, J., Magalhães, A., Zischler, L. F. C. M., Stuelp-Campelo, P. M., Elífio-Esposito, S. L., Roque-Barreira, M. C., Reis-Amaral, CA, & Moreno, A. N. (2012). BJcuL, a lectin purified from Bothrops jararacussu venom, induces apoptosis in human gastric carcinoma cells accompanied by inhibition of cell adhesion and actin cytoskeleton disassembly. *Toxicon*, 59(1), 81-85.

[90] Gabriel, L. M., Sanchez, E. F., Silva, S. G., & dos Santos, R. G. (2012). Tumor cytotoxicity of leucurolysin-B, a P-III snake venom metalloproteinase from Bothrops leucurus. *Journal of Venomous Animals and Toxins Including Tropical Diseases*, 18(1), 24-33.

[91] Nunes, E. S., Souza, M. A. A., Vaz, A. F. M., Silva, T. G., Aguiar, J. S., Batista, A. M., Guerra, M. M. P., Guarnieri, M. C., Coelho, L. C. B. B., & Correia, M. T. S. (2012). Cytotoxic effect and apoptosis induction by Bothrops leucurus venom lectin on tumor cell lines. *Toxicon*, 59(7-8), 667-671.

[92] Dehesa-Dávila, M., Martin, BM, Nobile, M., Prestipino, G., & Possani, L. D. (1994). Isolation of a toxin from Centruroides infamatus infamatus Koch scorpion venom that modifies Na^+ permeability on chick dorsal root ganglion cells. *Toxicon*, 32(12), 1487-1493.

[93] Chowell, G., Díaz-Dueñas, P., Bustos-Saldaña, R., Mireles, AA , & Fet, V. (2006). Epidemiological and clinical characteristics of scorpionism in Colima, Mexico (2000-2001). *Toxicon*, 47(7), 753-758.

[94] Goudet, C., Chi, C. W., & Tytgat, J. (2002). An overview of toxins and genes from the venom of the Asian scorpion Buthus martensi Karsch. *Toxicon*, 40(9), 1239-1258.

[95] Ferreira, L. A. F., Alves, E. W., & Henriques, O. B. (1993). Peptide T, a novel bradykinin potentiator isolated from Tityus serrulatus scorpion venom. *Toxicon*, 31(8), 941-947.

[96] Pimenta, A. M. C., & De Lima, M. E. (2005). Small peptides, big world: Biotechnological potential in neglected bioactive peptides from arthropod venoms. *Journal of Peptide Science*, 11(11), 670-676.

[97] Zeng, X. C., Li, W. X., Peng, F., & Zhu, Z. H. (2000). Cloning and characterization of a novel cDNA sequence encoding the precursor of a novel venom peptide (BmKbpp) related to a bradykinin- potentiating peptide from Chinese scorpion Buthus martensii Karsch. *IUBMB Life*, 49(3), 207-210.

[98] El -Saadani, M. A. M., & El -Sayed, M. F. (2003). A bradykinin potentiating peptide from Egyptian cobra venom strongly affects rat atrium contractile force and cellular calcium regulation. *Comparative Biochemistry and Physiology Part C: Toxicology and Pharmacology*, 136(4), 387-395.

[99] Bulet, P., Stöcklin, R., & Menin, L. (2004). Anti-microbial peptides: From invertebrates to vertebrates. *Immunological Reviews*, 198-169.

[100] Elgar, D., Du Plessis, J., & Du Plessis, L. (2006). Cysteine-free peptides in scorpion venom: Geographical distribution, structure-function relationship and mode of action. *African Journal of Biotechnology*, 5(25), 2495-2502.

[101] Corzo, G., Escoubas, P., Villegas, E., Barnham, K. J., He, W., Norton, R. S., & Nakajima, T. (2001). Characterization of unique amphipathic antimicrobial peptides from venom of the scorpion Pandinus imperator. *Biochemical Journal*, 359(1), 35-45.

[102] Cociancich, S., Goyffon, M., Bontems, F., Bulet, P., Bouet, F., Menez, A., & Hoffmann, J. (1993). Purification and Characterization of a Scorpion Defensin, a 4kDa Antibacterial peptide presenting structural similarities with insect defensins and scorpion toxins. *Biochemical and Biophysical Research Communications*, 194(1), 17-22.

[103] Ehret-Sabatier, L., Loew, D., Goyffon, M., Fehlbaum, P., Hoffmann, J. A., Van Dorsselaer, A., & Bulet, P. (1996). Characterization of novel cysteine-rich antimicrobial peptides from scorpion blood. *Journal of Biological Chemistry*, 271(47), 29537-29544.

[104] Conde, R., Zamudio, F. Z., Rodríguez, M. H., & Possani, L. D. (2000). Scorpine, an anti-malaria and anti-bacterial agent purified from scorpion venom. *FEBS Letters*, 471(2-3), 165-168.

[105] Dai, L., Corzo, G., Naoki, H., Andriantsiferana, M., & Nakajima, T. (2002). Purification, structure-function analysis, and molecular characterization of novel linear peptides from scorpion Opisthacanthus madagascariensis. *Biochemical and Biophysical Research Communications*, 293(5), 1514-1522.

[106] Moerman, L., Bosteels, S., Noppe, W., Willems, J., Clynen, E., Schoofs, L., Thevissen, K., Tytgat, J., Van Eldere, J., Van Der Walt, J., & Verdonck, F. (2002). Antibacterial

and antifungal properties of α-helical, cationic peptides in the venom of scorpions from southern Africa. *European Journal of Biochemistry*, 269(19), 4799-4810.

[107] Rodríguez La, Vega. R. C., García, B. I., D'Ambrosio, C., Diego-García, E., Scaloni, A., & Possani, L. D. (2004). Antimicrobial peptide induction in the haemolymph of the Mexican scorpion Centruroides limpidus limpidus in response to septic injury. *Cellular and Molecular Life Sciences*, 61(12), 1507-1519.

[108] Uawonggul, N., Thammasirirak, S., Chaveerach, A., Arkaravichien, T., Bunyatratchata, W., Ruangjirachuporn, W., Jearranaiprepame, P., Nakamura, T., Matsuda, M., Kobayashi, M., Hattori, S., & Daduang, S. (2007). Purification and characterization of Heteroscorpine-1 (HS-1) toxin from Heterometrus laoticus scorpion venom. *Toxicon*, 49(1), 19-29.

[109] Elgar, D., Verdonck, F., Grobler, A., Fourie, C., & Du, Plessis. J. (2006). Ion selectivity of scorpion toxin-induced pores in cardiac myocytes. *Peptides*, 27(1), 55-61.

[110] Torres-Larios, A., Gurrola, G. B., Zamudio, F. Z., & Possani, L. D. (2000). Hadrurin, a new antimicrobial peptide from the venom of the scorpion Hadrurus aztecus. *European Journal of Biochemistry*, 267(16), 5023-5031.

[111] Díaz, P., D'Suze, G., Salazar, V., Sevcik, C., Shannon, Sherman. N. E., & Fox, J. W. (2009). Antibacterial activity of six novel peptides from Tityus discrepans scorpion venom. A fluorescent probe study of microbial membrane Na^+ permeability changes. *Toxicon*, 54(6), 802-817.

[112] Shijin, Y., Hong, Y., Yibao, M., Zongyun, C., Han, S., Yingliang, W., Zhijian, C., & Wenxin, L. (2008). Characterization of a new Kv1.3 channel-specific blocker, J123, from the scorpion Buthus martensii Karsch. *Peptides*, 29(9), 1514-1520.

[113] Wang, Z., Wang, W., Shao, Z., Gao, B., Li, J., Che, J. H., & Zhang, W. (2009). Eukaryotic expression and purification of anti-epilepsy peptide of Buthus martensii Karsch and its protein interactions. *Molecular and Cellular Biochemistry*, 330(1-2), 97-104.

[114] Shao, J., Kang, N., Liu, Y., Song, S., Wu, C., & Zhang, J. (2007). Purification and characterization of an analgesic peptide from Buthus martensii Karsch. *Biomedical Chromatography*, 21(12), 1266-1271.

[115] Bai, Z. T., Liu, T., Pang, X. Y., Chai, Z. F., & Ji, Y. H. (2007). Suppression by intrathecal BmK IT2 on rat spontaneous pain behaviors and spinal c-Fos expression induced by formalin. *Brain Research Bulletin*, 73(4-6), 248-253.

[116] Gupta, S. D., Gomes, A., Debnath, A., & Saha, A. (2010). Apoptosis induction in human leukemic cells by a novel protein Bengalin, isolated from Indian black scorpion venom: Through mitochondrial pathway and inhibition of heat shock proteins. *Chemico-Biological Interactions*, 183(2), 293-303.

[117] Deshane, J., Garner, C. C., & Sontheimer, H. (2003). Chlorotoxin inhibits glioma cell invasion via matrix metalloproteinase-2. *Journal of Biological Chemistry*, 278(6), 4135-4144.

[118] Pessini, A. C., Kanashiro, A., Malvar, Dd. C., Machado, R. R., Soares, D. M., Figueiredo, MJ, Kalapothakis, E., & Souza, G. E. P. (2008). Inflammatory mediators involved in the nociceptive and oedematogenic responses induced by Tityus serrulatus scorpion venom injected into rat paws. *Toxicon*, 52(7), 729-736.

[119] Jaravine, V. A., Nolde, D. E., Reibarkh, M. J., Korolkova, Y. V., Kozlov, S. A., Pluzhnikov, K. A., Grishin, E. V., & Arseniev, A. S. (1997). Three-dimensional structure of toxin OSK1 from Orthochirus scrobiculosus scorpion venom. *Biochemistry*, 36(6), 1223-1232.

[120] Garcia-Calvo, M., Leonard, R. J., Novick, J., Stevens, S. P., Schmalhofer, W., Kaczorowski, G. J., & Garcia, M. L. (1993). Purification, characterization, and biosynthesis of margatoxin, a component of Centruroides margaritatus venom that selectively inhibits voltage-dependent potassium channels. *Journal of Biological Chemistry*, 268(25), 18866-18874.

[121] Crest, M., Jacquet, G., Gola, M., Zerrouk, H., Benslimane, A., Rochat, H., Mansuelle, P., & Martin-Eauclaire, M. F. (1992). Kaliotoxin, a novel peptidyl inhibitor of neuronal BK-type Ca^{2+}-activated K^+ channels characterized from Androctonus mauretanicus mauretanicus venom. *Journal of Biological Chemistry*, 267(3), 1640-1647.

[122] Garcia, ML. (1994). Purification and characterization of three inhibitors of voltage-dependent K^+ channels from Leiurus quinquestriatus var. Hebraeus venom. *Biochemistry*, 33(22), 6834-6839.

[123] Koschak, A., Bugianesi, R. M., Mitterdorfer, J., Kaczorowski, G. J., Garcia, M. L., & Knaus, H. G. (1998). Subunit composition of brain voltage-gated potassium channels determined by hongotoxin-1, a novel peptide derived from Centruroides limbatus venom. *Journal of Biological Chemistry*, 273(5), 2639-2644.

[124] Domingos, Possani. L., Martin, BM, & Svendsen, I. B. (1982). The primary structure of noxiustoxin: A K^+ channel blocking peptide, purified from the venom of the scorpion Centruroides noxius Hoffmann. *Carlsberg Research Communications*, 47(5), 285-289.

[125] Olamendi-Portugal, T., Gómez-Lagunas, F., Gurrola, G. B., & Possani, L. D. (1996). A novel structural class of K^+-channel blocking toxin from the scorpion Pandinus imperator. *Biochemical Journal*, 315(3), 977-981.

[126] Soroceanu, L., Manning Jr, T. J., & Sontheimer, H. (1999). Modulation of glioma cell migration and invasion using Cl^- and K^+ ion channel blockers. *Journal of Neuroscience*, 19(14), 5942-5954.

[127] Mamelak, A. N., & Jacoby, D. B. (2007). Targeted delivery of antitumoral therapy to glioma and other malignancies with synthetic chlorotoxin (TM-601). *Expert Opinion on Drug Delivery*, 4(2), 175-186.

[128] Jacoby, D. B., Dyskin, E., Yalcin, M., Kesavan, K., Dahlberg, W., Ratliff, J., Johnson, E. W., & Mousa, S. A. (2010). Potent pleiotropic anti-angiogenic effects of TM601, a synthetic chlorotoxin peptide. *Anticancer Research*, 30(1), 39-46.

[129] Wu, J. J., Dai, L., Lan, Z. D., & Chi, C. W. (2000). The gene cloning and sequencing of Bm-12, a Chlorotoxin-like peptide from the scorpion Buthus martensi Karsch. *Toxicon*, 38(5), 661-668.

[130] Fu, Y. J., Yin, L. T., Liang, A. H., Zhang, C. F., Wang, W., Chai, B. F., Yang, J. Y., & Fan, X. J. (2007). Therapeutic potential of chlorotoxin-like neurotoxin from the Chinese scorpion for human gliomas. *Neuroscience Letters*, 412(1), 62-67.

[131] D'Suze, G., Rosales, A., Salazar, V., & Sevcik, C. (2010). Apoptogenic peptides from Tityus discrepans scorpion venom acting against the SKBR3 breast cancer cell line. *Toxicon*, 56(8), 1497-1505.

[132] De Lima, ME, Figueiredo, S. G., Pimenta, A. M. C., Santos, D. M., Borges, M. H., Cordeiro, M. N., Richardson, M., Oliveira, L. C., Stankiewicz, M., & Pelhate, M. (2007). Peptides of arachnid venoms with insecticidal activity targeting sodium channels. *Comparative Biochemistry and Physiology Part C: Toxicology and Pharmacology*, 146(1-2), 264-279.

[133] Eitan, M., Fowler, E., Herrmann, R., Duval, A., Pelhate, M., & Zlotkin, E. (1990). A scorpion venom neurotoxin paralytic to insects that affects sodium current inactivation: purification, primary structure, and mode of action. *Biochemistry*, 29(25), 5941-5947.

[134] Karbat, I., Frolow, F., Froy, O., Gilles, N., Cohen, L., Turkov, M., Gordon, D., & Gurevitz, M. (2004). Molecular basis of the high insecticidal potency of scorpion alpha-toxins. *The Journal of Biological Chemistry*, 279(30), 31679-31686.

[135] Borchani, L., Stankiewicz, M., Kopeyan, C., Mansuelle, P., Kharrat, R., Cestèle, S., Karoui, H., Rochat, H., Pelhate, M., & El Ayeb, M. (1997). Purification, structure and activity of three insect toxins from Buthus occitanus tunetanus venom. *Toxicon*, 35(3), 365-382.

[136] Arnon, T., Potikha, T., Sher, D., Elazar, M., Mao, W., Tal, T., Bosmans, F., Tytgat, J., Ben-Arie, N., & Zlotkin, E. (2005). BjαIT: a novel scorpion α-toxin selective for insects- unique pharmacological tool. *Insect Biochemistry and Molecular Biology*, 35(3), 187-195.

[137] Jalali, A., Bosmans, F., Amininasab, M., Clynen, E., Cuypers, E., Zaremirakabadi, A., Sarbolouki, M. N., Schoofs, L., Vatanpour, H., & Tytgat, J. (2005). OD1, the first toxin isolated from the venom of the scorpion Odonthobuthus doriae active on voltage-gated Na^+ channels. *FEBS Letters*, 579(19), 4181-4186.

[138] Krimm, I., Gilles, N., Sautière, P., Stankiewicz, M., Pelhate, M., Gordon, D., & Lancelin-M, J. (1999). NMR structures and activity of a novel α-like toxin from the scorpion Leiurus quinquestriatus hebraeus. *Journal of Molecular Biology*, 285(4), 1749-1763.

[139] Cestèle, S., Stankiewicz, M., Mansuelle, P., De Waard, M., Dargent, B., Gilles, N., Pelhate, M., Rochat, H., Martin-Eauclaire-F, M., & Gordon, D. (1999). Scorpion α-like toxins, toxic to both mammals and insects, differentially interact with receptor site 3

on voltage-gated sodium channels in mammals and insects. *European Journal of Neuroscience*, 11(3), 975-985.

[140] Wang, C. G., Ling, M. H., Chi, C. W., Wang, D. C., Stankiewicz, M., & Pelhate, M. (2003). Purification of two depressant insect neurotoxins and their gene cloning from the scorpion Buthus martensi Karsch. The Journal of Peptide Research , 61(1), 7-16.

[141] Hamon, A., Gilles, N., Sautière, P., Martinage, A., Kopeyan, C., Ulens, C., Tytgat, J., Lancelin, J. M., & Gordon, D. (2002). Characterization of scorpion α-like toxin group using two new toxins from the scorpion Leiurus quinquestriatus hebraeus. *European Journal of Biochemistry*, 269(16), 3920-3933.

[142] Pelhate, M., & Zlotkin, E. (1982). Actions of insect toxin and other toxins derived from the venom of the scorpion Androctonus australis on isolated giant axons of the cockroach (Periplaneta americana). *The Journal of Experimental Biology*, 97-67.

[143] Pelhate, M., Stankiewicz, M., & Ben, Khalifa. R. (1998). Anti-insect scorpion toxins: historical account, activities and prospects. *Comptes Rendus des Séances de la Société de Biologie et de Ses Filiales*, 192(3), 463-484.

[144] Escoubas, P., Stankiewicz, M., Takaoka, T., Pelhate, M., Romi-Lebrun, R., Wu, F. Q., & Nakajima, T. (2000). Sequence and electrophysiological characterization of two insect-selective excitatory toxins from the venom of the Chinese scorpion Buthus martensi. *FEBS Letters*, 483(2-3), 175-80.

[145] Ori, M., & Ikeda, H. (1998). Spider venoms and spider toxins. *Journal of Toxicology-Toxin Reviews*, 17(3), 405-426.

[146] Rash, L. D., & Hodgson, W. C. (2001). Pharmacology and biochemistry of spider venoms. *Toxicon*, 40(3), 225-254.

[147] Bode, F., Sachs, F., & Franz, M. R. (2001). Tarantula peptide inhibits atrial fibrillation. *Nature*, 409(6816), 35-36.

[148] Mc Glasson, D. L., Babcock, J. L., Berg, L., & Triplett, D. A. (1993). ARACHnase: An evaluation of a positive control for platelet neutralization procedure testing with seven commercial activated partial thromboplastin time reagents. *American Journal of Clinical Pathology*, 100(5), 576-578.

[149] Futrell, J. M. (1992). Loxoscelism. *American Journal of the Medical Sciences*, 304(4), 261-267.

[150] Yan, L., & Adams, M. E. (1998). Lycotoxins, antimicrobial peptides from venom of the wolf spider Lycosa carolinensis. *Journal of Biological Chemistry*, 273(4), 2059-2066.

[151] Mazzuca, M., Heurteaux, C., Alloui, A., Diochot, S., Baron, A., Voilley, N., Blondeau, N., Escoubas, P., Gelot, A., Cupo, A., Zimmer, A., Zimmer, A. M., Eschalier, A., & Lazdunski, M. (2007). A tarantula peptide against pain via ASIC1a channels and opioid mechanisms. *Nature Neuroscience*, 10(8), 943-945.

[152] Van Meeteren, L. A., Frederiks, F., Giepmans, B. N. G., Fernandes, Pedrosa. M. F., Billington, S. J., Jost, B. H., Tambourgi, D. V., & Moolenaar, W. H. (2004). Spider and bacterial Sphingomyelinases D target cellular lysophosphatidic acid receptors by hydrolyzing lysophosphatidylcholine. *Journal of Biological Chemistry,* 279(12), 10833-10836.

[153] Fernandes, Pedrosa. M. F., Junqueira de, Azevedo. I. D. L. M., Gonçalves-de-Andrade, R. M., Van Den, Berg. C. W., Ramos, C. R. R., Lee, Ho. P., & Tambourgi, D. V. (2002). Molecular cloning and expression of a functional dermonecrotic and haemolytic factor from Loxosceles laeta venom. *Biochemical and Biophysical Research Communications,* 298(5), 638-645.

[154] Murakami, M. T., Fernandes-Pedrosa, M. F., Tambourgi, D. V., & Arni, R. K. (2005). Structural basis for metal ion coordination and the catalytic mechanism of sphingomyelinases D. *Journal of Biological Chemistry,* 280(14), 13658-13664.

[155] De Almeida, D. M., Fernandes-Pedrosa, M. F., Gonçalves de, Andrade. R. M., Marcelino, J. R., Gondo-Higashi, H., Junqueira de, Azevedo. I. D. L. M., Ho, P. L., Van Den, Berg. C., & Tambourgi, D. V. (2008). A new anti-loxoscelic serum produced against recombinant sphingomyelinase D: Results of preclinical trials. *American Journal of Tropical Medicine and Hygiene,* 79(3), 463-470.

[156] Bubien, J. K., Ji, H. L., Gillespie, G. Y., Fuller, C. M., Markert, J. M., Mapstone, T. B., & Benos, D. J. (2004). Cation selectivity and inhibition of malignant glioma Na+ channels by Psalmotoxin 1. American Journal of Physiology- Cell Physiology 56-5) , 287(5), C1282-C1291.

[157] Rodrigues, E. G., Dobroff, A. S. S., Cavarsan, C. F., Paschoalin, T., Nimrichter, L., Mortara, R. A., Santos, E. L., Fázio, MA, Miranda, A., Daffre, S., & Travassos, L. R. (2008). Effective topical treatment of subcutaneous murine B16F10-Nex2 melanoma by the antimicrobial peptide gomesin. *Neoplasia,* 10(1), 61-68.

[158] Khan, S. A., Zafar, Y., Briddon, R. W., Malik, K. A., & Mukhtar, Z. (2006). Spider venom toxin protects plants from insect attack. *Transgenic Research,* 15(3), 349-357.

[159] De Castro, C. S., Silvestre, F. G., Araújo, S. C., Yazbeck, G. D. M., Mangili, O. C., Cruz, I., Chávez-Olórtegui, C., & Kalapothakis, E. (2004). Identification and molecular cloning of insecticidal toxins from the venom of the brown spider Loxosceles intermedia. *Toxicon,* 44(3), 273-280.

[160] Figueiredo, S. G., Garcia, M. E. L. P., Valentim, A. D. C., Cordeiro, M. N., Diniz, C. R., & Richardson, M. (1995). Purification and amino acid sequence of the insecticidal neurotoxin Tx4(6-1) from the venom of the'armed' spider Phoneutria nigriventer (Keys). *Toxicon,* 33(1), 83-93.

[161] Zobel-Thropp, P. A., Kerins, A. E., & Binford, G. J. (2012). Sphingomyelinase D in sicariid spider venom is a potent insecticidal toxin. *Toxicon,* 60(3), 265-271.

[162] Ferrat, G., Bosmans, F., Tytgat, J., Pimentel, C., Chagot, B., Gilles, N., Nakajima, T., Darbon, H., & Corzo, G. (2005). Solution structure of two insect-specific spider toxins and their pharmacological interaction with the insect voltage-gated Na^{+} channel. *Proteins Structure, Function and Genetics*, 59(2), 368-379.

[163] Toledo, R. C., & Jared, C. (1995). Cutaneous granular glands and amphibian venoms. *Comparative Biochemistry and Physiology Part A: Physiology*, 111(1), 1-29.

[164] Tang, Y. Q., Tian, Sh., Hua, Jc., Wu, Sx., Zou, G., Wu, Gf., & Zhao, Em. (1990). Isolation, chemical and biological characterization of margaratensin, a neurotensin-related peptide from the skin of Rana margaratae. *Science in China (Scientia Sinica) Series B*, 33(7), 828-834.

[165] Wang, D. L., Qi, F. H., Tang, W., & Wang, F. S. (2011). Chemical constituents and bioactivities of the skin of Bufo bufo gargarizans cantor. *Chemistry and Biodiversity*, 8(4), 559-567.

[166] Cruz, J. S., & Matsuda, H. (1993). Arenobufagin, a compound in toad venom, blocks Na^{+}-K^{+} pump current in cardiac myocytes. *European Journal of Pharmacology*.

[167] Shindelman, J., Mosher, H. S., & Fuhrman, F. A. (1969). Atelopidtoxin from the Panamanian frog, Atelopus zeteki. *Toxicon*, 7(4), 315-319.

[168] Erspamer, G. F., Severini, C., Erspamer, V., & Melchiorri, P. (1989). Pumiliotoxin B-like alkaloid in extracts of the skin of the australian myobatrachid frog Pseudophryne coriacea: effects on the systemic blood pressure of experimental animals and the rat heart. *Neuropharmacology*, 28(4), 319-328.

[169] Zhang, Y., Yu, G., Wang, Y., Zhang, J., Wei, S., Lee, W., & Zhang, Y. (2010). A novel annexin A2 protein with platelet aggregation-inhibiting activity from amphibian Bombina maxima skin. *Toxicon*, 56(3), 458-465.

[170] Cunha, Filho. G. A., Schwartz, C. A., Resck, I. S., Murta, M. M., Lemos, S. S., Castro, M. S., Kyaw, C., Pires Jr, O. R., Leite, J. R. S., Bloch Jr, C., & Schwartz, E. F. (2005). Antimicrobial activity of the bufadienolides marinobufagin and telocinobufagin isolated as major components from skin secretion of the toad Bufo rubescens. *Toxicon*, 45(6), 777-782.

[171] Dourado, F. S., Leite, J. R. S. A., Silva, L. P., Melo, J. A. T., Bloch Jr, C., & Schwartz, E. F. (2007). Antimicrobial peptide from the skin secretion of the frog Leptodactylus syphax. *Toxicon*, 50(4), 572-580.

[172] Preusser, H. J., Habermehl, G., Sablofski, M., & Schmall, Haury. D. (1975). Antimicrobial activity of alkaloids from amphibian venoms and effects on the ultrastructure of yeast cells. *Toxicon*, 13(4), 285-289.

[173] Cui, X., Inagaki, Y., Xu, H., Wang, D., Qi, F., Kokudo, N., Fang, D., & Tang, W. (2010). Anti-hepatitis B virus activities of cinobufacini and its active components bufalin and cinobufagin in HepG2.2.15 Cells. *Biological and Pharmaceutical Bulletin*, 33(10), 1728-1732.

[174] Tempone, A. G., Pimenta, D. C., Lebrun, I., Sartorelli, P., Taniwaki, N. N., de Andrade Jr, H. F., Antoniazzi, MM, & Jared, C. (2008). Antileishmanial and antitrypanosomal activity of bufadienolides isolated from the toad Rhinella jimi parotoid macrogland secretion. *Toxicon*, 52(1), 13-21.

[175] Yogeeswari, P., Sriram, D., Bal, T. R., & Thirumurugan, R. (2006). Epibatidine and its analogues as nicotinic acetylcholine receptor agonist: an update. *Natural Product Research*, 20(5), 497-505.

[176] Erspamer, V., Melchiorri, P., Falconieri-Erspamer, G., Negri, L., Corsi, R., Severini, C., Barra, D., Simmaco, M., & Kreil, G. (1989). Deltrophins: a family of naturally occurring peptides with high affinity and selectivity for δ opioid binding sites. *Proceedings of the National Academy of Sciences of the United States of America*, 86(13), 5188-5192.

[177] Wang, X. L., Zhao, G. H., Zhang, J., Shi, Q. Y., Guo, W. X., Tian, X. L., Qiu, J. Z., Yin, L. Z., Deng, X. M., & Song, Y. (2011). Immunomodulatory effects of cinobufagin isolated from Chan Su on activation and cytokines secretion of immunocyte in vitro. *Journal of Asian Natural Products Research*, 13(5), 383-392.

[178] Qi, F., Inagaki, Y., Gao, B., Cui, X., Xu, H., Kokudo, N., Li, A., & Tang, W. (2011). Bufalin and cinobufagin induce apoptosis of human hepatocellular carcinoma cells via Fas- and mitochondria-mediated pathways. *Cancer Science*, 102(5), 951-958.

[179] Su, C. L., Lin, T. Y., Lin, C. N., & Won, S. J. (2009). Involvement of caspases and apoptosis-inducing factor in bufotalin-induced apoptosis of hep 3B cells. *Journal of Agricultural and Food Chemistry*, 57(1), 55-61.

[180] Balboni, F., Bernabei, P. A., Barberio, C., Sanna, A., Rossi, Ferrini. P., & Delfino, G. (1992). Cutaneous venom of Bombina variegata pachypus (Amphibia, anura): effects on the growth of the human HL 60 cell line. *Cell Biology International Reports*, 16(4), 329-338.

[181] Ghavami, S., Asoodeh, A., Klonisch, T., Halayko, A. J., Kadkhoda, K., Kroczak, T. J., Gibson, S. B., Booy, E. P., Naderi-Manesh, H., & Los, M. (2008). Brevinin-2R1 semi-selectively kills cancer cells by a distinct mechanism, which involves the lysosomal-mitochondrial death pathway. *Journal of Cellular and Molecular Medicine*, 12(3), 1005-1022.

[182] Marenah, L., Shaw, C., Orr, D. F., Mc Clean, S., Flatt, P. R., & Abdel-Wahab, Y. H. A. (2004). Isolation and characterisation of an unexpected class of insulinotropic peptides in the skin of the frog Agalychnis litodryas. *Regulatory Peptides*, 120(1-3), 33-38.

[183] Marsh, N. A., & Whaler, B. C. (1980). The effects of honey bee (Apis mellifera L.) venom and two of its constituents, melittin and phospholipase A2, on the cardiovascular system of the rat. *Toxicon*, 18(4), 427-435.

[184] Kaplinsky, E., Ishay, J., Ben-Shachar, D., & Gitter, S. (1977). Effects of bee (Apis mellifera) venom on the electrocardiogram and blood pressure. *Toxicon*, 15(3), 251-256.

[185] Vick, J. A., Shipman, W. H., & Brooks, R. Jr. (1974). Beta adrenergic and anti-arrhythmic effects of cardiopep, a newly isolated substance from whole bee venom. *Toxicon*, 12(2), 139-144.

[186] Ho, C. L., Hwang, L. L., Lin, Y. L., Chen, C. T., Yu, H. M., & Wang, K. T. (1994). Cardiovascular effects of mastoparan B and its structural requirements. *European Journal of Pharmacology*, 259(3), 259-264.

[187] Choo, Y. M., Lee, K. S., Yoon, H. J., Qiu, Y., Wan, H., Sohn, M. R., Sohn, H. D., & Jin, B. R. (2012). Antifibrinolytic role of a bee venom serine protease inhibitor that acts as a plasmin Inhibitor. *PLoS ONE*, 7(2).

[188] Choo, Y. M., Lee, K. S., Yoon, H. J., Kim, B. Y., Sohn, M. R., Roh, J. Y., Je, Y. H., Kim, N. J., Kim, I., Woo, S. D., Sohn, H. D., & Jin, B. R. (2010). Dual function of a bee venom serine protease: prophenoloxidase-activating factor in arthropods and fibrin(ogen)olytic enzyme in mammals. *PLoS ONE*, 5(5), 1.

[189] Qiu, Y., Choo, Y. M., Yoon, H. J., Jia, J., Cui, Z., Wang, D., Kim, D. H., Sohn, H. D., & Jin, B. R. (2011). Fibrin(ogen)olytic activity of bumblebee venom serine protease. *Toxicology and Applied Pharmacology*, 255(2), 207-213.

[190] Qiu, Y., Choo, Y. M., Yoon, H. J., & Jin, B. R. (2012). Molecular cloning and fibrin(ogen)olytic activity of a bumblebee (Bombus hypocrita sapporoensis) venom serine protease. *Journal of Asia-Pacific Entomology*, 15(1), 79-82.

[191] Han, J., You, D., Xu, X., Han, W., Lu, Y., Lai, R., & Meng, Q. (2008). An anticoagulant serine protease from the wasp venom of Vespa magnifica. *Toxicon*, 51(5), 914-922.

[192] Haim, B., Rimon, A., Ishay, J. S., & Rimon, S. (1999). Purification, characterization and anticoagulant activity of a proteolytic enzyme from Vespa orientalis venom. *Toxicon*, 37(5), 825-829.

[193] Yang, H., Xu, X., Zhang, D., Lai, K., & , R. (2008). A phospholipase A1 platelet activator from the wasp venom of Vespa magnifica (Smith). *Toxicon*, 51(2), 289-296.

[194] Xu, X., Li, J., Lu, Q., Yang, H., Zhang, Y., & Lai, R. (2006). Two families of antimicrobial peptides from wasp (Vespa magnifica) venom. *Toxicon*, 47(2), 249-253.

[195] Lazarev, V. N., Parfenova, T. M., Gularyan, S. K., Misyurina, O. Y., Akopian, T. A., & Govorun, V. M. (2002). Induced expression of melittin, an antimicrobial peptide, inhibits infection by Chlamydia trachomatis and Mycoplasma hominis in a HeLa cell line. *International journal of antimicrobial agents*, 19(2), 133-7.

[196] Choo, Y. M., Lee, K. S., Yoon, H. J., Je, Y. H., Lee, S. W., Sohn, H. D., & Jin, B. R. (2010). Molecular cloning and antimicrobial activity of bombolitin, a component of bumblebee Bombus ignitus venom. *Comparative Biochemistry and Physiology Part B: Biochemistry and Molecular Biology*, 156(3), 168-173.

[197] Stöcklin, R., Favreau, P., Thai, R., Pflugfelder, J., Bulet, P., & Mebs, D. (2010). Structural identification by mass spectrometry of a novel antimicrobial peptide from the

venom of the solitary bee Osmia rufa (Hymenoptera: Megachilidae). *Toxicon*, 55(1), 20-27.

[198] Chen, W., Yang, X., Yang, X., Zhai, L., Lu, Z., Liu, J., & Yu, H. (2008). Antimicrobial peptides from the venoms of Vespa bicolor Fabricius. *Peptides*, 29(11), 1887-1892.

[199] Baek, J. H., & Lee, S. H. (2010). Isolation and molecular cloning of venom peptides from Orancistrocerus drewseni (Hymenoptera: Eumenidae). *Toxicon*, 55(4), 711-718.

[200] Yang, E. J., Jiang, J. H., Lee, S. M., Yang, S. C., Hwang, H. S., Lee, M. S., & Choi-M, S. (2010). Bee venom attenuates neuroinflammatory events and extends survival in amyotrophic lateral sclerosis models. *Journal of Neuroinflammation*, 7(1), 69.

[201] Lee, J., Kim, S., Kim, T., Lee, S., Yang, H., Lee, D., & Lee, Y. (2004). Anti-inflammatory effect of bee venom on type II collagen-induced arthritis. *The American journal of Chinese medicine*, 32(3), 361-7.

[202] Park, J. H., Kim, K. H., Lee, W. R., Han, S. M., & Park, K. K. (2012). Protective effect of melittin on inflammation and apoptosis in acute liver failure. *Apoptosis*, 17(1), 61-69.

[203] Shkenderov, S., & Koburova, K. (1982). Adolapin- a newly isolated analgetic and anti-inflammatory polypeptide from bee venom. *Toxicon*, 20(1), 317-321.

[204] Haux, P. (1969). Amino acid sequence of MCD-peptide, a specific mast cell-degranulating peptide from bee venom. *Hoppe-Seyler's Zeitschrift fur Physiologische Chemie*, 350(5), 536-546.

[205] Kettner, A., Henry, H., Hughes, G. J., Corradin, G., & Spertini, F. (1999). IgE and T-cell responses to high-molecular weight allergens from bee venom. *Clinical & Experimental Allergy*, 29(3), 394-401.

[206] Kettner, A., Hughes, G. J., Frutiger, S., Astori, M., Roggero, M., Spertini, F., & Corradin, G. (2001). Api m 6: a new bee venom allergen. *Journal of Allergy and Clinical Immunology*, 107(5), 914-920.

[207] Pantera, B., Hoffman, D. R., Carresi, L., Cappugi, G., Turillazzi, S., Manao, G., Severino, M., Spadolini, I., Orsomando, G., Moneti, G., & Pazzagli, L. (2003). Characterization of the major allergens purified from the venom of the paper wasp Polistes gallicus. *Biochimica et Biophysica Acta (BBA)- General Subjects*, 1623(2-3), 72-81.

[208] An, S., Chen, L., Wei, J. F., Yang, X., Ma, D., Xu, X., He, S., Lu, J., & Lai, R. (2012). Purification and characterization of two new allergens from the venom of Vespa magnifica. *PLoS One*, 7(2), 27.

[209] Trindade, R. A., Kiyohara, P. K., de Araujo, P. S., & Bueno da. Costa, M. H. (2012). PLGA microspheres containing bee venom proteins for preventive immunotherapy. *International Journal of Pharmaceutics*, 423(1), 124-133.

[210] Dani, M. P., & Richards, E. H. (2010). Identification, cloning and expression of a second gene (vpr1) from the venom of the endoparasitic wasp, Pimpla hypochondriaca that displays immunosuppressive activity. *Journal of Insect Physiology*, 56(2), 195-203.

[211] Baptista-Saidemberg, N. B., Saidemberg, D. M., de Souza, B. M., Cesar-Tognoli, L. M., Ferreira, V. M., Mendes, M. A., Cabrera, M. P., Ruggiero, Neto. J., & Palma, M. S. (2010). Protonectin (1-6): a novel chemotactic peptide from the venom of the social wasp Agelaia pallipes pallipes. *Toxicon*, 56(6), 880-889.

[212] Souza, B. M., Mendes, M. A., Santos, L. D., Marques, M. R., Cesar, L. M., Almeida, R. N., Pagnocca, F. C., Konno, K., & Palma, M. S. (2005). Structural and functional characterization of two novel peptide toxins isolated from the venom of the social wasp Polybia paulista. *Peptides*, 26(11), 2157-2164.

[213] Graaf, D. C., Aerts, M., Danneels, E., & Devreese, B. (2009). Bee, wasp and ant venomics pave the way for a component-resolved diagnosis of sting allergy. *Journal of Proteomics*, 72(2), 145-154.

[214] Ownby, C. L., Powell, J. R., Jiang, M. S., & Fletcher, J. E. (1997). Melittin and phospholipase A2 from bee (Apis mellifera) venom cause necrosis of murine skeletal muscle in vivo. *Toxicon*, 35(1), 67-80.

[215] Hait, W. N., Grais, L., Benz, C., & Cadman, E. C. (1985). Inhibition of growth of leukemic cells by inhibitors of calmodulin: phenothiazines and melittin. *Cancer Chemotherapy and Pharmacology*, 14(3), 202-205.

[216] Moon, D. O., Park, S. Y., Heo, M. S., Kim, K. C., Park, C., Ko, W. S., Choi, Y. H., & Kim, G. Y. (2006). Key regulators in bee venom-induced apoptosis are Bcl-2 and caspase-3 in human leukemic U937 cells through downregulation of ERK and Akt. *International Immunopharmacology*, 6(12), 1796-1807.

[217] Orsolic, N., Sver, L., Verstovsek, S., Terzic, S., & Basic, I. (2003). Inhibition of mammary carcinoma cell proliferation in vitro and tumor growth in vivo by bee venom. *Toxicon*, 41(7), 861-870.

[218] Putz, T., Ramoner, R., Gander, H., Rahm, A., Bartsch, G., & Thurnher, M. (2006). Antitumor action and immune activation through cooperation of bee venom secretory phospholipase A_2 and phosphatidylinositol-(3,4)-bisphosphate. *Cancer Immunology Immunotherapy*, 55(11), 1374-1383.

[219] Cerovsky, V., Budesinsky, M., Hovorka, O., Cvacka, J., Voburka, Z., Slaninova, J., Borovickova, L., Fucik, V., Bednarova, L., Votruba, I., & Straka, J. (2009). Lasioglossins: three novel antimicrobial peptides from the venom of the eusocial bee Lasioglossum laticeps (Hymenoptera: Halictidae). *ChemBioChem*, 10(12), 2089-2099.

[220] Heinen, T. E., & da Veiga, A. B. (2011). Arthropod venoms and cancer. *Toxicon*, 57(4), 497-511.

[221] Pfeiffer, D. R., Gudz, T. I., Novgorodov, S. A., & Erdahl, W. L. (1995). The peptide mastoparan is a potent facilitator of the mitochondrial permeability transition. *The Journal of Biological Chemistry*, 270(9), 4923-4932.

[222] Souza, B. M., Silva, A. V., Resende, V. M., Arcuri, H. A., Santos, Cabrera. M. P., Ruggiero, Neto. J., & Palma, M. S. (2009). Characterization of two novel polyfunctional

mastoparan peptides from the venom of the social wasp Polybia paulista. *Peptides*, 30(8), 1387-1395.

[223] Wang, K. R., Zhang, B. Z., Zhang, W., Yan, J. X., Li, J., & Wang, R. (2008). Antitumor effects, cell selectivity and structure-activity relationship of a novel antimicrobial peptide polybia-MPI. *Peptides*, 29(6), 963-968.

[224] Kim, J. Y., Cho, S. H., Kim, Y. W., Jang, E. C., Park, S. Y., Kim, E. J., & Lee, S. K. (1999). Effects of BCG, lymphotoxin and bee venom on insulitis and development of IDDM in non-obese diabetic mice. *J Korean Med Sci*, 14(6), 648-652.

[225] Shin, Y., Moni, R. W., Lueders, J. E., & Daly, J. W. (1994). Effects of the amphiphilic peptides mastoparan and adenoregulin on receptor binding, G proteins, phosphoinositide breakdown, cyclic AMP generation, and calcium influx. *Cell Mol Neurobiol*, 14(2), 133-157.

[226] Straub, S. G., James, R. F., Dunne, M. J., & Sharp, G. W. (1998). Glucose augmentation of mastoparan-stimulated insulin secretion in rat and human pancreatic islets. *Diabetes*, 47(7), 1053-1057.

[227] Mc Gain, F., & Winkel, K. D. (2002). Ant sting mortality in Australia. *Toxicon*, 40(8), 1095-1100.

[228] Malta, M. B., Lira, MS, Soares, S. L., Rocha, G. C., Knysak, I., Martins, R., Guizze, S. P., Santoro, M. L., & Barbaro, K. C. (2008). Toxic activities of Brazilian centipede venoms. *Toxicon*, 52(2), 255-263.

[229] Carrijo-Carvalho, L. C., & Chudzinski-Tavassi, A. M. (2007). The venom of the Lonomia caterpillar: an overview. *Toxicon*, 49(6), 741-757.

[230] Veiga, A. B., Ribeiro, J. M., Guimaraes, J. A., & Francischetti, I. M. (2005). A catalog for the transcripts from the venomous structures of the caterpillar Lonomia obliqua: identification of the proteins potentially involved in the coagulation disorder and hemorrhagic syndrome. *Gene*, 355-11.

[231] Bohrer, C. B., Reck, Junior. J., Fernandes, D., Sordi, R., Guimaraes, J. A., Assreuy, J., & Termignoni, C. (2007). Kallikrein-kinin system activation by Lonomia obliqua caterpillar bristles: involvement in edema and hypotension responses to envenomation. *Toxicon*, 49(5), 663-669.

[232] Donato, J. L., Moreno, R. A., Hyslop, S., Duarte, A., Antunes, E., Le Bonniec, B. F., Rendu, F., & de Nucci, G. (1998). Lonomia obliqua caterpillar spicules trigger human blood coagulation via activation of factor X and prothrombin. *Thromb Haemost*, 79(3), 539-542.

[233] Chudzinski-Tavassi, A. M., Schattner, M., Fritzen, M., Pozner, R. G., Reis, C. V., Lourenco, D., & Lazzari, MA. (2001). Effects of lopap on human endothelial cells and platelets. *Haemostasis*, 31(3-6), 257-265.

[234] Pinto, A. F., Dobrovolski, R., Veiga, A. B., & Guimaraes, J. A. (2004). Lonofibrase, a novel alpha-fibrinogenase from Lonomia obliqua caterpillars. *Thrombosis Research*, 113(2), 147-154.

[235] Alvarez, Flores. M. P., Fritzen, M., Reis, C. V., & Chudzinski-Tavassi, A. M. (2006). Losac, a factor X activator from Lonomia obliqua bristle extract: its role in the pathophysiological mechanisms and cell survival. *Biochemical and Biophysical Research Communications*, 343(4), 1216-1223.

[236] Guerrero, B., Arocha-Pinango, C. L., Salazar, A. M., Gil, A., Sanchez-Acosta, EE, Rodriguez., A., & Lucena, S. (2011). The effects of Lonomin V, a toxin from the caterpillar (Lonomia achelous), on hemostasis parameters as measured by platelet function. *Toxicon*, 58(4), 293-303.

[237] Hink, W. F., Romstedt, K. J., Burke, J. W., Doskotch, R. W., & Feller, D. R. (1989). Inhibition of human platelet aggregation and secretion by ant venom and a compound isolated from venom. *Inflammation*, 13(2), 175-184.

[238] Orivel, J., Redeker, V., Le Caer, J. P., Krier, F., Revol-Junelles, A. M., Longeon, A., Chaffotte, A., Dejean, A., & Rossier, J. (2001). Ponericins, new antibacterial and insecticidal peptides from the venom of the ant Pachycondyla goeldii. *The Journal of Biological Chemistry*, 276(21), 17823-17829.

[239] Zelezetsky, I., Pag, U., Antcheva, N., Sahl, H. G., & Tossi, A. (2005). Identification and optimization of an antimicrobial peptide from the ant venom toxin pilosulin. *Archives of Biochemistry and Biophysics*, 434(2), 358-364.

[240] Peng, K., Kong, Y., Zhai, L., Wu, X., Jia, P., Liu, J., & Yu, H. (2010). Two novel antimicrobial peptides from centipede venoms. *Toxicon*, 55(2-3), 274-279.

[241] Altman, R. D., Schultz, D. R., Collins-Yudiskas, B., Aldrich, J., Arnold, P. I., & Brown, H. E. (1984). The effects of a partially purified fraction of an ant venom in rheumatoid arthritis. *Arthritis & Rheumatism*, 27(3), 277-284.

[242] Pan, J., & Hink, W. F. (2000). Isolation and characterization of myrmexins, six isoforms of venom proteins with anti-inflammatory activity from the tropical ant, Pseudomyrmex triplarinus. *Toxicon*, 38(10), 1403-1413.

[243] Hoffman, D. R. (1993). Allergens in Hymenoptera venom XXIV: the amino acid sequences of imported fire ant venom allergens Sol i II, Sol i III, and Sol i IV. *Journal of Allergy and Clinical Immunology*, 91(1), 71-78.

[244] Hoffman, D. R., Sakell, R. H., & Schmidt, M. (2005). Sol i 1, the phospholipase allergen of imported fire ant venom. *Journal of Allergy and Clinical Immunology*, 115(3), 611-616.

[245] Arbiser, J. L., Kau, T., Konar, M., Narra, K., Ramchandran, R., Summers, S. A., Vlahos, C. J., Ye, K., Perry, B. N., Matter, W., Fischl, A., Cook, J., Silver, P. A., Bain, J., Cohen, P., Whitmire, D., Furness, S., Govindarajan, B., & Bowen, J. P. (2007). Sole-

nopsin, the alkaloidal component of the fire ant (Solenopsis invicta), is a naturally occurring inhibitor of phosphatidylinositol-3-kinase signaling and angiogenesis. *Blood*, 109(2), 560-565.

[246] Sonoda, Y., Hada, N., Kaneda, T., Suzuki, T., Ohshio, T., Takeda, T., & Kasahara, T. (2008). A synthetic glycosphingolipid-induced antiproliferative effect in melanoma cells is associated with suppression of FAK, Akt, and Erk activation. *Biological and Pharmaceutical Bulletin*, 31(6), 1279-1283.

Chapter 3

Computer-Based Methods of Inhibitor Prediction

Silvana Giuliatti

Additional information is available at the end of the chapter

http://dx.doi.org/10.5772/ 52334

1. Introduction

This chapter presents *in silico* approaches used in protein structure prediction and drug discovery research.

The structural and functional diversity of animal toxins are interesting tools for therapeutic drug design. This diversity is also of great interest in the search for natural or synthetic inhibitors against these animal toxins.

Computational techniques are highly important in drug design. They are used in the search for candidate ligands binding to a receptor.

Drug design based on structure has become a highly developed technology and is used in large pharmaceutical companies. Firstly, the structure of the protein of interest must be known. Therefore, molecular modelling plays an important role in the discovery of new drugs.

If the structure of the receptor is known, then the application is essentially a problem of structure-based drug design. These methods have specific goals, such as attempting to identify the location of the active site of the ligand and the geometry of the ligand in the active site. Another goal is to select a number of related binders in terms of affinity or evaluation of the binding free energy.

The strategy of virtual screening has been used to contribute to the increase in hit rate in the selection of new drug candidates.

Virtual screening (VS) is a modern methodology that has been used in the identification of new bioactive substances. It is an *in silico* method that aims to identify small molecules contained in large databases of compounds with high potential for interaction with target proteins for subsequent biochemical analyses.

The strategy of VS can be divided into *ligand-based virtual screening* (LBVS), where a large number of molecules can be evaluated based on the similarity of known ligands, and *structure-based virtual screening* (SBVS), where a number of molecules can be evaluated for specifically binding to the active sites of target proteins (Figure 1).

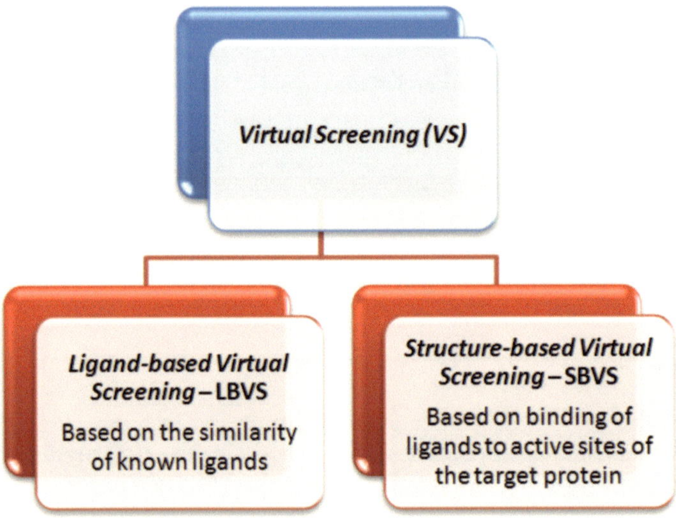

Figure 1. Virtual screening can be divided into ligand-based virtual screening (LBVS) and structure-based virtual screening (SBVS).

Molecular docking is used to determine the best orientation and conformation of a ligand in its receptor site. The aim is to generate a range of conformations of the protein-ligand complex and sort them according to their scores, which are based on their stabilities. In order to do this, the protein structure and a database of ligands (potential candidates) are used as inputs to the docking software. Thus, large collections of virtual compounds are subjected to docking into a protein-binding site and sorted according to their affinities for the macromolecular target, as suggested by the score function.

The focus of this chapter is to present the strategy of SBVS and the basic concepts of the methodologies involved. Examples of these approaches that have been applied to the identification of animal venom inhibitors have been presented at the end of the chapter.

2. Structure-Based Virtual Screening (SBVS)

SBVS involves the evaluation of databases based on the simulation of interactions between the ligands (small molecules) and receptors (target protein). The various steps in the process of SBVS are briefly shown in Figure 2. After obtaining the structure of the receptor and ligand, the next step in the process is molecular docking, which involves the coupling of the ligands with the receptor. At this stage, various conformations and orientations are generated and classified according to the score function. The target protein can be obtained from a database or by modelling.

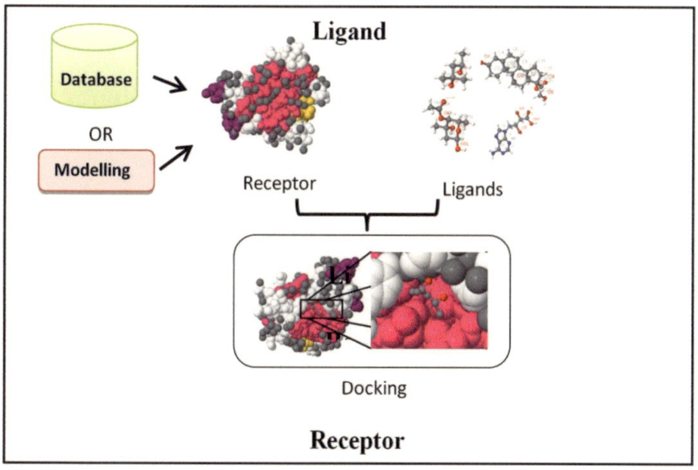

Figure 2. Stages of SBVS. The receptor (the target protein) can be obtained from a database or by modelling. Molecular docking completes the structure-based virtual screening.

2.1. Obtaining the Structure of the Protein Target

Knowledge of the target protein structure is essential for structure-based drug design. The determination of the 3-dimensional structure of the protein may be achieved experimentally by diffraction of X-rays or by magnetic resonance. If the structure of the target protein has already been solved, it can easily be found deposited in public databases such as PDB [37] which contains more than 80,000 experimentally solved structures.

However, sometimes the structure of the target is not known, and this poses a problem in the drug design process. This situation can be resolved by making use of computational methods for predicting protein structure.

Such methods are divided into 2 groups: those based on templates and those that are template-free. The first group includes comparative or homology modelling and threading. The second group includes methods that do not depend on templates to build the model, such as *ab initio* modelling (Figure 3).

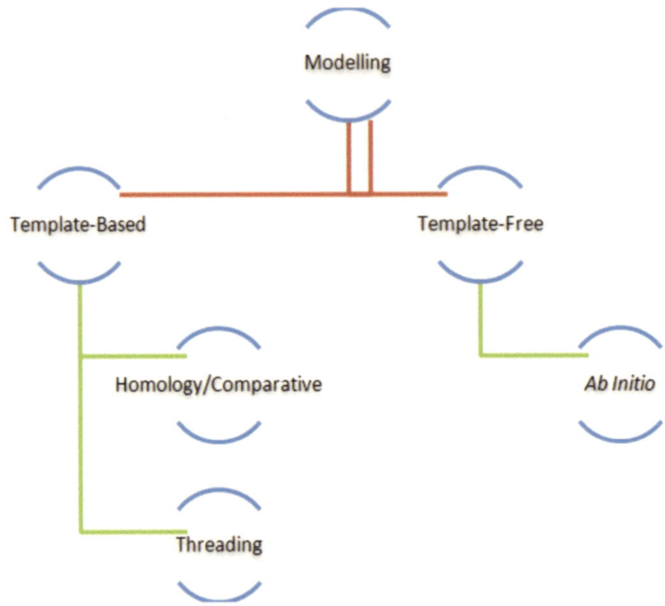

Figure 3. Modelling methods can be classified into template-based methods (homology/comparative modelling) and template-free methods (*ab initio*).

2.1.1. Template-Based Modelling

Homology modelling is based on the use of proteins that share an ancestral relationship with the target protein, that is, that they are evolutionarily related and tend to have similar structures. Thus, this method basically involves knowledge of the primary chain of the target protein and a search among databases for homologous proteins that have solved structures. These proteins are used as templates.

Threading modelling is based on the principle that proteins may have similar structures without sharing the same ancestral relationship because the structure tends to be more conserved than the primary sequence. In this case, these methods evaluate the primary chain of the target protein in relation to proteins that have solved structures.

2.1.1.1. Comparative/Homology Modelling

Comparative or homology modelling constructs a model structure of the target protein using its primary chain and the information obtained from homologous proteins that have solved structures. Therefore, this method depends on the availability of proteins that have structures similar to those of the target and can be used as templates. The whole process requires not only the construction of the model, but also the refinement and evaluation of the obtained model. The process can be divided into stages as follows: selection of the templates, which involves the identification of homologous sequences in a database of proteins that will be used as templates in the modelling process; sequence alignment between the target and the templates; refinement of the alignment; construction of the model, adding loops and side chains; and evaluation of the model (Figure 4).

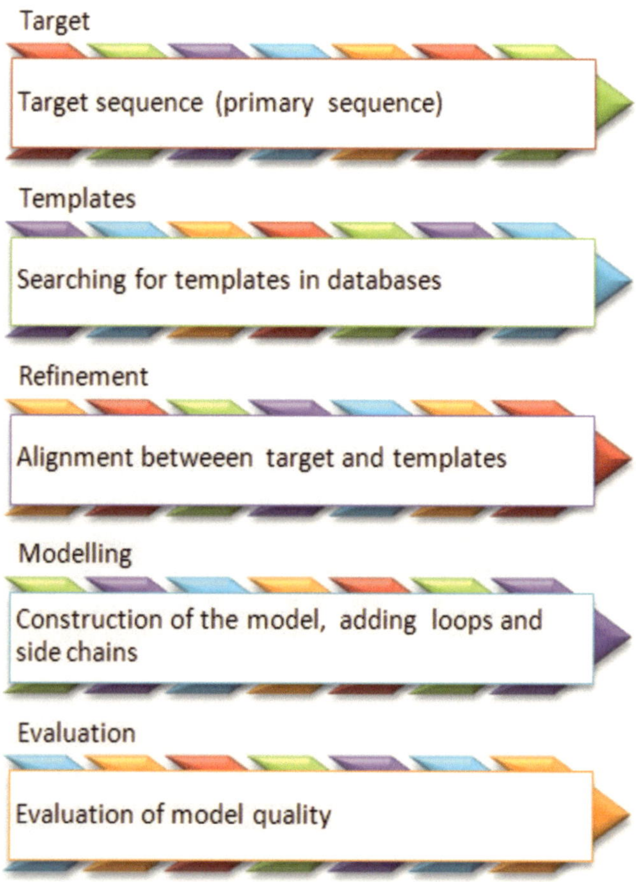

Figure 4. Steps in the comparative modelling process.

The construction of the model depends on the availability of templates. For this purpose, alignment of target and template sequences is widely used and is very efficient. Sequence alignments are typically generated by searching for the result that presents the largest region of identity and similarity. Generally, an identity percentage of at least 25% is considered significant.

There are several tools available for sequence alignment. They differ in the methods used, which can be exhaustive or heuristic, as well as the number of sequences involved in the alignment (multiple or pairwise comparisons). Among these tools, BLAST/PSIBLAST [1; 2] is a tool that performs local alignments based on the profiles between the target sequence and each sequence belonging to a known database.

The results of the alignment can be evaluated using the E-value. The E-value shows an inverse relationship with the identity/similarity between the sequences. Because it is a heuristic method, the results reported by BLAST are generally suboptimal.

If more than 1 template with similar scores is achieved, the best one can be selected as the template with the higher resolution.

Other methods such as HHpred [34] and Pyre [18] use Markov profiles (Hidden Markov models [HMMs]) combined with structural features.

When more than one template is selected, and taking into account that the results are usually suboptimal, there is a need for an alignment between the target protein and the selected templates. In this case, multiple alignments are indicated. There are several tools that perform multiple alignments, such as ClustalW [21]

After obtaining the alignments between the target and templates, the process of obtaining the model of the target protein begins. There are several software tools available, which differ with respect to the method applied. Prominent among these are MODELLER [9, 33] and SWISS-MODEL [3] The software that has shown the best performance is MODELLER. The program models the backbone using a homology-derived restraint method, which is based on the multiple alignment between the target and templates to differentiate between highly conserved and less conserved residues. The model is optimised by energy minimisation and molecular dynamics methods (Figure 5).

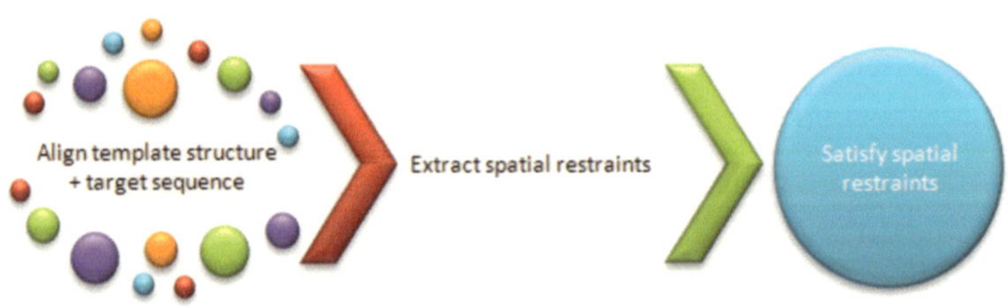

Figure 5. The template 3D structures are aligned with the target sequence to be modelled. Spatial features are transferred from the templates to the target and a number of spatial restraints on its structure are obtained. The 3D model is obtained by satisfying all the restraints as thoroughly as possible [33]

The regions of the target that are not aligned with the protein template generally represent loop regions. There are usually some regions caused by insertions and deletions producing gaps in the alignment. Closing these gaps requires modelling of the loops. The loops and the side chains are shaped during the refinement of the model. For this, methods that do not rely on templates can be applied. These include the use of physics parameters and knowledge-based data.

The loops are usually modelled using a database of fragments or by *ab initio* modelling. The use of a database involves finding parts of protein structures known to fit onto 2 regions (stems) of the target protein, which are the regions that precede and follow the loop to be modelled. The conformation of the best matching fragment is used to model the loop.

Ab initio methods generate many random loops and look for one that presents a low-energy state and includes conformational angles contained within the allowed regions of the Ramachandran plot [31] The software CODA [7] can be used for loop modelling.

The side chains can be modelled by programs that make use of libraries of rotamers, such as the software SCRWL4 [20]. The use of rotamer libraries reduces computational time because it reduces the number of favourable torsion angles being examined.

After obtaining the model, its quality must be evaluated. This should be done to make sure that the model has structural features consistent with the physical and chemical rules. Several errors in modelling can occur due to poor choice of template, bad alignment between the target and template, and incorrect determination of loops and side chains.

In the evaluation stage of the model, the structural characteristics as well as the stereochemistry accuracy of the model must be examined.

There are tools available for analysing stereochemical properties, such as PROCHECK [23]. PROCHECK checks the general physicochemical parameters such as phi-psi angles (Ramachandran plot) and chirality. The parameters of the model are compared with those already compiled.

To validate the model for chemical correctness, it is possible to use the software WHAT IF [39]. WHAT IF is a server that checks planarity and bond angles, among other parameters. It also displays the Ramachandran plot.

Verify3D [4, 26] can be used for the analysis of the pseudo-energy profile of the model. It has a database containing environmental profiles based on secondary structures, and the solvent exposure of solved structures at high resolution. It should be noted that the results may be different when different programs are used for verification.

To distinguish correct from incorrect regions, the ERRAT program [6] can be used; this is based on analysis of the characteristics of atomic interactions compared to the highly refined structures.

PROtein Volume Evaluation (PROVE; [30]) calculates the volume of the atoms in the macromolecules using an algorithm that treats the atoms as spheres, analysing the model in relation to the highly resolved and refined structures stored in the PDB.

These software tools are available on servers such as ModFold [27], ProQ (see Section 6 - Table 2), and SAVes (see Section 6 - Table 2).

2.1.1.2. Threading

Threading modelling is generally used when the template and target sequences share less than 30% identity. Thus, structures that do not share an evolutionary relationship with the target protein can be used as templates. However, the target protein has to adopt a fold similar to that of the protein that has had its structure solved. The method can be classified as a pairwise energy-based method.

Using the sequence of the target protein as input, a search is conducted on a database of structures in order to find the best structural match using the criterion of energy calculation. The process is accomplished through a search for solved structures that are most appropriate for the target protein. The comparison highlights secondary structures because they are evolutionarily conserved.

A model is constructed by placing aligned residues between the structure of the template and the target residues. In the next step, the energy of this model is calculated. This is done on various structures in the database. In the end, the models obtained are ranked based on the energy. The model presenting the lowest energy constitutes the most compatible folding model (Figure 6).

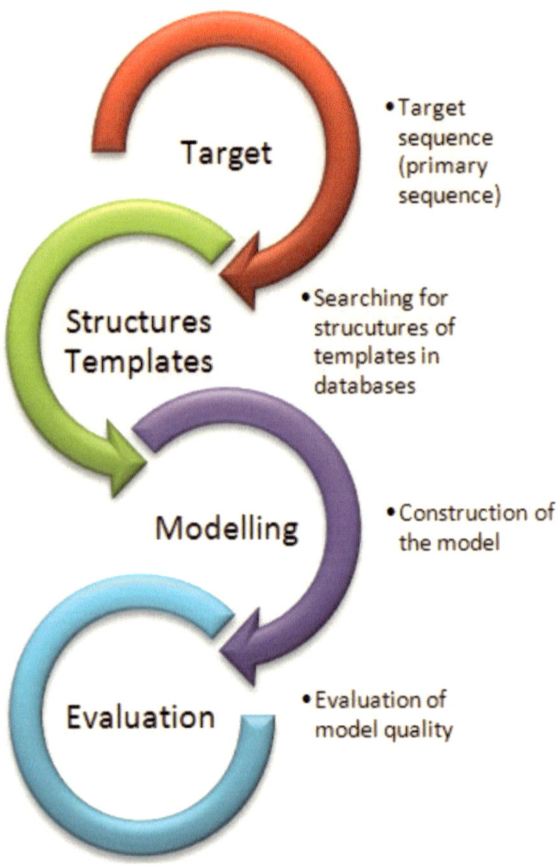

Figure 6. Steps in the threading modelling process.

Many programs such as THREADER [15, 28] and RAPTOR ([41, 42]) can be used to carry out this process.

2.1.2. Template-Free Modelling

One of the biggest problems in comparative modelling is the lack of templates. Template-free methods generate models based on the physicochemical properties and thermodynamic chain of the primary protein target. The processes are iterative. The conformation of the structure is altered until a configuration of lower potential energy is found.

Some methods use force fields based on knowledge as a scoring function. These methods are not strictly free of templates since they employ structures of small fragments of proteins such as, for example, ASTRO-FOLD [19, 35]. Others use energy functions based on first principles of energy and movement of atoms. Generally, these methods involve the calculation of energies of the structures, which has a high computational cost. They are therefore limited to small molecules (approximately 100 residues), as in the case of the software ROSETTA [32].

Firstly, ROSETTA breaks the sequence of the target protein into several short fragments and predicts the secondary structures of the fragments using HMMs. These fragments are then arranged (assembled) into a tertiary setting. Random combinations of these fragments generate a large number of models, which have their energies calculated. The conformation that presents the lowest global energy value is chosen as the best model (Figure 7).

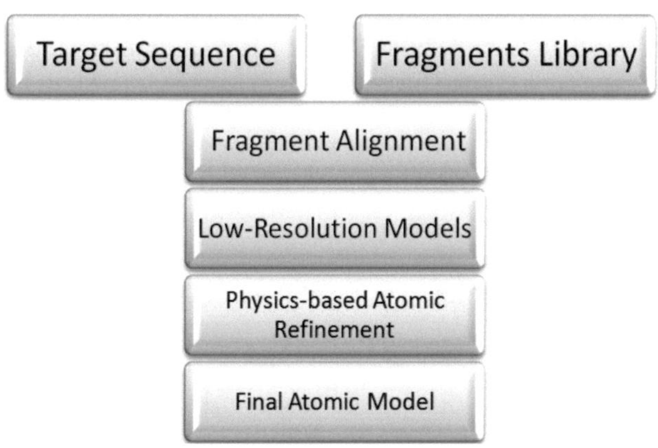

Figure 7. Steps in the ROSETTA process.

3. Molecular Docking

One application of molecular docking is virtual screening, in which a library of compounds is compared to one or more targets, thereby providing an analysis of compounds ranked by potential.

Virtual screening computational techniques are applied to the selection of compounds that can be active in a target protein.

In molecular docking, a ligand is usually placed in the binding site of a predetermined structure of a receptor (Figure 8). In other words, this is a method based on structure. The receptor is typically a protein and the ligand is a small molecule or a peptide. The optimal position and orientation of the ligand are determined using a search algorithm and a scoring function that ranks the solutions.

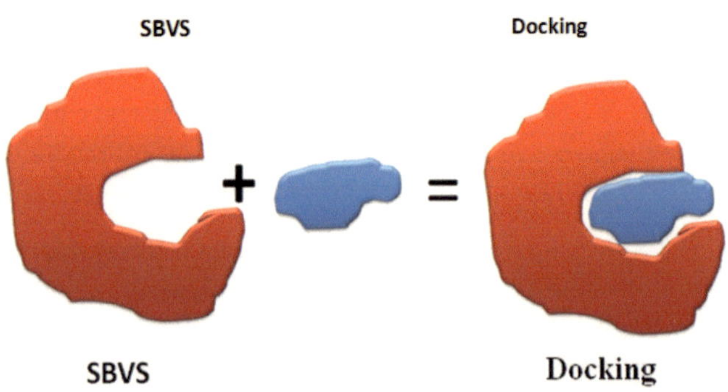

Figure 8. Diagram illustrating the docking of a ligand to a receptor to produce a complex.

The first step of the process of molecular docking is to determine the binding sites of the protein. This can be done by software programs such as Q-Sitefinder [24].

The metaPocket method [13] predicts binding sites using 4 methods: LIGSITEcs [12], PASS [5], Q-Sitefinder, and SURFnet [23] – which in combination increase the success rate of prediction. The methods LIGSITEcs, PASS, and SURFnet use only the geometrical characteristics of the protein structure, detecting regions that have the potential to be binding sites. Such methods do not require prior knowledge of the ligands.

In Q-Sitefinder, the surface of the protein is covered with a layer of methyl probes for the calculation of Van der Waals interactions between the protein and the probe. Probes with favourable interaction energies are retained, and are classified into groups based on the number of probes per group. The largest and most energetically favourable group is ranked first and considered the best potential binding site.

Another step is to define the position of the ligand in the pocket. This can be predicted by molecular docking algorithms.

Several methods have developed different scoring functions and different search methodologies.

The search algorithms have to be able to present different configurations and orientations of the ligand in a short time. Search algorithms, such as those used in molecular dynamics,

Monte Carlo simulations, and genetic algorithms, among others, are all suitable for molecular docking.

Scoring functions must be able to discriminate between different ligand-receptor interactions. These can be grouped into field-force, empirical, and knowledge-based methods.

The algorithms can be classified into rigid body docking and flexible docking algorithms. In rigid-body docking, both the ligand and receptor are rigid. These methods are faster, but do not allow ligand and receptor to adapt to the binding. In flexible methods, the computational cost is higher compared to rigid methods. However, in these cases, the flexibility of the ligand and/or receptor is considered.

Another important factor to be considered in ligand-receptor interactions is the presence of water. Some methods allow water molecules to be positioned. In cases where this is not possible, the position of water molecules can be predicted using a software program such as GRID [17].

GRID calculates the interactions between chemical groups and small molecules with known 3-dimensional structures. The energies are calculated using Lennard-Jones interactions, electrostatic and hydrogen bonding between the compounds, and 3-dimensional structures, using a position-dependent dielectric function.

Examples of tools available for docking proteins include AUTODOCK4.2 [29], GOLD [16], and GLIDE [10].

GOLD uses a genetic algorithm that seeks solutions through docking that propagates multiple copies of flexible models of the ligand in the active site of the receptor and recombining segments of copies at random until a converged set of structures is generated.

The process of searching the databases can be time consuming; a way to reduce the search space is filtering databases by performing a search with the fastest algorithms, selecting the best candidates ranked. Subsequently, within this selection, a search algorithm slowly generates a new ranking of the ligands. Another way to reduce the number of ligands being studied in the database is to perform a search for ligands that offer the greatest possibility of being used in drug design. In this case, it is possible to filter the database by using the ADMET (absorption, distribution, metabolism, excretion, and toxicity) filter.

Lipinski´s rule of 5 [25] can be used. The rule of 5 is a set of properties that characterise compounds that exhibit good oral bioavailability. It states that, in general, an orally active drug has no more than 1 violation of the rules (Table 1):

Lipinski´s Rule
Not more than 5 hydrogen bond donors (nitrogen or oxygen atoms with one or more hydrogen atoms
Not more than 10 hydrogen bond acceptors (nitrogen or oxygen atoms)
A molecular mass less than 500 daltons
An octanol-water partition coefficient log P not greater than 5

Table 1. Lipinski's Rule of Five

Analysis of the metabolic fate and chemical toxicity of the compounds can be accomplished using the software programs DEREK and METEOR [11]. DEREK predicts whether a given chemical is toxic to humans, mammals, and bacteria. METEOR uses the knowledge of metabolism rules to predict the metabolic fate of chemicals, assisting in the choice of more efficient molecules.

4. Ligand-Based Virtual Screening (LBVS)

Other methods can also be used for screening databases of compounds, such as those based on ligands (LBSV). In this case, a similarity search can be made between known bioactive compounds and molecules contained in databases. LBVS techniques include methods based on the pharmacophore and quantitative structure-activity relationship (QSAR) modelling.

In pharmacophore-based virtual screening, a hypothetical pharmacophore is taken as a template. The goal of screening is to identify molecules that show chemical similarities to the template [40].

QSAR is based on the similarity between structures. It is a quantitative relationship between a biological activity and the molecular descriptors that are used to predict the activity. QSAR searches for similarities between known ligands and each structure in a database, investigating how the biological activity of the ligands can be correlated to their structural features [8].

5. Examples of Virtual Screening / Molecular Docking in Animal Venom

[38] performed a virtual screening against α-Cobratoxin. The neurotoxin α-Cobratoxin (Cbtx), isolated from the venom of the Thai cobra *Naja kaouthia*, causes paralysis by preventing acetylcholine (ACh) binding to nicotinic acetylcholine receptors (nAChRs). A search for α- Cobratoxin structures was carried out in the PDB, and the virtual screening of 1990 compounds was performed using the program AutoDock. On [^{3}H]epibatidine and on [^{125}I] α-bungarotoxin, NSC121865 (compound 23) was most potent in binding with Ac (K*d* = 16.26 nM; K*d* = 36.63 nM). The results showed that, in clinical applications, NSC121865 would be a very useful potential lead in the development of a new treatment for snakebite victims. This inhibitor can be used for the development of a more potent and specific anti-cobratoxin.

[14] investigated the effects of protease inhibitors, including phenylmethylsulfonyl fluoride (PMSF), benzamidine (BMD), and their derivatives on the activity of recombinant gloshedobin, a snake venom thrombin-like enzyme (SVTLE), from the snake *Gloydius shedaoensis*. The structural model of gloshedobin was built by homology modelling using modelling package MODELLER. The stereochemical quality of the homology model was assessed using the PROCHECK program and the software AutoDock was used to dock inhibitors onto the structural model of gloshedobin. The docking results indicated that the strongest inhibitor, PMSF, bound covalently to the catalytic Ser195.

[36] evaluated the inhibitory effect of 1-(3-dimethylaminopropyl)-1-(4-fluorophenyl)-3-oxo-1,3-dihydroisobenzofuran-5-carbonitrile (DFD) on viper venom-induced haemorrhagic and PLA2 activities. Molecular docking studies of DFD and snake venom metalloproteases (SVMPs) were performed to understand the mechanism of inhibition by DFD, since SVMPs constitute one of the protein groups responsible for venom-induced haemorrhage. The docking results showed that DFD binds to a hydrophobic pocket in SVMPs with the *Ki* of 19.26×10^{-9} (kcal/mol) without chelating Zn^{2+} in the active site.

6. Conclusions

In silico approaches used in protein structure prediction and in drug discovery research have been presented in this chapter.

Computational methods used in the search for inhibitors play an essential role in the process of discovering new drugs.

The application of protein modelling methods has contributed significantly in cases where the structure of the target protein has not been solved, allowing the SBVS process be completed.

Good results obtained by virtual screening depend on the quality of structures, databases to be scanned, the search algorithms, and scoring functions. Therefore, there must be a good interaction and exchange of information between *in silico* and experimental methods. Careful application of these strategies is necessary for successful drug design.

Table 2 presents a list of software tools and server web sites.

	Summary Tools
PDB	http://www.rcsb.org/pdb/home/home.do
BLAST	http://blast.ncbi.nlm.nih.gov/
HHpred	http://toolkit.tuebingen.mpg.de/hhpred
ClustalW	http://www.ebi.ac.uk/Tools/msa/clustalw2/
SWISS-MODEL	http://swissmodel.expasy.org/
MODELLER	http://salilab.org/modeller/
SCRWL4	http://dunbrack.fccc.edu/scwrl4/
PROCHECK	http://www.ebi.ac.uk/thornton-srv/software/PROCHECK/
WHAT IF	http://swift.cmbi.ru.nl/whatif/
Verify3D	http://nihserver.mbi.ucla.edu/Verify_3D/
ERRAT	http://nihserver.mbi.ucla.edu/ERRATv2/
PROVE	http://www.doe-mbi.ucla.edu/Software/PROVE.html

Summary Tools	
modFold	https://www.reading.ac.uk/bioinf/ModFOLD/
ProQ	http://www.sbc.su.se/~bjornw/ProQ/ProQ.html
ROSETTA	http://www.rosettacommons.org/home
Q-sitefinder	http://www.modelling.leeds.ac.uk/qsitefinder/
SAVes	http://nihserver.mbi.ucla.edu/SAVES/
THREADER	http://bioinf.cs.ucl.ac.uk/software_downloads/threader/
metaPocket	http://projects.biotec.tu-dresden.de/metapocket/
PASS	http://www.ccl.net/cca/software/UNIX/pass/overview.shtml
SURFNET	http://www.ebi.ac.uk/thornton-srv/software/SURFNET/
AUTODOCK	http://autodock.scripps.edu/
GOLD	http://www.ccdc.cam.ac.uk/products/life_sciences/gold/
GLIDE	http://www.schrodinger.com/products/14/5/
Derek/Meteor	https://www.lhasalimited.org/
Raptorx	http://raptorx.uchicago.edu/
RAPTOR	http://www.bioinformaticssolutions.com/raptor/downloadpricing/freetrial.html
Phyre	http://www.sbg.bio.ic.ac.uk/~phyre/
MUSTER	http://zhanglab.ccmb.med.umich.edu/MUSTER/
I-TASSER	http://zhanglab.ccmb.med.umich.edu/I-TASSER/

Table 2. Software tools and server web sites.

Acknowledgements

The author would like to thank CAPES-PROEX and CNPq for financial support.

Author details

Silvana Giuliatti*

Address all correspondence to: silvana@fmrp.usp

Faculty of Medicine of Ribeirão Preto - University of São Paulo, Brazil

References

[1] Altschul, S. F., Madden, T. L., Schäffer, A. A., Zhang, J., Zhang, Z., Miller, W., & Lipman, D. (1997). Gapped BLAST and PSI-BLAST: A New Generation of Protein Database Search Programs. *Nucleic Acids Research,* 25(17), September, 3389-3402, 1362-4962.

[2] Altschul, S. F., Gish, W., Miller, W., Myers, E. W., & Lipman, D. J. (1990). Basic Local Alignment Search Tool. *Journal of Molecular Biology,* 215(3), October, 403-410, 0022-2836.

[3] Arnold, K., Bordoli, L., Kopp, J., & Schwede, T. (2006). The SWISS-MODEL Workspace: a Web-Based Environment for Protein Structure Homology Modelling. *Bioinformatics,* 22(2), January 2005, 195-201, 1460-2059.

[4] Bowie, J. U., Lüthy, R., & Eisemberg, D. (1991). A Method to Identify Protein Sequences that Fold into a Known Three-Dimensional Structure. *Science,* 253(5016), July, 164-170, 0036-8075.

[5] Brady, G., & Stouten, P. (2000). Fast Prediction and Visualization of Protein Binding Pockets with PASS. *Journal of Computer-Aided Molecular Design,* 14(4), May, 383-401, 1573-4951.

[6] Colovos, C., & Yeates, T. O. (1993). Verification of Protein Structures: Patterns of Nonbonded Atomic Interactions. *Protein Science,* 12(9), September, 1511-1519, 0036-8075.

[7] Deane, C. M., & Blundell, T. L. (2001). CODA: A Combined Algorithm for Predicting the Structurally Variable Regions of Protein Models. *Protein Science,* 10(3), March, 599-612, 0146-9896 X.

[8] Ebalunode, J. O., Zheng, W., & Tropsha, A. (2011). Application of QSAR and Shape Pharmacophore Modeling Approaches for Targeted Chemical Library Design. *Methods in Molecular Biology,* 685, 111-133, 1064-3745.

[9] Eswar, N., Marti-Renom, M. A., Webb, B., Madhusudhan, M. S., Eramian, D., Shen, M., Pieper, U., & Sali, A. (2007). Comparative Protein Structure Modelling With MODELLER. *Current Protocols in Bioinformatics,* 50, (November), unit 2.9.1-2.9.31, 1934-340X.

[10] Friesner, R. A., Banks, J. L., Murphy, R. B., Halgren, T. A., Klicic, J. J., Mainz, D. T., Repasky, M. P., Knoll, E. H., Shaw, D. E., Shelley, M., Perry, J. K., Francis, P., & Shenkin, P. S. (2004). Glide: A New Approach for Rapid, Accurate Docking and Scoring. 1. Method and Assessment of Docking Accuracy. *Journal of Medical Chemistry,* 47(7), March, 1739-1749, 1520-4804.

[11] Greene, N., Judson, P., Langowski, J., & Marchant, C. A. (1999). Knowledge-based expert Systems for Toxicity and Metabolism Prediction: DEREK, StAR and METEOR. *SAR QSAR Environmental Research,* 10(2-3), 299-313, 0013-9351.

[12] Huang, B., & Schroeder, M. (2006). LIGSITEcsc: Predictiong Ligand Binding Sites using the Connolly Surface and Degree of Conservation. *BMC Structural Biology*, 6, September, 19, 1472-6807.

[13] Huang, B. (2009). MetaPocket: A Meta Approach to Improve Protein Ligand Binding Site Prediction. *OMICS: A Journal of Integrative Biology*, 13(4), August, 325-330, 1557-8100.

[14] Jiang, X., Chena, L., Xua, J., & Yanga, Q. (2010). Molecular Mechanism Analysis of Gloydius Shedaoensis Venom Gloshedobin. *International Journal of Biological Macromolecules*, 48(1), January, 129-133, 0141-8130.

[15] Jones, D. T., Taylor, W. R., & Thornton, J. M. (1992). A New approach to Protein Fold Recognition. *Nature*, July, 358, 86-96, 0028-0836.

[16] Jones, G., Willett, P., Glen, R. C., Leach, A. R., & Taylor, R. (1997). Development and Validation of a Genetic Algorithm for Flexible Docking. *Journal of Molecular Biology*, 267(6381), July, 727-748, 0022-2836.

[17] Kastenholz, M. A., Pastor, M., Cruciani, G., Haaksma, E. E. J., & Fox, T. (2000). GRID/CPCA: A New Computational Tool to Design Selective Ligands. *Journal of Medical Chemistry*, 43(16), August, 3033-3044, 1520-4804.

[18] Kelley, L. A., & Stemberg, J. E. (2009). Protein Structure Predicition on the Web: a Case Study using the Phyre Server. *Nature Protocols*, 4(3), February, 363-371, 1754-2189.

[19] Klepeis, J. L., & Floudas, C. A. (2003). ASTRO-FOLD: A Combinatorial and Global Optimization Framework for Ab Initio prediction of Three-Dimensional Structures of Proteins from the Amino Acid Sequence. *Biophysical Journal*, 85(4), October, 2119-2146, 0006-3495.

[20] Krivov, G. G., Shapovalov, M. V., & Dunbrack, R. L. (2009). Improved Prediction of Protein Side-Chain Conformations with SCWRL4. *Proteins*, 77(4), December, 778-795, 1097-0134.

[21] Larkin, M. A., Blackshields, G., Brown, N. P., Chenna, R., Mc Gettigan, P. A., Mc William, H., Valentin, F., Wallace, I. M., Wilm, A., Lopez, R., Thompson, J. D., Gibson, T. J., & Higgins, D. G. (2007). Clustal W and Clustal X Version 2.0. *Bioinformatics*, 23(21), November, 2947-2948, 1460-2059.

[22] Laskowiski, R. (1995). SURFNET: a Program for Visualizing Molecular Surfaces, Cavities and Intermolecular Interactions. *Journal of Molecular Graphics*, 13(5), October, 323-330, 0263-7855.

[23] Laskowski, R. A., Macarthur, M. W., Moss, D. S., & Thornton, J. M. (1993). PROCHECK: a Program to Check the Stereochemical Quality of Protein Structures. *Journal of Applied Crystallography*, 26(2), April, 283-291, 1600-5767.

[24] Laurie, A., & Jackson, R. (2005). Q-SiteFinder: an Energy-based Method for the Prediction of Protein-Ligand Binding Sites. *Bioinformatics*, 21(9), May, 1908-1916, 1046-2059.

[25] Lipinski, C. A., Lombardo, F., Dominy, B. W., & Feeney, P. J. (2001). Experimental and Computational Approaches to Estimate Solubility and Permeability in Drug Discovery and Development Settings. *Advanced Drug Delivery Reviews*, 46(1-3), March, 3-26, 0016-9409 X.

[26] Lüthy, R., Bowie, J. U., & Eisemberg, D. (1992). Assessment of Protein Models with Three-Dimensional Profiles. *Nature*, 356(6364), March, 83-85, 0028-0836.

[27] Mc Guffin, L. J. (2008). The ModFOLD Server for the Quality Assessment of Protein Structural Models. *Bioinformatics*, 24, 586-587, 1460-2059.

[28] Milleer, R. T., Jones, D. T., & Thornton, J. M. (1996). Protein Fold Recognition by Sequence Threading: Tools and Assessment Techniques. *The FASEB Journal*, 10(1), January, 171-178, 1530-6860.

[29] Morris, G. M., Huey, R., Lindstrom, W., Sanner, M. F., Belew, R. K., Goodsell, D. S., & Olson, A. J. (2004). AutoDock4 and AutoDockTools4: Automated Docking with Selective Receptor Flexibility. *Journal of Computational Chemistry*, 30(16), December,2009, 2785-2791, 0109-6987 X.

[30] Pontius, J., Richelle, J., & Wodak, S. J. (1996). Deviations from Standard Atomic Volumes as a Quality Measure of Protein Crystal Structures. *Journal of Molecular Biology*, 264(1), November, 121-126, 0022-2836.

[31] Ramachandran, G. N., Ramakrishnan, C., & Sasisekharan, V. (1963). Stereochemistry of Polypeptide Chain Configurations. *Journal of Molecular Biology*, 7, July, 95-99, 0022-2836.

[32] Rohl, C. A., Strauss, C. E., Misura, K. M. S., & Baker, D. (2004). Protein Sructure Prediction using Rosetta. *Methods Enzymol*, 383, 66-93, 0076-6879.

[33] Sali, A. E., & Blundell, T. L. (1993). Comparative Protein Modelling by Satisfaction of Spatial Restraints. *Journal of Molecular Biology*, 234, 779-815, 0022-2836.

[34] Söding, J., Biegert, A., & Lupas, A. N. (2005). The HHpred Interactive Server for Protein Homology Detection and Structure Prediction. *Nucleic Acids Research*, 33(3), December, W244-W248, 1362-4962.

[35] Subramani, A., Wei, Y., & Floudas, C. A. (2012). ASTRO-FOLD 2.0: An Enhanced Framework for Protein Structure Prediction. *American Institute of Chemical Engineers Journal*, 58(5), May, 1619-1637, 1547-5905.

[36] Sunitha, K., Hemshekhar, M., Gaonkar, S. L., Santhosh, M. S., Kumar, M. S., Basappa Priya, B. S., Kemparaju, K., Rangappa, K. S., Swamy, S. N., & Girish, K. S. (2011). Neutralization of Hanemorrhagic Activity of Viper Venoms by 1-(3-Dimethylamino-

propyl)-1-(4-Fluorophenyl)-3-Oxo-1, 3-Dihydroisobenzofuran-5-Carbonitrile. *Basic & Clinical Pharmacology & Toxicology*, 109(4), October, 292-299, 1742-7843.

[37] Sussman, J. L., Lin, D., Jiang, J., Manning, N. O., Prilusky, J., Ritter, O., & Abola, E. E. (1998). Protein data bank (PDB): a Database of 3D Structural Information of Biological Macromolecules. *Acta Crystal*, D54, 1078-1084, 1600-5759.

[38] Utsintong, M., Talley, T. T., Taylor, P. W., Olson, A. J., & Vajragupta, O. (2009). Virtual Screening Against α-Cobratoxin. *Journal of Biomolecular Screening*, 14(9), October, 1109-1118, 1087-0571.

[39] Vriend, G. (1990). WHAT IF: A Molecular Modelling and Drug Design Program. *Journal of Molecular Graphics*, 8(1), March, 52-56, 0263-7855.

[40] Yang, U. S. (2010). Pharmacophore Modeling and Applications in Drug Discovery: Challenges and Recent Advances. *Drug Discovery Today*, 15(11-12), June, 446-450, 1359-6446.

[41] Peng , J., & Xu, J. (2010). Low-homology protein threading. *Bioinformatics*, 26, i294-i300, 10-1093.

[42] Peng , J., & Xu, J. (2011). RaptorX: Exploiting Structure Information for protein alignment by statistical inferenc. *Proteins: Structure, Functon, and Bioinformatics*, 79(S10), 167-171, 10-1002.

Chapter 4

New Perspectives in Drug Discovery Using Neuroactive Molecules From the Venom of Arthropods

Márcia Renata Mortari and
Alexandra Olimpio Siqueira Cunha

Additional information is available at the end of the chapter

http://dx.doi.org/10.5772/ 52382

1. Introduction

Arthropods are one of the most ancient groups of animals in earth and their venoms have been responsible for their chemical defense in a very efficient way. Resulting from an intense and elaborated evolutionary process, venoms produced by arthropods have a very complex repertoire of biologically active molecules. When inoculated in mammals these molecules induce a wide range of systemic effects, including actions in the CNS. In mammalian CNS, venom compounds may either inhibit or stimulate with affinity and specificity structures such as: ion channels, neurotransmitter receptors and transporters [1-3]. Not surprisingly, these actions have attracted the attention of many investigators in search of tools to help the understanding of neural mechanisms as well as those in search of novel probes in CNS drug design for the last 20 years [3,4]. In addition to the growing interest in finding new neuroactive compounds, the improvement of proteomic and transcriptome techniques has stimulated great progress in the bioprospecting, enabling and accelerating the testing of new toxins in several animal models. Animal research aiming at the efficacy of peptides and acylpoliamines, isolated from arthropod venoms, have revealed the great potential of these compounds to treat various diseases, such as epilepsy, Parkinson's, Alzheimer's, chronic pain and anxiety disorders

According to World Health Organization (WHO), neurological and mental disorders are one of the greatest threats to public health not only for its direct and immediate effects, but also for the progressive nature of these diseases, often leading to disability and death [5]. The symptoms of most of these diseases are often well treated with a several pharmaceuticals, such as antidepressants, anxiolytics, anticonvulsants and analgesics. However, it is well known that neuroactive drugs may induce a complex range of adverse effects that limit the usage in some patients or may even function as a factor of impairment in people's quality of life. According to [6], none of antiepileptic drugs discovered in the last 20 years, was efficient to cure or even suppress seizures in epileptic patients. Therefore, there is a continued need for the discovery of novel drugs to treat most neurological and mental disorders [7].

This chapter will target the discussion of recent contributions of research on the compounds of arthropod venom, for the discovery of novel tools to study the functioning of the structures of mammalian CNS, as well as the supply of novel alternatives to the treatment of neurological disorders. Among the major compounds, it will be highlighted those with the analgesic, anxiolytic, antiepileptic and neuroprotective effects, with emphasis on the most promising on preclinical or clinic evaluation.

2. Main targets of the neuroactive compounds isolated from arthropod venoms

Venom isolated from bee, scorpion and spider have been used to the treatment of various diseases in Chinese and Korean traditional medicine, such as epilepsy, stroke, facial paralysis, arthritis, rheumatism, back pain, cancerous, tumors, and skin diseases [8-10]. Moreover, venoms of arthropod animals have been used to study various physiopathological processes, and also offer opportunity to design and develop new therapeutic drugs [3,11,12] .

Arthropod venoms are rich in biologically active substances with different physiological actions, specially the neurotoxins. So far, identified neurotoxins generally comprise the classes of peptides or acylpolyamines, acting with affinity and specificity over excitatory or inhibitory neurotransmissions (for revision see [12]. The actions of these compounds include the interaction with Na^+, K^+ and Ca^{2+} ion channels, agonism or antagonism of metabotropic and ionotropic receptors for neurotransmitters as the excitatory neurotransmitter glutamate. At the presynaptic level, several studies have shown the interaction of arthropod neurotoxins with protein transporters of neurotransmitters, resulting in the facilitation or inhibition of their uptake.

3. Antinociceptive effects

Of extreme importance for the organism, pain is an indicator of corporal integrity and has been considered since January 2000, by the Joint Commission on Accreditation on Healthcare Organizations (JCAHO) as the fifth vital sign that should be assessed and recorded together with other signals immediately after birth. According to the International Association for the Study of Pain (IASP), pain is defined as an unpleasant sensation and emotional experience associated with actual or potential tissue damage. However, approximately one third of world population suffers from pathological persistent or recurrent pain, which is a common complaint in patients with different diseases, and exerts great impact on their social life [13]. In these cases, treatment is a challenge for researchers and health professionals who constantly seek new therapeutic strategies, since most of these are inadequate or cause serious side effects [14].

Analgesics and systemic conservative therapies are widely used for pain control. However, in many cases, especially in patients with neuropathic pain, more aggressive treatments are needed, which promote a significant clinical improvement but only in 30-50% of patients [15,16].

Although an injection of arthropod venoms is commonly reported to cause tonic pain and hyperalgesia, there is also evidence suggesting that these venoms might have antinociceptive effects on inflammation. Thus, nowadays, toxins isolated from arthropods are considered powerful tools, since they have congruent targets of the impulse transmission of pain, and may provide an attractive alternative to opioid treatments.

3.1. Polypeptide toxins from Scorpion

The most studied Arthropod venom is extracted from the Asian scorpion *Mesobuthus martensi* Karsch (BmK). It is composed of several toxins, and so far, ten have been described, which produce powerful antinociceptive effects. This is the case of the two β-excitatory anti-insect toxins BmK IT-AP (or Bm33-I) and BmK AngP1, two β- depressant anti-insect toxins BmK dITAP3 and BmK IT2, as well as six toxins yet without consensus classification, BmK AS, BmK AS1, BmK AGAP, BmK Ang M1, BmK AGP-SYPU1 and BmK AGP-SYPU2. These compounds probably belong to a family of peptides NaScTx that are composed of 60-76 amino acid residues with four disulfide bonds, the cysteine positions among these toxins are highly conserved [17,18]. Considering their structures, they might be able to bind to sodium channels impairing depolarization of the action potential in nerve and muscle, resulting in neurotoxicity [18], although it remains to be fully investigated.

The NaScTx family can be classified in at least two major families, α and β, according to the mode of action on Na^+ channels [19]. The binding of α-toxins delays Na_v channel inactivation, while that of β-toxins shifts the membrane potential dependence of channel activation to more negative potentials. α and β-toxins also exhibit pharmacological preferences for mammals or insects sodium channels. Therefore, considering their pharmacological activities, α and β NAScTx can be also divided into three groups:

i. "classic" highly specific for mammals;

ii. "α-like toxins" active both on mammals and insects, which are far less specific and less active than the "classical" ones;

iii. α-toxins only specific for insects and without any toxicity on mammals, even at high concentrations. Moreover, the insect selective β-toxins have been divided into two groups: the excitatory insect toxins and the depressant insect toxins.

Regarding the β-excitatory anti-insect toxins, BmK IT-AP (Insect Toxin-Analgesic Peptide), which was isolated in 1999, produces a potent antinociceptive effect in mouse-twisting model, after i.v. injection [20]. The same toxin has also been sequenced by another group and named Bm K 33-I [21]. Later, Guan and colleagues [22] identified a novel toxin with analgesic effects, BmK $AngP_1$, which shows an evident analgesic effect with simultaneous excitatory insect toxicity, but is devoid of any toxicity on mice even at high dosages. The analgesic effect was assessed with a mouse-twisting model. The analgesic effect on mice of the $AngP_1$ is at least 4-5 times weaker than that of IT-AP, but the toxicity to insects is twice as strong as that of IT-AP [20,22]

In relation of depressant toxins isolated from BmK venom, BmK IT2 has been more studied from the venom of BmK (Fig 1). Intraplantar injection of BmK IT2 inhibited thermal hyperalgesia in carrageenan-treated rats and significantly prolonged paw withdrawal latency in normal rats [23]. This toxin also displays an inhibitory effect on the C component of the rat nociceptive flexion reflex by subcutaneous injection in vivo [24]. Peripheral or spinal delivery of BmK IT2 suppressed formalin-induced nociceptive behaviors and c-Fos expression in spinal cord [25,26]. Both BmK IT2 and Bm K dIT-AP3 (depressant Insect Toxin-Analgesic Peptide 3) are toxic for insects, but not for mammals [27], and shows 86.7% of sequence similarity [23]. BmK dIT-AP3 also induces analgesia in the mouse-twisting model [18]. Using whole-cell patch clamp, it has been shown that BmK dIT-AP3 inhibits Na_v currents of rat dorsal root ganglion (DRG) neurons, blocking more selectively the tetrodotoxin-resistant (TTX-R) component of the Na^+ currents. These results suggest that the inhibition of the rat nociceptive flexion reflex by BmK dITAP3 may be attributed to modulation of the DRG's voltage-gated Na^+ channels [24].

Wang and colleagues [28] isolated a new antinociceptive peptide, named BmK AGP-SYPU1. Recombinant BmK AGP-SYPU1 showed similar analgesic effects on mice compared to natural when assayed using a mouse-twisting model [28]. More recently, BmK AGP-SYPU2 was purified and tested, also in mouse-twisting model. Sequence determination showed that the mature BmK AGP-SYPU2 peptide is composed of 66 amino acid residues, and BmK AGP-SYPU2 is identical to BmK alpha2 and BmK alphaTX11.

BmK AS had a strong analgesic effect on both visceral and somatic pain [29,30]. It relieves formalin-induced two-phase spontaneous flinching response and carrageenan-induced mechanical hyperalgesia, probably by modulating the voltage-gated Na^+ channels of sensory neurons [31,32]. Moreover, BmK AS showed activity nearly equivalent to that of morphine. Later, a new peptide that possesses 86.3% of similarity with BmK AS was identified. Both polypeptides have 66 amino acids cross-linked by four disulfide bridges [29]. In addition, these two peptides show a poor similarity with other known types of scorpion toxins. BmK AS and AS1 are not toxic against mammals and only have a weak toxicity to insects. BmK AS, then BmK AS1, have been found to significantly stimulate the binding of [3H]-ryanodine to partially purified ryanodine receptors [33]. More recently, electrophysiological studies have shown that they are able to inhibit Na^+ currents in NG108-15 cells [34] and to depress TTX-sensitive and TTX-resistant Na^+ currents in rat small DRG neurons. Interestingly, in rat models, BmK AS1 also displays antinociceptive effects according to [33]. These authors concluded that the effects could be mediated by the modulation of voltage-gated Na^+ channels and they also suggested that BmK AS and BmK AS1 could form a new family of scorpion insect toxins.

BmK AGAP (antitumor-analgesic peptide), isolated in 2003, had strong inhibitory effect on both viscera and soma pain [35]. To evaluate the extent to which residues of the toxin core contribute to its analgesic activity, nine mutants of BmK AGAP were produced and tested. However, further studies are necessarily to elucidate the mechanism of action as well as to exploit its analgesic activity [36]. In relation to BmK Ang M1 [37], it also was reported to exhibit potential analgesic effect. Moreover, electrophysiological studies showed that BmK AngM1 at the concentration of 1 μM inhibited voltage-dependent Na^+ current (I_{Na}) and voltage-dependent delayed rectifier K^+ current (I_K), but had no effects on transient K^+ current [37].

It is important to note that the excitatory and depressant anti-insect toxins belong to different groups, which have distinct modes of interaction with receptors. Thus, one can infer that the analgesic effect of these peptides may have a molecular mode and mechanism different from that of insect toxicity. Still, the mechanisms by which these scorpion toxins can modulate pain pathways remain to be clarified. According to [8], four different possibilities might be described:

i. peptides act directly Na^+ channels involved in the pathway of pain,

ii. peptides modulate indirectly the pain sensation,

iii. peptides also modulate other targets involved in pain pathway

iv. pain alleviation is only apparent and results from misinterpretations that might have occurred from animal models used.

3.2. Polypeptide toxins from Spider

Another group of arthropods that have very promising antinociceptive compounds are spiders [41]. In 1996, Roerig & Howse reported the effect of ω-agatoxina IVA (Fig 1) isolated from funnel spider *Agelenopsis aperta* venom, against thermal stimulation in the tail flick test, when co-administrated with morphine intrathecal. Intrathecal injection of ω-agatoxin IVA (0.2 nmol/kg) also decreased the licking time in both the early and late response phases in a dose-dependent manner in the Formalin test [42]. The use of this peptide as an analgesic could be of particular benefit in patients tolerant or opioid-dependent, since this compound exhibits selectivity for the P/Q Ca^{2+} channels [43]. Other spider venom very promissory is the venom of the Brazilian armed spider *Phoneutria nigriventer*, the purified fraction 3 (PhTx3) contains 6 toxin isoforms (Tx3-1 to -6) [44,45] that target Ca^{2+} channels with different affinity patterns. Moreover, one toxin, Tx3-6 (Phα1β), demonstrated that it preferentially blocks the N-type calcium current [46] and produce a potent antinociceptive effect with higher therapeutic index [44]. Dalmolin and colleagues [45] showed that Tx3-3 (purified the same fraction) caused a short-lasting antinociceptive effect in the nociceptive pain test and a long-lasting antinociceptive effect in neuropathic pain models, without producing detectable side effects. However, Tx3-3 did not change the inflammatory pain. Tx3-3 blockade of P/Q- and R-type Ca^{2+} channels and inhibit the glutamate release in rat brain cortical synaptosomes [47]. Other neurotoxin isolated from spider *Phoneutria nigriventer* is Phα1β, which is a potent toxin blocking neuronal voltage-sensitive Ca^{2+} channels. This peptide induced longer antiallodynic effect than μ-conotoxin MVIIA and morphine in mice [48].

In addition to toxins calcium modulators, compounds isolated from spider that interact with other ionic channels have shown great potential. A new class of peptide toxins named is the Huwentoxin I (HWTX-I, Fig 1) that is the most abundant toxic component in the crude venom of the Chinese bird spider *Ornithoctonus huwena*. Whole-cell patch clamp records revealed that HWTX-I selectively inhibits N-type Ca^{2+} channels in NG108-15 cells, and it also can block transmitter release from nerve endings by preventing depolarization induced by calcium influx [38] Antinociception effect of the HWTX-I in formalin test was greater and lasted two-fold longer time compared to morphine [39]. Furthermore, Tao and collaborators [40] demonstrated that intrathecal administration of HWTX-I is effective in antinociception in the rat model of rheumatoid arthritis more effective than ibuprofen.

Several studies have reported that intrathecal administration of non-selective blockers of Ca^{2+} channels shows antinociceptive effects in animals tested with thermal stimuli: hot plate and tail flick. According to [49], N and P/Q Ca^{2+} channels are probably involved in nociceptive behavior induced by formalin injection in rats, while the L-type channels has no effect. N- and P/Q-type Ca^{2+} channels are expressed specifically in the nervous system, and they have a major importance in controlling the excitation of spinal neurons from sensory afferents of inflamed tissues, relieving inflammatory pain.

A new class of peptide toxins named π-theraphotoxin-Pc1a (π-TRTX-Pc1a; also known as psalmotoxin-1 (PcTx1) was isolated from the venom of the spider neotropical *Psalmopoeus cambridgei* (Fig.1). π-TRTX-Pc1a is the most potent and selective blocker of ion channels sensitive to acid – ASICa [50]. These channels play important roles in pathological conditions such as cerebral ischemia or epilepsy, as well as being responsible for the sensation of pain that accompanies tissue acidosis and inflammation [51]. Since external acidification is a major factor in pain associated with inflammation (hematosis muscle and cardiac ischemia, or cancer), these neurotoxins can be used to control the pain sensation triggered by these channels [52]. π-TRTX-Pc1a was shown to be an effective analgesic, comparable to morphine, in rat models of acute and neuropathic pain when injected directly in Central Nervous System [53] and intranasal administration of this peptide resulted in neuroprotection of neurons in a mouse model of ischemic stroke even when administered hours after injury [54].

Other important target in the search for new analgesics isolated from spider venoms are Na_V channels, since modulatory compounds of these channels are the dominant pharmacological species in spider venoms, although still poorly characterized. In this context, Intrathecal administration of β-TRTX-Gr1b (formerly GsAFI), a peptide obtained from venom of *Grammostola spatulata*, the Chilean pink tarantula spider, induced analgesia in a variety of rat pain models such as the tail flick latency test, hot plate threshold test, von Frey threshold test, and formalin pain test, without any confounding side-effects. Moreover, the β-TRTX-Gr1b peptide did not exhibit cross tolerance with morphine [55].

Further on spider venoms, Purotoxin-1 (PT1) was recently isolated the, from the venom of the Central Asian spider *Geolycosa sp* [56]. PT1 is a 35-residue peptide with four disulfide bonds, and it exerts a potent analgesic effect in rat models of acute and chronic inflammatory pain by injection of either carrageenan or Freund's complete adjuvant, respectively. PT1 was also effective in reducing the number of nocifensive events triggered by the injection of capsaicin or formalin (only second phase) [56]. This molecule also inhibits P2X3 receptors in a powerful and selective manner. These ATP-activated receptors are largely expressed in mammalian sensory neurons play a key role in the pain perception. Thus, PT1 appears to be a promising lead compound for the development of analgesics that target these receptors [56].

3.3. Polypeptide toxins from Bees and Wasps

Bee venom has been traditionally used to relieve pain and treat chronic pain diseases (for revision see [57]). Moreover, acupoint stimulation into the subcutaneous region (acupuncture) rather than other injection sites may be important for the antinociceptive effects of this venom. There is increasing evidence suggesting that bee venom has antinociceptive effects on visceral nociceptive effects, mechanical and thermal hyperplasia, formalin-induced pain behavior and collagen-induced arthritic pain, as well as knee osteoarthritis (OA)-related pain [58-63]. BV contains at least 18 active components, including enzymes, peptides, and biogenic amines, which have a wide variety of pharmaceutical properties, and so multiple mechanisms associated to antinociceptive effects have been suggested, such as activation of the central and spinal opioid receptor and α_2-adrenergic receptor, as well as activation of the descending serotonergic pathways (for revision see [64]).

Melittin is a small protein containing 26 amino acid residues and is the major bioactive component in BV (Fig.1). This polypeptide readily integrates into and disrupts both natural and synthetic phospholipid bilayers [65,66]. Melittin also enhances the activity of PLA_2 [67] and has a variety of effects on living cells possibly through the disruption of the membrane [68]. The decrease in cyclooxygenase (COX)-2 and phospholipase PLA_2 expression and the decrease in the levels of tumor necrosis factor alpha (TNF-α), interleukin (IL)-1, IL-6, nitric oxide (NO) and oxygen reactive species (ROS) are suggested to be associated with the anti-arthritis effect of melittin [69]. This peptide has also been thought to play a role in production of anti-nociceptive and anti-inflammatory effects [64]. In addition, Merlo and colleagues [70] demonstrated the antinociceptive activity of the melittin in experimental models of nociceptive and inflammatory pain. Interestingly, melittin failed to increase the latency for the nociceptive response in the hot-plate model and in the first phase of the formalin test, revealing that melittin presents an activity that resembles more that of anti-inflammatory drugs and less that of centrally acting drugs [70]. Nevertheless, the molecular and cellular mechanisms underlying the anti-nociceptive effects of melittin are not entirely clear and remain to be further clarified by further experimental studies [57].

Addition of melittin, adolapin has been isolated from BV and it demonstrated a potent analgesic effect in mouse-twisting model and the Randall-Sellito's test [71]. The anti-inflammatory activity of adolapin was evaluated and it had a pronounced activity in the following tests: carrageenan, PG, adjuvant rat hind paw edema and adjuvant polyarthritis. The effects of adolapin are presumably due to its ability to inhibit the prostaglandin synthesis via inhibition of cyclooxygenase activity [71,72].

Venoms of wasps also have analgesic peptides. Mortari and colleagues [73] isolated a compound with antinociceptive activity from the venom of the Brazilian social wasp *Polybia occidentalis*. The isolated peptide is a neurokinin named Thr^6-Bradykinin. This neurokinin is a small peptide consisting of nine amino acid residues, Arg-Pro-Pro-Gly-Phe-Thr-Pro-Phe-Arg-OH, which exhibits a high degree of homology with bradykinin (BK), except for the substitution of Thr for Ser in position 6 at BK. As a result, small changes in their secondary structures are observed [74]. This modification has been regarded as responsible for increasing B_2 receptor affinity and potency of Thr^6-BK in relation to BK *in vitro* and *in vivo* [74,75]. Thr^6-BK antinociceptive effect was dose- and time- dependent, when injected directly into the CNS of rats in hot-plate and tail-flick tests, and it was three times more potent than morphine and 4 times more potent than BK in tail-flick test. Thr^6-BK induced antinociception by activating presynaptic B_2 receptors, which activate descending adrenergic pathways. Studies investigating the role of kinins in the CNS provide new information on the supraspinal system of the pain control, whose modulation may represent a new strategy to control pain-related pathologies [76].

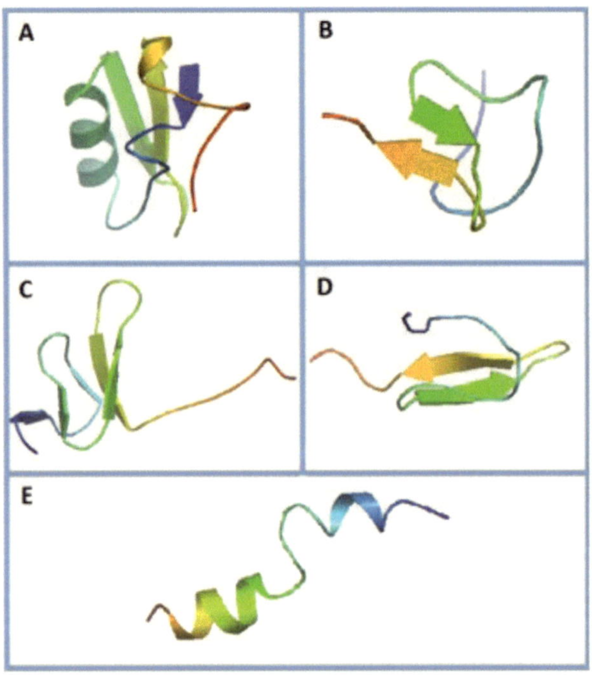

Figure 1. Tridimensional structure of antinociceptive peptides isolated from arthropod venoms. (A) BMK IT2; (B) HWTX 1; (C) ω-Agatoxin IVA; (D) π-Theraphotoxin-Pc1a; (E) Mellitin. Uniprot entry code: P68727, P56676, P30288, P60514 and P01501, respectively.

Besides peptides, some studies have evaluated the analgesic activity of acylpolyamines that can be used as new alternative drugs for the treatment of chronic pain, as well as tools for the study of the functional role of the AMPA/kainate receptors in the processing of nociceptive pain [77]. In this regard, intrathecal administration of different doses of these toxins blocked thermally induced allodynia [78] and hyperalgesia [79]. The effect of these neurotoxins may suggest a possible involvement of AMPA receptors in the spinal cord during the nociceptive excitatory stimulation [80,81].

4. Antiepileptic and neuroprotective effects

Neurodegenerative disorders comprise a wide range of conditions mostly characterized by a progressive loss of neuronal function and neuronal cell death. The incidence of these diseases in population differs greatly. In conditions such as Parkinson disease and Alzheimer, the number of cases significantly increases in elderly, whereas epileptic patients are mostly children and adolescents. Many processes may trigger neuronal cell death, such as trauma, stroke, tumors, infections, genetic factors and biochemical alterations. Among the latest, the alterations in Ca^{2+}-mediated signaling is thought to play a key role in many neurodegenerative disorders and the increase in intracellular Ca^{2+} concentration might alter neuronal membrane potential [82]. Moreover, the hyperactivation of excitatory transmission mediated mostly by L-glutamate and its ionotropic receptors; kainate, AMPA and NMDA, is responsible for the excessive cationic influx that depolarizes neuronal cells and lead to sustained hyperexcitation observed in brain pathologies such as epilepsy [83]. This increase in glutamatergic activity often referred to as glutamate excitotoxicity [84], might also involve non-receptor neurochemical events such as failure in glutamate uptake system, which ends with an increase in the availability of this neurotransmitter in the synaptic cleft [85,86]. The importance of L-glutamate in neurological disorders relies on the fact that this neurotransmitter is release in the great majority of fast synapses in CNS [84,83]. In this context, many molecules mostly peptides and acylpolyamines, acting on ion channels, receptors and transporters were isolated from arthropod venoms, remarkably spiders, scorpions and wasps [3]. According to [82], polyamines are non-specific antagonist of ligand-gated ion channels, acting at glutamatergic and Ach receptors in an uncompetitive way, that is, the receptor must be activated in order to occur the blockade. This mode of action might diminish the side effects of newly designed medicines, since it blocks only the activated receptors, but does not prevent their opening.

The venom of the orb-web spider *Nephilia clavata* was one of the first venoms studied during the 80s, which resulted in the identification of small compounds named acylpolyamines, among whose we may find jorotoxin (JSTX), one of the first glutamate receptor uncompetitive antagonists [83,84]. Together with JSTX, another polyamines such as argiopin from the venom of the spider *Argiope lobata* [85] and philantotoxin (PhTx) from the venom of the solitary wasp *Philanthus triangulum* [86]. Following the structural characterization and studies in insect or crustaceans, the reports on the action of these polyamines in mammalian CNS started to take place, mostly during the 90s [87]. JSTX-1 and JSTX-3 are synthetic analogues of JSTX. The first inhibits kainate-induced seizures, whereas the latter block glutamate release and hippocampal epileptic discharges [88,89]. Later, JSTX-3 was shown to inhibit the formation of superoxide dismutase-1 (SOD-1) aggregates that lead mutant motor neurons (mSOD-1) to death during the familiar form of the neurodegenerative disease, amyotrophic lateral sclerosis [90]. The authors concluded that increased Ca^{2+} influx mainly through AM-

PA/kainate glutamate receptors make mutant neurons more vulnerable to damage and therefore, JSTX-3 is an interesting neuroprotective agent in this model.

The fraction of the venom of the spider *Agelenopsis aperta* containing argiotoxin, was first demonstrated to have anticonvulsant in NMDA-induced and audiogenic seizures [91]. The synthetic analogue of argiotoxin, Arg-636, is a selective antagonist of NMDA receptors binding to the Mg^{2+} binding site at the receptor with anticonvulsant and neuroprotective actions. In addition, from the venom of *A. aperta,* another NMDA receptor blocker, Agatoxin 489 was reported as anticonvulsant against kainate-induced seizures and its synthetic analogue Agel-505, was able to block cationic currents in oocytes transfected with NMDA receptor cDNA [92].

Aside from antagonizing glutamate receptors, arthropod neurotoxins may exert anticonvulsant and neuroprotective effects targeting other neurotransmitter systems. The venom of the Brazilian spider *Phoneutria nigriventer* has been extensively studied over the past 20 years. Neurotoxins isolated from the venom of *P. nigriventer,* such as PhTx-3 (Tx-3) were reported to inhibit Ca^{2+} dependent-glutamate release [47]. Tx3-3 and Tx3-4 also inhibit voltage-activated Ca^{2+} channels of P/Q type [93] and recently their neuroprotective activity was tested. According to [94], Tx3-3 and Tx3-4 protected hippocampal slices against damage and cell death induced by ischemic insult resulted from low oxygen and low glucose. Moreover, PhTx3, Tx3-3, and Tx3-4, inhibited cell loss in retinal slices submitted to the same ischemic protocol [95]. Another Brazilian species lives in Cerrado, the colonial spider *Parawixia bistriata* and has many neuroactive molecules with different modes of action [96]. Parawixin-1 was the first isolated neurotoxin from *P. bistriata* venom. In experiments using rat retinas, submitted to ischemic insult, the intravitreal injection of Parawixin inhibited cell loss [97], probably through a potent and specific enhancing action on glutamate transporters type EAAT2 [98]. Another neurotoxin isolated from the venom of *P. bistriata,* Parawixin II, formerly, FrPbAII, inhibited GABA and glycine uptakes in synaptosomes from rat cerebral cortices. In addition, the administration of Parawixin II into the vitreous humor of Wistar rats protected retinal neurons against ischemic insult resulted from an increase in the intra ocular pressure [96]. Data also show that Parawixin II blocked seizures induced by the injection of GABAergic antagonists, bicuculline [99], pentylenetetrazole (PTZ) and picrotoxin, as well as pilocarpine and kainic acid [100]. It is worth noting that the acute injection of Parawixin II does not alter rat behavior in the open field and repeated central injection does not impair acquisition and learning in the Morris water maze. Finally, Parawixin II induces ataxia in the rotarod in doses far higher than effective doses, indicating good therapeutic indexes [100].

Also from South America, the Chilean giant pink tarantula *Grammostola spatulata* paralyzes its preys by injecting a mixture of toxins that blocks ion channels [101]. w-Grammotoxin SIA was isolated from the venom of *G. spatulata* and the potent blocking effect over N-, P-, and Q-type but not L-type of voltage gated calcium channels was reported [102]. The antagonistic activity of w-grammotoxin over voltage dependent calcium channels is considered a therapeutic option to be used in neurodegenerative disorders such as ischemia.

The African tarantula *Hysterocrates gigas* known as the giant baboon spider, inhabits the rain forests of West Africa. The isolation of the venom of *H. gigas,* resulted in the identification of the peptide SNX-482 that blocks R-type voltage dependent calcium channels [103].

The arboreal tarantula *Psalmopoeus cambridgei* is an aggressive spider that lives in the tropical forests of Trindad. As mentioned before, PcTx-1 (π-theraphotoxin-Pc1a) present in *P. cambridgei* venom is the only gating modifier of ASICs [50]. In addition to pain inhibitor, it exerts an interesting neuroprotective and a possible antidepressant activity due to the involvement of ASICs in cell excitability. A drop in pH from neutral 7.4 to more acid extracellular environments, lead to opening of ASICs Na^+ or Ca^{2+} permeable pore, membrane depolarization and increase in Ca^{2+} intracellular concentration [104].

In the light of these facts, Yang and coworkers [105] investigated the neuroprotective activity of PcTx in neurons from newborn piglets submitted to a model of asphyxia-induced cardiac arrest. Data show that the administration of PcTx before the hypoxia-ischemia insult partially prevents the death of neurons in putamen, the most vulnerable encephalic area in this model. The addition of MK-801, a NMDA antagonist, in combination with PcTx exerted better results in cell survival, but in low doses of MK-801. In addition to protection of neuronal cells, treatment with PcTx accelerated neurologic recovery. These results point PcTx as a very unique neurotoxin that should be used as tool in the investigation of processes underlying neuroprotection as well as the design of novel neuroprotective agents.

Bees and wasps are part of the group of the insects, whose stings release a cocktail of toxins, including enzymes, peptides and biogenic amines [106]. Toxins in bee venom have received attention for their properties as anti-inflammatory agents, and in many countries, physicians even prescribe bee stings as treatment of rheumatologic diseases. Recently, Doo and colleagues [107] showed that the bee venom when injected in rats with induced Parkinson disease prevent dopamine neurons cell death, possibly by the inhibition of Jun activation.

Regarding solitary wasps, the most studied wasp species is the European beewolf, *Philanthus triangulum,* the natural predators of honeybees. The adult individuals of this species are herbivores, whereas the larvae eat the paralyzed bees brought to the colony by foraging wasps. The isolation of venom contents begun in the early 80s and revealed that among other classes of molecules, *P. triangulum* venom contains potent acylpolyamines [86]. Philanthotoxins, like other acylpolyamines are mostly potent and selective antagonists of vertebrate and invertebrate glutamate receptors, particularly AMPA receptors [108]. The first isolated and most studied philathotoxin is PhTX-433 and its synthetic analogue, PhTx-343, which antagonize Ach and glutamate ionotropic receptors. The neuroprotective activity of PhTx-343 was tested in cerebellar granule cells culture challenged with NMDA and kainate toxicity and compared to that of Arg-636 [109]. Data showed that both polyamines protected cultures against damage, but Arg-636 was found to be less potent than PhTx-343 against kainate-induced damage. The structural change in PhTx-343 increased its potency, but in higher doses, toxic side effects, were observed.

Due to their lack of selectivity, the use of philanthotoxins as pharmaceuticals may have been limited, and so many modified synthetic analogues were designed for medical treatment purposes, so far [82]. However, the use of philanthotoxins and other polyamines as tools in research investigation has aided the understanding of several synaptic mechanisms. As it has been recently shown using Ca^{2+}-permeable AMPA receptors expressed in HEK cells. According to [110] the block of these AMPA receptors by PhTx-74, a synthetic analogue of PhTX-433 will reflect structural and biophysical parameters of the channel, such as its subunit composition and mean conductance, respectively. In addition, the investigation of the antagonistic activity of PhTx-343 over ACh receptors showed that the interaction of the toxin with nicotinic receptors is largely voltage dependent, slow and uncompetitive, a similar mode by which they block glutamate ionotropic channels [111].

Going further on wasp venoms, the anticonvulsant and/or neuroprotective effects of molecules in the venom of two Brazilian social species of the genus *Polybia,* were investigated. According to Cunha and co-workers [112] and Mortari and co-workers [113], the non-enzymatic fraction of the venoms of *Polybia ignobilis* and *Polybia occidentalis* inhibit seizures evoked by the injection of several chemoconvulsants in Wistar rats. The neuroactive molecules present in the venom of *P. ignobilis* and *P. occidentalis* are now in phase of structure-function investigation.

Finally, neurotoxins from scorpion venoms have been subject of a wide range of works, mostly approaching the identification of voltage-dependent ion channel activators/blockers. The neuroprotective and/or anticonvulsant activity of these peptides, in turn have received a few lines of investigation [3] despite the ancient use of these animals whole or parts, in the popular medicine in oriental countries, like China [20]. One of the most studied species is the Asian scorpion *Buthus martensi Karsch* whose venom has several neuroactive peptides, among whose, we may find BmK AEP, which was the first anticonvulsant peptide isolated from scorpion venoms. According to [28], the injection of BmK AEP blocked seizures induced by the injection of coriaria lactone in doses causing no visible side effects [114]. Further isolation of venom of *B. martensi* led to the identification of other peptides, such as BmK AS and BmK Ts and other mostly with analgesic activity. According to Zhao and co-workers [115] BmK AS, a sodium channel modulator at site-4 receptor, inhibited PTZ induced behavioral and electroencephalographic seizures and decreased mean score of pilocarpine-induced seizures. Moreover, these authors showed that BmK AS does not impair locomotion or motor behavior.

The venom of the Mexican scorpion *Centruroides limpidus limpidus,* was fractionated and many activators of voltage-gated ion channel ligands were identified [116]. An exception is Cll9, which stands for *Centruroides limpidus limpidus* toxin nr 9. Cll9 is a 63-residue peptide that has a divergent mode of action; it inhibits sodium channels in superior cervical ganglion neurons and [117]. When injected in Wistar rats via i.c.v., Cll9 inhibited behavioral and electroencephalographic seizures evoked by the microinjection of penicillin into the basolateral amygdala. It is worth noticing that Cll9 has no effect on arthropods such as crickets or crayfish like many sodium channels modulators found in scorpion venoms.

5. Actions on mood disorders

According to the World Health Organization, depression, one of the most important mood disorders, affects up to 5-10% of people worldwide at any time of their lives. Patients with a diagnosed mood disorder are more likely to be women, in productive years, 20 to 40 year-old, and will need in most cases, psychotherapy and/or pharmacological intervention. The costs of these psychiatric and/or psychological disorders are immense, since they affect people regardless of education or socioeconomic status, accounting in the worse cases, for a huge number of suicides. In the United States up to 95% of all suicides, involve mentally ill people, accounting for 1.3% of all deaths [118]. A recent survey shows that generalized anxiety disorder, posttraumatic stress disorder, social anxiety disorder and panic disorder are highly predictive of suicidal idealization [118]. Many aspects of the pathophysiology of mood disorders, as well as the regulation of normal mood states remain unknown. However, with the improvement of techniques for research and diagnosis, such as positron emission tomography, magnetic resonance and multiple channels recording electroencephalogram, soon researchers will be capable to identify structures and neurochemical mechanism involved in the regulation of mental states, including mood. So far, we know that limbic structures, such as the amygdala, hippocampus, hypothalamus and prefrontal cortex control the emotional aspects of brain function. There are plenty of connections among these structures, which might be involved in the onset of mood disorders [119].

Pharmacological treatment of mood disorders consists in daily intake of anti-depressants, anxiolytics or anti-psychotics, most of which cause a wide set of undesired side effects that impose restrictions to patients quality of life. In this regard novel drugs prescribed for mood disorder, such as serotonin uptake inhibitors might be better tolerated and safer than classical drugs, such as monoamine oxidase inhibitors. Among the observed undesired effects we can cite; dizziness, sedation, sexual dysfunction and suicidal though, a paradoxical effect of serotonin uptake inhibitors [119]. Aside from tolerability, medicines used as treatment of depression for example, take too long to produce effect in only a minority of patients; 35-45% of treated patients [120]. Therefore, there is a still great need for novel alternatives to be used both, in basic and clinical science.

The neurochemistry of mood disorders is complex and there is a list of candidates for targets of mood stabilizers, such as adrenaline, GABA, serotonin and glutamate receptors and transporters. There is not many works relating neurotoxins from arthropods and mood disorders, but the few works available showed that in some cases, these molecules might contribute for the development of novel drugs.

The venom of the Brazilian colonial spider *Parawixia bistriata* was fractionated and tested in many animal models of epilepsy, neurodegeneration and anxiety. According to [121], the microinjection of Parawixin 2 (formerly FrPbAII) in the dorsal hippocampus of male Wistar rats increased the time spent in the open arms of the elevated plus maze. Moreover, rats exposed to the light-dark choice apparatus spent more time in the light side of the box, similarly to what observed for diazepam or nipecotic acid, a GABA transporter-1 (GAT-1) inhibitor [121]. In another investigation of *P. bistriata* venom contents, Saidemberg and co-workers

[122] isolated PwTx-I and tested the inhibitory activity of this neurotoxin and its enantiomers on mammalian monoamine oxidases (MAO)-A and -B. According to these authors, PwTx-I, acted as non-competitive inhibitors of MAO-A and MAO-B. MAO metabolizes monoamines dopamine, serotonin and adrenaline, terminating monoaminergic transmission. Inhibitors or MAO (MAOi) have been extensively used as mood stabilizers and currently they have received attention due to their protective activity against age-induced neurodegenerative disorders [123].

Considering alternative targets for mood stabilizers, interesting results were obtained with PcTx, isolated from the venom of the spider *P. cambridgei,* a selective blocker of ASICs. Data showed that both PcTx and amiloride attenuated the stress-induced hyperthermia, whereas only the administration of PcTx increased number of punished crosses measured in the four-plate test. These results indicate that both blockers could attenuate autonomic anxiety parameters, but only PcTx exerted effects on the behavioral anxiety parameters [124].

The aggressive Brazilian social wasp *Agelaia vicina,* builds huge nests where with over a million of individuals. The neurobiological activity of the venom of *A. vicina,* was investigated. Oliveira and colleagues [125] showed that the central injection of the non-enzymatic fraction of the venom induced catalepsy in Wistar compared to the neuroleptic drug haloperidol, a nonselective D2 dopamine antagonist. This effect was reversed by the injection of theophylline or ketamine. The fractionation of the venom led to the identification of two peptides, AvTx-7, mastoparan, and AvTx-8. The investigation of AvTx-8 mode of action in vivo, was performed in a model of panic induction through the activation of GABAergic pathways connecting mesencephalic substantia nigra pars reticulate to superior colliculus [126]. These experiments showed that intranigral microinjection of AvTx-8 inhibited the panic like response induced by the GABAergic blockade of superior colliculus. These effects were similar to those of baclofen, a $GABA_B$ agonist, but differed from the effects of muscimol, a $GABA_A$ agonist. Since post-synaptic $GABA_B$ is a metabotropic receptor complex with a potassium channel, AvTx-8 could act in many different sites that would end in channels opening and hyperpolarization of neuronal membrane.

6. Tools for the study of the functioning of the CNS: learning and memory

Neurotoxins isolated from arthropod are important tools to study of the normal function of the CNS, especially in the structure-function research of the ion channels and the interaction the blockers and modulators in the regulation of the learning and memory (for revision see [127]). In this context, the principal compound used in study of the mechanism of the learning and memory in models of experimental animals is the apamin. Apamin is a short peptide (18 aa) isolated from the venom of honeybee, *Apis mellifera*. It is generally accepted that apamin selectively blocks small conductance calcium-activated potassium channels (SK or K_{ca}), although evidences point to an allosteric modulation of opening rather than the block of the pore [128]. Upon an increase in intracellular calcium, SK channels will open and allow an outward current of potassium ions that is responsible for the hyperpolarization phase of the action potentials. Most studies on structure-function of SK channels were conducted using apamin blockade. The homomeric or heteromeric expression of these channels occurs in higher brain areas such as the neocortex, hippocampus and sub-cortical areas such as thalamus and basal ganglia as well as in cerebellum and brainstem. Substantial data SK channels show the involvement of SK channels in processes of learning and memory, and apamin blockade of SK lead to an increase in cellular excitability, facilitates synaptic plasticity and memory processes run by the hippocampus. In addition, apamin induces alterations in dendritic morphology that might counteract aging and neurodegenerative processes that lead to cognitive and memory impairment [129]. In fact, SK channels co-localize with Ca^{2+}-permeable NMDA receptors in the CA1 region of the hippocampus and the entry of calcium in the cell through these receptors might activate SK that will hyperpolarize membrane. The blockade of SK channels will modulate hippocampal excitability that is essential in memory processes such as long-term potentiation a commonly observed event of synaptic plasticity. Due to its actions, the use of apamin as a tool in research has been consolidated. In addition, the therapeutic use of apamin, in order to maintain hippocampal function and avoid the deleterious effects of aging in memory and cognitive processes have also been proposed [129].

Besides apamin, modulators peptides of the potassium channel isolated from scorpion also have been tested in models of the learning and memory. The good examples are: Charybdotoxin isolated from scorpion *Leiurus quinquestriatus*, Kaliotoxin isolated from *Androctonus mauretanicus* and Iberiotoxin from *Buthus tasmulus*. Charybdotoxin is a potent selective inhibitor of high (large or big) conductance Ca^{2+}-activated potassium channels (KCa1.1, BK, or maxi-K), as well as a Kv1.3 channel [130]. Kaliotoxin is a specific inhibitor of Kv1.1 and Kv1.3 [131] and Iberiotoxin is a selective inhibitor of KCa1.1 channels (formerly BK) [132]. These peptides induced an improvement effect in passive avoidance test and olfactory discrimination task [133,134].

7. Final remarks

The stories of voltage-gated, ligand-gated ion channels and venom toxins are very closely tied. Indeed, the isolation and structural characterization of venom molecules provided a plethora of tools that have been used in the investigation of ion channels structure-function relationships. With the aid of arthropod toxins, remarkably, scorpionic toxins, the characterization of sodium channels was possible. Spider and wasps polyamines, in turn are considered unique ligands of glutamatergic and cholinergic ionotropic receptors. Regarding to peptides and small proteins, arthropod venoms possess an arsenal of these molecules that remain largely unknown and consequently, their pharmacological potential is left unexplored.

Due to the mode of action of neurotoxins, their affinity and selectivity for neuronal structures, many researchers consider them as probes to novel drugs design and development. However, despite of the thousands of patents made with neurotoxins in the past 30 years, very few molecules came to commercialization.

Acknowledgements

The authors thank Msc Juliana Castro e Silva for help in preparing the figure.

Author details

Márcia Renata Mortari[1*] and Alexandra Olimpio Siqueira Cunha[2]

*Address all correspondence to: mmortari@unb.br

1 Department of Physiological Sciences, Institute of Biological Sciences, University of Brasília, Brazil

2 Department of Physiology, FMRP, University of São Paulo, Brazil

References

[1] Zhijian, C., Chao, D., Dahe, J., & Wenxin, L. (2006). The effect of intron location on the splicing of BmKK2 in 293T cells. *J Biochem Mol Toxicol*, 20(3), 127-32.

[2] Estrada, G., Villegas, E., & Corzo, G. (2007). Spider venoms: a rich source of acylpolyamines and peptides as new leads for CNS drugs. *Nat Prod Rep*, 24(1), 145-61.

[3] Mortari, M. R., Cunha, A. O., Ferreira, L. B., & dos, Santos. W. F. (2007). Neurotoxins from invertebrates as anticonvulsants: from basic research to therapeutic application. *Pharmacol Ther.*, 114(2), 171-83.

[4] Rogoza, L. N., Salakhutdinov, N. F., & Tolstikov, G. A. (2005). Polymethyleneamine alkaloids of animal origin. I. Metabolites of marine and microbial organisms]. *Bioorg Khim*, 31(6), 563-77.

[5] WHO. (2007). Neurological Disorders:. *Public Health Challenges.*

[6] Bialer, M., & White, H. S. (2010). Key factors in the discovery and development of new antiepileptic drugs. *Nature reviews Drug discovery*, 9(1), 68-82.

[7] Blier, P. (2010). The well of novel antidepressants: running dry. *J Psychiatry Neurosci*, 35(4), 219-20.

[8] Goudet, C., Chi, C. W., & Tytgat, J. (2002). An overview of toxins and genes from the venom of the Asian scorpion Buthus martensi Karsch. *Toxicon official journal of the International Society on Toxinology*, 40(9), 1239-58.

[9] Cherniack, E. P. (2011). Bugs as drugs, part two: worms, leeches, scorpions, snails, ticks, centipedes, and spiders. *Alternative medicine review : a journal of clinical therapeutic*, 16(1), 50-8.

[10] Ratcliffe, N. A., Mello, C. B., Garcia, E. S., Butt, T. M., & Azambuja, P. (2011). Insect natural products and processes: new treatments for human disease. *Insect Biochem Mol Biol*, 41(10), 747-69.

[11] Monteiro, M. C., Romao, P. R., & Soares, A. M. (2009). Pharmacological perspectives of wasp venom. *Protein and peptide letters*, 16(8), 944-52.

[12] Beleboni, R. D., Pizzo, A. B., Fontana, A. C. K., Carolino, R. D. O. G., Coutinho-Netto, J., & dos, Santos. W. F. (2004). Spider and wasp neurotoxins: pharmacological and biochemical aspects. *Eur J Pharmacol*, 493(1-3), 1-17.

[13] Ashburn, M. A., & Staats, P. S. (1999). Management of chronic pain. *Lancet*, 353(167), 865-869.

[14] Stucky, C. L., Gold, M. S., & Zhang, X. (2001). Mechanisms of pain. *Proc Natl Acad Sci U S A.*, 98(21), 11845-6.

[15] Sindrup, S. H., & Jensen, T. S. (1999). Efficacy of pharmacological treatments of neuropathic pain: an update and effect related to mechanism of drug action. *Pain*, 83(3), 389-400.

[16] Villetti, G., Bergamaschi, M., Bassani, F., Bolzoni, P. T., Maiorino, M., Pietra, C., et al. (2003). Antinociceptive activity of the N-methyl-D-aspartate receptor antagonist N-(2-Indanyl)-glycinamide hydrochloride (CHF3381) in experimental models of inflammatory and neuropathic pain. *J Pharmacol Exp Ther*, 306(2), 804-14.

[17] Ji, Y. H., Mansuelle, P., Terakawa, S., Kopeyan, C., Yanaihara, N., Hsu, K., et al. (1996). Two neurotoxins (BmK I and BmK II) from the venom of the scorpion Buthus martensi Karsch: purification, amino acid sequences and assessment of specific activity. *Toxicon : official journal of the International Society on Toxinology*, 34(9), 987-1001.

[18] Guan, R., Wang, C. G., Wang, M., & Wang, D. C. (2001). A depressant insect toxin with a novel analgesic effect from scorpion Buthus martensii Karsch. *Biochim Biophys Acta*, 1549(1), 9-18.

[19] Rodriguez dela Vega, R. C., & Possani, L. D. (2005). Overview of scorpion toxins specific for channels and related peptides: biodiversity, structure-function relationships and evolution. *Toxicon : official journal of the International Society on Toxinology*, 46(8), 831-44.

[20] Xiong, Y. M., Lan, Z. D., Wang, M., Liu, B., Liu, X. Q., Fei, H., et al. (1999). Molecular characterization of a new excitatory insect neurotoxin with an analgesic effect on mice from the scorpion Buthus martensi Karsch. *Toxicon*, 37(8), 1165-80.

[21] Escoubas, P., Stankiewicz, M., Takaoka, T., Pelhate, M., Romi-Lebrun, R., Wu, F. Q., et al. (2000). Sequence and electrophysiological characterization of two insect-selec-

tive excitatory toxins from the venom of the Chinese scorpion Buthus martensi. *FEBS Lett*, 483(2-3), 175 -80 .

[22] Guan, R. J., Wang, M., Wang, D., & Wang, D. C. (2001). A new insect neurotoxin AngP1 with analgesic effect from the scorpion Buthus martensii Karsch: purification and characterization. *The journal of peptide research official journal of the American Peptide Society*, 58(1), 27-35.

[23] Wang, C. Y., Tan, Z. Y., Chen, B., Zhao, Z. Q., & Ji, Y. H. (2000). Antihyperalgesia effect of BmK IT2, a depressant insect-selective scorpion toxin in rat by peripheral administration. *Brain research bulletin*, 53(3), 335-8.

[24] Tan, Z. Y., Xiao, H., Mao, X., Wang, C. Y., Zhao, Z. Q., & Ji, Y. H. (2001). The inhibitory effects of BmK IT2, a scorpion neurotoxin on rat nociceptive flexion reflex and a possible mechanism for modulating voltage-gated Na(+) channels. *Neuropharmacology*, 40(3), 352-7.

[25] Bai, Z. T., Liu, T., Pang, X. Y., Chai, Z. F., & Ji, Y. H. (2007). Suppression by intrathecal BmK IT2 on rat spontaneous pain behaviors and spinal c-Fos expression induced by formalin. *Brain Res Bull*, 73(4-6), 248 -253 .

[26] Zhang, X. Y., Bai, Z. T., Chai, Z. F., Zhang, J. W., Liu, Y., & Ji, Y. H. (2003). Suppressive effects of BmK IT2 on nociceptive behavior and c-Fos expression in spinal cord induced by formalin. *J Neurosci Res*, 74(1), 167-73.

[27] Li, Y. J., Tan, Z. Y., & Ji, Y. H. (2000). The binding of BmK IT2, a depressant insect-selective scorpion toxin on mammal and insect sodium channels. *Neurosci Res*, 38(3), 257-64.

[28] Wang, Y., Wang, L., Cui, Y., Song, Y. B., Liu, Y. F., Zhang, R., et al. (2011). Purification, characterization and functional expression of a new peptide with an analgesic effect from Chinese scorpion Buthus martensii Karsch (BmK AGP-SYPU1). *Biomed Chromatogr*, 25(7), 801-7.

[29] Ji-H, Y., Li-J, Y., Zhang-W, J., Song-L, B., Yamaki, T., Mochizuki, T., et al. (1999). Covalent structures of BmK AS and BmK AS-1, two novel bioactive polypeptides purified from Chinese scorpion Buthus martensi Karsch. *Toxicon*, 37(3), 519-36.

[30] Lan-D, Z., Dai, L., Zhuo-L, X., Feng-C, J., Xu, K., & Chi-W, C. (1999). Gene cloning and sequencing of BmK AS and BmK AS-1, two novel neurotoxins from the scorpion Buthus martensi Karsch. *Toxicon*, 37(5), 815-23.

[31] Chen, B., & Ji, Y. (2002). Antihyperalgesia effect of BmK AS, a scorpion toxin, in rat by intraplantar injection. *Brain Res*, 952(2), 2322-6.

[32] Chen, J., Feng, X. H., Shi, J., Tan, Z. Y., Bai, Z. T., Liu, T., et al. (2006). The anti-nociceptive effect of BmK AS, a scorpion active polypeptide, and the possible mechanism on specifically modulating voltage-gated Na+ currents in primary afferent neurons. *Peptides*, 27(9), 182-92.

[33] Tan, Z. Y., Mao, X., Xiao, H., Zhao, Z. Q., & Ji, Y. H. (2001). Buthus martensi Karsch agonist of skeletal-muscle RyR-1, a scorpion active polypeptide: antinociceptive effect on rat peripheral nervous system and spinal cord, and inhibition of voltage-gated Na(+) currents in dorsal root ganglion neurons. *Neurosci Lett*, 297(2), 65-8.

[34] Wu, Y., Ji, Y. H., & Shi, Y. L. (2001). Sodium current in NG108-15 cell inhibited by scorpion toxin BmKAS-1 and restored by its specific monoclonal antibodies. *J Nat Toxins*, 10(3), 193-8.

[35] Liu, Y. F., Ma, R. L., Wang, S. L., Duan, Z. Y., Zhang, J. H., Wu, L. J., et al. (2003). Expression of an antitumor-analgesic peptide from the venom of Chinese scorpion Buthus martensii karsch in Escherichia coli. *Protein Expr Purif*, 27(2), 253-8.

[36] Cui, Y., Guo, G. L., Ma, L., Hu, N., Song, Y. B., Liu, Y. F., et al. (2010). Structure and function relationship of toxin from Chinese scorpion Buthus martensii Karsch (BmKAGAP): gaining insight into related sites of analgesic activity. *Peptides*, 31(6), 995-1000.

[37] Cao, Z. Y., Mi, Z. M., Cheng, G. F., Shen, W. Q., Xiao, X., Liu, X. M., et al. (2004). Purification and characterization of a new peptide with analgesic effect from the scorpion Buthus martensi Karch. *J Pept Res*, 64(1), 33-41.

[38] Peng, K., Chen, X. D., & Liang, S. P. (2001). The effect of Huwentoxin-I on Ca(2+) channels in differentiated NG108-15 cells, a patch-clamp study. *Toxicon : official journal of the International Society on Toxinology*, 39(4), 491-8.

[39] Chen, J. Q., Zhang, Y. Q., Dai, J., Luo, Z. M., & Liang, S. P. (2005). Antinociceptive effects of intrathecally administered huwentoxin-I, a selective N-type calcium channel blocker, in the formalin test in conscious rats. *Toxicon : official journal of the International Society on Toxinology*, 45(1), 15-20.

[40] Wen, Tao. Z., Gu, Yang. T., Ying, R., Mao, Cai. W., Lin, L., Chi, Miao. L., et al. (2011). The antinociceptive efficacy of HWTX-I epidurally administered in rheumatoid arthritis rats. *Int J Sports Med*, 32(11), 869-74.

[41] Saez, N. J., Senff, S., Jensen, J. E., Er, S. Y., Herzig, V., Rash, L. D., et al. (2010). Spider-venom peptides as therapeutics. *Toxins*, 2(12), 2851-71.

[42] Murakami, M., Nakagawasai, O., Suzuki, T., Mobarakeh, I. I., Sakurada, Y., Murata, A., et al. (2004). Antinociceptive effect of different types of calcium channel inhibitors and the distribution of various calcium channel alpha 1 subunits in the dorsal horn of spinal cord in mice. *Brain Res*, 1024(1-2), 122 -9.

[43] Rajendra, W., Armugam, A., & Jeyaseelan, K. (2004). Toxins in anti-nociception and anti-inflammation. *Toxiconofficial journal of the International Society on Toxinology*, 44(1), 1-17.

[44] Souza, A. H., Ferreira, J., Cordeiro, Mdo. N., Vieira, L. B., De Castro, C. J., Trevisan, G., et al. (2008). Analgesic effect in rodents of native and recombinant Ph alpha 1beta

toxin, a high-voltage-activated calcium channel blocker isolated from armed spider venom. *Pain*, 140(1), 115-26.

[45] Dalmolin, G. D., Silva, C. R., Rigo, F. K., Gomes, G. M., Cordeiro, Mdo. N., Richardson, M., et al. (2011). Antinociceptive effect of Brazilian armed spider venom toxin Tx3-3 in animal models of neuropathic pain. *Pain*, 152(10), 2224-32.

[46] Vieira, L. B., Kushmerick, C., Hildebrand, M. E., Garcia, E., Stea, A., Cordeiro, M. N., et al. (2005). Inhibition of high voltage-activated calcium channels by spider toxin PnTx3-6. *J Pharmacol Exp Ther*, 314(3), 1370-7.

[47] Prado, MA, Guatimosim, C., Gomez, M. V., Diniz, C. R., Cordeiro, M. N., & Romano-Silva, MA. (1996). A novel tool for the investigation of glutamate release from rat cerebrocortical synaptosomes: the toxin Tx from the venom of the spider Phoneutria nigriventer. *Biochem J*, 314(Pt1), 145-50.

[48] De Souza, A. H., Lima, M. C., Drewes, C. C., da, Silva. J. F., Torres, K. C., Pereira, E. M., et al. (2011). Antiallodynic effect and side effects of Phalpha1beta, a neurotoxin from the spider Phoneutria nigriventer: comparison with omega-conotoxin MVIIA and morphine. *Toxicon : official journal of the International Society on Toxinology*, 58(8), 626-33.

[49] Malmberg, A. B., & Yaksh, T. L. (1994). Voltage-sensitive calcium channels in spinal nociceptive processing: blockade of N- and P-type channels inhibits formalin-induced nociception. *J Neurosci*, 14(8), 4882-90.

[50] Saez, N. J., Mobli, M., Bieri, M., Chassagnon, I. R., Malde, A. K., Gamsjaeger, R., et al. (2011). A dynamic pharmacophore drives the interaction between Psalmotoxin-1 and the putative drug target acid-sensing ion channel 1a. Mol Pharmacol Epub 2011/08/10., 80(5), 796-808.

[51] Mc Cleskey, E. W., & Gold, M. S. (1999). Ion channels of nociception. *Annu Rev Physiol*, 61, 835-56.

[52] Waldmann, R., Champigny, G., Lingueglia, E., De Weille, J. R., Heurteaux, C., & Lazdunski, M. (1999). H(+)-gated cation channels. *Ann N Y Acad Sci*, 868, 67-76.

[53] Mazzuca, M., Heurteaux, C., Alloui, A., Diochot, S., Baron, A., Voilley, N., et al. (2007). A tarantula peptide against pain via ASIC1a channels and opioid mechanisms. *Nat Neurosci*, 10(8), 943-5.

[54] Pignataro, G., Simon, R. P., & Xiong, Z. G. (2007). Prolonged activation of ASIC1a and the time window for neuroprotection in cerebral ischaemia. *Braina journal of neurology*, 130(Pt 1), 151 -158 .

[55] Lampe, R. A. (1999). Analgesic peptides from venom of grammostola spatulata and use thereof. http://www.patentgenius.com/patent/5776896.html.

[56] Grishin, E. V., Savchenko, G. A., Vassilevski, A. A., Korolkova, Y. V., Boychuk, Y. A., Viatchenko-Karpinski, V. Y., et al. (2010). Novel peptide from spider venom inhibits 2X3receptors and inflammatory pain. *Ann Neurol*, 67(5), 680-3.

[57] Chen, J., & Lariviere, W. R. (2010). The nociceptive and anti-nociceptive effects of bee venom injection and therapy: a double-edged sword. *Prog Neurobiol*, 92(2), 151-83.

[58] Kwon, Y. B., Kang, M. S., Kim, H. W., Ham, T. W., Yim, Y. K., Jeong, S. H., et al. (2001). Antinociceptive effects of bee venom acupuncture (apipuncture) in rodent animal models: a comparative study of acupoint versus non-acupoint stimulation. *Acupunct Electrother Res*, 26(1-2), 59-68.

[59] Kwon, Y. B., Kim, J. H., Yoon, J. H., Lee, JD, Han, H. J., Mar, W. C., et al. (2001). The analgesic efficacy of bee venom acupuncture for knee osteoarthritis: a comparative study with needle acupuncture. *Am J Chin Med*, 29(2), 187-99.

[60] Lee-H, J., Kwon-B, Y., Han-J, H., Mar-C, W., Lee-J, H., Yang-S, I., et al. (2001). Bee Venom Pretreatment Has Both an Antinociceptive and Anti-Inflammatory Effect on Carrageenan-Induced Inflammation. *J Vet Med Sci*, 63(3), 251-9.

[61] Lee, J. D., Park, H. J., Chae, Y., & Lim, S. (2005). An Overview of Bee Venom Acupuncture in the Treatment of Arthritis. *Evidence-based complementary and alternative medicine : eCAM*, 2(1), 79-84.

[62] Kwon, Y. B., Kang, M. S., Han, H. J., Beitz, A. J., & Lee, J. H. (2001). Visceral antinociception produced by bee venom stimulation of the Zhongwan acupuncture point in mice: role of alpha(2) adrenoceptors. *Neurosci Lett*, 308(2), 133-7.

[63] Baek, Y. H., Huh, J. E., Lee, J. D., Choi do, Y., & Park, D. S. (2006). Antinociceptive effect and the mechanism of bee venom acupuncture (Apipuncture) on inflammatory pain in the rat model of collagen-induced arthritis: Mediation by alpha2-Adrenoceptors. *Brain Res*, 073-074, 305-10.

[64] Son, D. J., Kang, J., Kim, T. J., Song, H. S., Sung, K. J., Yun, Y., et al. (2007). Melittin, a major bioactive component of bee venom toxin, inhibits PDGF receptor beta-tyrosine phosphorylation and downstream intracellular signal transduction in rat aortic vascular smooth muscle cells. *Journal of toxicology and environmental health Part A*, 70(15-16), 1350 -5 .

[65] Lauterwein, J., Bosch, C., Brown, L. R., & Wuthrich, K. (1979). Physicochemical studies of the protein-lipid interactions in melittin-containing micelles. *Biochim Biophys Acta*, 556(2), 244-64.

[66] Lavialle, F., Levin, I. W., & Mollay, C. (1980). Interaction of melittin with dimyristoyl phosphatidylcholine liposomes: evidence for boundary lipid by Raman spectroscopy. *Biochim Biophys Acta*, 600(1), 62-71.

[67] Shier WT. (1979). Activation of high levels of endogenous phospholipase A2 in cultured cells. *Proc Natl Acad Sci U S A*, 76(1), 195-9.

[68] Lad, P. J., & Shier, W. T. (1979). Activation of microsomal guanylate cyclase by a cytotoxic polypeptide: melittin. *Biochem Biophys Res Commun*, 89(1), 315-21.

[69] Park, H. J., Lee, H. J., Choi, M. S., Son, D. J., Song, H. S., Song, M. J., et al. (2008). JNK pathway is involved in the inhibition of inflammatory target gene expression and NF-kappaB activation by melittin. *J Inflamm (Lond).*, 5, 7.

[70] Merlo, L. A., Bastos, L. F., Godin, A. M., Rocha, L. T., Nascimento, E. B. Jr, Paiva, A. L., et al. (2011). Effects induced by Apis mellifera venom and its components in experimental models of nociceptive and inflammatory pain. *Toxicon : official journal of the International Society on Toxinology*, 57(5), 764-71.

[71] Shkenderov, S., & Koburova, K. (1982). Adolapin- A newly isolated analgetic and anti-inflammatory polypeptide from bee venom. *Toxicon*, 20(1), 317-21.

[72] Koburova, K. L. S. G., & Michailova, S. V. (1985). Shkenderov Further investigation on the antiinflammatory properties of adolapin--bee venom polypeptide. *Acta Physiol Pharmacol Bulg*, 11(2), 50-5.

[73] Mortari, M. R., Cunha, A. O., Carolino, R. O., Coutinho-Netto, J., Tomaz, J. C., Lopes, N. P., et al. (2007). Inhibition of acute nociceptive responses in rats after i.c.v. injection of Thr6-bradykinin, isolated from the venom of the social wasp, Polybia occidentalis. *Br J Pharmacol*, 151(6), 860-9.

[74] Pellegrini, M., Mammi, S., Peggion, E., & Mierke, D. F. (1997). Threonine6-bradykinin: structural characterization in the presence of micelles by nuclear magnetic resonance and distance geometry. *J Med Chem*, 40(1), 92-8.

[75] Pellegrini, M., & Mierke, D. F. (1997). Threonine6-bradykinin: molecular dynamics simulations in a biphasic membrane mimetic. *J Med Chem*, 40(1), 99-104.

[76] Nagy, I., Paule, C., White, J., & Urban, L. (2007). Taking the sting out of pain. *Br J Pharmacol*, 151(6), 721-2.

[77] Kawai, N., Shimazaki, K., Sahara, Y., Robinson, H. P., & Nakajima, T. (1991). Spider toxin and the glutamate receptors. *Comp Biochem Physiol C*, 98(1), 87-95.

[78] Sorkin, L. S. Y. T., & Doom, C. M. (1999). Mechanical allodynia in rats is blocked by a Ca2+ permeable AMPA receptor antagonist. *Neuroreport*, 10(17), 3523-6.

[79] Stanfa, L. C., Hampton, D. W., & Dickenson, A. H. (2000). Role of Ca2+-permeable non-NMDA glutamate receptors in spinal nociceptive transmission. Neuroreport Epub 2000/10/24., 11(14), 3199-202.

[80] Jones, M. G., & Lodge, D. (1991). Comparison of some arthropod toxins and toxin fragments as antagonists of excitatory amino acid-induced excitation of rat spinal neurones. *Eur J Pharmacol*, 204(2), 203-9.

[81] Sorkin, L. S., Yaksh, T. L., & Doom, C. M. (2001). Pain models display differential sensitivity to Ca2+-permeable non-NMDA glutamate receptor antagonists. *Anesthesiology*, 95(4), 965-73.

[82] Andersen, T. F., Vogensen, S. B., Jensen, L. S., Knapp, K. M., & Stromgaard, K. (2005). Design and synthesis of labeled analogs of PhTX-56, a potent and selective AMPA receptor antagonist. *Bioorg Med Chem*, 13(17), 5104-12.

[83] Dingledine, R., Borges, K., Bowie, D., & Traynelis, S. F. (1999). The glutamate receptor ion channels. *Pharmacol Rev*, 51(1), 7-61.

[84] Rajendra, W., Armugam, A., & Jeyaseelan, K. (2004). Neuroprotection and peptide toxins. *Brain Res Brain Res Rev*, 45(2), 125-41.

[85] Grishin, E. V., Volkova, T. M., & Arseniev, A. S. (1989). Isolation and structure analysis of components from venom of the spider Argiope lobata. *Toxicon*, 27(5), 541-9.

[86] Clark, R. B., Donaldson, P. L., Gration, K. A., Lambert, J. J., Piek, T., Ramsey, R., et al. (1982). Block of locust muscle glutamate receptors by delta-philanthotoxin occurs after receptor activations. *Brain Res*, 241(1), 105-14.

[87] Usherwood, P. N., & Blagbrough, I. S. (1991). Spider toxins affecting glutamate receptors: polyamines in therapeutic neurochemistry. Pharmacol Ther Epub 1991/11/01., 52(2), 245-68.

[88] Herold, E. E., & Yaksh, T. L. (1992). Anesthesia and muscle relaxation with intrathecal injections of AR636 and AG489, two acylpolyamine spider toxins, in rat. *Anesthesiology*, 77(3), 507-12.

[89] Kanai, H., Ishida, N., Nakajima, T., & Kato, N. (1992). An analogue of Joro spider toxin selectively suppresses hippocampal epileptic discharges induced by quisqualate. *Brain Res*, 581(1), 161-4.

[90] Roy, J., Minotti, S., Dong, L., Figlewicz, D. A., & Durham, H. D. (1998). Glutamate potentiates the toxicity of mutant Cu/Zn-superoxide dismutase in motor neurons by postsynaptic calcium-dependent mechanisms. *J Neurosci*, 18(23), 9673-84.

[91] Seymour, P. A. M. E. (1989). In vivo antagonist activity of the polyamine spider venom component, Argiotoxin-636. *Soc Neurosci Abs*, 15, 463-24.

[92] K, W. (1993). Effects of Agelenopsis aperta toxins on the N-methyl-D-aspartate receptor: polyamine-like and high-affinity antagonist actions. *J Pharmacol Exp Ther*, 266(1), 231-6.

[93] Miranda, D. M., Romano-Silva, M. A., Kalapothakis, E., Diniz, C. R., Cordeiro, M. N., Moraes-Santos, T., et al. (2001). Spider neurotoxins block the beta scorpion toxin-induced calcium uptake in rat brain cortical synaptosomes. *Brain Res Bull*, 54(5), 533-6.

[94] Pinheiro, A. C., da Silva, A. J., Prado Cordeiro, MA, Mdo, N., Richardson, M., Batista, M. C., et al. (2009). Phoneutria spider toxins block ischemia-induced glutamate release, neuronal death, and loss of neurotransmission in hippocampus. *Hippocampus*, 19(11), 1123-9.

[95] Agostini, R. M., Nascimento do Pinheiro, A. C., Binda, N. S., Romano, Silva., Nascimento do, Cordeiro. M., Richardson, M., et al. (2011). Phoneutria spider toxins block

ischemia-induced glutamate release and neuronal death of cell layers of the retina. *Retina*, 31(7), 1392-9.

[96] Beleboni, R. O., Guizzo, R., Fontana, A. C., Pizzo, A. B., Carolino, R. O., Gobbo-Neto, L., et al. (2006). Neurochemical characterization of a neuroprotective compound from Parawixia bistriata spider venom that inhibits synaptosomal uptake of GABA and glycine. *Mol Pharmacol*, 69(6), 1998-2006.

[97] Fontana, A. C., Guizzo, R., de Oliveira, Beleboni. R., Meirelles, E. S. A. R., Coimbra, N. C., Amara, S. G., et al. (2003). Purification of a neuroprotective component of Parawixia bistriata spider venom that enhances glutamate uptake. *Br J Pharmacol*, 139(7), 1297-309.

[98] Fontana, A. C., de Oliveira, Beleboni. R., Wojewodzic, M. W., Ferreira, Dos., Santos, W., Coutinho-Netto, J., Grutle, N. J., et al. (2007). Enhancing glutamate transport: mechanism of action of Parawixin1, a neuroprotective compound from Parawixia bistriata spider venom. *Mol Pharmacol*, 72(5), 1228-37.

[99] Cairrão, M. A. R. R. A., Pizzo, A. B., Fontana, A. C. K., Beleboni, R. O., Coutinho-Neto, J., Miranda, A., & Santos, W. F. (2002). Anticonvulsant and GABA uptake inhibition properties of P. bistriata and S. raptoria spider venom fractions. *Pharm Biol*, 40(6), 472-7.

[100] Gelfuso, E. A., Cunha, A. O., Mortari, M. R., Liberato, J. L., Paraventi, K. H., Beleboni, R. O., et al. (2007). Neuropharmacological profile of FrPbAII, purified from the venom of the social spider Parawixia bistriata (Araneae, Araneidae), in Wistar rats. *Life Sci*, 80(6), 566-72.

[101] Lampe, R. A., Defeo, P. A., Davison, Young. J., Herman, J. L., Spreen, R. C., et al. (1993). Isolation and pharmacological characterization of omega-grammotoxin SIA, a novel peptide inhibitor of neuronal voltage-sensitive calcium channel responses. *Mol Pharmacol*, 44(2), 451-60.

[102] Piser, T. M., Lampe, R. A., Keith, R. A., & Thayer, S. A. (1995). Complete and reversible block by ω-grammotoxin SIA of glutamatergic synaptic transmission between cultured rat hippocampal neurons. *Neurosci Lett*, 201(2), 135-8.

[103] Newcomb, R. P. A., Szoke, B. G., Tarczy-Hornoch, K., Hopkins, W. F., Cong, R. L., Miljanich, G. P., Dean, R., Nadasdi, L., Urge, L., & Bowersox, S. S. (2005). inventor; Elan Pharmaceuticals Inc US, assignee. Class e voltage-gated calcium channel antagonist and methods patent 0920504

[104] Chu, X. P., Papasian, C. J., Wang, . J. Q., & Xiong, Z. G. (2011). Modulation of acid-sensing ion channels: molecular mechanisms and therapeutic potential. *International journal of physiology, pathophysiology and pharmacology*, 3(4), 288-309.

[105] Yang, Z. J., Ni, X., Carter, E. L., Kibler, K., Martin, L. J., & Koehler, R. C. (2011). Neuroprotective effect of acid-sensing ion channel inhibitor psalmotoxin-1 after hypoxia-ischemia in newborn piglet striatum. *Neurobiol Dis*, 43(2), 446-54.

[106] Libersat, F. (2003). Wasp uses venom cocktail to manipulate the behavior of its cockroach prey. *Journal of comparative physiology A, Neuroethology, sensory, neural, and behavioral physiology*, 189(7), 497-508.

[107] Doo, A. R., Kim, S. T., Kim, S. N., Moon, W., Yin, C. S., Chae, Y., et al. (2010). Neuroprotective effects of bee venom pharmaceutical acupuncture in acute 1-methyl-4-phenyl-1,2,3,6-tetrahydropyridine-induced mouse model of Parkinson's disease. *Neurol Res*, 32(1), 88-91.

[108] Stromgaard, K. (2005). Natural products as tools for studies of ligand-gated ion channels. *Chem Rec*, 5(4), 229-39.

[109] Green, A. C., Nakanishi, K., & Usherwood, P. N. (1996). Polyamine amides are neuroprotective in cerebellar granule cell cultures challenged with excitatory amino acids. *Brain Res*, 717(1-2), 135 -46 .

[110] Jackson, A. C., Milstein, A. D., Soto, D., Farrant, M., Cull-Candy, S. G., & Nicoll, R. A. (2011). Probing TARP modulation of AMPA receptor conductance with polyamine toxins. *J Neurosci*, 31(20), 7511-20.

[111] Brier, T. J., Mellor, I. R., Tikhonov, D. B., Neagoe, I., Shao, Z., Brierley, MJ, et al. (2003). Contrasting actions of philanthotoxin-343 and philanthotoxin-(12) on human muscle nicotinic acetylcholine receptors. *Mol Pharmacol*, 64(4), 954-64.

[112] Cunha, A. O., Mortari, M. R., Oliveira, L., Carolino, R. O., Coutinho-Netto, J., & dos Santos, W. F. (2005). Anticonvulsant effects of the wasp Polybia ignobilis venom on chemically induced seizures and action on GABA and glutamate receptors. *Comparative biochemistry and physiology Toxicology & pharmacology : CBP*, 141(1), 50-7.

[113] Mortari, M. R., Cunha, A. O., de Oliveira, L., Vieira, E. B., Gelfuso, E. A., Coutinho-Netto, J., et al. (2005). Anticonvulsant and behavioural effects of the denatured venom of the social wasp Polybia occidentalis (Polistinae, Vespidae). *Basic & clinical pharmacology & toxicology*, 97(5), 289-95.

[114] Wang, C. G., He, X. L., Shao, F., Liu, W., Ling, M. H., Wang, D. C., et al. (2001). Molecular characterization of an anti-epilepsy peptide from the scorpion Buthus martensi Karsch. *Eur J Biochem*, 2268(8), 480-5.

[115] Zhao, R., Weng-C, C., Feng, Q., Chen, L., Zhang-Y, X., Zhu-Y, H., et al. (2011). Anticonvulsant activity of BmK AS, a sodium channel site 4-specific modulator. *Epilepsy & Behavior*, 20(2), 267-76.

[116] Martin, BM R. A., Gurrola, G. B., Nobile, M., Prestipino, G., Possani, L. D., & Novel, K. (1994). channel-blocking toxins from the venom of the scorpion Centruroides limpidus limpidusKarsch. *Biochem J*, 15(304), 51-6.

[117] Corona, M., Coronas, F. V., Merino, E., Becerril, B., Gutiérrez, R., Rebolledo-Antunez, S., et al. (2003). A novel class of peptide found in scorpion venom with neurodepressant effects in peripheral and central nervous system of the rat. *Biochimica et Biophysica Acta BBA)- Proteins & Proteomics*, 1649(1), 58-67.

[118] Cougle, J. R., Keough, Riccardi. C. J., & Sachs-Ericsson, N. (2009). Anxiety disorders and suicidality in the National Comorbidity Survey-Replication. *J Psychiatr Res*, 43(9), 825-9.

[119] Hatcher, S., & Arroll, B. (2012). Newer antidepressants for the treatment of depression in adults. *BMJ*, 344, d8300.

[120] Nemeroff, C. B., & Owens, M. J. (2002). Treatment of mood disorders. *Nat Neurosci. Suppl*, 5, 1068-70.

[121] Liberato, J. L., Cunha, A. O., Mortari, M. R., Gelfuso, E. A., Beleboni, Rde. O., Coutinho-Netto, J., et al. (2006). Anticonvulsant and anxiolytic activity of FrPbAII, a novel GABA uptake inhibitor isolated from the venom of the social spider Parawixia bistriata (Araneidae: Araneae). *Brain Res*, 1124(1), 19-27.

[122] Saidemberg, D., Ferreira, M., Takahashi, M. A., Gomes, T. N., Cesar-Tognoli, P. C., da, L. M., Silva-Filho, L. C., et al. (2009). Monoamine oxidase inhibitory activities of indolylalkaloid toxins from the venom of the colonial spider Parawixia bistriata: functional characterization of PwTX-I. *Toxicon*, 54(6), 717-24.

[123] Maruyama, M., & Na, W. Monoamine Oxidase Inhibitors as Neuroprotective Agents in Age-Dependent Neurodegenerative Disorders. *Curr Pharm Des*, 19, 799-817.

[124] Dwyer, J. M., Rizzo, S. J., Neal, S. J., Lin, Q., Jow, F., Arias, R. L., et al. (2009). Acid sensing ion channel (ASIC) inhibitors exhibit anxiolytic-like activity in preclinical pharmacological models. *Psychopharmacology (Berl)*, 203(1), 41-52.

[125] de Oliveira, L., Cunha, A. O., Mortari, M. R., Coimbra, N. C., & Dos, Santos. W. F. (2006). Cataleptic activity of the denatured venom of the social wasp Agelaia vicina (Hymenoptera, Vespidae) in Rattus norvegicus (Rodentia, Muridae). *Prog Neuropsychopharmacol B ol Psychiatry*, 30(2), 198-203.

[126] de Oliveira, L., Cunha, A. O., Mortari, M. R., Pizzo, A. B., Miranda, A., Coimbra, N. C., et al. (2005). Effects of microinjections of neurotoxin AvTx8, isolated from the social wasp Agelaia vicina (Hymenoptera, Vespidae) venom, on GABAergic nigrotectal pathways. *Brain Res*, 1031(1), 74-81.

[127] Gati, C. D., Mortari, M. R., & Schwartz, E. F. (2012). Towards therapeutic applications of arthropod venom k(+)-channel blockers in CNS neurologic diseases involving memory acquisition and storage. *Journal of toxicology*, 756358.

[128] Dilly, S., Lamy, C., Marrion, N. V., Liegeois, . J. F., & Seutin, . V. (2011). Ion-channel modulators: more diversity than previously thought. *Chembiochem : a European journal of chemical biology*, 12(12), 1808-12.

[129] Romero-Curiel, A., Lopez-Carpinteyro, D., Gamboa, C., De la Cruz, F., Zamudio, S., & Flores, G. (2011). Apamin induces plastic changes in hippocampal neurons in senile Sprague-Dawley rats. *Synapse*, 65(10), 1062-72.

[130] Gimenez-Gallego, G., Navia, MA, Reuben, J. P., Katz, G. M., Kaczorowski, G. J., & Garcia, M. L. (1988). Purification, sequence, and model structure of charybdotoxin, a

potent selective inhibitor of calcium-activated potassium channels. *Proc Natl Acad Sci U S A*, 85(10), 3329-33.

[131] Crest, M., Jacquet, G., Gola, M., Zerrouk, H., Benslimane, A., Rochat, H., et al. (1992). Kaliotoxin, a novel peptidyl inhibitor of neuronal BK-type Ca(2+)-activated K+ channels characterized from Androctonus mauretanicus mauretanicus venom. *J Biol Chem*, 267(3), 1640-7.

[132] Galvez, A., Gimenez-Gallego, G., Reuben, J. P., Roy-Contancin, L., Feigenbaum, P., Kaczorowski, G. J., et al. (1990). Purification and characterization of a unique, potent, peptidyl probe for the high conductance calcium-activated potassium channel from venom of the scorpion Buthus tamulus. *J Biol Chem*, 265(19), 11083-90.

[133] Kourrich, S., Mourre, C., & Soumireu-Mourat, B. (2001). Kaliotoxin, a Kv1.1 and Kv1.3 channel blocker, improves associative learning in rats. *Behav Brain Res*, 120(1), 35-46.

[134] Edwards, T. M., & Rickard, N. S. (2006). Pharmaco-behavioural evidence indicating a complex role for ryanodine receptor calcium release channels in memory processing for a passive avoidance task. *Neurobiol Learn Mem*, 86(1), 1-8.

Chapter 5

Venom Bradykinin-Related Peptides (BRPs) and Its Multiple Biological Roles

Claudiana Lameu, Márcia Neiva and
Mirian A. F. Hayashi

Additional information is available at the end of the chapter

http://dx.doi.org/10.5772/52872

1. Introduction

The kallikrein-kinin system is an extensively studied biological pathway and involves a multi-protein complex, which includes serine proteinases from tissue and plasma. These proteinases act on substrates as kininogens (high and low molecular weight), releasing the active kinins. The main kinin is the nonapeptide bradykinin (BK).

Several studies aiming to evaluate the biological activities of the kinins revealed that this peptide is implicated in diverse physiological processes as regulation of blood pressure, cardiac, and renal function. Due to its ability to increase the vascular permeability by acting on endothelial cells, BK is correlated to several pathological processes including inflammation. These actions have been observed and described in both mammals and rodents [1].

The knowledge on the role of BK in various biological pathways as coagulation cascade, blood pression regulation, and central nervous system modulation and signaling has been significantly improved, leading to the identification of BK receptors and posterior development of drugs targeting its pathways [2].

This research was mainly driven by scientific studies on animal venoms, which lead to the identification of the BK-related peptides (BRPs). The best, and maybe also the first, example of such contribution was the discovery of the bradykinin-potentiating peptides (BPPs), first described in *Bothrops jararaca* venom [3, 4]. The BPPs are proline-rich oligopeptides that inhibit the angiotensin-converting enzyme (ACE), and that are responsible for the hypotensive effect of the *Bothrops* genus snake venoms. The pharmacological effects of these peptides have been studied since 70's [3, 4], and allowed not only to the discovery of the neuropeptide BK [5], but also to the development of the first active site-directed inhibitor of ACE as drug for the treatment of human hypertension [6]. In fact, several other drugs derived from venom toxins, with or without modifications, are also commercially available (*e.g*. Captopril, Ancrod, and Prialt) [7]. Moreover, the study of toxins has widely contributed to the identification of new targets with therapeutic potential in mammals, as well as it has allowed to the understanding and discovery of the biochemical pathways involving these targets.

Since then, the BPPs/BRPs have been found in several snake venoms, and also in wasps and frogs, by using either biochemical or/and recombinant DNA techniques [8-11]. For instance, molecular cloning studies using cDNA libraries of four species of snakes from Crotalinae family showed evidences that these bioactive peptides are expressed by orthologous genes [12]. The cloning of orthologous precursors from different snakes from *Bothrops* and *Crotalus* genus allowed the identification of several new BPPs sequences [13-15], and some of them was shown to display different specificity toward each active sites of the somatic ACE ectoenzyme [16]. This was believed to be a great opportunity for the development of a new generation of antihypertensive drugs.

The employment of recombinant DNA techniques were also fundamental to first determine the structure of the precursor protein of BPPs, which was found to contain several sequences of BPPs distributed as tandem repeats, followed by a C-type natriuretic peptide (CNP) at the C-terminus of this precursor molecule [15]. In contrast to other members of the natriuretic peptide (NP) family, CNP is synthesized in the brain and has hypotensive effect with no significant diuretic or natriuretic actions [17]. Moreover, Northern blot analysis of several snake tissues demonstrated the presence of similar BPPs-CNP precursor mRNA in non-venomous tissues, such as the central nervous system (CNS) [14]. In *situ* hybridization studies also detected the presence of the BPP/CNP-precursor mRNA in regions of snake brain correlated with neuroendocrine functions, such as the ventromedial hypothalamus, paraventricular nuclei, paraventricular organ, and subcommissural organ [14]. Analogous CNP precursor mRNAs was also described in similar regions in rat and human brains [18].

These studies suggesting the potential expression of BPPs in snake CNS stimulated us to investigate the putative target(s) of these peptides. Based on the *in vivo* biodistribution studies showing the preferential accumulation of BPPs in the rat kidney, and also a significant presence in the brain, the first studies were conducted in theses tissues leading to the description of several completely new potential targets and pathways, as the nicotinic acetylcoline receptors [19], L-argininosuccinate synthase [20], and an orphan G protein-coupled receptor (GPCR) [20]. The importance of both NO release for the antihypertensive effects of BPPs [20-22], and also the involvement of the GPCRs, namely B2 receptor and M1 muscarinic receptor (mACh-M1), in vasodialtion were demonstrated [23].

Together all these data collected during the last decade showed the pharmacologial significance of the BPPs and, more importantly, that the biological effects of these peptides, although first believed, are not limited to the inhibiton of the somatic ACE [2]. The high variability of molecular structures of these peptides reflecting in different specifities is an indicative that there are still more to be discovered regarding the biological effects of this peptides family.

In this book chapter, we intend to gather the most important results obtained up to now, thanks to the isolation and characterization of BPPs from diverse organisms and to the knowledge accumulated, while searching for new targets for these molecules.

2. The discovery of the snake venom BK and BRPs

The main function of snake venoms is still believed to be the immobilization of preys to ensure feeding. The snake venoms are composed of a complex mixture of proteins and biologically active peptides [24, 25]. The study of the pathophysiological mechanisms of poisoning and molecular characterization of toxins from the venom of *Bothrops jararaca* resulted in many scientific contributions of great importance, and among them, stand out the discovery of BK [5] and the discovery of the first BRPs, more specifically the BPPs produced by the snake venom glands, [4, 26] whose synergistic action is capable of causing a sharp drop in blood pressure of small animals, for instance mammalian preys.

The BPPs are molecules able to enhance some pharmacological activities of BK, as the action of contractile smooth muscle of guinea pig ileum evaluated in *ex vivo* assays [26], and also *in vivo*, acting in the CNS, cardiovascular, and antinociceptive systems [27, 28]. The isolation of the first BPPs expressed by the *Bothrops jararaca* venom glands was described in the early 60's, and they were initially coined as Bradykinin Potentiating Factors (BPF) due to their ability to potentiate the effects of BK ignoring at that time the fact that these molecules were composed by amino acid residues [26]. Only in early 70's, when their primary sequence were determined, which allowed to characterize them as peptide molecules, they were re-named as BPPs [3]. Since then, several peptides presenting similar structural characteristics have been identified from the venom of these snakes and also from other snakes belonging to several different genus [12, 13, 29-31]. Interestingly, they had also been described in wasps and frogs [8-11]. Typically, the BPPs are peptides of 5-14 amino acid residues [32]. In general, all known naturally occuring BPPs could be classified into two groups: (i) peptides of small molecular size like BPP-5a from the venom of *Bothrops jararaca,* whose structural characteristic is a pyroglutamic acid at the N-terminal and a proline residues at the C-terminal of molecule, and (ii) peptides consisting of about ten amino acid residues, with a pyroglutamic acid at the N-terminal and a notable high content of proline residues [32], which gives to them some resistance to hydrolysis by amino-peptidases, carboxypeptidases, and also endopeptidases [33].

2.1. cDNA cloning, identification and characterization of BRPs

The BK and its related peptides, *e.g.* the BRPs, are widely found in venomous animals, for instance in snakes, lizards, frogs, and insects [10, 13, 34]. In general, they include several sequences, either showing only one single amino acid substitution compared to BK or, in some cases, presenting just a frugal sequence similarity, but with unquestionable biological/ functional correlation, for instance, acting on the same pathway or even same target protein. In fact, these sequence variations were verified either by *de novo* sequencing of several BRPs found in snake venoms [32] or by analysis of the deduced amino acid sequences of cDNAs cloned from venomous glands [12, 14, 15], and in some cases by using both strategies [30, 34].

The pharmacological evaluations revealed that even acting in the same pathway, they can show distinct biological activities compared to BK, including potentiating its effects by inhibition of its degradation or by acting on receptors and/or molecules involved in the BK signaling pathway, including activating or blocking the BK receptors [10, 35]. As such, the BRPs also include BPPs and the Bradykinin Inhibitor Peptides (BIPs) [13, 29, 32, 36].

2.2. BPPs and BIPs

Helokinestatins are a family of proline-rich peptides (PRPs) found originally in the lizard venom (*Heloderma suspectum*) that display the function of inhibiting the BK actions on the vascular smooth muscle [35]. Synthetic replicates of all helokinestatins were found to antagonize the relaxation effect observed following BK application to a rat arterial smooth muscle preparation, and hence, represent a family of BRPs also known as BIPs [34].

In contrast, BPPs firstly described and isolated from the venom of the Brazilian snake *Bothrops jararaca* are mainly known due to their ability to potentiate the biological effects of BK [3, 26]. These BRPs are one of the most outstanding group of PRPs, as they were used as structural and functional template/model for the development of a drug employed up to now for the treatment of human hypertension [6].

Although functionally related to the BK and also present with the NPs in the same precursor protein, the helokinestatins are quite different from the snake venom BPPs [12, 30, 31, 37-39]. PRPs with the same BK inhibitory characteristics have also been described in the 'venomous' secretion of two species of anguid lizards, the *Texas alligator* (*Gerrhonotus infernalis*) and the *Giant Hispanolian galliwasp* (*Celestus warreni*) [38]. Although the primary structural variation of the peptides from these species, they share several common features [34]. For instance, they are peptides rich in prolyl residues (30-50%), which confer rigidity and order to the spatial structure features, and also a measure of resistance to generalized proteolysis. They all possess a Pro-Arg dipeptide motif at the C-terminus, which is quite different from the C-terminal Ile/Val-Pro-Pro motif present in most BPPs C-terminus extremity [12]. The high degree of conservation of these structural core features across phylogeny suggest a fundamental biological function for this group of peptides in the lizards venoms. Among the two closely-related species of helodermatid lizards, several helokinestatins have fully-conserved primary structure, while several others present different sequences. Similarly to the BRPs from amphibian skin [40] and snakes venom [13, 14, 30], helokinestatins compose tandem repeat domains in their respective precursor proteins, probably reflecting discrete exons within the genomic DNA. As already mentioned, some tandem repeats are composed by identical primary structure, while some others exhibit significant amino acid substitutions. prominent And this process of exon multiplication might facilitate the molecular diversity, by permitting the expression of site-mutated isoforms, which is a phenomenon often described for bioactive peptide-encoding genes, as also observed for the glucagon gene in vertebrates [41].

Cloning and alignment of cDNAs encoding BRPs precursors from the venom gland and brain of a pit viper have allowed observing a higher degree of sequence consevation for the regions not including the bioative peptides, and a higher variation in the primary structure of these biological active peptides [14]. These results were shown to be in good agreement with the accelerated evolution hypothesis suggested by Ohno and colleagues [42]. According to this hypothesis, the more frequent occurrence of nucleotide nonsynonymous substitutions in the coding regions compared to the untranslated regions (UTRs) of the genes allows specific genes to evolve in an accelerated fashion to attain unique physiological activity. On the other hand, despite the consequent changes in the BRPs sequences observed, both the high content of proline residues and the biological activities correlated to BK effects are still maintained (Figure 1). Another highly conserved region involves the sequence of the NPs always present in C-terminus extremity of all known BRPs precursor proteins [12-15, 30, 31, 34, 36].

2.3. BRPs and NPs

The NP system consists of three types of hormones [atrial NP (ANP), brain or B-type NP (BNP), and C-type NP (CNP)], and three types of receptors [NP receptor (R)-A, NPR-B, and NPR-C]. Both ANP and BNP are circulating hormones secreted from the heart, whereas CNP is basically a neuropeptide. The NP system plays pivotal roles in cardiovascular and body fluid homeostasis. The ANP is secreted in response to an increase in blood volume, and acts on various organs to decrease both water and Na^+, resulting in restoration of blood volume. The family of NPs were originally Na^+-extruding hormones in fishes; however, they evolved to be volume-depleting hormones promoting the excretion of both Na^+ and water in tetrapods, in which both are always regulated in the same direction. Vertebrates expanded their habitats from fresh water to the sea or to land during evolution. The structure and function of osmoregulatory hormones have also undergone evolution during this ecological evolution [43].

Members of the NPs family have been detected in several snake venoms, and they have been shown to be located in the same precursor protein containing multiple BRPs sequences. While this organization was demonstrated for many species of viperid snakes, including members of the genera *Bothrops, Crotalus, Lachesis, Agkistrodon,* and *Trimeresurus* [12, 13, 15, 30, 31], it may extend to some other taxa such as *Bitis gabonica,* that was also shown to have BPPs in their venom [12, 13, 15, 30, 31, 44]. The presence of NPs in some elapid snakes venom (*Dendroaspis*) has also been described [45]. It has been shown that the venom-derived NP precursors from helodermatid lizard have a structural organization similar to that found in many BRPs precursors from viperid snake venoms. However, the additionally encoded tandem-repeat peptides are non-canonical BPPs, based on their primary structural characteristics or in terms of the amino acid cleavage site, presenting characteristics of a recognition site typical of propeptide convertase enzymes, that eventually might be the potential responsible for the release of the mature BIPs from the respective biosynthetic precursors [36]. However, the BPP/CNP biosynthetic precursors of the bushmaster (*Lachesis muta*), the tropical rattlesnake (*Crotalus durissus terrificus*), and the massasauga rattlesnake from desert (*Sistrurus catenatus ewardsi)* showed that, in addition to the classical BPPs and a NP sequence, they all also encode single copies of a BIP exhibiting a closer structural similarity, and a propeptide convertase cleavage site that allows the release of the BIP helokinestatins, whose sequences are [TPPAGPDVGPR] or [TPPAGPDGGPR] [36] (Figure 1). On the other hand, putative helokinestatins peptides could not be identified in the BPP/CNP precursor of snakes as *Bothrops jararaca, Bothrops jararacussu,* and *Agkistrodon blomhoffi* (Figure 1). The phylogenetic analysis

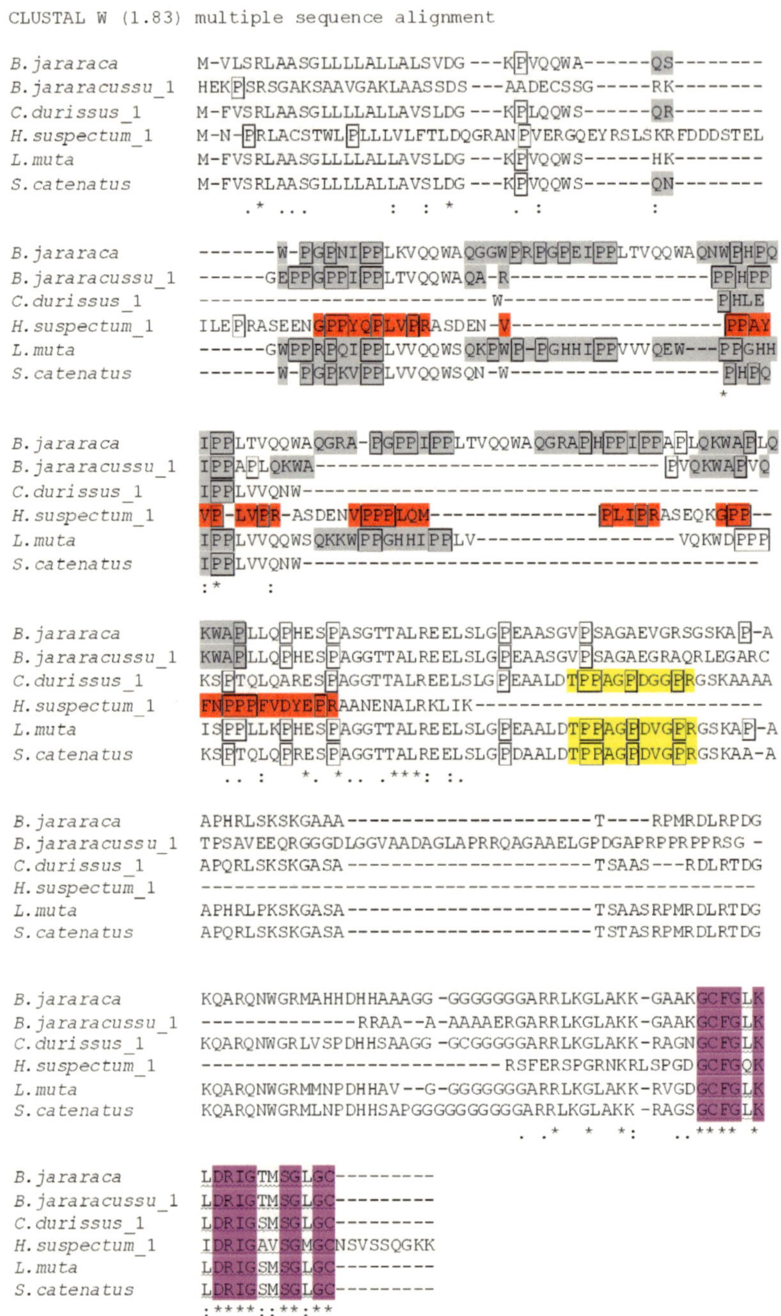

Figure 1. Alignment of the amino acid sequences of BRPs precursors. Organization of the BPP/CNP and helokinestatin/CNP precursor from venoms, indicating the mature BPPs (grey), helokinestatins, BIPs (red), and CNP (underlined) Note that precursors of *C. durissus*, *L. muta*, and *S. catenatus* present both mature BPPs and BIPs in their sequences. The conserved amino acid seqeunces compared to fragments involving the CNP region are highlighted (pink) and the proline residues are indicated by boxes.

presented here separates NPs precursor of different species into three distinct groups, those which contain in their precursor sequence (i) only BPPs, (ii) only BIPs, and/or (iii) both BRPs, *i.e.* BPPs and BIPs (Figure 1 and 2), suggesting that mutations in the coding regions of BRPs were important for the adaptative changes along evolution of the venom system [40].

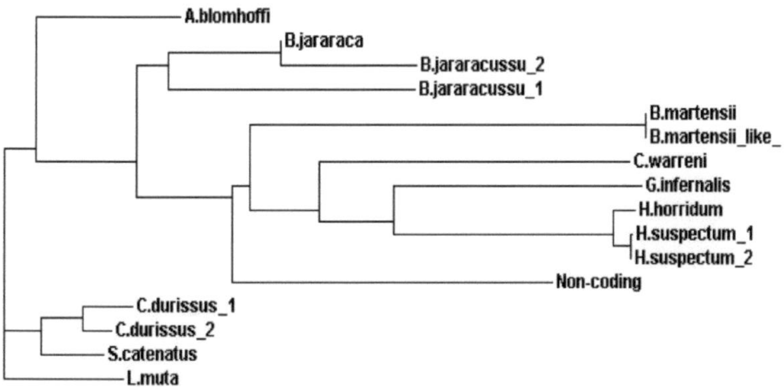

Figure 2. Phylogenetic tree based on BRP/NPs precursors. The phylogenetic analysis was performed using T-Coffee - Multiple Sequence Alignment avaiable at http://www.ebi.ac.uk/Tools/msa/tcoffee/. In this analysis, protein sequences of BRP/CNP precursors from reptiles were used. The NPs precursor of *A. blomhoffi. B. jararaca,* and *B. jararacussu* contain only BPP sequences; *C. warreni, G. infernalis, H. suspectum,* and *H. horridum* contain only BIP sequences and, *C. durrissus*, *L. mutta*, and *S. catenatus* contain both BRPs sequences, *i.e.* BPP and BIP. Despite the aligned *B. martensii* sequence was partial, and therefore does not contain the sequence coding for BRPs, this species was found to express the closest related precursor sequence to those containing only BIPs and to the *B. jararaca* non-coding RNA homologous to BPP/CNP precursor.

2.4. Molecular evolution of genes encoding BRPs

Here, we take BPP/CNP and helokinestatin/CNP precursors as examples to illustrate the evolution of a gene, since BPP/CNP precursor is also expressed in other tissues of *Bothrops jararaca* besides the venom gland, incluing brain and spleen [14, 15]. A high similarity was oberved for the BPP/CNP cDNAs isolated from brain and venom gland, although they are not identical to each other as it should be expected [14]. Three out of the five BPP isoforms present in the brain precursor (BPPs of 5, 10 and 13 amino acid residues) were identical to those found in the venom gland precursor [14]. Moreover, most of insertions/deletions and point mutations were observed within the BPP/CNP coding region, suggesting an effect of a Darwinian-type accelerated evolution frequently observed intra-specie [42, 46] This process has been widely observed, since a number of neuropeptides and hormones, such as the NPs [15, 47] and the vascular endothelium growth factor [48] evolved into toxins in the venom gland of poisonous animals.

It is believed that BRPs from the venom may be considered the toxin counterparts of endogenous peptides. It has also been suggested that both CNP and BPPs could be physiologically associated, to perform fluid homeostasis and regulation of the vascular tonus, since BPP/CNP precursor are present in regions of the snake brain showed to be involved in the control of these activities, as described for the mammalian CNS [14].

It is known that in the process of evolution, several mutations may occur in the genes, some of which not affecting the mature protein sequence, while others might lead even to the generation of messenger RNAs that are not translated into proteins. In 2000's it was first shown that non-coding RNAs can be involved in several roles including repression of genes, catalysis, regulation of the development process, among others [49]. A non-coding mRNA showing a sequence similarity to the BPPs precursor of the pit viper *Bothrops jararaca* was cloned by us from the venom gland [Genbank Acc. No. AY310916.1]. This long RNA sequence does not encode a protein, since several stop codons were observed for all possible reading frames (Figure 3).

```
G T R Stop K L P N N Stop S N S L I V L T I R T I N Q R N C L S S E F V G A S S L E A F E K R L D R H L S E
Met V P S N S I I I L V Y Stop L T P I E I L C K T Q L W T R L Q Stop R F Y L F Y L L I K F L C R S S P K T
R S G Stop Q H K Stop N N I S T F Q N Stop N Q S Stop K A Y N F Y Y I A F A P V S E G A Met S Y I A L P K L
T L S K S H K S H R R K N S E Q A Met L I Stop S A W R S E V N F V W K T L S L E A K Met A Met G I H L D Met
Y Met S R Y S I N Q S N K E I R K Y S F S N F P S I L N S H R C T S G E R S K F K N S D I Stop F Y L R L Y F
Y L F F F F S N L S C C L Stop G I I S K E V L L A I L Q L F Y W V T P A V V E V G K K K I S V I Y F W N R E
D N A I Q W Met I V F S N N N Stop T A F Stop C N F L F S I L F F Stop F Q A Y L E S V R A H R V G L L R V P
S V R Q C H L A G P R A R A F S V A A P A L W N Q L P S E V H T A S S L L A F R K L L K T H L C R Q V W G V
Stop A A L C P W A F D C D C V W C E Stop N K L R S F Y T V N Stop Stop F Stop L I Y V Met F F I L V L L L
Stop T A L S L V R R A A Y K F N K Stop Stop Stop Stop Y S L T N V V V F Y K Q Stop E L H A Q S Stop V V K
Met Stop N V S Stop A D S W L G E F K F L L I S E K K F C F L E V F A G F Y C W H I Met Stop I P Q Stop S A
G D G Met Stop P F S K V L P F Stop C S T G H I N F P L D C R I S W Q K V I S R Q P D R T L Q Q F F Met V Y
S H G I S S L Q K V K K N N N S H K R A Stop H Stop K S E F F Stop N E A L S Y L N V L S L H G G Met E N P P
Met G I Q S L L P Y H R L G P K F S S A S W L P P Q F F D R R S S S S G R T V Stop L L F H V L Stop E N Y L
P R P V R G G R G F S I P P C R E R T S G K T T L L S P A W V D S E S T N G T Y P S P Q K S P W E G V Stop A
I S Y Stop A S T I C C R D L L P N E P S A A A N Stop S I L Stop F L T K E D G E A H V A A L Q I S L Q R R L
R A P S C R R R H L A A V F E L R P H P I R G H F W T S P A I H P G I P G P H S L S P V G T S T Stop R S H F
S V G E V L G R G W T E F C A P K S S Y L T Stop Y I P R C H I Y I D R Y K Y T Q H K K T R P P T T S S P R Q
R T V S G N G E N Q L R Met P S R L L F V H S C H A Stop Met Y L S C K S Y L Y I V Y K E I F I K K N F I Y V
N Stop T K R G R A L Stop T F F F S P F S S Stop I V G R K E K K I Met D D L I T C L A F Stop S D A V F L S
E Met G G L N K A F R Y H G Stop E Stop K Met H L Stop R N R T L S T K G V K E P D A P F L Met F L A E I K K
P L F K E V L R I K K K K K K K K K K K K K K K K K K K K K K K K K
```

Figure 3. Potential deduced amino acid sequences from the all possible frames of the non-coding RNA homologous to the BPP/CNP precursor coding RNA both from *Bothrops jararaca*. Total mRNA obtained from *Bothrops jararaca* venom gland higher than 2 Kb length was used to construct the long cDNA library. The complete cDNA sequence of the BPP/CNP precursor (clone NM 96) was used as template to screen about 2 x 10^6 clones, allowing the identification of four independent positive clones containing identical inserts of approximately 3.5 Kb [15]. All potential frames of the *Bothrops jararaca* BPP/CNP-related pseudogene mRNA presents a high content of stop codons (bold), as shown by the representative amino acid deduced sequence from one of the possible reading frames. No signal peptide could observed, although several methionine (Met) residues (underlined) that does not seem to represent an initial of translation were found.

These non-coding RNAs are usually transcribed by a gene known as a pseudogene, which are often found in the genomes of several life forms, including bacteria, plants, insects, and vertebrates [50]. The pseudogene is a sequence that is present in the genome, and it is typically characterized by presenting high similarity with one or more functional gene paralogs. The pseudogene can be derived from gene duplication occurred by two different pathways: retrotransposition or duplication of genomic DNA [50].

The regulation of the expression of a functional gene showing sequence similarity to a pseudogene has been reported [51]. Generally, the sequence similarity between functional genes and pseudogenes is observed at the 5' UTR fragment. However, for the comparison of the non-coding RNA and the RNA coding for BPP/CNP precursor, a high similarity was observed only for the 3' UTR sequence (Figure 4). Moreover, the non-coding RNA is of approximately 3.5 Kb, while the RNA coding for the BPPs precursor is of about 1.8 Kb, and its RNA expression was found to be about 6-fold higher than that of the 3.5 Kb non-coding RNA.

Nevertheless, it is also possible that non-coding RNA of 3.5 Kb [GenBank Acc. No. AY310916.1] may also ensures the stability of the functional coding messenger RNA, since the stability of messenger RNAs is preferably controlled by factors present in the 3' UTR region [52].

```
non-coding   TATCTCTTACTAGGCCTCTACTATCTGCTGCAGGGACCTTCTACCAAACGAACCCTCAGC
BPP-coding   TGCTTT------GGCCT----------------GAAGCT---------CGA--CCGCATC
             *   *       *****                * * **         ***  ** ** *

non-coding   TGCAGCGAATTGATCGATCTTGTAATTTCTAACGAAGGAGGACGGAGAGGCCCACGTGGC
BPP-coding   GGCACCA---TGAGCGGCCT------------------GGGCTGCTGAAGCCGTCGAGG-
              *** *    *** **  **                   **  *  ** ***  ** **

non-coding   CGCTCTGCAAATTTCTCTCCAGCGGCGCCTGCGTGCGCCAAGCTGCCGAAGGCGACACCT
BPP-coding   ---------------------GCGGCGC-------------------GAAGGCGACACCT
                                  *******                   *************

non-coding   GGCGGCGGTCTTTGAACTGAGACCCCACCCCATCCGCGGACATTTCTGGACATCCCCTGC
BPP-coding   GGCGGCGGTCTTTGAACTGAGACCCCACCCCATCCGCGGACATTTCTGGACATCCCCTGC
             ************************************************************

non-coding   AATTCATCCAGGGATCCCAGGCCCACACAGCCTGTCTCCTGTTGGTACGAGCACTTGAAG
BPP-coding   AATTCATCCAGGGATCCCAGGCCCACACAGCCTGTCTCCTGTTGGTACGAGCACTTGAAG
             ************************************************************

non-coding   AAGCCATTTTTCAGTGGGAGAGGTTCTGGGTAGAGGTTGGACTGAGTTTTGCGCCCCCAA
BPP-coding   AAGCCATTTTTCAGTGGGAG-GGTTCTGGGTAG-GGTTGGACTGAGTTTTGCGCCCCCAA
             ******************** ************ **************************

non-coding   ATCTTCCTATCTTACCTAATATATACCTAGATGCCATATATATATCGATAGATACAAGTA
BPP-coding   ATCTTCCTATCTTACCTAATATATACCTAGATGCCATATATAT ATCGATAGATACAAGTA
             ************************************************************

non-coding   CACCCAACACAAAAAAACACGCCCGCCCACAACTTCTTCCCCGCGACAAAGGACGGTGTC
BPP-coding   CACCCAACACAAAAAA-CACGCCCGCCCACAACTTCTTCCCCGCGACAAAGGACGGTGTC
             **************** *******************************************

non-coding   GGGAAACGGAGAGAACCAGCTGCGTATGCCATCGAGATTGCTGTTTGTACATTCGTGTCA
BPP-coding   GGGAGACGGAGAGAACCAGCTGCGTATGCCATCGAGATTGCTGTTTGTACATTCGTGTCA
             **** *******************************************************

non-coding   CGCATAAATGTATTTAAGTTGTAAAAGCTATTTATATATTGTTTATAAAGAGATATTTAT
BPP-coding   CGCATAAATGTATTTAAGTTGTAAAAGCTATTTATATATTGTTTATAAAGAGATATTTAT
             ******************************** ***************************

non-coding   AAAAAAAAATTTATTTATGTAAACTAAACGAAAAGGGGTCGAGCATTGTAAACTTTTTT
BPP-coding   AAAAAAAAATTTATTTATGTAAACTAAACGAAAAGGGGTCGAGCATTGTAAACTTTTTT
             ************************************************************

non-coding   TTTTTCCCCTTTCTCATCCTGAATAGTCGGAAGGAAAGAAAAAAAAA-TCATGGACGATT
BPP-coding   TTT--CCCCTTTCTCATCCTGAATAGTCGGAAGGAAAGAAAAAAAAAATCATGGACGATT
             ***  ****************************************** ************

non-coding   TGATAACCTGTCTTGCATTTTAATCGGATGCAGTCTTTCTTTCCGAAATGGGTGGTTTGA
BPP-coding   TGATAACCTGTCTTGCATTTTAATCGGATGCAGTCTTTCTTTCCGAAATGGGTGGTTTGA
             ******************************** ***************************

non-coding   ACAAGGCTTTTAGATACCACGGATAAGAGTAAAAAATGCATTTGTAAAGAAATCGCACGC
BPP-coding   ACAAGGCTTTTAGATACCACGGATAAGAGTAAAAAATGCATTTGTAAAGAAATCGCACGC
             ******************************************************* ****

non-coding   TATCTACCAAAGGTGTAAAAGAACCCGACGCGCCGTTTTTGATGTTTTTAGCAGAAATAA
BPP-coding   TATCTACCAAAGGTGTAAAAGAACCCGACGCGCCGTTTTTGACGTTTTTAGCAGAAATAA
             ****************************************** *****************

non-coding   AAAAA-CCACTTTTCAAAGAGGTCCTCAGAATT
BPP-coding   AAAAAACCACTTTTCAAAGAGGTCCTCAGAATT
             ***** ***************************
```

Figure 4. Partial sequence alignment of the*Bothrops jararaca* BPP/C NP-related pseudogene mRNA and mRNA coding for BPP/CNP precursor. Alignment of the nucleotide sequences of a segment of the pseudogene mRNA (non-coding: upper sequence) and the mRNA coding for BPP/CNP precursor (BPP-coding: lower sequence) was performed using the Clustaw W program, available at http://www2.ebi.ac.uk/clustalw/. Identical nucleotides are indicated by "*" and insertions or deletions are represented by gaps (-).The boldface type letters indicate the region with higher similarity between the RNA sequences, corresponding to about 97% identity in this region.

In the BPP/CNP precursor of *Bothrops jararaca*, the pentapeptide BPP-5a [QKWAP] that was used as template for the development of the antihypertensive drug captopril, is found duplicated, *i.e.*, there are two copies of the same peptide in a single precursor protein. It is believed that this peptide might have a special importance in the venom of snakes belonging to the *Bothrops* genus, since it is also found repeated three times in isoform 1 [GenBank Acc. No. AY310914.1], and four times in isoform 2 [Genbank Acc. No. AY310915.1] of the precursors isolated from *Bothrops jararacussu* venom glands (Figure 5). In fact, BPP-5a is a potent potentiator of the BK effects in isolated guinea pig ileum, and also *in vivo* [29].

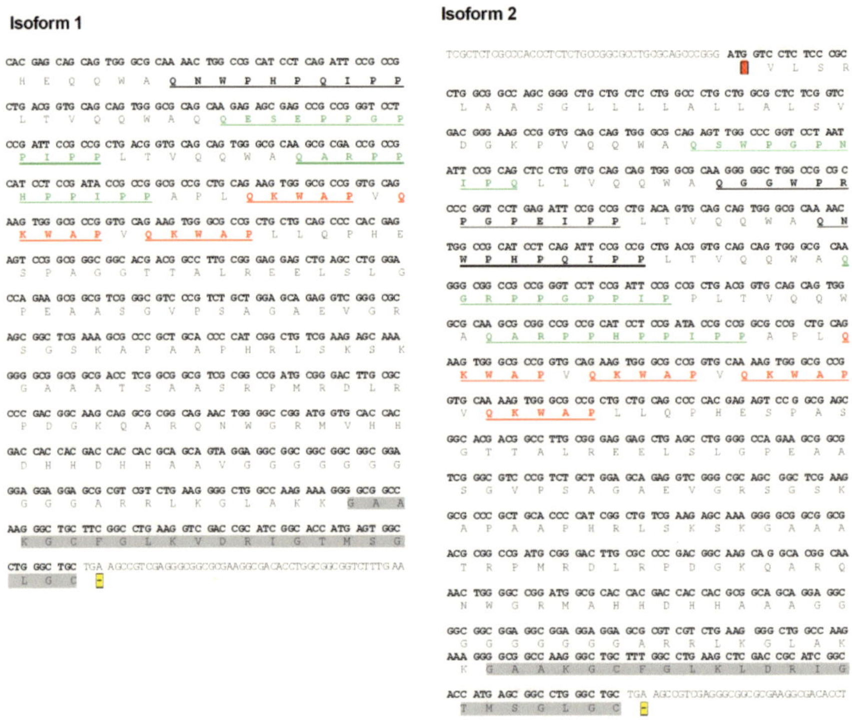

Figure 5. Partial nucleotide and amino acid sequences of the BPP/CNP of precursor from*Bothrops jararacussu* (isoform 1 and 2). Shaded in grey, the amino acid sequences of the C-type natriuretic peptide (CNP). Sequences of new putative BPPs are shown in green, and the underlined sequences correspond to other previously known BPPs. In red, the pentapeptide BPP-5a that was found in duplicate in the pit viper precursor and, triplicate and quadruplicate in the isoforms 1 and 2, respectively, of the precursor from *Bothrops jararacussu*. Symbol "M" represents the initial methionine and (-) the stop codon.

3. BRPs as structural model for drug development

The discovery of the potential inhibitory action of BPPs on ACE brought a great interest in these natural peptides, since the importance of ACE in blood pressure control and the urge to develop a therapy for cardiovascular disease, as hypertension, was iminent [2].

http://dx.doi.org/10.5772/52872

At that time, among the identified peptides were BPP-9a, under the generic name of teprotide, and the BPP-5a, which was also one of first BPP to be characterized. Assays using these peptides showed that BPP-9a was more effective and had a longer lasting effect in blood pressure compared to BPP-5a [53]. Therefore, BPP-9a was used in the first clinical demonstration of the potential use of BPPs for the hypertension control in humans, showing a significant antihypertensive effect [54, 55].

However, on that time it was demonstrated that the therapeutic utility of BPP-9a was limited by the lack of activity by oral administration and the high cost of its synthesis [54, 56, 57]. Therefore, the pharmaceutical development of a non-peptide inhibitor of ACE orally effective was essential. Thus, molecular structure of the BRPs, namely BPP-5a and BPP-9a, were studied by Cushman and Ondetti [3, 58], who suggested specific interaction of the proline, present at the C-terminal of these peptides, with the ACE active site [59]. Thus, captopril was synthetized by simple addition of a chelator radical to a dipeptide containing a proline residue (BPP carboxy-terminal amino acid) [59]. Unodoubtely captopril was a blockbuster drug that inspired the creation of generations of mimetic antihypertensive compounds [2].

4. Biological activities of BRPs

4.1. Interference of BRPs in the renin-angiotensin and kallikrein-kinin system

The ACE (EC 3.4.15.1) is mainly expressed in vascular endothelium in epithelial cells of the proximal tubules of the kidney, brain, and intestinal cells [60]. This enzyme is responsible for conversion of angiotensin I (Ang I) to angiotensin II (Ang II), and for the degradation of BK. Therefore, this enzyme has roles in both renin-angiotensin and kallikrein-kinin system [61].

The renin-angiotensin system (RAS) is composed by a set of peptides, enzymes, and receptors, that are involved in the control of the extracellular fluid and blood pressure [62]. The formation of the effector peptide of this system occurs initially by the action of the renin released by the kidneys [62] that acts on the angiotensinogen produced in the liver [63]. This leads to the generation of the decapeptide Ang I, which then is cleaved by ACE to form the octapeptide Ang II, a potent antihypertensive molecule [64]. Ang II actions is mediated by the angiotensin receptors AT1 and AT2. The binding of Ang II to the AT1 receptor triggers several cellular processes, among them vasoconstriction, protein synthesis, cell growth, regulation of renal function, and electrolyte balance [65]. Ang II also acts as a neurotransmitter and as a neuro-regulador, modulating the central control of the blood pressure, influencing the sympathetic activity, salt appetite, and thirst [65].

The kallikrein-kinin system (KKS) is a metabolic cascade in which the tissue and plasma kallikrein release vasoactive kinins from both high and low molecular weight kininogens. The nonapeptide BK, derived from the cleavage of the high molecular weight kininogen by kallikrein, is the major plasma kinin playing a role in the KKS [66].

Kinins are involved in various physiological and pathological processes, including vasodilation, increased vascular permeability, release of plasminogen activator of tissue type (t-PA), and nitric oxide (NO) and arachidonic acid metabolism, mainly due to their ability to activate endothelial cells [66]. Thus, the kinins participate in the physiologically regulation of blood pressure, cardiac and renal functions, and also in pathological processes as inflammation [66].

The several pharmacological activities of kinins are mediated basically by the their binding to two types of specific receptors (B1 and B2 receptors), prior to their fast metabolization by various peptidases [67].

Actions such as vasodilation and hypotension are mediated by the B2 receptor by releasing of NO, prostacyclin, and endothelium-derived hyperpolarizing factor (EDHF). On the other hand, the actions mediated by the B1 receptors include important roles in angiogenesis, inflammation, and septic shock [68]. Moreover, unlike B2 receptor, B1 receptor is not constitutively expressed, and its expression is induced by mediators of inflammation in conditions of injury [68].

The primarily responsible for the degradation of BK are the peptidases (zinc metallopeptidases) including ACE [67]. Since the early 90's, it is well known that somatic ACE has two active sites, the N-terminus (N-site) and the C-terminus (C-site) active sites [69]. Although *in vitro*, the two active sites are equally effective to convert Ang I to Ang II, as well as to degrade the BK into BK_{1-7} and BK_{1-5} [70], the N-site is several times more effective to hydrolyze other bioactive peptides, such as the AcSDKP, a negative regulatory factor for differentiation and proliferation of hematopoietic stem cells [71].

Thus, ACE inhibitors as BPPs inhibit not only the generation of Ang II, but also potentiate the effects of BK, by inhibiting its degradation. Therefore, the physiological effects of the angiotensin system are decreased (since there is no formation of Ang II), and the physiological effects of KKS are potentiated (due to inhibition of the BK degradation). In contrast, the BIPs, most known as helokinestatins, inhibit KKS by blocking the B2 receptor (Figure 6).

4.2. Mechanisms of action underlying the antihypertensive effect of BRPs

Although ACE inhibition is a relevant mechanism to explain the activity of most BPPs, and despite of their high primary sequence similarity [53, 72], as previously suggested, the BPPs show remarkable wide variety of mechanistic pathways that could explain the antihypertensive activity of BPPs at molecular level [13, 14, 19, 20, 22, 23, 29, 73-76]. Definitely the biological effects of BPPs and the consequent pharmacological importance of their activity are not limited to and it cannot be explained solely based on their ability to inhibit ACE [2].

The differences were first observed when comparing the selectivity of the BPPs encoded by the neuronal BPP/CNP precursor protein [*e.g.* BPP-5a, BPP-10c, BPP-11e, BPP-12b, and BPP-13a] [14] by the different active sites of the somatic ACE and the corresponding biological activity of these peptides evaluated by their ability to potentiate the contractile effect triggered by BK in isolated guinea pig ileum. For instance, the BPP-5a was shown to be much less effective ACE inhibitor compared to BPP-13a, although presenting one of the most potent potentiator effects of BK in *ex vivo* experiments. In contrast, BPP-10c is an excellent selective inhibitor of the C-terminal active site of somatic ACE, and its BK potentiating effect is very similar to that observed for both BPP-5a and BPP-12b, which were shown to be selective for

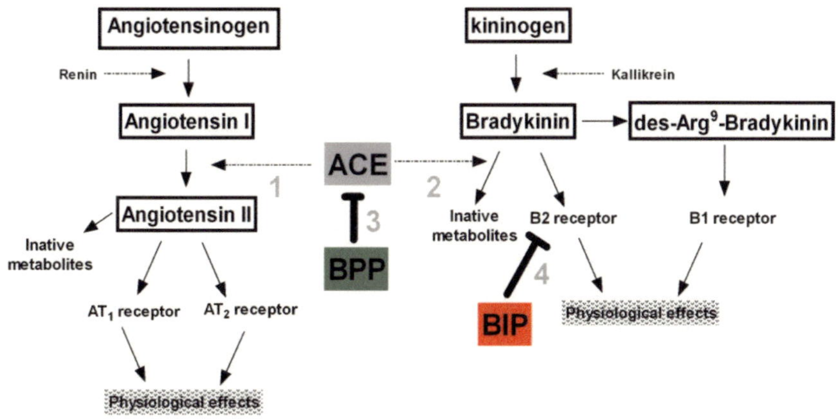

Figure 6. Schematic representation of ACE roles on the renin-angiotensin and kallikrein-kinin systems, and the potential sites for interference by BRPs (BPPs and BIPs). A) *Conversion of angiotensin I into angiotensin II*, 2) *BK degradation* 3) *ACE inhibition by BPPs*. 4) *B2 receptor antagonism by BIPs*. Physiological effects on the renin-angiotensin system mediated by AT1 receptors include vasoconstriction, sodium and water retention, release of aldosterone, increased sympathetic nerve activity, among others, while those mediated by AT2 receptors include cell differentiation, vasodilation, among others. The effects on the kallikrein-kinin system, mediated by kinins action on B2 receptor include vasodilation and hypotension via release of NO, prostacyclins and endothelium-derived hyperpolarizing factor (EDHF). Due to the ACE inhibition by BPPs, the physiological effects of angiotensin system are decreased (with no formation of angiotensin II) and the physiological effects of kallikrein-kinin are potentiated (by inhibition of BK degradation). In contrast, BIPs action on B2 receptor blocked BK effects. Adapted from [132-134].

the ACE N-terminal active site. In the same way, besides the weak BK potentiation effects of BPP-11e, it is also not among the best inhibitors of ACE, and no preference for any of the active sites of ACE was observed for this peptide [29].

Later on, in 2007, molecular studies of the antihypertensive activity of the BPPs, namely BPP-7a and BPP-10c, brought noteworthy information on the molecular mechanism underlying the action of these peptides at cellular level. In fact, these BPPs have a strong and sustained antihypertensive activity in awake spontaneously hypertensive rats (SHRs), but they do not prevent the formation of Ang II from Ang I *in vivo*, showing that they do not need to affect the physiological functions of ACE to promote the decrease of the blood pressure in these animals. Furthermore, for BPP-10c, we have also shown that the dose necessary to produce the antihypertensive effect is lower than that required to inhibit ACE *in vivo* [77], suggesting the participation of other putative targets determining this particular pharmacological effect.

This finding was reinforced by the studies conducted to clarify the biological distribution of BPP-10c using a I^{125} labeled analog, which showed that this peptide accumulated in various rat organs such as brain, liver, testis, and kidney, even after pre-saturation of the potential active sites of ACE with a specific inhibitor of this enzyme, namely captopril [78].

This stimulated us to conduct studies aiming to identify new potential molecular targets for snake BPPs. So, it was shown that at least three BPPs, namely BPP-10c, BPP-12b, and BPP-13a, are able to bind to the enzyme argininosuccinate synthase (AsS) modulating positively its activity [20, 75].

The AsS is the rate-limiting step enzyme responsible for providing the substrate for the nitric oxide synthase (NOS) that produces NO [79, 80]. Guerreiro and colleagues also demonstrated that blood pressure decrease promoted in SHRs by BPP-10c administration is due to the increased bioavailability of L-arginine required for the production of NO [20], which is a potent vasodilator agent [81]. Later it was demonstrated that other BPPs also induces NO production to determine the antihypertensive effect [21, 75].

Moreover, at least for the BPP-5a-induced NO production, the involvement of both B2 receptor and mACh-M1, without any involvement of AsS, was recently demonstrated [23]. BPP-13a induces NO production through a mechanism that involves activation of subtype M3 muscarinic receptor (mACh-M3), triggering the raise of the free intracellular calcium concentration ($[Ca^{2+}]_i$) that is able to activate NOS and to provide the substrate for NO production by modulating the AsS activity [75].

Both BPP-11e and BPP-12b do not stimulate NO production, but the $[Ca^{2+}]_i$ mobilization assays suggest that these peptides are agonists of a membrane receptor involved in the release of EDHF, and other functions involving the modulation of gene expression and activation of different NOS enzymes is expected [82]. As BPP-12b modulates positively AsS activity only at very high concentrations, this should not be its main mechanism of action [75].

Since the BPP-9a has ACE as main target for its biological actions, based on its potent inhibitory activity against this enzyme also showing selectivity for the C-terminal active site [73], we suggest that it is possible to suggest this pathway to explain the antihypertensive effect and BK potentiation of BPP-9a (teprotide). Moreover, it has no effect on the AsS induced intracellular calcium and it also does not interfere with NO production.

Apparently all BPPs share the ability to decrease arterial pressure [21, 56, 75, 77, 83], through the amplitude of the antihypertensive effect caused by BK, each related peptides is different. But, unfortunately, the mechanisms of action of other BPPs are still less understood up to now [75].

4.3. Peripheral and central biological activities of BPPs

Changes in mean arterial pressure (MAP) promoted by some BPPs are accompanied by a significant reduction in heart rate (HR) [23, 75, 77] rather than by an HR increase, as it would be expected by the response of the baroreceptors to the hypotension [84]. The fact is that *in bolus* injections of BPPs decrease both MAP and HR of awake SHRs, and BPPs expression in the same precursor protein of a brain expressed peptide as CNP suggests a CNS role for these peptides. In fact, recently it was shown that the BPP-10c is able to promote the release of the neurotransmitters GABA and glutamate, which are known to participate in the regulation of cardiac and vascular autonomic systems, leading to decline MAP and HR of SHRs [22]. According to Lameu and collaborators, BPP-10c-induced decrease of MAP results from this BRP-induced interference in the autonomic nervous system, provoking subsequent changes in HR and baroreflex control [22, 74].

Arterial baroreflex is one of the most important regulatory mechanisms in the cardiovascular system, mainly by triggering a coordinated sympathetic and parasympathetic tone response on the heart and vessels [85-90].

The CNS is connected to the heart through two different groups of nerves, the parasympathetic and sympathetic systems. Stimulation of parasympathetic nerves determines the decrease of HR, of contraction force of atrial muscle, and of conduction of impulses through the atrioventricular node, and at the same time, it also causes the increase of the time delay between the atrial and ventricular contraction, and the reduction of blood flow through the coronary arteries, which maintains the nutrition of the myocardium. All these effects can be summarized by saying that the parasympathetic stimulation decreases all the activities of the heart. On the other hand, the stimulation of sympathetic nerves has exactly the opposite effects on the heart, leading to an increased HR, increased contraction force, and increased blood flow through the blood vessels [87, 91].

It was observed that BPP-11e causes a slight reduction in MAP, but surprisingly with a strong reduction in HR [75], suggesting a BPPs action in specialized muscle cells located in the sinoatrial region (pacemaker) of the heart, which is a special region of the heart that controls the cardiac frequency [92]. Although the heart has its own intrinsic control systems, it can operate under neural influences, therefore effectiveness of the cardiac action can be significantly modified by regulatory pulses from the CNS [92]. Thus there is also possible that the BPP-11e has an effect on the stimulation of the parasympathetic system and/or in the decreasing of the sympathetic system stimulation, leading to a reduction of the HR and a slight decrease in MAP, observed after *in vivo* injection of this peptide [75].

A more detailed study of the BPPs effects on the CNS was performed for the BPP-10c, in which intracerebroventricular administration was shown to produce similar effects to those observed for higher doses injections of this peptide by intravenous route. In our interpretation, this data suggested the involvement of the CNS in the pathway underlying these biological effects [74].

Aiming to explain tbe BPPs effects on CNS, *Lameu et al.* have also conducted studies to demonstrate that the BPP-10c acts through activation of an unidentified $G_{i/o}$-coupled receptor present in neuronal cells, and that this effect was independent of both ACE inhibition and B2 receptor activation. Peptide–receptor binding resulted in the activation of calcium influx and release of intracellular calcium by calcium-induced calcium release (CICR) mechanism, which was shown to involve the activation of the ryanodine- or IP3-sensitive calcium stores and also the inhibition of adenylate cyclase [74]. However the specific target GPCR could not be identified yet.

On the other hand, affinity chromatography, using immobilized BPP-10c, associated with mass spectrometric and immunoblot analyses, allowed the identification of two important targets of BPP-10c, namely the AsS in the kidney cytosol [20] and the synapsin in the brain (Figure 7) [93]. AsS, together with argininosuccinate lyase (AsL), is part of the urea cycle in the liver and of the arginine-citrulline cycle, the major source of arginine in the renal cells and citrulline–NO cycle, which is the main source of NO in other cells, including endothelial and neuronal cells [94].

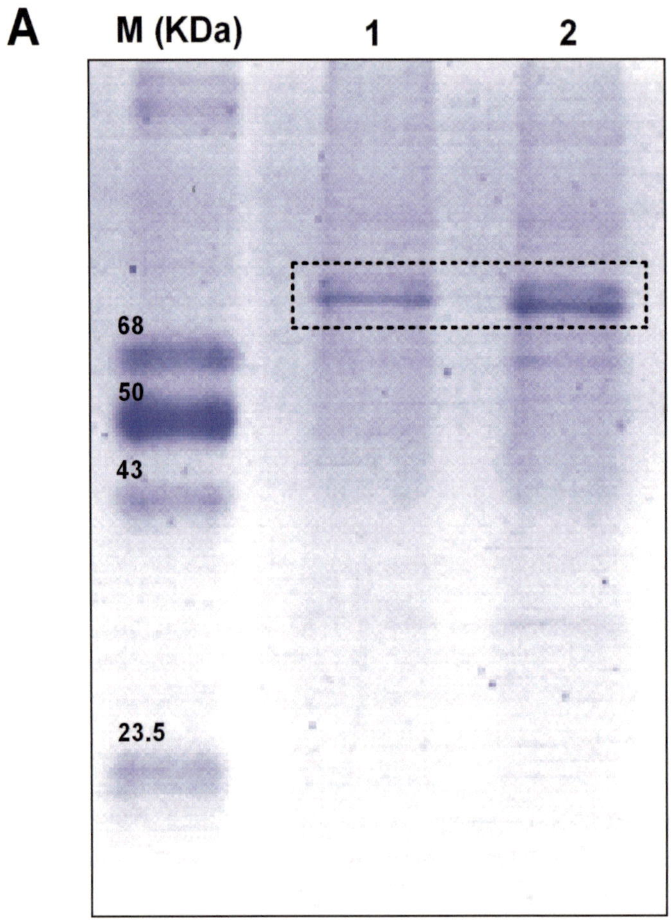

B

Lane	Elution type	Protein	Molecular Mass	Swiss Protein Database	Covarage (%)
1	Competition	Synapsin	74.1	NP_062006	43
2	Lowering of pH	Synapsin	74.1	NP_062006	57

Figure 7. Synapsin binds to BPP-10c. (**A**) SDS-PAGE analysis of brain rat cytosolic proteins submitted to HiTrap-BPP-10c affinity chromatography. Rat brain cytosol preparation to affinity chromatography using the HiTrap NHS-activated HP resin to which BPP-10c was immobilized by chemical conjugation **M (KDa)**, molecular mass markers; **lane 1**, protein eluted by competition using 5 mg of BPP-10c; **lane 2**, protein eluted with 100 mM glycine, 0.5 M NaCl pH 3.0 (elution buffer: by lowering the pH). (**B**) protein identification by mass spectrometric analysis of the bands enclosed in the box in the panel **A**. The 74-kDa major protein that bounds to BPP-10c was identified as synapsin, by trypsin digestion and peptide mass fingerprint analysis.

AsS is a ubiquitously expressed enzyme, present in many tissues, including brain and kidney [94]. *In vivo* BPP-10c administration in SHRs animal models results in increase of plasma arginine level [20] and augmented NO production in brain tissues, as well as in neuronal and endothelial cells [20, 22].

NO is generated in the citrulline-NO cycle by NO synthase (NOS) using L-arginine as a substrate. Three isoforms of NOS have been described: Ca^{2+}-dependent endothelial (eNOS) and neuronal (nNOS) isoforms [95] and inducible NOS. The expression and activity of the latter are induced by inflammatory stimuli, independent of the cytosolic Ca^{2+} concentration [96].

NO is mainly involved in the regulation of local and systemic vascular resistance in sodium balance, and hence in blood pressure control [97], since it is one of the smooth muscle relaxing factors released by the endothelium, which diffuses to the adjacent smooth muscle cells promoting vasodilatation [98, 99].

Nevertheless, NO has been attributed to other various functions, including non-cholinergic and non-adrenergic smooth muscle relaxation, reduction of arterial pressure, and signal transmission in the CNS [100]. NO-mediated actions in the CNS include central vascular regulation [101] and baroreflex control of HR [102]. Antihypertensive activity, based on the facilitated release of both GABA and glutamate in the CNS and NO production, is suggested to result in the diminished transmission of sympathetic tone to the periphery [101, 103].

Treatments with BPP-10c also induced an increase in AsS gene expression [22]. In contrast, nNOS was not found differentially expressed in the brains of SHRs treated with BPP-10c compared to vehicle-treated animals. On the other hand, the gene expression levels of eNOS, similarly to those of AsS, were found increased in the brains of SHRs animals treated with BPP-10c [22]. This data is in line with the results obtained by Kishi and colleagues [104] who were able to show that the overexpression of eNOS in the rostral ventrolateral medulla and the nucleus of the solitary tract of hypertensive rats results in reduced systolic arterial pressure and reduced HR.

However, the specificity of NO reactions with neuronal targets is determined in part by the precise localization of NOS within the cell. The targeting of NOS to discrete nuclei of neurons, mediated by adapter proteins, allowed to suggest that both synapsin and NOS participate of a ternary complex, which changes in the subcellular localization of NOS [105].

Knowing that the BPP-10c binds to synapsin in the CNS, we hypothesized the formation of a quaternary complex upon binding of BPP-10c with synapsin. The formation of this complex would direct the reactions of NO in neural targets, which would be determined in part by the location of this complex and by targeting NOS to specific sites of neurons [105].

We were able to show that BPP-10c is capable to induce intracellular Ca^{2+} signaling that involves the activation of GPCRs, NO production, and release of neurotransmitters, such as GABA and glutamate [22, 74]. The amino acid glutamate is the major excitatory neurotransmitter in the CNS of mammals, whereas GABA is the main mediator of sympathetic inhibitory currents. Both glutamate and GABA play key roles in the control of cardiovascular function in the CNS [103]. Excitatory amino acid neurotransmitters, like glutamate and aspartate, generally cause pressure responses and tachycardia, while inhibitory amino acid neurotransmitters, namely GABA and glycine, are responsible for depressing bradycardia [104]. It is well established that the excitatory amino acid glutamate is considered the main neurotransmitter of primary afferent fibers of baroreceptors to the nucleus tractus solitarii (NTS) [106]. Furthermore, an excitatory projection from NTS to the caudal ventrolateral medulla (CVLM) is an essential part of the circuit of baroreflex control. The CVLM communicates with the rostral ventrolateral medulla (RVLM) by secretion of GABA. In addition to GABAergic inhibition of RVLM, excitatory amino acids are also known to exert important roles in cardiovascular regulation [107]. These neurotransmitters can regulate vasodilatation through reduction of both sympathetic activity and baroreflex sensitivity control, by acting on regulation of both sympathetic and parasympathetic systems. Therefore, the augmented baroreflex sensitivity by i.v. injection of BPP-10c is attributted to the release of these neurotransmitters [22, 74]. These data is summarized in Figure 8.

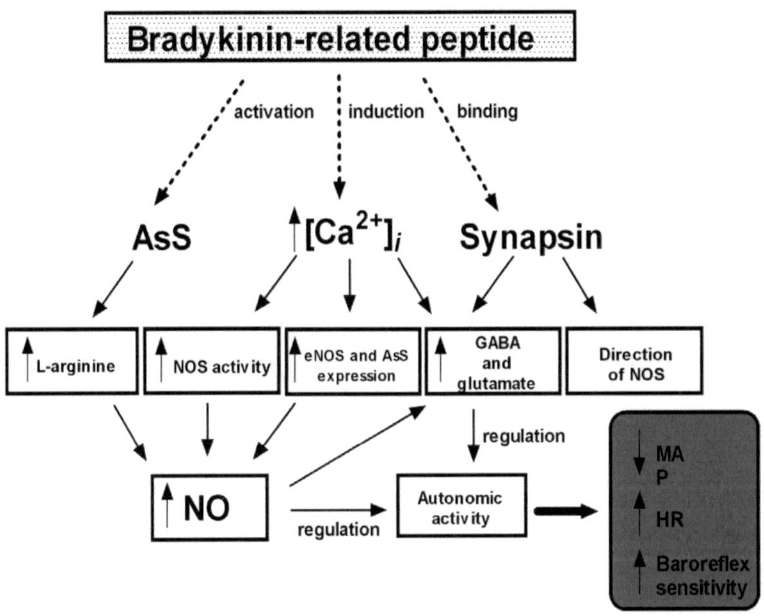

Figure 8. Schematic representation of BPP-10c mechanism of action in the CNS. According to [22, 74, 93], the proposed mechanism to explain the BPP-10c effects on the blood pressure (BP) and heart rate (HR) in spontaneously hypertensive rats (SHRs) was summarized in this figure. First, BPP-10c-induced $[Ca^{2+}]_i$ elevations activates signal transduction pathways responsible for the increased nitric oxide synthase (NOS) activity and the expression of the enzymes, namely endothelial NOS (eNOS) and argininosuccinate synthase (ASS). It also triggers the release of the neurotransmitters GABA and glutamate. After the BPP-10c internalization by neuronal cells, this peptide binds to synapsin to control the release of GABA and glutamate, and to direct the NOS to discrete cores of the neurons. Furthermore, BPP-10c can positively activate the AsS functions to increase the levels of L-arginine. NO production due to increased concentration of L-arginine, NOS activation, and increased expression of eNOS and AsS should contribute for the release of neurotransmitters and also for the regulation of autonomous activity. Likewise GABA and glutamate determine the reduction of both blood pressure and heart rate, and the increases of the baroreflex sensitivity in SHRs.

The fact of BPPs decrease the HR does not mean that its action is limited to the CNS. Taking the example of BPP-10c, *in vivo* biodistribution studies showed a significant presence of this peptide in the brain, however accumulation was also observed in the rat kidney [78]. Considering its high accumulation in kidneys with the fact that BPP-10c induces NO production in endothelial cells [20, 108] and the increase of plasma L-arginine level *in vivo* [20], we conclude that this peptide, and also potentially the other BPPs, may display both peripheral and central actions.

Moreover, there might exhist BPPs with exclusive peripheral action. As suggested for BPP-9a that promotes discret decrease of MAP and does not affect HR [75], whose effects were possible to be explained solely based on the classical mechanism of action suggested for the BPPs, *i.e.*, relying in the selective inhibition of the somatic ACE [73].

The pharmaceutical compositions for the applications in chornic-degenerative diseases and hypertension of the BPPs and their structural and/or conformational analogs, as well as the isolation and purification of BRPs secreted by snake venom glands are protected by the patents US20050031604 and US20080199503. The inventions further refer to pharmaceutical compositions that increase the biodisponibility and efficacy of BRPs peripheral and central biological activities. BRPs allowed the development a successful oral drug to treat human hypertension, but they also have the potential to become a drug by itself or a drug model to develop compouds devoted to treat central nervous system diseases, once pharmaceutical compositions that allow efficient delivery *in vivo* of these BRPs is achieved.

4.4. Mechanism of action that underlies the hyperalgesia and inflammatory responses

For many years it has been known that BK is an inflammatory mediator involved in the nociceptive process [109]. BK and also the BRPs produce pain and hyperalgesia due to their ability to excite and/or sensitize nociceptors [10].

In particular, two novel BRPs named fulvonin [SIVLRGKAPFR] and cyphokinin [DTRPPGFTPFR] were recently described in wasp (*Cyphononyx fulvognathus*). They could be structurally and functionally considered as BRPs, since they both are able to inhibit ACE as well as to induce the hyperalgesic effect in living rats after intraplantar injection, mostly due to the agonist action of these peptides on distinct B2 or B1 receptors, respectively [10].

5. Potential and effective pharmaceutical applications

5.1. Application of BPPs to treat CNS disorders and hypertension

In the last few years, as presented here, it was possible to describe a number of new mechanisms of action for BRPs previously known only as potent ACE inhibitors. Taking this into account, many pharmaceutical applications could be possible suggested for these peptides solely based on the treatment of pathologies related with their targets, for instace the somatic ACE, AsS and so on.

Regarding AsS as a novel potential target for the development of new drugs based on BPPs structural model, it is worth mentioning that its action on L-arginine metabolims contributes to three main functions in the organism, depending on the cell or tissue type involved, including effects on detoxification of ammonia in the liver, production of L-arginine in the kidney to be distributed to the whole organism, and the synthesis of L-arginine for the production of NO in several other cells [94]. In addition to these three major functions, it has also been suggested that AsS plays an important role in neuromodulation by producing argininosuccinate [110].

Due to its involvement in biochemical processes that generate physiological impacts on the organism, AsS is of great clinical value since its deficiency or excessive expression has been associated with some diseases, such as citrullinemia [111], hypertension [112, 113], and Alzheimer's disease [114, 115].

Since, AsS also participates in the L-arginine recycling, which contributes to the maintenance of NOS substrate,and AsS catalytic activity is considered the limiting step for NO production [116], the upregulation of this enzyme restores the balance of that system with consequent reduction in blood pressure [20].

Moreover, the identification of acetylcholine receptors as novel putative targets responsible for the vasodilatation promoted by the BRPs [19, 23, 75] also opens new avenues to the development of possible future therapeutic applications of BRPs related compounds for CNS diseases treatment.

Different experimental approaches demonstrate that acetylcholine muscarinic receptors are present in virtually all organs, tissues and cell types. The muscarinic receptors in the CNS are involved in the regulation of an extraordinary number of cognitive, behavioral, sensory, motor, and autonomous functions. Reduced or increased signalling of different subtypes of muscarinic receptors are involved in the pathophysiology of several diseases of the CNS including Alzheimer's and Parkinson's diseases, depression, schizophrenia, and epilepsy [117].

The contribution of the muscarinic acetylcholine receptor, mAchR-M1, in the NO production stimulated by BPP-5a is therapeutically and scientifically interesting, since much effort has been undertaken in the search for mAchR-M1 agonists to treat cognitive disorders including the Alzheimer’s disease [118, 119].

On other hand, the mAchR-M3 is mainly involved in the control of vascular tone. The main actions mediated by these peripheral muscarinic receptors include the reduction of HR, stimulation of glandular secretion, and smooth muscle relaxation [117]. Compounds that activate this receptor to promote vasorelaxation, such as pilocarpine, are used for the treatment of glaucoma, ocular hypertension [120, 121]. However, the BRPs as BPP-13a is not only able to activate mAchR-M3, but in the same time it acts modulating the AsS activity. Since both pathways contribute to the antihypertensive effects by controlling the NO production, BPP-13a represents a potent vasodilator compound with potential broader applications in the medicine [75].

Taking together, the comparison of the biological actions of BRPs found in the venom and brain of the pit viper *Bothrops jararaca* with those from different species, allowed us to describe that, contrary to what was thought for several decades, these peptides have different biological effects and therefore are an inexhaustible source of powerful biological tools not only for the study and discovery of new physiological pathways, but also as potentially useful compounds for new drug development.

Therefore, a patent protecting the use of these oligopeptides capable of binding to diverse targets, determining the increase and the sustenance of nitric oxide (NO) production in mammalian cells by potentiating the endogenous argininosuccinate synthase activity present in animal cells and/or by increasing the intracellular bivalent free calcium ion in the cytosol of cells was filed (US20100035822). Pharmaceutical compositions containing one or more of these peptides is also described and also disclosed in this same patent.

5.2. Application of BIPs in the treatment of pain and inflammation

NO is involved in vasodilatation and in many other physiological processes. Several lines of evidence have indicated that NO plays a complex and diverse role in the modulation of pain [122]. It has been shown that NO mediates the analgesic effect of opioids and other analgesic substances, opening opportunities of potential use of molecules able to regulate NO production in pain therapy. Modification of pre-existing analgesic and anti-inflammatory drugs by addition of NO-releasing moieties has been shown to improve the analgesic efficacy of these drugs, and also to reduce their side effects [123].

NO donors have also been used with opioids to reduce pain in patients with cancer [124]. This strategy enhances the analgesic efficacy of morphine in patients with cancer pain, delaying the morphine tolerance and decreasing the incidence of the adverse effects of opioids [88, 125].

Nevertheless, the use of NO donors should be carefully evaluated, since the excessive levels of NO production can be deleterious to the organism [126]. Soon, keeping NO production at a safe level, avoiding the deleterious threshold, is of particular interest.

Therefore, the BRPs that modulate AsS activity [20, 75] could be considered for pain treatment. The fact that this AsS activity interferes with L-arginine metabolism, a source of NO synthesis that has its own levels subjected to very precise mechanisms of physiological control, represents the most likely target able to regulate NO production without generating undesired reactive by-products (review by [127]).

Other family of BRPs, which should be considered in the treatment of pain and inflammation, are the antagonists of BK receptors (BIPs), namely helokinestatins. Although these BRPs were described as vasoactive peptides, due to their ability to antagonize the relaxation effect induced by BK [35, 36], they could potencially be employed in the therapy of hyperalgesia.

Kinins formed following tissue trauma and in inflammatory processes, acting by means of the activation of B2 receptors, are among the most potent endogenous algogenic mediators. Kinins through action on BK receptors can release a large number of inflammatory mediators, such as prostaglandins and neuropeptides such as neurokinins [128], that in turn amplify the nociceptive response. Therefore, these receptors play an important role in pain transmission. BK produces a short-lived hyperalgesia, while des-Arg9-BK causes a long-lasting hyperalgesia [1].

However, most of the B2 receptor antagonists present partial agonist activity and fail to produce antinociception when given orally [1]. Non-peptide B2 receptor antagonists, although they are generally less potent when compared with Hoe 140, for instance, produce long-lasting oral antinociception with no evidence of partial agonistic activity [129-131]. In this way, further studies of BRPs applied in the pain treatment could provide valuable information for the development of novel peptidic or non-peptidic molecules to effectively relieve the pain of human patients.

The BRPs isolated from toad (*Bombina maxima*) defensive skin secretion, and their analogs thereof, prodrugs including the peptides, pharmaceutical compositions are protected by patent WO2004/068928. These BRPs and analogs thereof are antagonists of B2 receptor and they can be used to treat and/or prevent disorders associated with BK, including cardiovascular disorders, inflammation, asthma, allergic rhinitis, angiogenesis, pain and related pathologies.

Author details

Claudiana Lameu[1], Márcia Neiva[2] and Mirian A. F. Hayashi[2]

1 Departamento de Bioquímica, Instituto de Química, Universidade de São Paulo, Brazil

2 Departamento de Farmacologia, Escola Paulista de Medicina (EPM), Universidade Federal de São Paulo (UNIFESP), Brazil

References

[1] Calixto JB, Cabrini DA, Ferreira J, Campos MM. Kinins in pain and inflammation. Pain. 2000 Jul;87(1):1-5.

[2] Camargo AC, Ianzer D, Guerreiro JR, Serrano SM. Bradykinin-potentiating peptides: beyond captopril. Toxicon. 2012 Mar 15;59(4):516-23.

[3] Ferreira SH, Bartelt DC, Greene LJ. Isolation of bradykinin-potentiating peptides from Bothrops jararaca venom. Biochemistry. 1970 Jun 23;9(13):2583-93.

[4] Ferreira SH, Greene LH, Alabaster VA, Bakhle YS, Vane JR. Activity of various fractions of bradykinin potentiating factor against angiotensin I converting enzyme. Nature. 1970 Jan 24;225(5230):379-80.

[5] Rocha ESM, Beraldo WT, Rosenfeld G. Bradykinin, a hypotensive and smooth muscle stimulating factor released from plasma globulin by snake venoms and by trypsin. The American Journal of Physiology. 1949 Feb;156(2):261-73.

[6] Ondetti MA, Cushman DW. Design of protease inhibitors. Biopolymers. 1981 Sep; 20(9):2001-10.

[7] Hayashi MAF, Kerkis I. Toxinas como terapêuticos. São Paulo: Roca 2008.

[8] Bekheet SH, Awadalla EA, Salman MM, Hassan MK. Bradykinin potentiating factor isolated from Buthus occitanus venom has a protective effect against cadmium-induced rat liver and kidney damage. Tissue & Cell. 2011 Dec;43(6):337-43.

[9] Conceicao K, Konno K, de Melo RL, Antoniazzi MM, Jared C, Sciani JM, et al. Isolation and characterization of a novel bradykinin potentiating peptide (BPP) from the skin secretion of Phyllomedusa hypochondrialis. Peptides. 2007 Mar;28(3):515-23.

[10] Picolo G, Hisada M, Moura AB, Machado MF, Sciani JM, Conceicao IM, et al. Bradykinin-related peptides in the venom of the solitary wasp Cyphononyx fulvognathus. Biochemical Pharmacology. 2010 Feb 1;79(3):478-86.

[11] Zeng XC, Li WX, Peng F, Zhu ZH. Cloning and characterization of a novel cDNA sequence encoding the precursor of a novel venom peptide (BmKbpp) related to a bradykinin-potentiating peptide from Chinese scorpion Buthus martensii Karsch. IUBMB Life. 2000 Mar;49(3):207-10.

[12] Higuchi S, Murayama N, Saguchi K, Ohi H, Fujita Y, Camargo AC, et al. Bradykinin-potentiating peptides and C-type natriuretic peptides from snake venom. Immunopharmacology. 1999 Oct 15;44(1-2):129-35.

[13] Gomes CL, Konno K, Conceicao IM, Ianzer D, Yamanouye N, Prezoto BC, et al. Identification of novel bradykinin-potentiating peptides (BPPs) in the venom gland of a rattlesnake allowed the evaluation of the structure-function relationship of BPPs. Biochemical Pharmacology. 2007 Nov 1;74(9):1350-60.

[14] Hayashi MA, Murbach AF, Ianzer D, Portaro FC, Prezoto BC, Fernandes BL, et al. The C-type natriuretic peptide precursor of snake brain contains highly specific inhibitors of the angiotensin-converting enzyme. Journal of Neurochemistry. 2003 May;85(4):969-77.

[15] Murayama N, Hayashi MA, Ohi H, Ferreira LA, Hermann VV, Saito H, et al. Cloning and sequence analysis of a Bothrops jararaca cDNA encoding a precursor of seven bradykinin-potentiating peptides and a C-type natriuretic peptide. Proceedings of the National Academy of Sciences of the United States of America. 1997 Feb 18;94(4): 1189-93.

[16] Fernandez JJ, Li S. An improved algorithm for anisotropic nonlinear diffusion for denoising cryo-tomograms. Journal of Structural Biology. 2003 Oct-Nov;144(1-2): 152-61.

[17] Cho Y, Somer BG, Amatya A. Natriuretic peptides and their therapeutic potential. Heart Disease (Hagerstown, Md. 1999 Nov-Dec;1(5):305-28.

[18] Komatsu Y, Nakao K, Suga S, Ogawa Y, Mukoyama M, Arai H, et al. C-type natriuretic peptide (CNP) in rats and humans. Endocrinology. 1991 Aug;129(2):1104-6.

[19] Nery AA, Trujillo CA, Lameu C, Konno K, Oliveira V, Camargo AC, et al. A novel physiological property of snake bradykinin-potentiating peptides-reversion of MK-801 inhibition of nicotinic acetylcholine receptors. Peptides. 2008 Oct;29(10): 1708-15.

[20] Guerreiro JR, Lameu C, Oliveira EF, Klitzke CF, Melo RL, Linares E, et al. Argininosuccinate synthetase is a functional target for a snake venom anti-hypertensive peptide: role in arginine and nitric oxide production. The Journal of Biological Chemistry. 2009 Jul 24;284(30):20022-33.

[21] Ianzer D, Xavier CH, Fraga FC, Lautner RQ, Guerreiro JR, Machado LT, et al. BPP-5a produces a potent and long-lasting NO-dependent antihypertensive effect. Therapeutic Advances in Cardiovascular Disease. 2011 Dec;5(6):281-95.

[22] Lameu C, Pontieri V, Guerreiro JR, Oliveira EF, da Silva CA, Giglio JM, et al. Brain nitric oxide production by a proline-rich decapeptide from Bothrops jararaca venom improves baroreflex sensitivity of spontaneously hypertensive rats. Hypertens Res. 2010 Dec;33(12):1283-8.

[23] Morais KL, Hayashi MA, Bruni FM, Lopes-Ferreira M, Camargo AC, Ulrich H, et al. Bj-PRO-5a, a natural angiotensin-converting enzyme inhibitor, promotes vasodilatation mediated by both bradykinin B(2)and M1 muscarinic acetylcholine receptors. Biochemical Pharmacology. 2011 Mar 15;81(6):736-42.

[24] Tanen DA, Ruha AM, Graeme KA, Curry SC, Fischione MA. Rattlesnake envenomations: unusual case presentations. Archives of Internal Medicine. 2001 Feb 12;161(3): 474-9.

[25] Walter FG, Bilden EF, Gibly RL. Envenomations. Critical care clinics. 1999 Apr;15(2): 353-86, ix.

[26] Ferreira SH. A Bradykinin-Potentiating Factor (BPF) Present in the venom of Bothrops jararaca. British Journal of Pharmacology and Chemotherapy. 1965 Feb; 24:163-9.

[27] Camargo AC, Graeff FG. Subcellular distribution and properties of the bradykinin inactivation system in rabbit brain homogenates. Biochemical Pharmacology. 1969 Feb;18(2):548-9.

[28] Ribeiro SA, Corrado AP, Graeff FG. Antinociceptive action of intraventricular bradykinin. Neuropharmacology. 1971 Nov;10(6):725-31.

[29] Hayashi MA, Camargo AC. The Bradykinin-potentiating peptides from venom gland and brain of Bothrops jararaca contain highly site specific inhibitors of the somatic angiotensin-converting enzyme. Toxicon. 2005 Jun 15;45(8):1163-70.

[30] Soares MR, Oliveira-Carvalho AL, Wermelinger LS, Zingali RB, Ho PL, Junqueira-de-Azevedo IL, et al. Identification of novel bradykinin-potentiating peptides and C-type natriuretic peptide from Lachesis muta venom. Toxicon. 2005 Jul;46(1):31-8.

[31] Murayama N, Michel GH, Yanoshita R, Samejima Y, Saguchi K, Ohi H, et al. cDNA cloning of bradykinin-potentiating peptides - C-type natriuretic peptide precursor, and characterization of the novel peptide Leu3-blomhotin from the venom of Agkistrodon blomhoffi. European Journal of Biochemistry / FEBS. 2000 Jul;267(13):4075-80.

[32] Ianzer D, Konno K, Marques-Porto R, Vieira Portaro FC, Stocklin R, Martins de Camargo AC, et al. Identification of five new bradykinin potentiating peptides (BPPs) from Bothrops jararaca crude venom by using electrospray ionization tandem mass spectrometry after a two-step liquid chromatography. Peptides. 2004 Jul;25(7): 1085-92.

[33] Cheung HS, Cushman DW. Inhibition of homogeneous angiotensin-converting enzyme of rabbit lung by synthetic venom peptides of Bothrops jararaca. Biochimica et Biophysica Acta. 1973 Feb 15;293(2):451-63.

[34] Ma C, Yang M, Zhou M, Wu Y, Wang L, Chen T, et al. The natriuretic peptide/helokinestatin precursor from Mexican beaded lizard (Heloderma horridum) venom: Amino acid sequence deduced from cloned cDNA and identification of two novel encoded helokinestatins. Peptides. 2011 Jun;32(6):1166-71.

[35] Kwok HF, Chen T, O'Rourke M, Ivanyi C, Hirst D, Shaw C. Helokinestatin: a new bradykinin B2 receptor antagonist decapeptide from lizard venom. Peptides. 2008 Jan;29(1):65-72.

[36] Zhang Y, Wang L, Zhou M, Zhou Z, Chen X, Chen T, et al. The structure of helokinestatin-5 and its biosynthetic precursor from Gila monster (Heloderma suspectum) venom: evidence for helokinestatin antagonism of bradykinin-induced relaxation of rat tail artery smooth muscle. Peptides. 2010 Aug;31(8):1555-61.

[37] Fry BG, Roelants K, Winter K, Hodgson WC, Griesman L, Kwok HF, et al. Novel venom proteins produced by differential domain-expression strategies in beaded lizards and gila monsters (genus Heloderma). Molecular Biology and Evolution. 2010 Feb;27(2):395-407.

[38] Fry BG, Winter K, Norman JA, Roelants K, Nabuurs RJ, van Osch MJ, et al. Functional and structural diversification of the Anguimorpha lizard venom system. Molecular Cell Proteomics. 2010 Nov;9(11):2369-90.

[39] Higuchi S, Murayama N, Saguchi K, Ohi H, Fujita Y, da Silva NJ, Jr., et al. A novel peptide from the ACEI/BPP-CNP precursor in the venom of Crotalus durissus collili-

neatus. Comparative Biochemistry and Physiology - Part C: Toxicology & Pharmacology. 2006 Oct;144(2):107-21.

[40] Fry BG, Vidal N, Norman JA, Vonk FJ, Scheib H, Ramjan SF, et al. Early evolution of the venom system in lizards and snakes. Nature. 2006 Feb 2;439(7076):584-8.

[41] Irwin DM. cDNA cloning of proglucagon from the stomach and pancreas of the dog. DNA Sequence. 2001 Nov;12(4):253-60.

[42] Ohno M, Menez R, Ogawa T, Danse JM, Shimohigashi Y, Fromen C, et al. Molecular evolution of snake toxins: is the functional diversity of snake toxins associated with a mechanism of accelerated evolution? Progress in Nucleic Acid Research and Molecular Biology. 1998;59:307-64.

[43] Takei Y. Structural and functional evolution of the natriuretic peptide system in vertebrates. International Review of Cytology. 2000;194:1-66.

[44] Sanz L, Ayvazyan N, Calvete JJ. Snake venomics of the Armenian mountain vipers Macrovipera lebetina obtusa and Vipera raddei. Journal of Proteomics. 2008 Jul 21;71(2):198-209.

[45] Schweitz H, Vigne P, Moinier D, Frelin C, Lazdunski M. A new member of the natriuretic peptide family is present in the venom of the green mamba (Dendroaspis angusticeps). The Journal of Biological Chemistry. 1992 Jul 15;267(20):13928-32.

[46] Nakashima K, Nobuhisa I, Deshimaru M, Nakai M, Ogawa T, Shimohigashi Y, et al. Accelerated evolution in the protein-coding regions is universal in crotalinae snake venom gland phospholipase A2 isozyme genes. Proceedings of the National Academy of Sciences of the United States of America. 1995 Jun 6;92(12):5605-9.

[47] Ho PL, Soares MB, Maack T, Gimenez I, Puorto G, Furtado MF, et al. Cloning of an unusual natriuretic peptide from the South American coral snake Micrurus corallinus. European Journal of Biochemistry / FEBS. 1997 Nov 15;250(1):144-9.

[48] Junqueira de Azevedo IL, Farsky SH, Oliveira ML, Ho PL. Molecular cloning and expression of a functional snake venom vascular endothelium growth factor (VEGF) from the Bothrops insularis pit viper. A new member of the VEGF family of proteins. The Journal of Biological Chemistry. 2001 Oct 26;276(43):39836-42.

[49] Eddy SR. Non-coding RNA genes and the modern RNA world. Nature Reviews. 2001 Dec;2(12):919-29.

[50] Mighell AJ, Smith NR, Robinson PA, Markham AF. Vertebrate pseudogenes. FEBS Letters. 2000 Feb 25;468(2-3):109-14.

[51] Hirotsune S. [An expressed pseudogene regulates mRNA stability of its homologous coding gene]. Tanpakushitsu Kakusan Koso. 2003 Nov;48(14):1908-12.

[52] Mignone F, Pesole G. rRNA-like sequences in human mRNAs. Applied Bioinformatics. 2002;1(3):145-54.

[53] Greene LJ, Camargo AC, Krieger EM, Stewart JM, Ferreira SH. Inhibition of the conversion of angiotensin I to II and potentiation of bradykinin by small peptides present in Bothrops jararaca venom. Circulation Research. 1972 Sep;31(9):Suppl 2:62-71.

[54] Gavras H, Brunner HR, Laragh JH, Sealey JE, Gavras I, Vukovich RA. An angiotensin converting-enzyme inhibitor to identify and treat vasoconstrictor and volume factors in hypertensive patients. The New England Journal of Medicine. 1974 Oct 17;291(16): 817-21.

[55] Gavras H, Gavras I, Textor S, Volicer L, Brunner HR, Rucinska EJ. Effect of angiotensin converting enzyme inhibition on blood pressure, plasma renin activity and plasma aldosterone in essential hypertension. The Journal of Clinical Endocrinology and Metabolism. 1978 Feb;46(2):220-6.

[56] Gavras H, Brunner HR, Laragh JH, Gavras I, Vukovich RA. The use of angiotensin-converting enzyme inhibitor in the diagnosis and treatment of hypertension. Clinical Science and Molecular Medicine. 1975 Jun;2:57s-60s.

[57] Krieger EM, Salgado HC, Assan CJ. Greene LL, Ferreira SH: Potential screening test for detection of overactivity of renin-angiotensin system. Lancet. 1971 Feb 6;1(7693): 269-71.

[58] Stewart JM, Ferreira SH, Greene LJ. Bradykinin potentiating peptide PCA-Lys-Trp-Ala-Pro. An inhibitor of the pulmonary inactivation of bradykinin and conversion of angiotensin I to II. Biochemical Pharmacology. 1971 Jul;20(7):1557-67.

[59] Cushman DW, Cheung HS, Sabo EF, Ondetti MA. Design of potent competitive inhibitors of angiotensin-converting enzyme. Carboxyalkanoyl and mercaptoalkanoyl amino acids. Biochemistry. 1977 Dec 13;16(25):5484-91.

[60] Turner AJ, Hooper NM. The angiotensin-converting enzyme gene family: genomics and pharmacology. Trends in Pharmacological Sciences. 2002 Apr;23(4):177-83.

[61] Acharya KR, Sturrock ED, Riordan JF, Ehlers MR. Ace revisited: a new target for structure-based drug design. Nat Rev Drug Discov. 2003 Nov;2(11):891-902.

[62] Kurtz A, Wagner C. Cellular control of renin secretion. The Journal of Experimental Biology. 1999 Feb;202(Pt 3):219-25.

[63] Ben-Ari ET, Garrison JC. Regulation of angiotensinogen mRNA accumulation in rat hepatocytes. The American Journal of Physiology. 1988 Jul;255(1 Pt 1):E70-9.

[64] Ng KK, Vane JR. Conversion of angiotensin I to angiotensin II. Nature. 1967 Nov 25;216(5117):762-6.

[65] de Gasparo M, Catt KJ, Inagami T, Wright JW, Unger T. International union of pharmacology. XXIII. The angiotensin II receptors. Pharmacological Reviews. 2000 Sep; 52(3):415-72.

[66] Moreau ME, Garbacki N, Molinaro G, Brown NJ, Marceau F, Adam A. The kallikrein-kinin system: current and future pharmacological targets. Journal of Pharmacological Sciences. 2005 Sep;99(1):6-38.

[67] Margolius HS. Theodore Cooper Memorial Lecture. Kallikreins and kinins. Some unanswered questions about system characteristics and roles in human disease. Hypertension. 1995 Aug;26(2):221-9.

[68] Marceau F, Bachvarov DR. Kinin receptors. Clinical Reviews in Allergy & Immunology. 1998 Winter;16(4):385-401.

[69] Wei L, Alhenc-Gelas F, Corvol P, Clauser E. The two homologous domains of human angiotensin I-converting enzyme are both catalytically active. The Journal of Biological Chemistry. 1991 May 15;266(14):9002-8.

[70] Jaspard E, Wei L, Alhenc-Gelas F. Differences in the properties and enzymatic specificities of the two active sites of angiotensin I-converting enzyme (kininase II). Studies with bradykinin and other natural peptides. The Journal of Biological Chemistry. 1993 May 5;268(13):9496-503.

[71] Rousseau A, Michaud A, Chauvet MT, Lenfant M, Corvol P. The hemoregulatory peptide N-acetyl-Ser-Asp-Lys-Pro is a natural and specific substrate of the N-terminal active site of human angiotensin-converting enzyme. The Journal of Biological Chemistry. 1995 Feb 24;270(8):3656-61.

[72] Camargo A, Ferreira SH. Action of bradykinin potentiating factor (BPF) and dimercaprol (BAL) on the responses to bradykinin of isolated preparations of rat intestines. British Journal of Pharmacology. 1971 Jun;42(2):305-7.

[73] Cotton J, Hayashi MA, Cuniasse P, Vazeux G, Ianzer D, De Camargo AC, et al. Selective inhibition of the C-domain of angiotensin I converting enzyme by bradykinin potentiating peptides. Biochemistry. 2002 May 14;41(19):6065-71.

[74] Lameu C, Hayashi MA, Guerreiro JR, Oliveira EF, Lebrun I, Pontieri V, et al. The central nervous system as target for antihypertensive actions of a proline-rich peptide from Bothrops jararaca venom. Cytometry A. 2010 Mar;77(3):220-30.

[75] Morais KLP, Ianzer D, Santos RAS, Miranda JRR, Melo RL, Guerreiro JR, et al. The structural diversity of proline-rich oligopeptides from Bothrops jararaca (Bj-PROs) provides synergistic cardiovascular actions Hypertension Research. submitted.

[76] Mueller S, Gothe R, Siems WD, Vietinghoff G, Paegelow I, Reissmann S. Potentiation of bradykinin actions by analogues of the bradykinin potentiating nonapeptide BPP9alpha. Peptides. 2005 Jul;26(7):1235-47.

[77] Ianzer D, Santos RA, Etelvino GM, Xavier CH, de Almeida Santos J, Mendes EP, et al. Do the cardiovascular effects of angiotensin-converting enzyme (ACE) I involve ACE-independent mechanisms? new insights from proline-rich peptides of Bothrops

jararaca. The Journal of Pharmacology and Experimental Therapeutics. 2007 Aug; 322(2):795-805.

[78] Silva CA, Portaro FC, Fernandes BL, Ianzer DA, Guerreiro JR, Gomes CL, et al. Tissue distribution in mice of BPP 10c, a potent proline-rich anti-hypertensive peptide of Bothrops jararaca. Toxicon. 2008 Mar 15;51(4):515-23.

[79] Flam BR, Eichler DC, Solomonson LP. Endothelial nitric oxide production is tightly coupled to the citrulline-NO cycle. Nitric Oxide. 2007 Nov-Dec;17(3-4):115-21.

[80] Shen LJ, Beloussow K, Shen WC. Accessibility of endothelial and inducible nitric oxide synthase to the intracellular citrulline-arginine regeneration pathway. Biochemical Pharmacology. 2005 Jan 1;69(1):97-104.

[81] Ignarro LJ, Byrns RE, Wood KS. Endothelium-dependent modulation of cGMP levels and intrinsic smooth muscle tone in isolated bovine intrapulmonary artery and vein. Circulation Research. 1987 Jan;60(1):82-92.

[82] Finkbeiner S, Greenberg ME. Spatial features of calcium-regulated gene expression. Bioessays. 1997 Aug;19(8):657-60.

[83] Bianchi A, Evans DB, Cobb M, Peschka MT, Schaeffer TR, Laffan RJ. Inhibition by SQ 20881 of vasopressor response to angiotensin I in conscious animals. European Journal of Pharmacology. 1973 Jul;23(1):90-6.

[84] Bunag RD, Walaszek EJ, Mueting N. Sex differences in reflex tachycardia induced by hypotensive drugs in unanesthetized rats. The American Journal of Physiology. 1975 Sep;229(3):652-6.

[85] Krieger EM. Neurogenic Hypertension in the Rat. Circulation research. 1964 Dec; 15:511-21.

[86] Chapleau MW, Li Z, Meyrelles SS, Ma X, Abboud FM. Mechanisms determining sensitivity of baroreceptor afferents in health and disease. Annals of the New York Academy of Sciences. 2001 Jun;940:1-19.

[87] Michelini LC. Regulação neuro-humoral da pressão arterial. Rio de Janeiro: Ghuanabar Kogan 1999.

[88] Lanfranchi PA, Somers VK. Arterial baroreflex function and cardiovascular variability: interactions and implications. American Journal of Physiology. 2002 Oct; 283(4):R815-26.

[89] Irigoyen MC, Moreira ED, Werner A, Ida F, Pires MD, Cestari IA, et al. Aging and baroreflex control of RSNA and heart rate in rats. American Journal of Physiology. 2000 Nov;279(5):R1865-71.

[90] Schlaich MP, Lambert E, Kaye DM, Krozowski Z, Campbell DJ, Lambert G, et al. Sympathetic augmentation in hypertension: role of nerve firing, norepinephrine reuptake, and Angiotensin neuromodulation. Hypertension. 2004 Feb;43(2):169-75.

[91] Velden M, Karemaker JM, Wolk C, Schneider R. Inferring vagal effects on the heart from changes in cardiac cycle length: implications for cycle time-dependency. Int J Psychophysiol. 1990 Nov;10(1):85-93.

[92] Somsen RJ, Jennings JR, Van der Molen MW. The cardiac cycle time effect revisited: temporal dynamics of the central-vagal modulation of heart rate in human reaction time tasks. Psychophysiology. 2004 Nov;41(6):941-53.

[93] Lameu C. The central nervous system as target for anti-hypertensive actions of a proline-rich peptide from Bothrops jararaca venom [PhD thesis, Tese para obtenção do título doutor em ciências (bioquímica)]. São Paulo: Universidade de São Paulo; 2009.

[94] Husson A, Brasse-Lagnel C, Fairand A, Renouf S, Lavoinne A. Argininosuccinate synthetase from the urea cycle to the citrulline-NO cycle. European Journal of Biochemistry / FEBS. 2003 May;270(9):1887-99.

[95] Bredt DS, Snyder SH. Isolation of nitric oxide synthetase, a calmodulin-requiring enzyme. Proceedings of the National Academy of Sciences of the United States of America. 1990 Jan;87(2):682-5.

[96] Sears CE, Ashley EA, Casadei B. Nitric oxide control of cardiac function: is neuronal nitric oxide synthase a key component? Philosophical transactions of the Royal Society of London. 2004 Jun 29;359(1446):1021-44.

[97] Umans JG, Levi R. Nitric oxide in the regulation of blood flow and arterial pressure. Annual Review of Physiology. 1995;57:771-90.

[98] Bolotina VM, Najibi S, Palacino JJ, Pagano PJ, Cohen RA. Nitric oxide directly activates calcium-dependent potassium channels in vascular smooth muscle. Nature. 1994 Apr 28;368(6474):850-3.

[99] Murphy ME, Brayden JE. Nitric oxide hyperpolarizes rabbit mesenteric arteries via ATP-sensitive potassium channels. The Journal of Physiology. 1995 Jul 1;486 (Pt 1): 47-58.

[100] Garthwaite J, Boulton CL. Nitric oxide signaling in the central nervous system. Annual Review of Physiology. 1995;57:683-706.

[101] Patel KP, Li YF, Hirooka Y. Role of nitric oxide in central sympathetic outflow. Experimental Biology and Medicine (Maywood, NJ. 2001 Oct;226(9):814-24.

[102] Pontieri V, Venezuela MK, Scavone C, Michelini LC. Role of endogenous nitric oxide in the nucleus tratus solitarii on baroreflex control of heart rate in spontaneously hypertensive rats. Journal of Hypertension. 1998 Dec;16(12 Pt 2):1993-9.

[103] Gordon FJ, Sved AF. Neurotransmitters in central cardiovascular regulation: glutamate and GABA. Clinical and Experimental Pharmacology & Physiology. 2002 May-Jun;29(5-6):522-4.

[104] Kishi T, Hirooka Y, Sakai K, Shigematsu H, Shimokawa H, Takeshita A. Overexpression of eNOS in the RVLM causes hypotension and bradycardia via GABA release. Hypertension. 2001 Oct;38(4):896-901.

[105] Jaffrey SR, Erdjument-Bromage H, Ferris CD, Tempst P, Snyder SH. Protein S-nitrosylation: a physiological signal for neuronal nitric oxide. Nature Cell Biology. 2001 Feb;3(2):193-7.

[106] Lawrence AJ, Jarrott B. Neurochemical modulation of cardiovascular control in the nucleus tractus solitarius. Progress in Neurobiology. 1996 Jan;48(1):21-53.

[107] Ito S, Sved AF. Tonic glutamate-mediated control of rostral ventrolateral medulla and sympathetic vasomotor tone. The American Journal of Physiology. 1997 Aug; 273(2 Pt 2):R487-94.

[108] Benedetti G, Morais KL, Guerreiro JR, de Oliveira EF, Hoshida MS, Oliveira L, et al. Bothrops jararaca peptide with anti-hypertensive action normalizes endothelium dysfunction involved in physiopathology of preeclampsia. PloS One. 2011;6(8):e23680.

[109] Dray A, Perkins M. Bradykinin and inflammatory pain. Trends in Neurosciences. 1993 Mar;16(3):99-104.

[110] Nakamura H, Saheki T, Ichiki H, Nakata K, Nakagawa S. Immunocytochemical localization of argininosuccinate synthetase in the rat brain. The Journal of Comparative Neurology. 1991 Oct 22;312(4):652-79.

[111] Curis E, Nicolis I, Moinard C, Osowska S, Zerrouk N, Benazeth S, et al. Almost all about citrulline in mammals. Amino Acids. 2005 Nov;29(3):177-205.

[112] Dusse LM, Lwaleed BA, Silva RM, Cooper AJ, Carvalho MG. Nitric oxide in preeclampsia: be careful with the results! European Journal of Obstetrics, Gynecology, and Reproductive Biology. 2008 Jun;138(2):242-3.

[113] Panza JA. Endothelial dysfunction in essential hypertension. Clinical Cardiology. 1997 Nov;20(11 Suppl 2):II-26-33.

[114] Haas J, Storch-Hagenlocher B, Biessmann A, Wildemann B. Inducible nitric oxide synthase and argininosuccinate synthetase: co-induction in brain tissue of patients with Alzheimer's dementia and following stimulation with beta-amyloid 1-42 in vitro. Neuroscience Letters. 2002 Apr 5;322(2):121-5.

[115] Wiesinger H. Arginine metabolism and the synthesis of nitric oxide in the nervous system. Progress in Neurobiology. 2001 Jul;64(4):365-91.

[116] Solomonson LP, Flam BR, Pendleton LC, Goodwin BL, Eichler DC. The caveolar nitric oxide synthase/arginine regeneration system for NO production in endothelial cells. The Journal of Experimental Biology. 2003 Jun;206(Pt 12):2083-7.

[117] Wess J. Muscarinic acetylcholine receptor knockout mice: novel phenotypes and clinical implications. Annual Review of Pharmacology and Toxicology. 2004;44:423-50.

[118] Conn PJ, Jones CK, Lindsley CW. Subtype-selective allosteric modulators of muscarinic receptors for the treatment of CNS disorders. Trends in Pharmacological Sciences. 2009 Mar;30(3):148-55.

[119] Fisher A, Pittel Z, Haring R, Bar-Ner N, Kliger-Spatz M, Natan N, et al. M1 muscarinic agonists can modulate some of the hallmarks in Alzheimer's disease: implications in future therapy. J Mol Neurosci. 2003;20(3):349-56.

[120] Costagliola C, dell'Omo R, Romano MR, Rinaldi M, Zeppa L, Parmeggiani F. Pharmacotherapy of intraocular pressure: part I. Parasympathomimetic, sympathomimetic and sympatholytics. Expert opinion on Pharmacotherapy. 2009 Nov;10(16): 2663-77.

[121] Hurvitz LM, Kaufman PL, Robin AL, Weinreb RN, Crawford K, Shaw B. New developments in the drug treatment of glaucoma. Drugs. 1991 Apr;41(4):514-32.

[122] Cury Y, Picolo G, Gutierrez VP, Ferreira SH. Pain and analgesia: The dual effect of nitric oxide in the nociceptive system. Nitric Oxide. 2011 Oct 30;25(3):243-54.

[123] Stefano F, Distrutti E. Cyclo-oxygenase (COX) inhibiting nitric oxide donating (CINODs) drugs: a review of their current status. Current topics in Medicinal Chemistry. 2007;7(3):277-82.

[124] Toda N, Kishioka S, Hatano Y, Toda H. Modulation of opioid actions by nitric oxide signaling. Anesthesiology. 2009 Jan;110(1):166-81.

[125] Lauretti GR, Lima IC, Reis MP, Prado WA, Pereira NL. Oral ketamine and transdermal nitroglycerin as analgesic adjuvants to oral morphine therapy for cancer pain management. Anesthesiology. 1999 Jun;90(6):1528-33.

[126] Ridnour LA, Thomas DD, Mancardi D, Espey MG, Miranda KM, Paolocci N, et al. The chemistry of nitrosative stress induced by nitric oxide and reactive nitrogen oxide species. Putting perspective on stressful biological situations. Biological Chemistry. 2004 Jan;385(1):1-10.

[127] Lameu C, de Camargo AC, Faria M. L-arginine signalling potential in the brain: the peripheral gets central. Recent Patents on CNS Drug Discovery. 2009 Jun;4(2):137-42.

[128] Dray A, Perkins M. Kinins and pain.: London: Academic Press 1997.

[129] Burgess GM, Perkins MN, Rang HP, Campbell EA, Brown MC, McIntyre P, et al. Bradyzide, a potent non-peptide B(2) bradykinin receptor antagonist with long-lasting oral activity in animal models of inflammatory hyperalgesia. British Journal of Pharmacology. 2000 Jan;129(1):77-86.

[130] de Campos RO, Alves RV, Ferreira J, Kyle DJ, Chakravarty S, Mavunkel BJ, et al. Oral antinociception and oedema inhibition produced by NPC 18884, a non-peptidic

bradykinin B2 receptor antagonist. Naunyn-Schmiedeberg's Archives of Pharmacology. 1999 Sep;360(3):278-86.

[131] Griesbacher T, Amann R, Sametz W, Diethart S, Juan H. The nonpeptide B2 receptor antagonist FR173657: inhibition of effects of bradykinin related to its role in nociception. British Journal of Pharmacology. 1998 Jul;124(6):1328-34.

[132] Burnett JC, Jr. Vasopeptidase inhibition: a new concept in blood pressure management. J Hypertens Suppl. 1999 Feb;17(1):S37-43.

[133] Couture R, Girolami JP. Putative roles of kinin receptors in the therapeutic effects of angiotensin 1-converting enzyme inhibitors in diabetes mellitus. European Journal of Pharmacology. 2004 Oct 1;500(1-3):467-85.

[134] Santos RA, Frezard F, Ferreira AJ. Angiotensin-(1-7): blood, heart, and blood vessels. Current Medicinal Chemistry. 2005 Oct;3(4):383-91.

Chapter 6

Serine proteases — Cloning, Expression and Potential Applications

Camila Miyagui Yonamine, Álvaro Rossan de Brandão Prieto da Silva and Geraldo Santana Magalhães

Additional information is available at the end of the chapter

http://dx.doi.org/10.5772/53063

1. Introduction

1.1. Snake venom serine proteases

Serine proteases have been isolated from the venoms of viperidae snakes [1, 2] and affect several physiological processes such as the coagulation cascade. These enzymes are called snake venom serine proteases (SVSPs), they are multi-functional proteins with a catalytic triad formed by HDS amino acids [3].

The SVSPs resembles at least in part thrombin, a multifunctional protease that plays a key role in coagulation. Therefore these enzymes are denominated snake venom thrombin-like enzymes (SVTLEs), and are widely distributed in the venoms of several genera [4,5]. While thrombin is able to cleave both fibrinopeptide A (FPA) and fibrinopeptide B (FPB) from fibrinogen leading the formation of fibrin and activating factor XIII, some actions of SVTLEs usually cleave FPA alone and only a few cleave FPB. Thus, without cleavage of both FPA and FPB they are unable to activate factor XIII producing fibrin monomers that are not cross-linked, leading to clots markedly susceptible to digestion by plasmin and are rapidly removed from circulation by either reticuloendothelial phagocitosis and/or normal fibrinolysis. This process causes a breakdown in the fibrinolytic system and effective removal of fibrinogen from the plasma [6].

2. Body

There are three groups of snake venom fibrinogen clotting enzymes based on the rates of release of fibrinopeptides A and/or B from fibrinogen. In addition to SVLTEs, other SVSPs groups are active in other parts of the coagulation cascade, such as kallikrein-like enzymes (KN); plasminogen activators (PA); protein C like enzyme and factor V activators. One group releases fibrinopeptide A preferentially (the venombin A group including ancrod from venom of the Malayan pit viper, *Calloselasma rhodostoma*); another group releases both fibrinopeptides A and B (the venombin AB group including halystase and calobin from *Agkistrodon halys blomhoffii* and *Agkistrodon caliginosus*, respectively) and the third group releases fibrinopeptide B preferentially (the venombin B group including v enzyme from venom of the southern copperhead, *Agkistrodon contortrix contortrix*) [5,7,8]. Figure 1 summarizes some snake toxins that affect the blood coagulation cascade, based on [6].

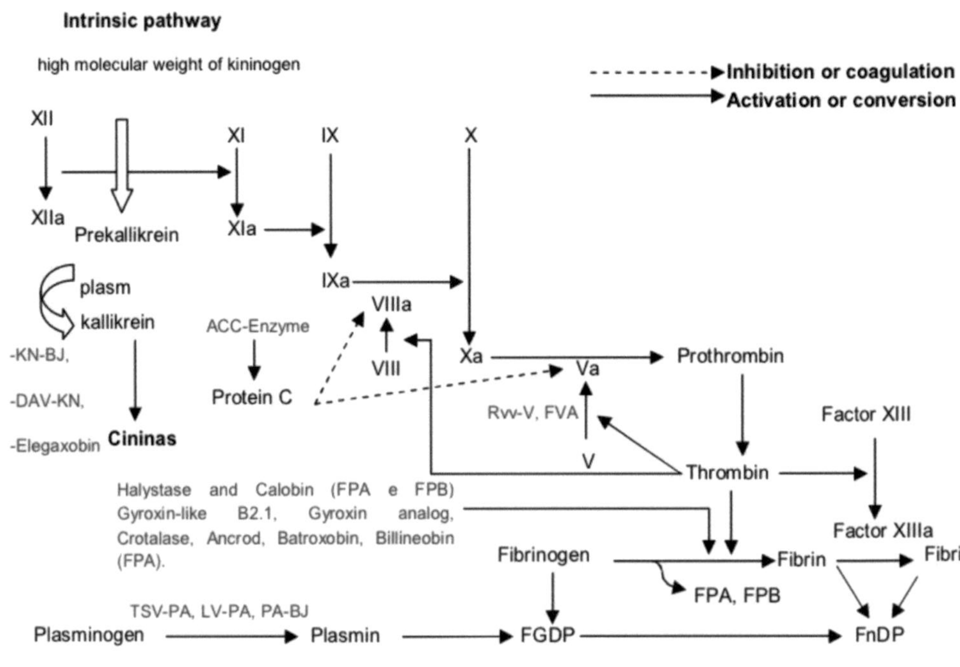

Figure 1. Some SVSPs acting in blood system. FGDP: Fibrinogen degradation products; FNDP: Fibrin degradation products; FPA: Fibrinopeptide A; FPB: Fibrinopeptide B. **KN-BJ**, *Bothrops jararaca* (O13069) [9]; **Dav-KN**, *Agkistrodon acutus* (Q9I8X0) [10]; **Elegaxobin-1**, *Trimeresurus elegans* (P84788) [11]; **ACC-C Protein C activator;** *Agkistrodon contortrix contortrix* (P09872) [12]; **RVV-Vα** Russel's viper venom FV activator alpha, *Daboia russelli siamensis* (P18964) [13]; **FVA Factor V-activating enzyme**, *Vipera lebetina* (Q9PT41) [14]; **Halystase**, *Agkistrodon halys blomhoffii* (P81176) [15]; **Calobin**, *Agkistrodon caliginosus* (Q91053) [16], **Gyroxin-like B2.1**, *Crotalus durissus terrificus* (Q58G94) [17]; **Gyroxin analog**, *Lachesis muta muta* (P33589) [18]; **Crotalase**, *Crotalus adamanteus* [19]; **Ancrod**, *Agkistrodon rhodostoma* (P26324) [20]; **Batroxobin**, *Bothrops atrox* (P04971) [21]; **Bilineobin**, *Agkistrodon bilineatus* (Q9PSN3) [22];**TSV-PA**, *Trimeresurus stejnegeri* (Q91516) [23]; **LV-PA**, *Lachesis muta muta* (P84036) [24]; **PA-BJ**, *Bothrops jararaca* (P81824) [25]. Toxin names were indicated in bold followed by snake species in italic and the Swissprot accession numbers were represented in parenthesis.

The major symptoms from snakebite affecting the haemostatic system are: (a) reduced coagulability of blood, resulting in an increased tendency to bleed, (b) bleeding due to the damage to blood vessels, (c) secondary effects of increased bleeding, ranging from hypovolaemic shock to secondary-organ damage, such as intracerebral haemorrhage, anterior pituitary haemorrhage or renal damage and (d) direct pathologic thrombosis and its sequelae, particularly pulmonary embolism [26].

The venom fibrinogenolytic serine proteases as well as the venom plasminogen activator, share extensive sequence homology with the thrombin-like venom serine proteases [27] such as ancrod [20, 28], batroxobin [21, 29], crotalase [30,31], gyroxin-like serine proteases [17], kallikrein-like enzyme from *Crotalus atrox* [32] and the protein C activator from *A. c. contortrix* [33] venoms.

The SVSPs share the conserved catalytic triad formed by the amino acids His, Asp and Ser, six disulfide bonds and global highly similarities, as seen in Figure 2. In this alignment, the deduced amino amino acid sequences of gyroxin-like B2.1, B1.3, B1.4, and B1.7 are highly similar to other SVSPs with several biological functions [17].

In order to predict the biological function of SVSPs, a functional dendrogram was generated based on the amino acid sequence alignment from Figure 2. Clearly there are subtle differences among these homologous enzymes that may explain different functions such as: fibrinogenolytic (group I), Aα fibrinogenases (subgroup I a), Protein C activator and CPI-enzyme (subgroup I b), kininogenases (subgroup I c), plasminogen activator (group II), factor V activators (group III) thrombin-like, or other specific enzymatic activities (Figure 3) [17].

Despite significant sequence identity (50–70%), SVSPs display high specificity toward distinct macromolecular substrates. Based on their biological roles, they have been classified as activators of the fibrinolytic system, procoagulant, anticoagulant and platelet-aggregating enzymes [34]. The procoagulant SVSPs activate FVII, FX and prothrombin [35] and shorten the coagulation times, while the anticoagulants inactivates factors Va and VIIIa and plays a key role in controlling haemostasis, Ancrod (from the Malayan pit viper, *Calloselasma rhodostoma*), in particular, has been used as an anticoagulant to achieve "therapeutic defibrination" [34].

As it can be seen in Figure 4 (top), the 3D model of gyroxin-like B2.1 shows the catalytic site (Ser184, His43 and Asp88) superimposed with the catalytic site of thrombin (Ser_{195}, His_{57} and Asp_{102}) [36]. The overall structure (bottom) show the typical fold of a serine proteinase in which the active-site cleft is located at the junction of the two six-stranded β-barrels. Among the conserved 3D structural features between trypsin-like enzyme and SVSPs are the two β-barrel subdomains, the orientation of catalytic site and the pattern of Cys residues. In contrast with other serine proteases, a unique long C-terminal tail of gyroxin are highly conserved only on SVSPs. In addition, SVSPs are active only as a single chain enzyme while prothrombin is activated by Factor Xa generating the Light (L) and Heavy (H) chains of active thrombin.

2.1. The role of Protease Activated Receptor (PAR) on serine protease coagulation

Protease-activated receptors (PARs) are members of family of seven-transmembrane G-protein-coupled receptors (GPCRs). The activation is triggered by the cleavage of the N-terminus of the receptor by a serine protease, resulting in the generation of a new tethered ligand that interacts with the receptor within its extracellular loop-2. This ligand binding to

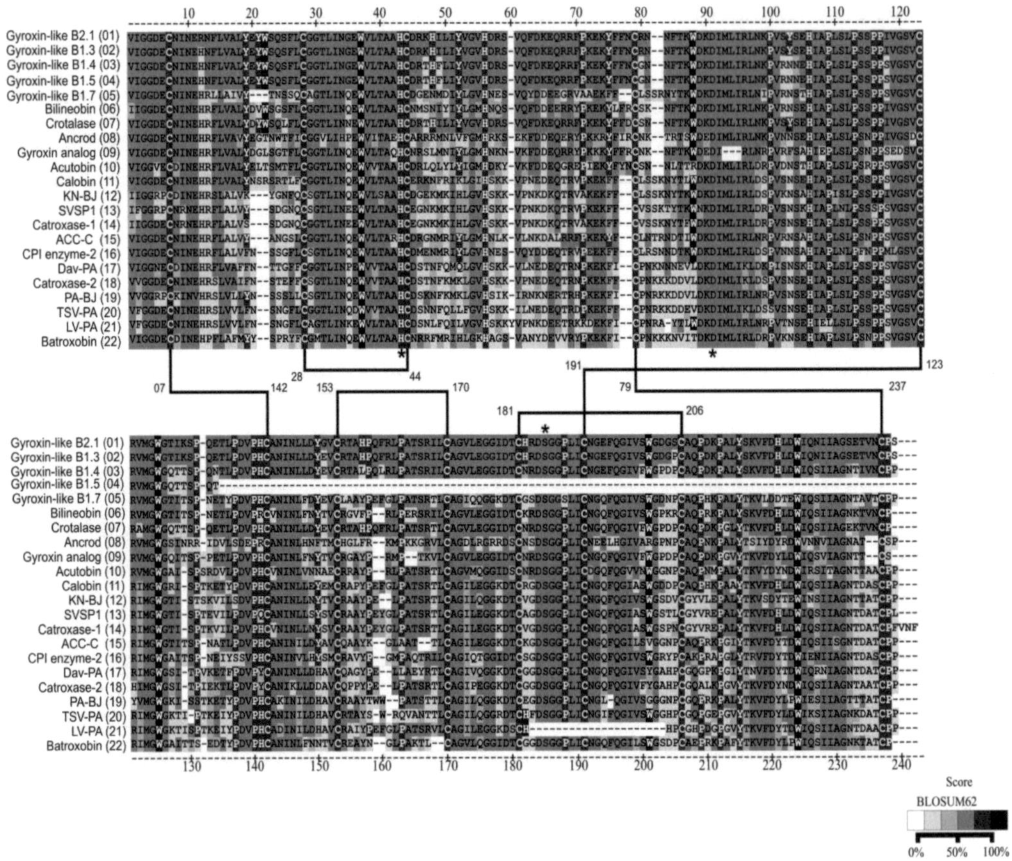

Figure 2. Alignment of snake venom serine proteases 1-5) Gyroxin-like B2.1, B1.3, B1.4, B1.5, B1.7 from *Crotalus durissus terrificus* (Q58G94, B0FXM1, B0FXM2, EU360953, B0FXM3, respectively). 6) Bilineobin from *Agkistrodon bilineatus* (Q9PSN3). 7) Crotalase from *Crotalus adamanteus*. 8) Ancrod from *Agkistrodon rhodostoma* (P26324). 9) Gyroxin analog from *Lachesis muta muta* (P33589). 10) Acutobin from *Agkistrodon acutus* (Q9I8X2). 11) Calobin from *Agkistrodon caliginosus* (Q91053). 12) KN-BJ from *Bothrops jararaca* (O13069). 13) SVSP-1 Venom serine proteinase from *Crotalus adamanteus* (Q8UUK2). 14) Catroxase-1 from *Crotalus atrox* (Q8QHK3). 15) ACC-C Protein C activator from *Agkistrodon contortrix contortrix* (P09872). 16) CPI enzyme from *Agkistrodon caliginosus* (O42207). 17) Dav-PA from *Agkistrodon acutus* (Q9I8X1). 18) Catroxase-2 from *Crotalus atrox* (Q8QHK2). 19) PA-BJ from *Bothrops jararaca* (P81824). 20) TSV-PA from *Trimeresurus stejnegeri* (Q91516). 21) LV-PA from *Lachesis muta muta* (P84036). 22) Batroxobin from *Bothrops atrox* (P04971). Indicated accession numbers are from Swissprot. The lines indicate the disulfide bonds and the catalytic triad (His, Asp and Ser) are represented by *. Toxin names were indicated in bold followed by snake species in italic and the Swissprot accession numbers were represented in parenthesis.

the core of PARs initiates an intracellular signal transduction pathway, which stimulates phosphoinositide breakdown and cytosolic calcium mobilization [37].

There are four PARs (PAR-1, PAR-2, PAR-3 and PAR-4), PAR-1, PAR-3 and PAR-4 can be activated by thrombin while PAR-2 is activated by trypsin and trypsin-like proteases, but not by thrombin [38]. PAR-1 is important for activation of human platelets by thrombin, but plays no apparent role in mouse platelet activation [39]. The consensus sequence among all the

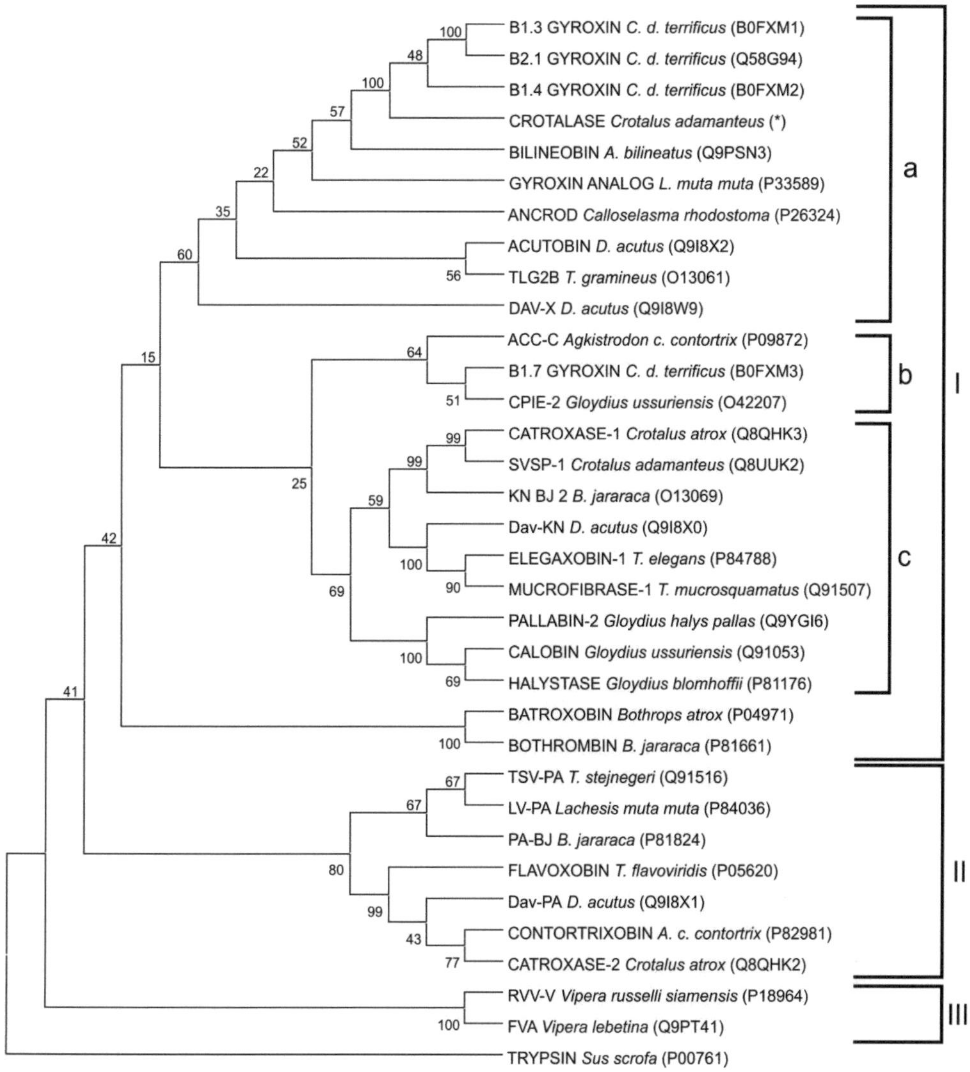

Figure 3. Dendrogram of 34 mature snake venom serine proteases. Toxin names were indicated in bold followed by snake species in italic and the Swissprot accession numbers were represented in parenthesis. (*) Crotalase toxin sequence was based on [19]. All positions containing gaps and missing data were eliminated from the dataset. There were a total of 188 positions in the final dataset. The distance was calculated by number of amino-acid differences. The optimal tree with the sum of branch length = 796.39 and the percentage of replicate trees in which the associated taxa clustered together in the bootstrap test (500 replicates) are shown next to the branches. Fibrinogenolytic (group I), Aα fibrinogenases (subgroup I a), Protein C activator and CPI-enzyme (subgroup I b), kininogenases (subgroup I c), plasminogen activator (group II), factor V activators (group III).

human PAR-1 activating peptides is XFXXR, indicating that the second residue (Phe) and fifth residue (Arg) are critical for the agonist binding and activation [40].

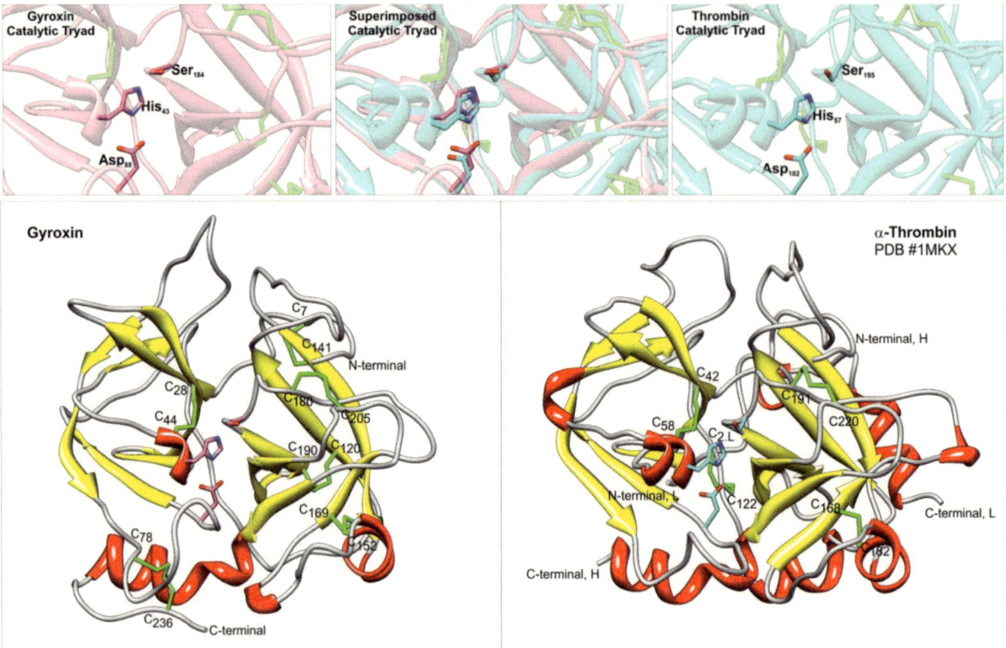

Figure 4. Gyroxin and bovine a-Thrombin (1mkx). The gyroxin homology model was based on crystallographic structures of *Trimeresurus stejnejeri* TSV-PA (1bqy), *Agkistrodon acutus* AaV-SP I (1op0) and *Agkistrodon acutus* AaV-SP II- DAV-PA (1op2). Top: Catalytic tryad superimposition of gyroxin residues (pink) and α-thrombin (blue). Bottom: Two β-barrel domains formed by β-sheets are depicted in yellow and α-helixes in red. Disulfid bridges are depicted in green. The residues from active site are showed in pink to gyroxin molecule and blue to activated thrombin.The C-teminus and N-terminus are indicated to both thrombin heavy (H) and ligth (L) chains and to gyroxin model.

It is known that the inhibitory effects of PAR1 antagonists on platelet aggregation caused by high concentrations of thrombin are limited but can be enhanced by combination with PAR4-blocking antibody, suggesting that simultaneous blockade of PAR1 and PAR4 may provide more effective antithrombotic therapy [41].

An example of snake venom serine protease that acts on coagulation through PAR is gyroxin (serine protease from *C.d.terrificus*) that promotes platelet aggregation through its involvement with PAR 1 and 4 [42]. In fact, a significant inhibition of the maximum platelet aggregation effect induced by gyroxin was observed in the presence of inhibitors of both PAR-1 [SCH79797] and PAR-4 [tcY-NH_2]. PAR-1 inhibitor was effective at concentration of about two orders of magnitude below than that required for PAR-4 inhibitor, and the combination of these two inhibitors were not capable to completely inhibit the platelet aggregation induced by gyroxin [42].

2.2. Molecular biology of SVSPs

Batroxobin (*Bothrops atrox* serine protease, E 3C.4.21.29) is a thrombin-like enzyme derived from *Bothrops atrox, moojeni* venom. In contrast to thrombin which converts fibrino-

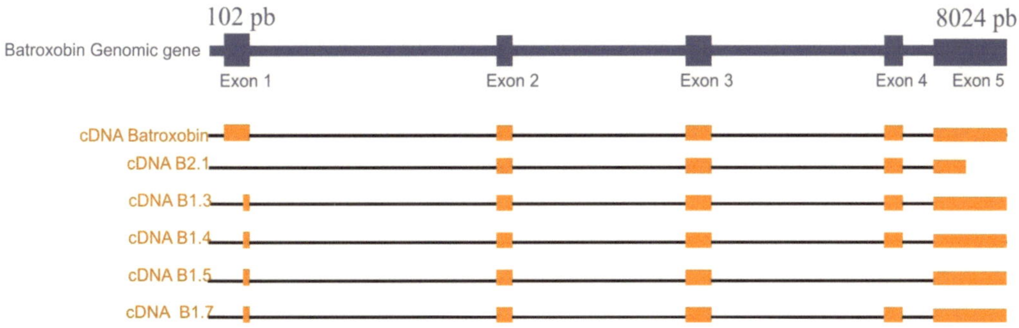

Figure 5. Organization of the batroxobin genomic gene, cDNA of Batroxobin and gyroxin-like B2.1, B.1.3, B1.4, B1.5 and B1.7 from *C.d.terrificus.*Blue boxes denote the location of exons of batroxobin genomic gene (X12747), the blue bars denote noncoding regions of introns. Orange boxes denote the location of exons of cDNA of Batroxobin (J02684) and gyroxin-like B1.3, B1.4, B1.5, B1.7 from *C.d.terrificus* (EU360951; EU360952; EU360953 and EU360954, respectively). In case of clone B2.1, only a partial sequence was obtained (GenBank accession number AY954040). The lack of exon 4 in B1.5 clone is because this clone is truncated by the insertion of a stop codon in translated sequence at the position 472 pb due to the joining of the exon 3 and exon 5.

gen into fibrin by splitting off fibrinopeptides A and B, batroxobin only splits off fibrinopeptide A [43].

Batroxobin gene spans 8 kilobase pairs and contains five exons and its mature form is encoded by exons 2 to 5. The catalytic residues of batroxobin, His-41, Asp-86, and Ser-178, are encoded by separate exons, exons 2, 3, and 5, respectively [44].

The exon/intron organization of the batroxobin gene is different from that of the prothrombin gene but very similar to those of the trypsin and kallikrein genes. These results indicate that batroxobin is not a member of the prothrombin family but one of the trypsin kallikrein family. The snake venom gland is assumed to originate from the submaxillary gland. Therefore, batroxobin is expected to be a member of the glandular kallikrein family [44].

cDNA libraries of snake venom glands have been constructed from various species and several clones encoding SVSPs have been isolated and sequenced. SVSPs are one chain proteins encoded by cDNAs containing an open reading frame (ORF) around 800 bp. The 5′UTRs (5 ′untranslated region) are usually short while the 3′UTRs (3′untranslated region) vary in length and may contain more than 1200 nucleotides [3].

Snake venom serine protease are synthesized as zymogens of ~256–257 amino acids with a putative signal peptide of 18 amino acids and a proposed activation peptide of six amino acid residues [3]. In the process of protein export, a central role is played by the signal sequence: an N-terminal segment that somehow initiates export whereupon it is cleaved from the zymogen. Three structurally dissimilar regions have been recognized so far: a positively charged N-terminal region, a central hydrophobic region and a more polar C-terminal region that seems to define the cleavage site [45].

The organization of batroxobin gene, batroxobin cDNA and gyroxin-like B2.1, B1.3, B1.5 and B1.7 [17, 36, 44] are shown in Figure 5.

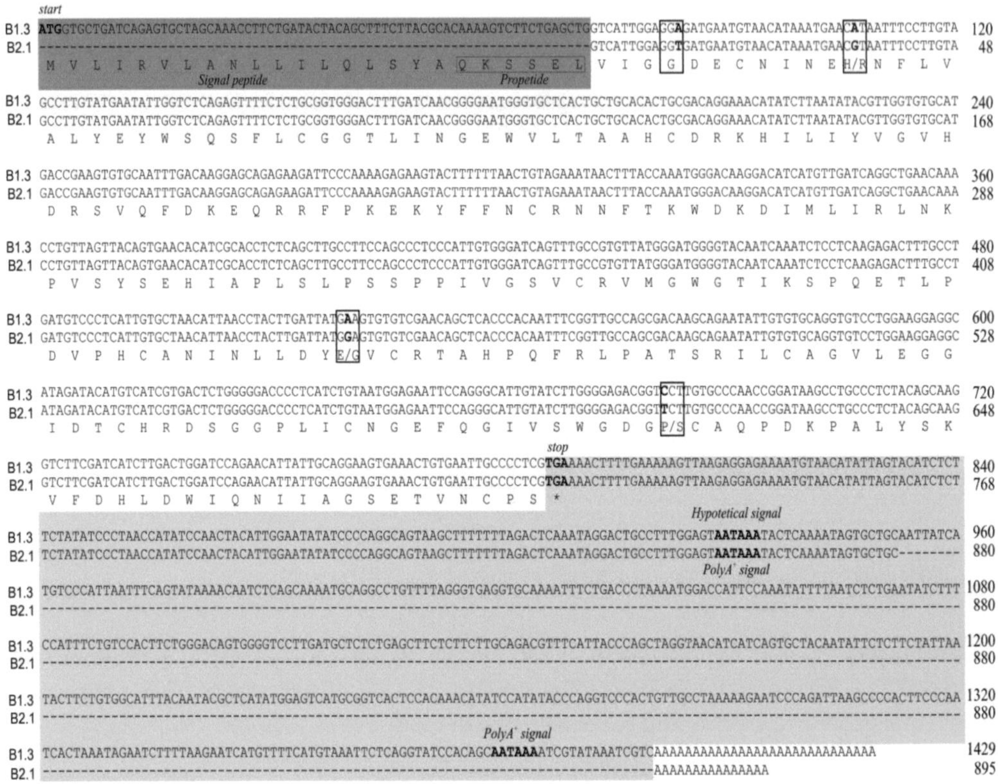

Figure 6. Alignment of nucleotide sequences from gyroxin-like B1.3 (EU360951) and B2.1 (AY954040). Coding region for signal peptide and propeptide is indicated in dark grey. Start codon and stop codons are in bold. The mature coding region is indicated in white. The mutations between B1.3 and B2.1 sequences are indicated by a box line and differences in nucleotides are in bold. Light grey encompasses the 3′ UTR. B1.3 hypothetical poly A+ signal (929–934 bp), B1.3 poly A+ signal (1380–1385 bp) and B2.1 poly A+ signal (857–862 bp) are in bold. Dashes represent gaps introduced for optimal sequence alignment.

Gyroxin-like B2.1 has a shorter 3′UTR compared with other clones. The lack of exon 4 in gyroxin-like B1.5 is because this clone is truncated by the insertion of a stop codon in translated sequence at the position 472 pb due to the joining of the exon 3 and exon 5 [17].

In Figure 6, the alignment of nucleotide sequences from gyroxin-like B1.3 and B2.1 revealed that clone B1.3 contains two consensus motifs for hypothetical poly(A^+) signals (5′- AATAAA -3′) at positions 929 and 1380 bp, whereas the B2.1 sequence contains only the first poly(A^+) signal at the position 857 bp and has a shorter 3′UTR and poly(A^+) tail [17].

The transcription of mRNA can be related with polyadenilation sites on 3′UTR (3′untranslated region). The presence of short and long 3′UTRs was also described for myogenin, Xmyog U_1 and Xmyog U_2 from *Xenopus laevis* (Xmyog U_2) [46] that contains one and two consensus motifs for a poly(A^+) signal, respectively. These results suggest the presence of at least, two different poly(A^+) signals in Xmyog U_2, generating two transcripts with different 3′ ends.

Similarly, the presence of two signals of polyadenylation in gyroxin-like B1.3, suggests that two mRNAs could be transcripted with longer or smaller 3′ UTR. Gyroxin-like B2.1 has only one signal of polyadenilation, showing a shorter 3′UTR than gyroxin-like B1.3 (Figure 5) [17].

2.3. Recombinant serine protease expression

Due to the great biotechnological potential of toxins present in the snakes venoms, many efforts have been made in order to clone and express those toxins in order to study its biological activity. However, the study of their properties is often hampered due to the small amount obtained and the difficulty of getting the animals to extract the poison, and when these are not the case, many toxins require several purification steps that result in a lower final yield. For these reasons, many toxin genes have been isolated, cloned and expressed in heterologous systems. This methodology not only make possible to obtain a large amount of toxins, but also enable amino acids modification by specific mutations in their DNA sequence. Thus, whole molecules may be broken down in order to study the function of its domains [47, 48], as well as amino acid residues may be exchanged for to study its role in substrate binding [49, 50].

2.3.1. Expression of serine protease on prokaryotic cells

Currently, the most used system to express snake toxins has been bacteria. However, the expression of recombinant SVSPs using *E. coli* as a host may result in expression of insoluble proteins that must be refolded *in vitro* in order to be activated. Batroxobin, for example, was the first SVSP to be expressed in insoluble form in *E. coli* and subsequently refolded to yield an active enzyme [51]. The plasminogen activator from *T. stejnegeri* was expressed in *E. coli*, but had to undergo a a denaturation-renaturation process in appropriate redox conditions to allow for the correct formation of disulfide bridges. Using an innovative method, a kallikrein-like protease (Tm-5) from the snake venom Taiwan habu (*Trimeresurus mucrosquamatus*), was expressed in *E.coli* by placing a polyhistidine-tag linked to an autocatalyzed site based on the cleavage specificity of the serine protease. The autocatalytic cleavage of Tm-5 from the polyhistidine-tagged fusion protein resulted in an active recombinant enzyme [53].

Acutin and mucrosobin, enzymes with fibrinogen-clotting and β-fibrinogenase activities respectively, were successfully expressed in *E. coli* [54,55]. The expression of a SVSP in *E.coli*, rCC-PPP, an isoform of cerastocytin from *Cerastes cerastes* with platelet-aggregating activity was reported [56]. After refolding, the recombinant enzyme showed to be a potent platelet proactivator and to clot fibrinogen.

2.3.2. Expression of serine protease on eukaryotic cells

In general SVSPs are glycosylated and this post-translational modification is important to the toxin activity, besides that, when expressed in *E. coli* those toxins frequently results in insoluble or inactive forms. Therefore the eukaryotic system such as yeast, mammalian cells and baculovirus expression system in insect cells have been explored, and although the number of works using this systems are small, they are growing substantially, mainly because of its superior refolding machinery and post-translational modifications (e.g. phosphorylation and glycosylation) [57].

The recombinant Haly-PA was successfully expressed using the baculovírus expression system, displayed an indirect fibrinogenolytic activity depending on the presence of plasminogen and cleaved the plasminogen to generate the active plasmin. These results indicate that Haly-PA is a plasminogen activator and displays fibrinogenolytic activity through conversion of plasminogen to plasmin [58].

The recombinant Batroxobin from *Bothrops atrox moojeni* venom –expressed in *Pichia pastoris,* was able to coagulate plasma in a dose dependent manner. However, its molecular weight was higher than the native protein, indicating yeast-type carbohydrate in its structure [59].

The expression of a glycoprotein Gyroxin-like B2.1 from *Crotalus durissus terrificus* venom was reported in COS-7. In order to promote the secretion of this toxin to the culture medium it was fused to the IgK-chain secretion signal peptide at the N terminus [17]. The recombinant Gyroxin expressed in COS-7 cell (Figure 7-Western blot, lane 1) showed the same electrophoretic pattern of the native Gyroxin purified from the venom (Figure 7-Western blot, lane 2). Recombinant Gyroxin-like B2.1 was successfully achieved with esterase activity in the conditioned culture medium, as revealed by immunoblot of secreted protein and standard anti-crotalic serum from Butantan Institute (Figure 7).

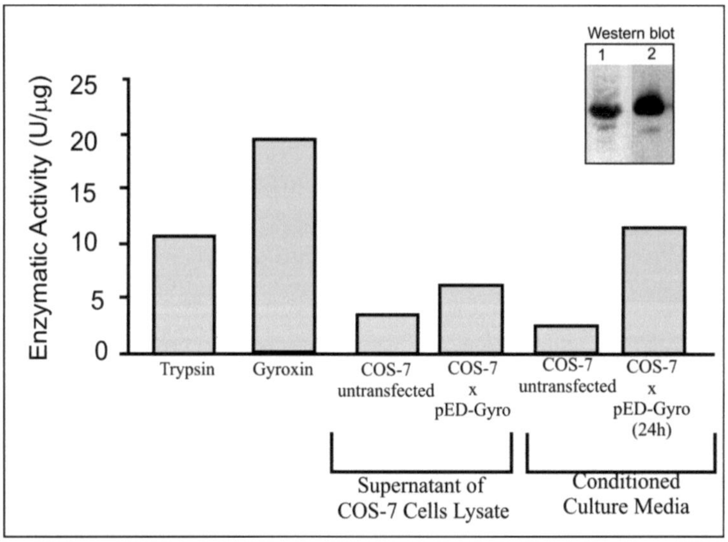

Figure 7. Esterase activity assay of recombinant Gyroxin purified by Benzamidine Sepharose from the supernatant of lysate and conditioned culture medium over 24 h of transfected COS-7 cells with pED-Gyro. Supernatant lysate and conditioned culture medium of untransfected COS-7 cells were used as negative controls. Porcine pancreas Trypsin and purified Gyroxin from *C.d.terrificus* venom were used as positive controls. 1- Western blot of COS-7 cells extract transfected with pED-Gyro., 2- 0.05 mg of Gyroxin purified from *C.d.terrificus* (positive control). The primary antibody was anti-crotalic serum from Butantan Institute and the reaction was detected with secondary antibody conjugated to horseradish peroxidase.

Drug/trade name®	Target and function/treatment	Source
Ancrod (Viprinex)	Fibrinogen inhibitor/stroke	*Agkistrodon rhodostoma* (Malayan pit viper)
Batroxobin (Defibrase)	thrombin and protrhombin inhibitor/acute cerebral infarction, unspecific angina pectoris	*Bothrops moojeni*
Hemocoagulase	thrombin-like effect and thromboplastin activity/ prevention and treatment of haemorrhage	*Bothrops atrox*
Protac/protein C activator	protein C activator/clinical diagnosis of haemostatic disorder	*Agkistrodon contortix contortix* (American copperhead)
Reptilase	diagnosis of blood coagulation disorder	*Bothrops jararaca* (South American lance adder)
RVV-V	Proteolytic activation of factor V	*Daboia ruselli*

Table 1. Clinical applications and diagnostic kits from snake venom serine proteases.

2.4. Therapeutic and diagnostic use

Due to the properties of SVTLEs, they have been extensively investigated over the last decade for potential therapeutic and diagnostic use and some of them are summarized in Table 1, based on [6, 60-62].

In this regard, ancrod [63] from *Calloselasma rhodostoma* venom, whose current brand name is Viprinex™, was approved in 2005 in the fast track program of United States Food and Drug Administration (FDA) for investigating its use in patients suffering from acute ischemic stroke [64].

This program is currently undergoing phase III, where the patients received a one-time, 2-3 hour infusion of ancrod or placebo within six hours of the initial symptom onset of their ischemic stroke, and are then followed for three months to collect information on their functional status. Since then, many research articles about the use of ancrod in ischaemic stroke has been published [63,65-68].

Another thrombin-like enzyme that has been used clinically is Batroxobin (Defibrase®) from *Bothrops atrox* venom. In a randomized clinical trial using this toxin in association with aspirin indicated a reduced rate of restenosis in patients with diabetes undergoing angioplasty for lower-limb ischemia [69]. In another experiment, the combination of batroxobin and tranexamic acid in 80 adolescent patients undergoing scheduled idiopathic scoliosis surgery was able to markedly reduce blood loss and allogeneic blood transfusion [70]. Others trials involving batroxobin include deep vein thrombosis [71] treatment of hyperfibrinogenemia for secondary stroke prevention [72] and acute ischemic stroke [73].

Since SVSPs shortens the bleeding time and clotting time, by promoting coagulation locally at the site of bleeding, combination of enzymes is also employed for the prevention or treatment of hemorrhage such as might be encountered in surgeries. In this regard, hemocoagulase, a mixture of purified enzymes isolated from the venom of *Bothrops atrox* is another example in clinical trials [74,75]. It has two different enzymatic activities, one which promotes blood coagulation by converting prothrombin to thrombin (thromboplastin like enzymes) and the other that causes a direct transformation of fibrinogen to fibrin monomer.

Despite its use in clinical application, some SVSPs have also been explored as a diagnostic tool, mainly because they are not inhibited by heparin and therefore they can be used to test plasma samples containing this anticoagulant or to remove fibrinogen from samples containing heparin. In this context, Reptilase®, a thrombin-like serine protease isolated from the venom of *Bothrops atrox* is used to assess blood fibrinogen and fibrinogen degradation products [76,77]. It is useful to check whether a prolonged thrombin time is caused by the presence of heparin in the sample. However, the reptilase time is rarely performed in isolation and therefore, the results of this test should be considered together with other tests and in particular the thrombin time.

It is important to point out that the name "reptilase" was first described in 1958 [78] for an extract with the fibrinogen clotting activity from the venom of *Bothrops jararaca* and sometimes t his term has also been described as a synonymous of "batroxobin" from the venom of *Bothrops moojeni* and *Bothrops atrox*.

Protac®, a serine protease from *Agkistrodon contortrix* venom is another example that has found a broad application in diagnostic practice for the determination of disorders in the protein C (PC) pathway. Unlike thrombin-catalyzed PC activation reaction which requires thrombomodulin as a cofactor, Protac® directly converts the zymogen PC into the catalytically active form which can easily be determined by means of coagulation or chromogenic substrate techniques [79-81].

Due to the capability of a serine protease extracted from Russels´s viper (*Daboia ruselli*) venom (RVV-Vα) to activate Factor V, and since activated factor V is not stable and loses its activity within 20 hours at 37° C, RVV-V has been used to destabilize and selectively inactivate factor V in plasma. Therefore, it has been used to prepare a routine reagent for factor V determination. Studies have demonstrated the ability of the Prothrombinase-induced clotting time (PiCT) assay, which uses RVV-V among its components, to determine activities of both direct and indirect thrombin inhibitors in a linear manner over a wide concentration range [60-62].

While the original native snake venom compounds are usually unsuitable as therapeutics, interventions by medicinal chemists as well as scientists and clinicians in pharmaceutical R&D have made it possible to use snake toxins as therapeutics for multiple disorders based on the available structural and functional information. Therefore, snake venoms, with their cocktail of individual components, have great potential as therapeutic agents for human diseases [6].

2.4.1. Serine protease inhibitors

Most animal species synthesize a variety of protease inhibitors with different specificities, whose function is to prevent unwanted proteolysis. They generally act by unabling access of substrates to the proteases'active site through steric hindrance. Proteases are also involved in various disease states such as the destruction of the extracellular matrix of articular cartilage and bone in arthritic joints is thought to be mediated by excessive proteolitic activity [82]. Among the enzymes involved in extracellular matrix degradation, a few serine proteases (elastase, collagenase, cathepsin G) are able to solubilize fibrous proteins such as elastin and collagen [83,84].

Given the specific recognition by proteases of defined amino acid sequences, it may be possible to inhibit these enzymes when they are involved in pathological processes. Potent inhibitors have the potential to be developed as new therapeutic agents. In vertebrates for example serine protease inhibitors, have been studied for many years and they are known to be involved in phagocytosis, coagulation, complement activation, fibrinolysis, blood pressure regulation. Moreover, some of the protease inhibitors isolated from invertebrate sources are quite specific towards individual mammalian serine proteases. This also offers huge opportunities for medicine. Thus, the development of non-toxic protease inhibitors extracted from invertebrates for *in vivo* application may be quite important [82].

The last decade, drug discovery in leeches has opened the gate for new molecules to treat emphysema, coagulation, inflammation, dermatitis and cancer. Also other invertebrates, such as insects, harvest potential interesting molecules, such as serine protease inhibitors that can be exploited by the medical industry [85].

3. Conclusions

Snake venom serine proteases have several different functions and have found most use in medicine in blood coagulation system. These enzymes are used in several ways as tools in basic research helping to elucidate the relation of structure- function of coagulant proteins and their interactions with platelets or in experimental models of haemostatic alterations.

Some SVSPs have already been found to be a commercial use in coagulation diagnostic and some of them are used either to influence physiological homeostasis or as a form of supportive treatment in haemostatic disorders and micro vascular surgery promoting cicatrization.

Despite the high homology of serine proteases and even sharing the same target, small differences in their amino acids composition may lead significant binding intensity causing differences in their biological effects. Therefore, even isoforms of those molecules in the same organism must be explored. Many animals besides snakes also possess serine proteases that are used for attack or defense purposes, such as scorpions, bees, spiders and even the exotic platypuses which make 26 different kinds of serine proteases [86].

Therefore, the diversity of those toxins is extensive and demand many research to elucidate their function and potential clinical applications

Acknowledgements

Financial support by FAPESP and CNPq.

Author details

Camila Miyagui Yonamine[1], Álvaro Rossan de Brandão Prieto da Silva[2] and Geraldo Santana Magalhães[3]

1 Department of Pharmacology, Federal University of São Paulo, Brazil

2 Department of Genetic, Butantan Institute, Brazil

3 Department of Immunology, Butantan Institute, Brazil

References

[1] Kornalik F. Toxins affecting blood coagulation and fibrinolysis. In: Shier W. T. and Meb D. (eds.) Handbook of Toxicology. New York: Marcel Dekker; 1990. p.697-709.

[2] Matsui T, Fujimura Y, Titani K. Snake venom proteases affecting hemostasis and thrombosis. Biochim. Biophys.Acta 2000;1477(1-2) 146–156.

[3] Serrano S, Mauron RC. Snake venom serine proteinases: sequence homology vs. Substrate specificity, a paradox to be solved. Toxicon 2005;45(8) 1115-1132.

[4] Bell WRJr. Defibrinogenating enzymes. Drugs 1997;54(3) 18–30,discussion 30-1.

[5] Pirkle H. Thrombin-like enzymes from snake venoms: an update inventory. Thromb. Haemost. 1998;79(3) 675–683.

[6] Koh DCI, Armugan A, Jeyaseelan K. Snake venom components and their applications in biomedicine. Cell. Mol. Life Sci. 2006;63(24) 3030-3041.

[7] Stocker K, Fischer H, Meier J. Thrombin-like snake venom proteinases. Toxicon 1982;20(1) 265-273.

[8] Pirkle H, Theodor I. Thrombin-like venom enzymes: Structure and function. Adv. Exp. Med.Biol. 1990;281: 165-175.

[9] Serrano SMT, Hagiwara Y, Murayama N, Higuchi S, Mentele R, Sampaio CA, Camargo AC, Fink E. Purification and characterization of a kinin-releasing and fibrinogen-clotting serine proteinase (KN-BJ) from the venom of *Bothrops jararaca* and

molecular cloning and sequence analysis of its cDNA. Eur.J.Biochem. 1998;251(3) 845-853.

[10] Wang YM, Wang SR, Tsai IH. Serine protease isoforms of *Deinagkistrodon acutus* venom: cloning, sequencing and phylogenetic analysis. Biochem.J. 2001;354(Pt 1) 161-168.

[11] Oyama E, Takahashi H. Amino acid sequence of a thrombin like enzyme, elegaxobin, from the venom of *Trimeresurus elegans* (Sakishima-habu). Toxicon 2002;40(7) 959-970.

[12] Mcmullen BA, Fujikawa K, Kisiel W. Primary structure of a protein C activator from *Agkistrodon contortrix contortrix* venom. Biochemistry 1989;28(2) 674-679.

[13] Tokunaga F, Nagasawa K, Tamura S, Miyata T, Iwanaga S, Kisiel W. The factor V-activating enzyme (RVV-V) from Russell's viper venom. Identification of isoproteins RVV-V alpha, -V beta, and -V gamma and their complete amino acid sequences. J. Biol. Chem. 1988;263(33) 17471-17481.

[14] Siigur E, Aaspõllu A, Siigur J. Molecular cloning and sequence analysis of a cDNA for factor V activating enzyme. Biochem. Biophys. Res. Commun. 1999;262(2) 328-332.

[15] Matsui T, Sakurai Y, Fujimura Y, Hayashi I, Oh-Ishi S, Suzuki M, Hamako J, Yamamoto Y, Yamazaki J, Kinoshita M, Titani K. Purification and amino acid sequence of halystase from snake venom of *Agkistrodon halys blomhoffii*, a serine protease that cleaves specifically fibrinogen and kininogen. Eur.J.Biochem. 1998;252(3) 569-575.

[16] Hahn BS, Yang KY, Park EM, Chang IM, Kim YS. Purification and molecular cloning of calobin, a thrombin-like enzyme from *Agkistrodon caliginosus* (Korean viper). J. Biochem. 1996;119(5) 835-843.

[17] Yonamine CM, Prieto-da-Silva ARB, Magalhães GS, Rádis-Baptista G, Morganti L, Ambiel FC, Chura-Chambi RM, Yamane T, Camillo MAP. Cloning of serine protease cDNAs from *Crotalus durissus terrificus* venom gland and expression of a functional Gyroxin homologue in COS-7 cells. Toxicon 2009;54(2) 110-120.

[18] Magalhaes A, Da Fonseca BC, Diniz CR, Richardson M. The complete amino acid sequence of a thrombin-like enzyme/gyroxin analogue from venom of the bushmaster snake (*Lachesis muta muta*).FEBS Lett. 1993;329(1-2) 116-120.

[19] Henschen-Edman AH, Theodor I, Edwards BF, Pirkle H. Crotalase, a fibrinogen-clotting snake venom enzyme: primary structure and evidence for a fibrinogen recognition exosite different from thrombin. Thromb. Haemost. 1999;81(1) 81-86.

[20] Burkhart W, Smith GFH, SU JL, Parikh I, Levine HIII. Amino acid sequence determination of ancrod, the thrombin-like alpha-fibrinogenase from the venom of *Akistrodon rhodostoma*. FEBS Lett. 1992;297(3) 297-301.

[21] Itoh N, Tanaka N, Mihashi S, Yamashina I. Molecular cloning and sequence analysis of cDNA for batroxobin, a thrombin-like snake venom enzyme J. Biol. Chem. 1987;262(7) 3132-3135.

[22] Nikai T, Ohara A, Komori Y, Fox JW, Sugihara, H. Primary structure of a coagulant enzyme, bilineobin, from *Agkistrodon bilineatus* venom. Arch. Biochem. Biophys. 1995;318(1) 89-96.

[23] Zhang Y, Wisner A, Xiong YL, Bon C. A novel plasminogen activator from snake venom. Purification, characterization, and molecular cloning. J. Biol. Chem. 1995;270(17) 10246-10255.

[24] Sanchez EF, Santos CI, Magalhaes A, Diniz CR, Figueiredo S, Gilroy J, Richardson M. Isolation of a proteinase with plasminogen-activating activity from *Lachesis muta muta* (bushmaster) snake venom. Arch. Biochem. Biophys. 2000;378(1) 131-141.

[25] Serrano SMT, Mentele R, Sampaio CAM, Fink E. Purification, characterization, and amino acid sequence of a serine proteinase, PA-BJ, with platelet-aggregating activity from the venom of *Bothrops jararaca*. Biochemistry 1995;34 (21) 7186-7193.

[26] Numeric P, Moravie V, Didier M, Chatot-Henry D, Cirille S, Bucher B, Thomas L. Multiple cerebral infarctions following snakebite by *Bothrops carribbaeus*. Am. J. Trop. Med. Hyg.2002;67(3) 287–288.

[27] Markland FS. Snake venom and the hemostatic system. Toxicon 1998;36(12) 1749-1800.

[28] Nolan C, Hall LS, Barlow GH. Ancrod, the coagulating enzyme from Malayan pit viper (*Agkistrodon rhodostoma*) venom. Methods Enzymol. 1976;45: 205-213.

[29] Stocker K, Barlow GH. The coagulant enzyme from *Bothrops atrox* venom (Batroxobin). Methods Enzymol.1976;45: 214-223.

[30] Markland FS, Damus PS. Purification and properties of a thrombin-like enzyme from the venom of *Crotalus adamanteus* (Eastern diamondback rattlesnake). J. Biol. Chem. 1971;246(21) 6460-6473.

[31] Markland, FS. Crotalase. Methods Enzymol.1976;45: 223-236.

[32] Bjarnason JB, Barish A, Direnzo GS, Campbell R, Fox JW. Kallikrein-like enzymes from *Crotalus atrox* venom. J. Biol. Chem.1983;258(20) 12566-12573.

[33] Stocker K, Fischer H, Meier J, Brogli M, Svendsen L. Characterization of protein C activator Protac from venom of the southern copperhead (*Agkistrodon contortrix*) snake. Toxicon 1987;25(3) 239-252.

[34] Marsh N, Williams V. Practical applications of snake venom toxins in haemostasis. Toxicon 2005;45(8) 1171–1181.

[35] Kini RM.The intriguing world of prothrombin activators from snake venom. Toxicon 2005;45(8) 1133-1145.

[36] Yonamine, CM. Cloning of serine proteases from the venom of rattlesnake Crotalus durissus terrificus and expression of a Gyroxin in mammalian cells. Master of science disertation. IPEN (Nuclear and Energy Research Institute); 2007.

[37] Gratio V, Walker F, Lehy T, Laburthe M, Darmoul D. Aberrant expression of proteinase-activated receptor 4 promotes colon cancer cell proliferation through a persistent signaling that involves Src and ErbB-2 kinase. Int. J. Cancer 2009;124(7) 1517–1525.

[38] Coughlin, SR. How the protease thrombin talks to cells. Proc Natl Acad Sci USA 1999;96(20) 11023–11027.

[39] Kahn ML, Zheng YW, Huang W, Bigornia V, Zeng D, Moff S, Farese RVJr, Tam C, Coughlin SR. A dual thrombin receptor system for platelet activation. Nature 1998;394(6694) 690–694.

[40] Mao Y, Jin J, Kunapuli SP. Characterization of a new peptide agonist of the protease-activated receptor-1. Biochem. Pharmacol. 2008;75(2) 438-447.

[41] Kahn ML, Nakanishi-Matsui M, Shapiro MJ, Ishihara H, Coughlin SR. Protease-activated receptors 1 and 4 mediate activation of human platelets by thrombin. J. Clin. Invest. 1999;103(6) 879–887.

[42] Da Silva JAA, Spencer P, Camillo MAP, de Lima VMF. Gyroxin and its biological activity: effects on CNS basement membranes and endothelium and protease-activated receptors. Curr. Med. Chem.2012;19(2) 281-291.

[43] Stocker K. *Defibrinogenation* with *thrombin-like snake venom enzymes*. In Markwardt F. (ed) Handbook of Experimental Pharmacology. Berlin: Springer-Verlag; 1978. p. 451-484.

[44] Itoh N, Tanaka N, Funakoshi I, Kawasaki T, Mihashi S, Yamashina I. The complete nucleotide sequence of the gene for batroxobin, a thrombin-like snake venom enzyme. Nucleic Acids Res.1988;16(21) 10377-10378.

[45] Von Heijne G. Signal sequences.The limits of variation. J. Mol. Biol.1985;184(1) 99-105.

[46] Charbonnier F, Gaspera BD, Armand AS, Van der Laarse WJ, Launay T, Becker C, Gallien CL, Chanoine C. Two myogeninrelated genes are differentially expressed in *Xenopus laevis* myogenesis and differ in their ability to transactivate muscle structural genes. J. Biol. Chem.2002;277(2) 1139–1147.

[47] Assakura MT, Silva CA, Mentele R, Camargo AC, Serrano SM. Molecular cloning and expression of structural domains of bothropasin, a P-III metalloproteinase from the venom of Bothrops jararaca. Toxicon 2003;41(2) 217-227.

[48] Moura-da-Silva AM, Línica A, Della-Casa MS, Kamiguti AS, Ho PL, Crampton JM, Theakston RD. Jararhagin ECD-containing disintegrin domain: expression in Escherichia coli and inhibition of the platelet-collagen interaction. Arch Biochem Biophys. 1999;369(2) 295-301.

[49] Tian J, Paquette-Straub C, Sage EH, Funk SE, Patel V, Galileo D, McLane MA. Inhibition of melanoma cell motility by the snake venom disintegrin eristostatin. Toxicon. 2007;49(7) 899-908.

[50] Sanz L, Chen RQ, Pérez A, Hilario R, Juárez P, Marcinkiewicz C, Monleón D, Celda B, Xiong YL, Pérez-Payá E, Calvete JJ. cDNA cloning and functional expression of jerdostatin, a novel RTS-disintegrin from *Trimeresurus jerdonii* and a specific antagonist of the alpha1beta1 integrin. J Biol Chem. 2005;280(49) 40714-40722.

[51] Maeda M, Satoh S, Suzuki S, Niwa M, Itoh N, Yamashina I. Expression of cDNA for batroxobin, a thrombin-like snake venom enzyme. J. Biochem. 1991;109(4) 632-637.

[52] Zhang Y, Wisner, A, Maroun, R.C, Choumet V, Xiong Y, Bon C. *Trimeresurus stejnegeri* Snake Venom Plasminogen Activator SITE-DIRECTED MUTAGENESIS AND MOLECULAR MODELING. J. Biol. Chem 1997; 272(33) 20531-20537.

[53] Hung CC, Chiou SH. Expression of a kallikrein-like protease from the snake venom: engineering of autocatalytic site in the fusion protein to facilitate protein refolding. Biochem. Biophys. Res. Commun.2000;275(3) 924–930.

[54] Pan H, Du X, Yang G, Zhou Y, Wu X. cDNA cloning and expression of acutin. Biochem. Biophys. Res. Commun.1999;255(2) 412–415.

[55] Guo YW, Chang TY, Lin KT, Liu HW, Shih KC, Cheng SH. Cloning and functional expression of the mucrosobin protein, a beta-fibrinogenase of *Trimeresurus mucrosquamatus* (Taiwan Habu). Protein Exp. Purif.2001;23(3) 483–490.

[56] Dekhil H, Wisner A, Marrakchi N, El Ayeb M, Bon C, Karoui H. Molecular cloning and expression of a functional snake venom serine proteinase, with platelet aggregating activity, from the *Cerastes cerastes* viper. Biochemistry 2003;42(36) 10609–10618.

[57] Butler M. Animal cell cultures: recent achievements and perspectives in the production of biopharmaceuticals. Appl. Microbiol. Bioftechnol. 2005,68(3) 283-291.

[58] Park D, Kim H, Chung K, Kim DS, Yun Y. Expression and characterization of a novel plasminogen activator from *Agkistrodon Halys* venom. Toxicon 1998;36(12) 1807-1819.

[59] You WK, Choi WS, Koh YS, Shin HC, Jang Y, Chung KH. Functional characterization of recombinant batroxobin, a snake venom thrombin-like enzyme, expressed from *Pichia pastoris*. FEBS letters 2004;571(1-3) 63-73.

[60] Korte W, Jovic R, Hollenstein M, Degiacomi P, Gautschi M, Ferrández A. The uncalibrated prothrombinase-induced clotting time test. Equally convenient but more pre-

cise than the aPTT for monitoring of unfractionated heparin. Hamostaseologie. 2010;30(4) 212-6.

[61] Calatzis A, Peetz D, Haas S, Spannagl M, Rudin K, Wilmer M. Prothrombinase-induced clotting time assay for determination of the anticoagulant effects of unfractionated and low-molecular-weight heparins, fondaparinux, and thrombin inhibitors. Am. J. Clin. Pathol. 2008;130(3) 446-54.

[62] Fenyvesi T, Jorg I, Harenberg J. Effect of phenprocoumon on monitoring of lepirudin, argatroban, melagatran and unfractionated heparin with the PiCT method. *Pathophysiol. Haemost. Thromb.* 2002;32(4) 174-179.

[63] Nolan C, Hall LS, Barlow GH. Ancrod, the coagulating enzyme from Malayan pit viper (*Agkistrodon rhodostoma*) venom. Methods Enzymol. 1976;45: 205–213.

[64] The Internet Strocke Center. http://www.strokecenter.org/trials/clinicalstudies/asp-ii-ancrod-stroke-program-ancrod-viprinex%E2%84%A2-for-the-treatment-of-acute-ischemic-stroke (accessed 2 July 2012).

[65] Liu S, Marder VJ, Levy DE, Wang SJ, Yang F, Paganini-Hill A, Fisher MJ. Ancrod and fibrin formation: perspectives on mechanisms of action. Stroke 2011;42(11) 3277-3280.

[66] Levy DE, del Zoppo GJ, Demaerschalk BM, Demchuk AM, Diener HC, Howard G, Kaste M, Pancioli AM, Ringelstein EB, Spatareanu C, Wasiewski WW. Ancrod in acute ischemic stroke: results of 500 subjects beginning treatment within 6 hours of stroke onset in the ancrod stroke program. Stroke. 2009;40(12) 3796-3803.

[67] Hyperfibrinogenemia and functional outcome from acute ischemic stroke. del Zoppo GJ, Levy DE, Wasiewski WW, Pancioli AM, Demchuk AM, Trammel J, Demaerschalk BM, Kaste M, Albers GW, Ringelstein EB. Stroke. 2009;40(5) 1687-1691.

[68] Hennerici MG, Kay R, Bogousslavsky J, Lenzi GL, Verstraete M, Orgogozo JM, ESTAT investigators. Intravenous ancrod for acute ischaemic stroke in the European Stroke Treatment with Ancrod Trial: a randomised controlled trial. Lancet. 2006;368(9550) 1871-1878.

[69] Wang J, Zhu YQ, Li MH, Zhao JG, Tan HQ, Wang JB, Liu F, Cheng YS.Batroxobin plus aspirin reduces restenosis after angioplasty for arterial occlusive disease in diabetic patients with lower-limb ischemia. J Vasc Interv Radiol. 2011;22(7) 987-994.

[70] Xu C, Wu A, Yue Y. Which is more effective in adolescent idiopathic scoliosis surgery: batroxobin, tranexamic acid or a combination? Arch. Orthop. Trauma Surg. 2012;132(1) 25-31.

[71] Lei Z, Shi Hong L, Li L, Tao YG, Yong LW, Senga H, Renchi Y, Zhong CH. Batroxobin mobilizes circulating endothelial progenitor cells in patients with deep vein thrombosis. Clin Appl Thromb Hemost. 2011;17(1) 75-79.

[72] Xu G, Liu X, Zhu W, Yin Q, Zhang R, Fan X. Feasibility of treating hyperfibrinogenemia with intermittently administered batroxobin in patients with ischemic stroke/

transient ischemic attack for secondary prevention. Blood Coagul Fibrinolysis. 2007;18(2) 193-197.

[73] Gusev EI, Skvortsova VI, Suslina ZA, Avakian GN, Martynov MIu, Temirbaeva SL, Tanashian MA, Kamchtnov PR, Stakhovskaia LV, Efremova NM. Batroxobin in patients with ischemic stroke in the carotid system (the multicenter study). Zh. Nevrol. Psikhiatr. Im. S. S. Korsakova. 2006;106(8) 31-34.

[74] Lodha A, Kamaluddeen M, Akierman A, Amin H. Role of hemocoagulase in pulmonary hemorrhage in preterm infants: a systematic review. Indian J. Pediatr. 2011;78(7) 838-844.

[75] Kim SH, Cho YS, Choi YJ. Intraocular hemocoagulase in human vitrectomy. Jpn. J. Ophthalmol. 1994;38(1) 49–55.

[76] Funk C, Gmür J, Herold R, Straub PW. Reptilase-R--a new reagent in blood coagulation. Br. J. Haematol. 1971;21(1) 43-52

[77] Van Cott EM, Smith EY, Galanakis DK. Elevated fibrinogen in an acute phase reaction prolongs the reptilase time but typically not the thrombin time. Am. J. Clin. Pathol. 2002;118(2) 263-268.

[78] Blomback B, Blomback M, Nilsson IM. Coagulation studies on reptilase, an extract of the venom from Bothrops jararaca. Thromb. Diath. Haemorrh. 1958;1(1) 76-86.

[79] Green L, Safa O, Machin SJ, Mackie IJ, Ryland K, Cohen H, Lawrie AS. Development and application of an automated chromogenic thrombin generation assay that is sensitive to defects in the protein C pathway. Thromb. Res. 2012 Jan 18. [Epub ahead of print].

[80] Tripodi A, Legnani C, Lemma L, Cosmi B, Palareti G, Chantarangkul V, Mannucci PM. Abnormal Protac-induced coagulation inhibition chromogenic assay results are associated with an increased risk of recurrent venous thromboembolism. J. Thromb. Thrombolysis. 2010;30(2) 215-219.

[81] Stocker K, Fischer H, Meier J. Practical application of the protein C activator Protac from *Agkistrodon contortrix* venom. Folia Haematol. Int. Mag. Klin. Morphol. Blutforsch. 1988;115(3) 260-264.

[82] Royston D. Preventing the inflammatory response to open heart surgery; the role of aprotinin and other protease inhibitors. Int J Cardiol 1996;53: S11-S37.

[83] Sloane BF, Rozhin J, Johnson K, Taylor H, Crissman JD, Honn KV. Cathepsin B: Association with plasma membrane in metastatic tumor. Proc. Natl. Acad. Sci. USA 1986;83(8) 2483-2487.

[84] Berquin IM; Sloane BF. Cathepsin B expression in human tumors. Adv.Exp Med Biol 1996,389: 281-94.

[85] Clynen E., Schoofs L and Salzet M. A. Review of the Most Important Classes of Serine Protease Inhibitors in Insects and Leeches. Med. Chem. Rev. online 2005,2(3)

197-206. http://www.ingentaconnect.com/content/ben/mcro/2005/00000002/00000003/art00003 (acessed 2 July 2012).

[86] Whittington CM, Papenfuss AT, Locke DP, Mardis ER, Wilson RK, Abubucker S, Mitreva M, Wong ES, Hsu AL, Kuchel PW, Belov K, Warren WC. Novel venom gene discovery in the platypus.Genome Biol. 2010;11(9) R95.

Chapter 7

Toxins from *Lonomia obliqua* — Recombinant Production and Molecular Approach

Ana Marisa Chudzinski-Tavassi,
Miryam Paola Alvarez-Flores,
Linda Christian Carrijo-Carvalho and
Maria Esther Ricci-Silva

Additional information is available at the end of the chapter

http://dx.doi.org/10.5772/53697

1. Introduction

Few species of butterflies and moths (order Lepidoptera) are involved in human envenoming [1]. Caterpillars are the larval forms of moths and butterflies. Toxins are usually found in the caterpillar's hairs and spines with defense purposes. The majority of medically important encounters with lepidopterans occur with exposure to the caterpillar's urticating hairs or spines, but hemolymph can also have toxic properties [1, 2]. A variety of clinical effects have been described, which depend on the family and species involved, ranging from local to systemic reactions [3, 4].

In most occasions, the adverse effects caused by caterpillars are self-limited and can be treated with topical antipruritics [4]. However, for the envenoming by the South American *Lonomia obliqua* caterpillars (Figure 1), named lonomism, the antilonomic serum produced at the Butantan Institute in Brazil is the only effective treatment to reestablish the coagulation parameters in poisoned patients and to avoid the complications seen in severe cases such as intracerebral hemorrhage and acute renal failure [5-10].

In 1989, an outbreak of accidents with this species became a serious public health threat in southern Brazil, with high fatality rates [5, 11-15]. Since then, many studies have been carried out to understand the pathophysiological mechanisms of envenoming [14] and to identify the toxins responsible for adverse reactions.

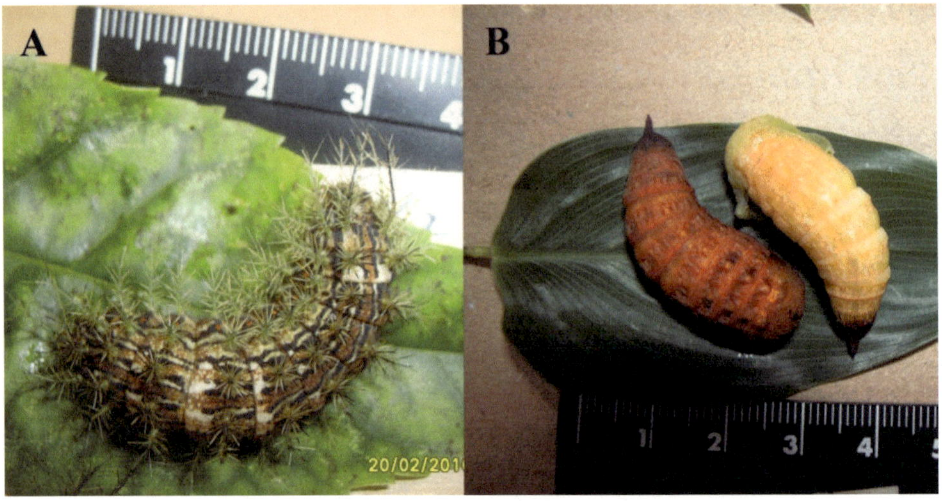

Figure 1. A) *Lonomia obliqua* caterpillar (5th instar) and B) pupa.

L. obliqua is the caterpillar that has the most studied venom, which main components have been isolated and characterized [14, 16, 17]. Table 1 lists the biological activities and toxins isolated and characterized from the bristle extract or hemolymph of *L. obliqua*. *In vivo* studies reported an antithrombotic effect caused by the bristle extract, while most *in vitro* studies reported procoagulant activities [14, 16-23]. It is well known, for a wide range of animal venoms, that procoagulant toxins can cause *in vivo* activation of the coagulation system. The hemostatic disturbances observed in the envenoming by *L. obliqua* caterpillars, result in a consumption coagulopathy (resembling a disseminated intravascular coagulation) and secondary fibrinolysis, which can lead to the hemorrhagic syndrome [6].

The principal components in the caterpillar's venom have been initially identified by isolating toxins through classical purification methods and following the main activities observed in the whole bristle extract (Figure 2). However, this approach provides knowledge restricted only to the most abundant toxins, and usually reveals that activities which are directly associated to the main symptoms and effects observed in the envenoming outcomes. Experimental assays were specifically developed to test the hemostatic and enzymatic activities of *Lonomia* toxins and their actions on the coagulation cascade. This knowledge has been valuable for description and management of the envenoming syndrome, but with the classical approach, low abundant components and unexpected effects are usually overlooked. Possible interaction of venom components, cross-reactions and secondary effects, useful to provide a systemic view of the pathways involved in the toxin's effects are often unnoticed.

In the last years, methods applied in genomic, transcriptomic and proteomic analyses have been applied with the aims of cataloging and classifying the toxins based on their structure and activity (Figure 3). Thus, it was possible to analyze the envenoming processes at the molecular level. For example, significant advance was achieved through two independent transcriptome studies, which generated a list of putative toxic proteins from *L. obliqua* bristles

Activity (toxin)	Source	MW (kDa)	Characteristics and observed effects	Reference
Prothrombin activation (Lopap)	Bristle extract	21	Serine protease, activity increased by Ca^{2+}; consumption coagulopathy *in vivo;* cell survival in endothelial cell culture. Recombinant form produced in bacteria and yeast.	[18, 19, 21, 24-26]
FXa-like	Bristle extract	21	Hydrolytic activity on S-2222 chromogenic substrate, Ca^{2+}-independent; N-terminal sequence similar to Lopap.	[27]
Factor X activation (Losac)	Bristle extract	45	Serine protease, Ca^{2+}-independent; Cell survival in HUVEC. Recombinant form produced in bacteria.	[20-22, 28]
Phospholipase A_2-like	Bristle extract	15	Indirect hemolytic activity in human and rat red blood cells *in vitro*, Ca^{2+}-independent; intravascular hemolysis *in vivo*.	[29-31]
Fibrinogenolytic (Lonofibrase)	Hemolymph	35	αβ fibrinogenase activity; enable to affect fibrin cross-linked.	[32-34]
Hyaluronidase (Lonoglyases)	Bristle extract	49 53	β-endohexosaminidase activity; degradation of extracellular matrix.	[35]
Antiapoptotic	Hemolymph	51	Activity on *Spodoptera frugiperda* (Sf-9) cell culture.	[36]
Antiviral	Hemolymph	20	Antiviral activity against measles, influenza and polio viruses. Recombinant form produced in baculovirus/insect.	[37, 38]
Nociceptive and Edematogenic	Bristle extract	NI	Nociception facilitated by prostaglandin production; edematogenic response facilitated by prostanoids and histamine.	[39]
Kallikrein-kinin system activation	Bristle extract	NI	Kinin release from low molecular weight kininogen; edema formation and fall in arterial pressure.	[40]
Platelet adhesion and aggregation	Bristle extract	NI	Direct platelet aggregation and ATP secretion; activity inhibited by *p*-bromophenacyl bromide, a specific PLA_2 inhibitor.	[41, 42]

NI: None isolated, studies carried out using the whole venom

Table 1. Toxins and activities described in *L. obliqua* venom.

and hemolymph [20, 43]. In addition, significant advance was achieved as a result of microarray study [44]. Moreover, by coupling proteomics and immunochemical approaches, some immunogenic components were identifying in the bristle extract, especially those related to hemostasis [9]. These components were detected by the antilonomic hyperimmune serum produced at the Butantan Institute, and abundant proteins were identified.

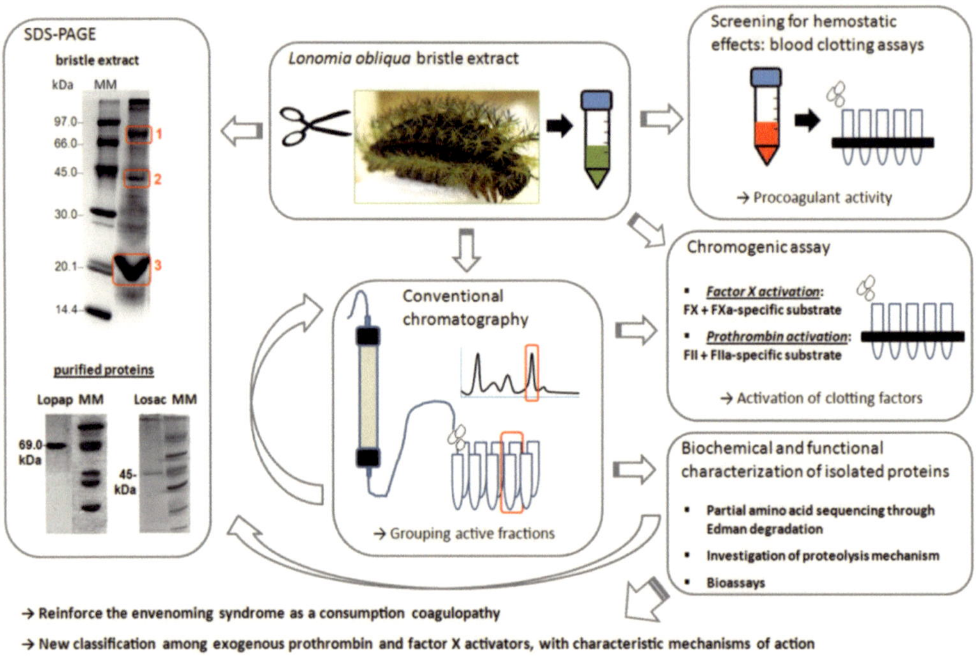

Figure 2. Schematic representation of the classical strategy employed in initial studies of the *Lonomia obliqua* venom. The bristle extract was analyzed through denaturing electrophoresis (SDS-PAGE) which showed the venom is a complex mixture of proteins. Screening assays were carried out to investigate possible effects on blood coagulation and fibrinolysis. The venom showed procoagulant activity by decreasing blood clotting time. Two procoagulant components (Lopap, a prothrombin activator and Losac, a factor X activator) were identified and isolated from the bristle extract for further characterization. The specific activity of Lopap and Losac were observed on purified coagulation factor zymogens (FII or FX) using chromogenic substrates to detect generation of active forms of clotting factors (FIIa and FXa) by these toxins. This assay was used in the purification process to identify the active fractions containing each toxin. SDS-PAGE profile shows Lopap (1- multimer, 3- monomer) and Losac (2) are abundant components in the venom. MM: molecular markers.

Production of recombinant forms of *Lonomia* toxins and discovery of new molecules are opening perspectives in the scientific area for basic and applied researches. These molecules can point out novel mechanisms of action, undiscovered molecular interactions and new classes of enzymes and inhibitors. Interesting, some venom toxins have shown multifunctional properties [19, 22, 28]. The best examples are Lopap (a prothrombin activator with high similarity with lipocalins) and Losac (a factor X activator highly similar to hemolins). Besides activation of blood coagulation, Lopap and Losac can modulate cellular functions and promote cell survival [22, 45]. Both molecules were cloned and produced in its recombinant form in yeast and/or bacteria [19, 25, 28].

Additional studies will be conducted to determine the involvement of the venom components in the envenoming syndrome and their biological significance for physiological processes of the animal, such as insect metamorphosis, which is a combination of growth/activation/differentiation/programmed cell death signals. Thus, this chapter reviews the currently

http://dx.doi.org/10.5772/53697

available information about *L. obliqua* venom, and focus on strategies to unveil molecular aspects of toxins and the perspectives for therapeutic and biotechnological applications.

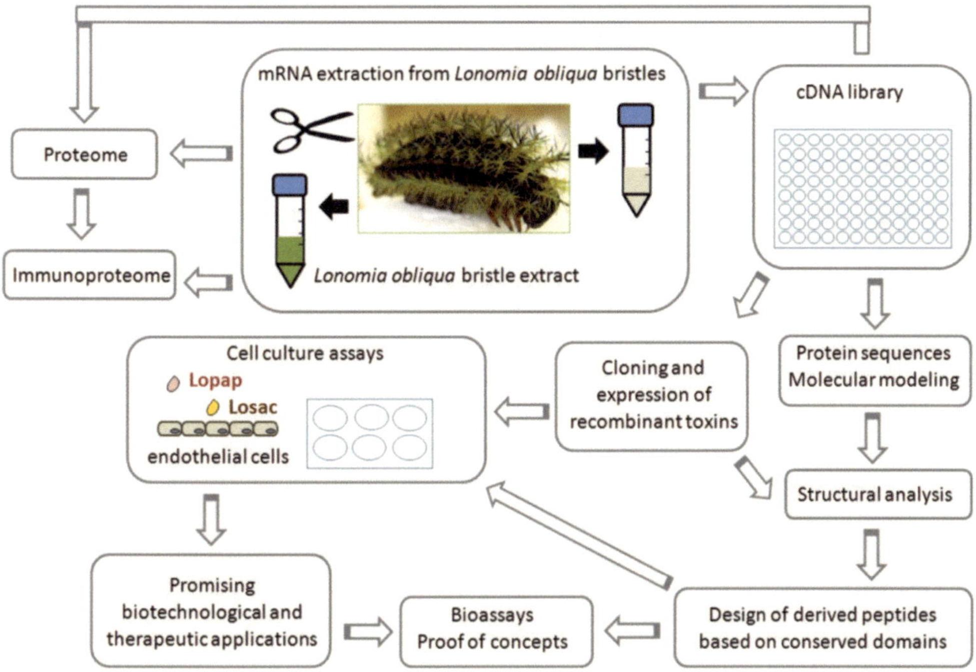

Figure 3. Schematic representation of the strategies to explore the Lonomia obliqua venom and toxins based on cellular and molecular approaches. Results obtained indicate promising applications for these proteins and derived peptides.

2. Molecular approach

For many years, direct purification of toxins from venoms was the best procedure to characterize them with regard to their primary structure. Then, the development of molecular approaches to characterize toxin genes represented an expansion in the understanding of the structure and function of toxin, critical for the development of new treatments directed against the venom toxins (antivenoms). Cloning of cDNAs coding for biochemically isolated toxins has improved their characterization. *Transcriptomic* allows the identification of cellular transcripts in a given cell population, while proteomic studies protein's properties and functions (expression level, structure, post-translational modification, etc.) of proteins expressed by the genome of an organism at a certain point of time. The availability of technologies for high throughput analysis has led to integrate toxin expression at mRNA and protein level. This flow of genetic information from DNA to proteins is the base of the central dogma of molecular biology [46].

2.1. Transcriptomics of *Lonomia obliqua* bristle extract

Expressed Sequence Tags strategy is an approach to characterize the transcriptome of a cell, gland or organism and is based in all the transcript (the most abundant are the mRNAs) produced at a specific time and fully sequenced to create a representative catalogue of expressed genes [47]. Hundreds to a thousand of sequences are grouped into *contigs* or clusters based on DNA sequence information and bioinformatics analysis (Figure 4). Nowadays, the EST-based strategy is commonly employed for identifying expressed genes in species of interest [48, 49]. This approach has been successfully used to compile a lists of genes expressed in venom's glands of a wide range of animals [50-53].

EST-strategy was used to identify the major transcripts present in *L. obliqua* bristle extract [19, 20, 43]. About 702 clusters (representing 1,278 independent clones) were assembled and characterized as lipocalins, hemolins, serine proteases, serine protease inhibitors, serpins, tumor suppressors, ribosomal, structural and cell cycle proteins as shown in Table 2 [20]. Most of the transcripts represent proteins involved in the animal physiology. Those sequences were deposited in data bank (NCBI GenBank accession numbers: CX815710–CX817210, CX820335–CX820336, AY908986) [20]. A pool of DNA sequences showed no similarities with well-known sequences in data bank. The most abundant toxin was a lipocalin of 21 kDa, and analysis of its N-terminal sequence shows 100% homology with Lopap (GenPept accession number: AAW88441). The Lopap whole sequence (accounting for 1.6% of the total clones) was identified in this cDNA library (accession number: AY908986).

Functional categories	No. of clusters	No. of clones	Clones/ clusters	% of Total	% of Hits
General Metabolism	72	94	1.30	6.1	7.0
Transcriptional and translational	165	462	2.80	30.7	37.0
Processing and sorting	10	13	1.30	0.8	1.0
Degradation	9	20	2.22	1.3	2.0
Structural functions	47	243	5.17	16.2	19.0
Cell regulation	26	82	3.15	5.4	6.0
Other functions	138	244	1.77	16.2	19.0
Conserved unknown proteins	42	120	2.86	8.0	9.0
TOTAL	509	1278	2.51	85.0	100.0

Table 2. Major transcripts present in the *Lonomia obliqua* bristle extract identified by EST-based strategy. Adapted from EST data-bank of NCBI deposited by Reis and colleagues in 2004 [19, 20].

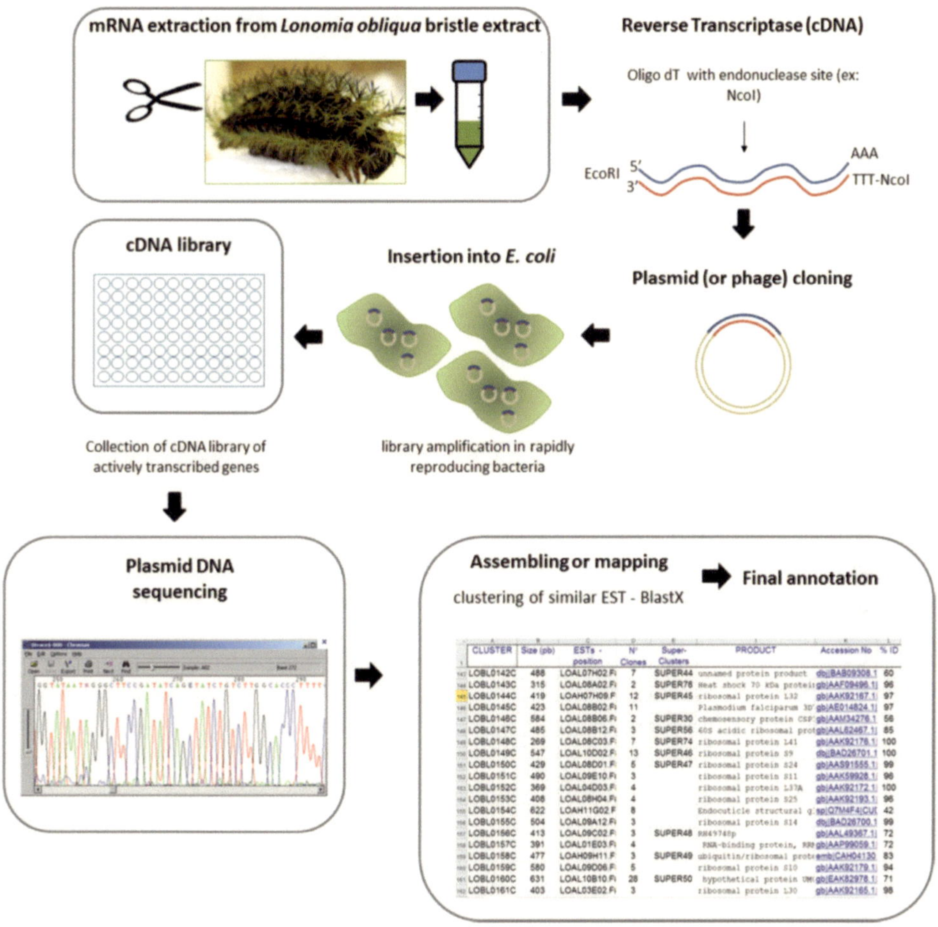

Figure 4. Schematic view of a transcriptomic approach based on EST-strategy. The strategy of construction of the cDNA library starts by the extraction of total RNA from a sample (ex. *L. obliqua* bristle extract). After purification of the mRNAs with an oligo (dT)-cellulose column, the cDNAs are synthesized (reverse transcription) by using synthetic oligonucleotides containing a restriction sites (in figure: NcoI and EcoRI for sense and antisense primers, respectively). The cDNA obtained can be inserted into a vector (plasmids or phages), generating a cDNA library. The library can be perpetuated by transforming the clones (plasmids) or infecting themselves (in the cases of phages) in *E. coli*. Based on DNA sequence information, bioinformatics tools predict the amino acid sequence of the corresponding gene products and their similarity to known genes. The redundant EST data sets are organized and integrated into cluster [54, 55].

Other cDNA libraries were constructed from bristles and integument [43]. The transcripts of those libraries revealed the presence of sequences related to trypsin-like enzymes, blood coagulation factors, prophenoloxidase cascade activators, cysteine proteases, phospholipase A2, serpins, cystatins, antibacterial proteins, lipocalins, and others (GenBank accession number: AY829732–AY829859) [43]. Sequences deposited independently in gene banks from both cDNA libraries are complementary. Apart from new venom component precursors, both libraries describe gene products related to cellular processes important for venom production, including high protein synthesis, tuned post-translational processing and trafficking. Those important projects contributed significantly to the characterization of this venom, which showed to be a rich source of proteins and active principles. Further studies about the biological and pharmacological properties of these molecules are necessary to understand its involvement in the envenoming process. Recently, the next-generation of sequencing methods - for example, pyrosequencing - have improved and increased the sequencing reducing time and cost compared to the traditional Sanger method [47, 56].

2.2. Microarray analysis

The identification of genes expressed in cells of a tissue is a basic step to provide essential information about gene function and tissue physiology. The gene expression analysis through the microarray technology (cDNA arrays) has become a powerful tool for rapid analysis of the functional effects of toxins on cells and tissues [57]. The main application of cDNA arrays is to compare the expression of known genes in different physiological situations, for example, tissues in normal and pathological conditions [58]. Thus, analyses of array data contribute to a better understanding of complex gene expression patterns related to physiology and metabolism, unveiling networks or pathways previously unknown.

A study of the effects of *L. obliqua* bristle extract on the gene expression profile of cultured human fibroblasts showed that many genes are up- and down-regulated, especially those related to the inflammatory processes such as IL-8, IL-6, CXCL1 and CCL2 [44]. Other changes in the expression pattern of some genes, such as prostaglandin-endoperoxide synthase 2, urokinase-type plasminogen activator receptor and tissue factor, were also observed, which could contribute to the pathological effects of lonomism. The authors suggest that the clinical manifestations may be a result of the direct action of *L. obliqua* venom on the host cells allied to an indirect effect caused by alteration in the gene expression pattern in host tissues.

2.3. Immunoproteome of *Lonomia obliqua* bristle extract

The identification of antigens eliciting an immune response by applying proteomic technologies can be defined as *Immunoproteomics*. Some usual immunoproteomics approaches are shown in Figure 5. Here, the perspective for its application regards the improvement of serum therapy by the selection of antigens for toxin-specific immunization of horses. Furthermore, some applications correlate the identification of antigens with certain diseases, such as infectious, autoimmune or cancer, providing diagnostic and monitoring informations. In this way, these methodologies are good choices in developing clinical applications and also to discover biomarkers. [59].

In classical gel-based strategy, the isolation and identification of proteins/antigens comprises a combination of bidimensional electrophoresis, immunoblotting and mass spectrometry. The aim of bidimensional electrophoresis is to isolate proteins based on their charge and mass [60, 61]. The first step is isoelectric focusing (IEF), where proteins migrate to reach their isoelectric point in an immobilized pH gradient gel under high voltage. All proteins are given negative charge by addition of SDS detergent. This step also includes denaturation of proteins by reduction and alkylation. The second step is SDS-polyacrylamide gel electrophoresis (SDS-PAGE), where smaller proteins migrate faster through the gel to the anode than larger ones. Detection of proteins can be performed by gel staining or immunoblotting.

Immunoblotting involves the transfer of proteins from gel to a nitrocellulose or PVDF membrane in an electric field [62]. The immobilized proteins in the membrane are subsequently incubated with antibodies that have affinity for the proteins of interest. Detection is carried out by enzyme-labelled secondary antibodies against the constant region of the primary IgG antibody, followed by the addition of a chemilluminescent substrate. The substrate reaction can be visualized by fluorescence.

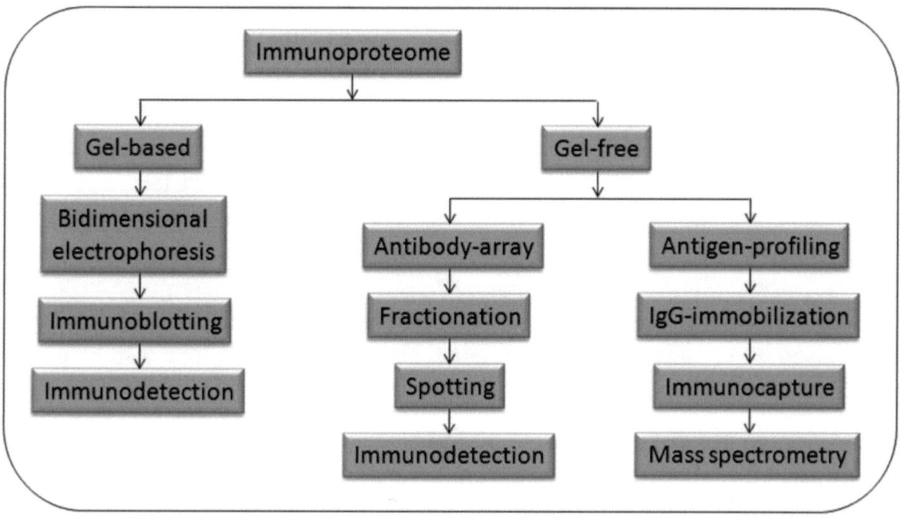

Figure 5. General approaches in Immunoproteomics. **Gel-based approach**: Bidimensional electrophoresis is based on protein separation on their pI and molecular mass. Then, the proteins are transferred from gel and immobilized on membrane (Western blotting). Antigens will be detected after serum incubation, followed by addition of secondary labelled antibodies and their substrates. **Gel-free approaches**: Antigen array: Proteins are fractionated (pI, hydrophobicity,etc) and spotted in a solid support. After that, antigenic fractions can be detected using patient serum and secondary labelled antibodies. Antigen profiling: Immunocapture is based on immobilization of patient immunoglobulins G, which are directly used to capture and isolate antigenic proteins from a complex mixture of proteins. Captured antigens are profiled by mass spectrometry (modified from 66).

Following this, the immunogenic proteins are removed from the gel and enzymatically digested for further mass spectrometry analyses [63]. Trypsin is generally used, cleaving an amide bond on the C-terminal side of lysine and arginine residues, which will be protonated and analyzed in positive-ion mode. Addition of diluted acid (0.1% formic acid or 1% trifluoracetic acid) to the sample contributes to the ionization process.

The ionization methods that are most often used for peptides and proteins are Matrix Assisted Laser Desorption Ionization (MALDI) and Electrospray Ionization (ESI). Peptides and proteins can be identified by Peptide mass fingerprinting (PMF) or *de novo* sequencing [63]. PMF is based on their fragmentation pattern, considering that identical peptide maps have identical amino acid sequences. For *de novo* sequencing analyses, the precursor ion is selected for fragmentation and the product ions are evaluated by mass differences between successive peaks in the spectrum, which are related to the individual mass of their residues.

The identification of immunogenic compounds from *L. obliqua*'s bristle extract was performed on gel-based approach using the polyclonal horse anti-Lonomic hyperimmune serum and anti-Lopap specific rabbit serum produced by the Butantan Institute [9]. Bidimensional electrophoresis of bristle extract revealed 157 silver stained spots, under non-reducing conditions (without DTT and iodoacetamide addition), providing an overview protein mapping (Figure 6A). However, 153 spots were immunodetected using anti-Lonomic serum (Figure 6B) and 30 spots detected using anti-Lopap serum (Figure 6C). Abundant proteins from 24 selected colloidal Coomassie Blue gel spots, corresponding to immunogenic proteins, were digested with trypsin and analysed by tandem mass spectrometry. The identification searches were carried out using the *L. obliqua* bristle EST databank. Lipocalins (spots 05, 09, 10, 14, 15, 16, 18, 24), cuticle protein (spots 05, 06, 07, 08, 11, 12, 13) and serpins (spot 21) were amongst the proteins identified (Figure 6A) [9]. Lipocalins can play a role in homeostasis and inflammation, as a defense mechanism in haematophagous arthropods. Lopap, characterized as a lipocalin protein member, and its all isoforms were highly represented as immunogenic proteins, revealed by the specific anti-Lopap serum (Figure 6C). The bristle' cDNA libraries also confirm the high abundance of lipocalins. As previously described [9, 19], these proteins have important role in envenoming. The cuticle proteins identified can be related to the inflammatory response caused by macerated spicule proteins. The serpin protein may also be involved in the defense mechanism.

Besides the biochemical and pharmacological tests, the quality control of serum and vaccine production can be monitored by proteomic technologies [64], such as chromatographic analyses, bidimensional electrophoresis and immunoblotting, once they are able to detect protein degradation and also confirm the presence of specific antibodies. However, immunotherapy can be more effective if a better characterization of venom composition is performed, improving immunization procedures, increasing its specificity and reducing side effects. The new generation of high affinity antibodies against low abundant immunogenic toxins can be evaluated by an antivenomic approach [64, 65].

A novel approach is the investigation of post-translational modifications (PTM) that affect antigen recognition, given that many peptides presented to T cells by the major histocompability complex are post-translationally modified [66]. Glycosylation and phosphorylation are important PTMs of proteins, playing crucial roles in several biological processes, including cell recognition and signalling pathway [67, 68]. Some potential targets for cancer therapy are based on glycosylated and phosphorylated epitopes discoveries [59].

Otherwise, phosphorylated proteins are usually enriched by immunoprecipitation (mainly for phosphotyrosine peptides) or by chromatographic procedures, such as Strong Cation eXchange (SCX), Hydrophilic Interaction Liquid Chromatography (HILIC), Immobilized Metal Affinity Chromatography (IMAC) or Metal Oxide Affinity Chromatography (MOAC).

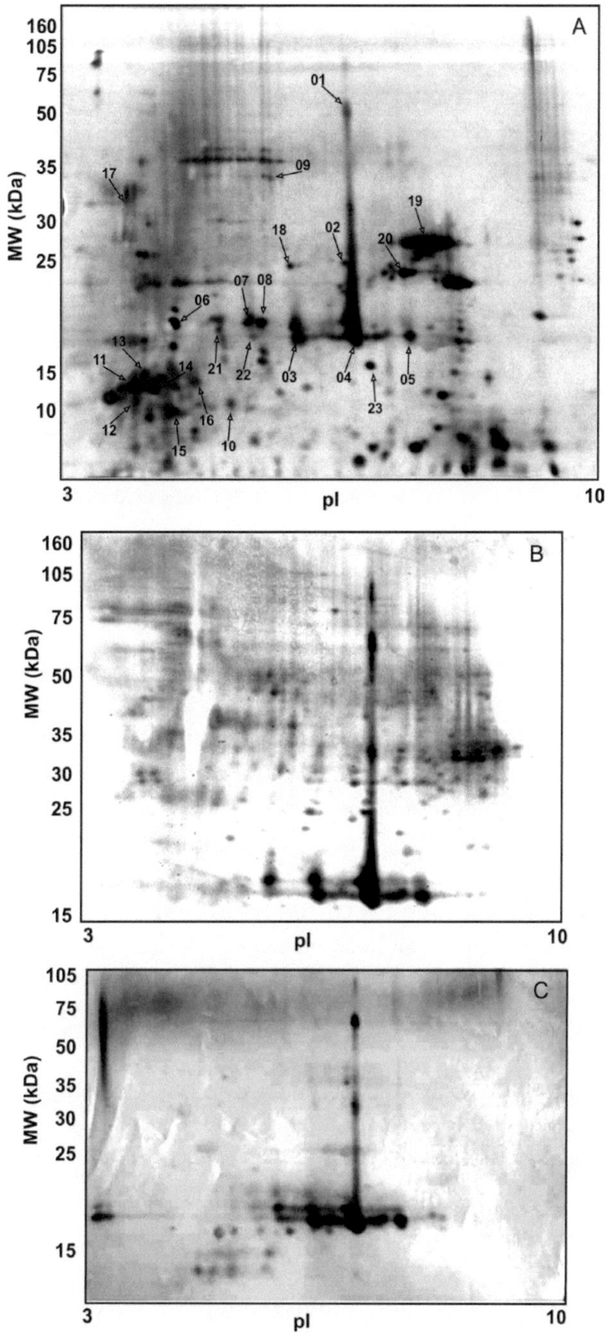

Figure 6. Bidimensional electrophoresis and immunoblotting from *Lonomia obliqua*'s bristle extract. (A): silver stained bidimensional gel (100 µg of protein applied) under non-reducing condition. Panels (B) and (C): PVDF immunoblotted 2D gels incubated with anti-Lonomic horse serum diluted 1:500 (B) or with anti-Lopap rabbit serum diluted 1:250 (C) [9].

Different metals may be used (iron, zirconium, gallium, etc) and peptides eluted by acidic or basic conditions, releasing mono-phosphorylated and multi-phosphorylated peptides, respectively [67].

The simultaneous screening of thousands of proteins from complex samples in a fast and sensitive manner can be performed using protein arrays. Amongst the different protein microarray applications are biomarker discovery, protein interaction studies, enzyme-substrate profiling, immunological profiling and vaccine development. As our interest is in the immune response, an antibody microarray can be used for identification of antigens that react specifically with the antibodies spotted on a solid support, with the complex formed then detected by fluorescence [59].

A large number of not yet identified proteins are considered as unknowns, but higher probabilities of identifications are reached when different methodologies are applied for analysis of complex samples. The combination of several proteomic techniques described here could improve the detection of immunogenic compounds and create new perspectives for effective immunotherapies.

3. *Lonomia obliqua* toxins

The *L. obliqua* caterpillar venom contain non-protein and protein components [21]. The procoagulant proteins present in the venom cause hemostatic disturbances mainly mediated by thrombin formation, the key enzyme of blood coagulation. Physiologically, thrombin generation from prothrombin occurs by assembling of the prothrombinase complex, which consists of factor Xa (catalytic factor), factor Va (non-enzymatic cofactor), calcium and a phospholipid membrane surface. Despite figured as a cascade of subsequent activation of coagulation factors, blood coagulation is currently conceived in a cell based-model [69]. In Figure 7 a simplified cascade model of hemostasis is illustrated, showing the known interactions of the *L. obliqua* venom and toxins.

Several molecules and activities were reported in bristles or hemolymph (Table 1). Some of them are related to the pathophysiology of the envenoming others to the development process of the animal such as regulation of the cell cycle [16]. Donato and colleagues [70] identified in the bristle extract a direct factor X activator which is calcium-independent, and a prothrombin activator. The prothrombin and factor X activators were later isolated and named Lopap and Losac, respectively [22, 24]. Interestingly, both molecules are no longer similar with any well-known procoagulant molecule from human or any other species.

3.1. Lopap: Functional characterization, recombinant production and bioinformatics analysis

Lopap (*Lonomia obliqua* Prothrombin Activator Protease) was purified from the bristle extract as a 69-kDa protein through gel filtration followed by reverse-phase chromatography. The purified protein was subjected to trypsin hydrolysis and partial amino acid sequences of N-terminal and internal fragments were obtained through Edman degradation [24].

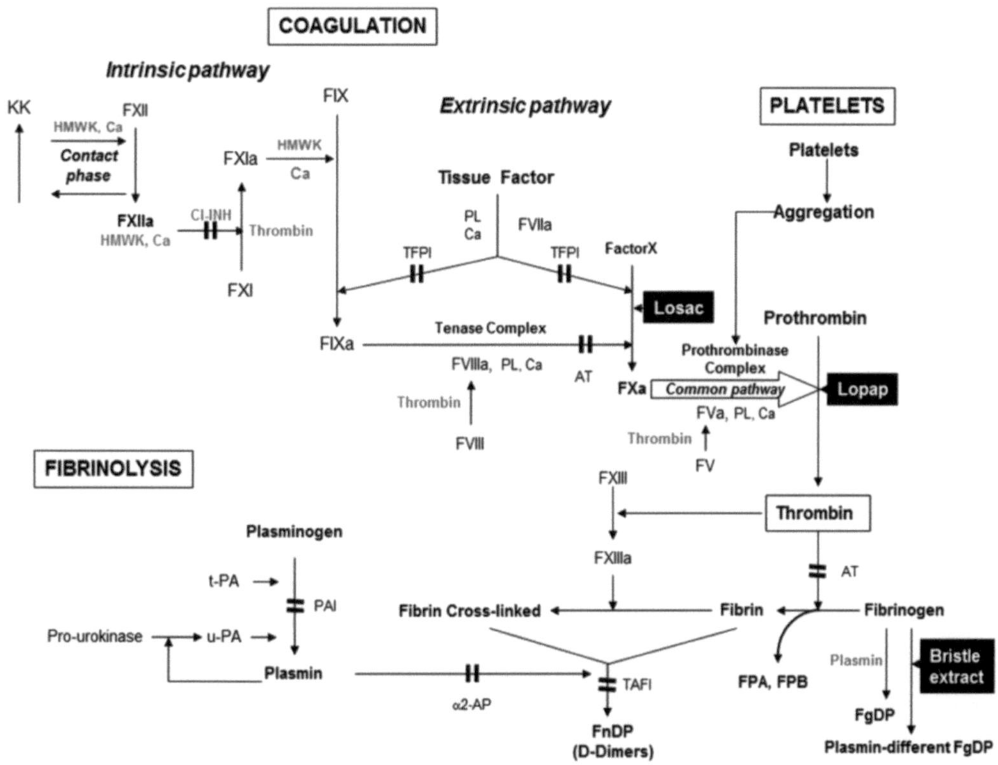

Figure 7. Schematic overview of hemostasis. Dark double-bars indicate where inhibitors act. HMWK = high molecular-weight-kininogen. PK = Prekallikrein. KK = Kallikrein. CI-INH = CI-inhibitor. TFPI = tissue factor pathway inhibitor. PL = phospholipids. Ca = calcium ions. AT = antithrombin. FDA = Fibrinopeptide A. FDB = Fibrinopeptide B. TAFI = Thrombin-activatable fibrinolysis inhibitor. FnDP = Fibrin degradation products. FgDP = Fibrinogen degradation products. α_2-AP = α_2-antiplasmin. Known interactions of the *L. obliqua* venom are indicated in the black boxes. Losac = *L. obliqua* Stuart factor activator. Lopap = *L. obliqua* prothrombin activator protease.

The recombinant protein (rLopap) was obtained in enzymatically active form as monomer of 21 kDa with a polyhistidine tag after purification by immobilized metal-chelate affinity chromatography. Partial amino acid sequences of native Lopap lead to identification of its respective clone from the cDNA library of *L. obliqua* bristles [20], encoding for a signal peptide (16 aa residues) and the mature protein (185 aa residues). cDNA of mature protein, consisting in a transcript with 603 bp open reading frame, was subcloned into the pAE vector and expressed in the bacteria E. coli BL21(DE3) with a fusion tag (His6). Protein was recovered in inclusion bodies after cell lysis and subjected to refolding and purification after solubilization in urea [71].

Interestingly, the deduced amino acid sequence of Lopap showed no similarity with other prothrombin activators or serine proteases, but was similar to lipocalin family members, either from insects or mammals [71]. Lopap sequence alignment with other lipocalins is shown in Figure 8. Members of lipocalin family usually share only about 30% of similarity in amino acid sequence, despite showing conserved secondary and tertiary structures. Furthermore, these proteins have in primary structure three characteristic conserved motifs [72].

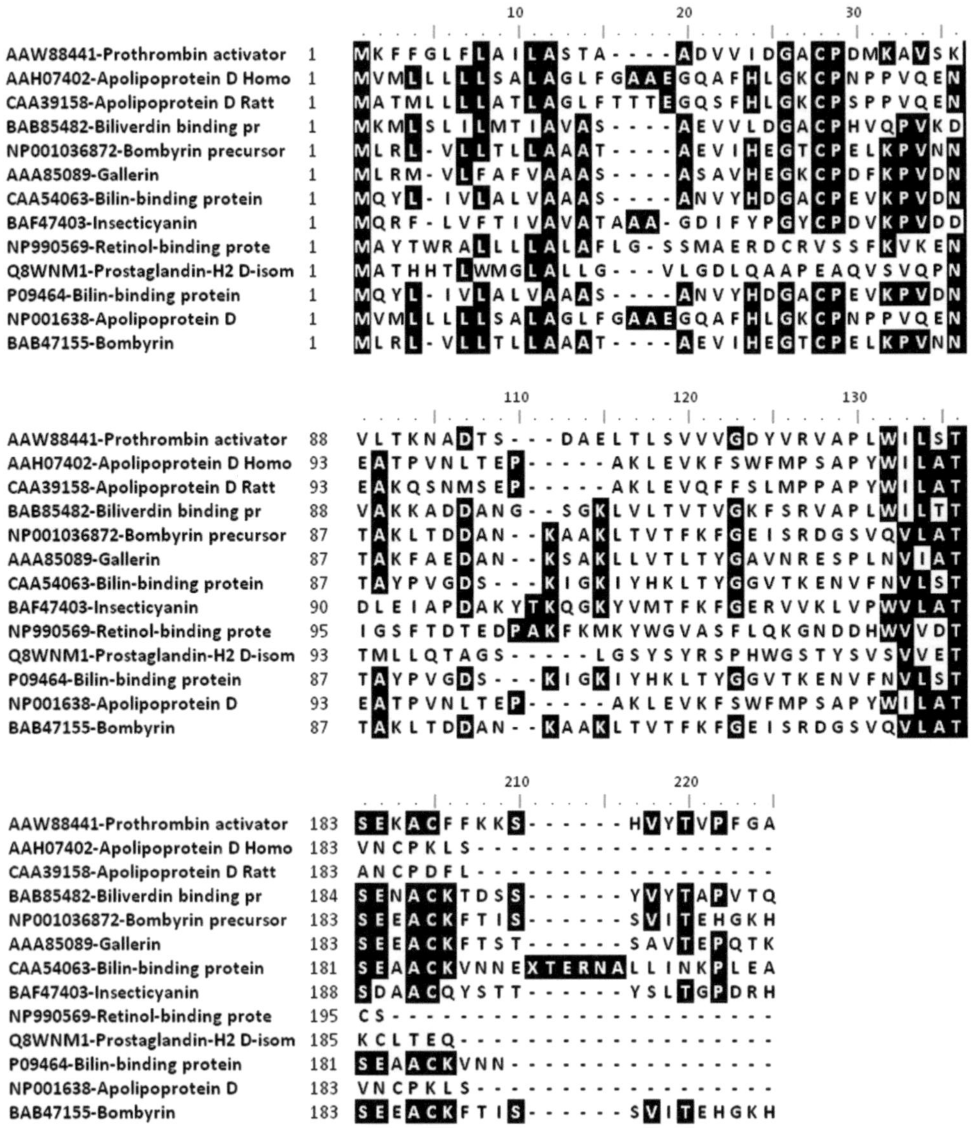

Figure 8. Amino acid sequence alignment of Lopap and other lipocalins. Sequences were accessed from protein data bank at NCBI and aligned using BioEdit [80].

Lopap's tridimensional structure obtained by molecular modeling has the characteristic fold of lipocalins, consisting in an eight stranded antiparallel β-barrel (Figure 9) with a hydrophobic pocket for binding of hydrophobic ligands. A serine protease catalytic triad was also predicted

http://dx.doi.org/10.5772/53697

[19]. Lopap is the first lipocalin described that displays proteolytic activity. On the other hand, through a peptide mapping approach based on lipocalin conserved motifs found in the Lopap's primary structure, a synthetic peptide was obtained (Figure 10), which has been proposed as a sequence signature among lipocalins, sharing a common role in cell protection and development process [73]. Other lipocalins that have been described with antiapoptotic activity share similar sequences, which have similar conformations in their tridimensional structures [73].

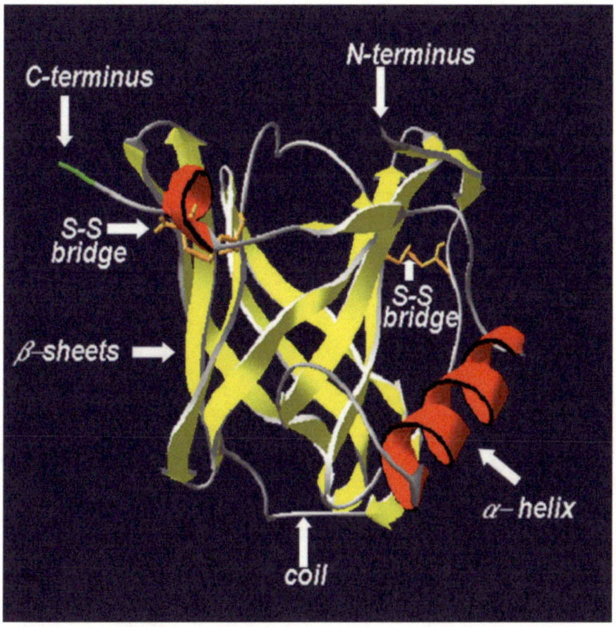

Figure 9. Model of the tridimensional structure of Lopap [81].

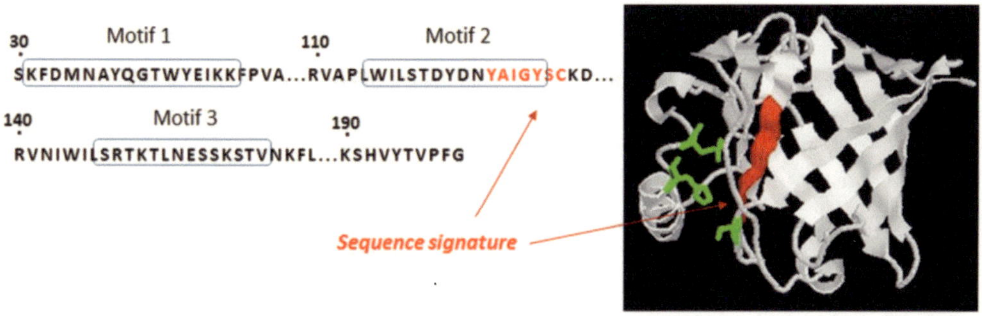

Figure 10. Lipocalin sequence signature highlighted among lipocalin conserved motifs identified in Lopap sequence [19] and in the model of tridimensional structure. Residues predicted in the catalytic triad are shown in green [25].

Lopap shows specific proteolytic activity towards prothrombin. It displays serine protease-like activity and activates human prothrombin through hydrolysis of Arg^{284}-Thr^{285} and Arg^{320}-Ile^{321} peptide bounds, generating active thrombin, without formation of the intermediate meizothrombin [24]. This mechanism is similar to prothrombin activation by FXa in absence of the prothrombinase complex (Figure 11), previously described [74]. This is the unique prothrombin activation mechanism described for an exogenous serine protease, which is independent of prothrombinase complex components. All other exogenous prothrombin activators (metalloproteases and serine proteases) currently described from snake venoms fit into four groups, sharing similar mechanisms of action [75].

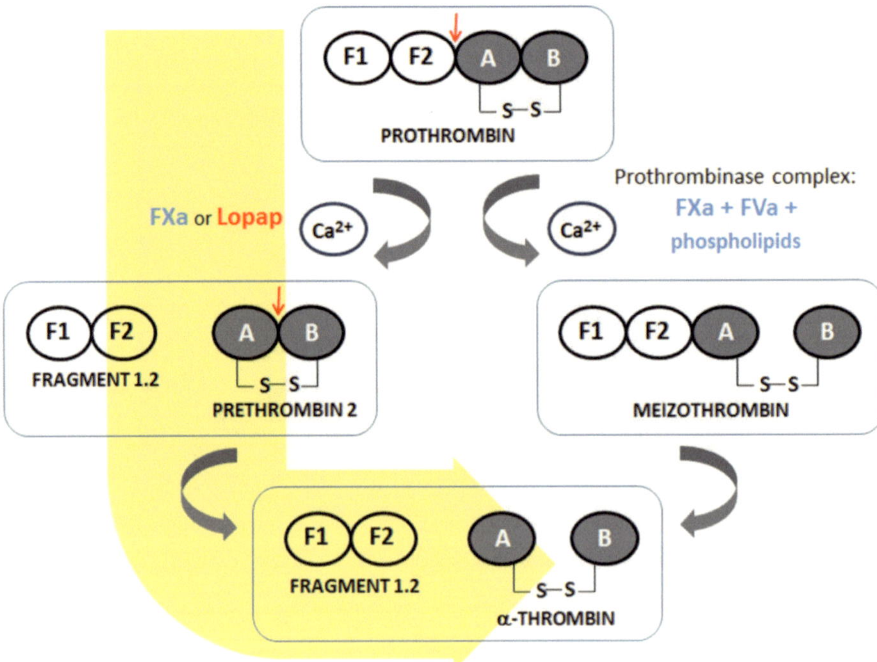

Figure 11. Prothrombin activation mechanisms indicating the Lopap hydrolysis sites and its generated products.

When administered *in vivo*, Lopap induces blood clotting into microvessels, resulting in fibrinogen consumption and blood incoagulability [76]. These effects resemble the consumption coagulopathy triggered by the whole venom, indicating the involvement of this prothrombin activator as a key toxin in envenoming [26]. In addition, Lopap is able to modulate endothelial cell responses promoting cell survival, IL-8, nitric oxide (NO) and PGI_2 release, expression of the cell adhesion molecules ICAM-1 and E-selectin, but not VCAM-1 and PCAM-1 [45, 77, 78]. Lopap also displays cytoprotective activity in neutrophils and do not modify expressions of L-selectin and β2 integrin. Secretion of the proinflammatory cytokines IL-6 and TNF-α is not changed by Lopap treatment in both cell cultures [78]. Lopap seems to have no effect on modulation of coagulation and fibrinolysis through endothelial cell response, since it does not modify von Willebrand factor (vWF) and tissue plasminogen activator (t-PA) release or tissue factor procoagulant activity on endothelial cell surface [45, 77].

The Lopap-derived peptide obtained through chemical synthesis (Survicalin) reproduces the Lopap's modulation on endothelial cells and neutrophils cell, triggering antiapoptotic activity [73]. Survicalin also induces fibroblast responses, decreasing caspase-3 and increasing Bcl-2, Ki-67, IL-1β and the receptors for IL-8 and IL-6. Enhanced production of extracellular matrix proteins, such as collagen, fibronectin, tenascin and laminin is also induced by Survicalin in fibroblast culture [79].

3.2. Losac: Functional characterization

Losac is the first factor X activator purified from a lepidopter secretion. It was obtained from caterpillar's bristle extract as a single polypeptide chain protein of about 45 kDa [22]. Some years later, from a cDNA library of *L. obliqua* bristle transcripts [19], the specific clone encoding for Losac was identified and the recombinant protein produced in bacteria system (for details, see section 3.3). Studies using the native or recombinant form of Losac (rLosac) revealed specificity toward factor X [20, 22, 28]. Moreover, Losac had no effect on fibrin or fibrinogen, indicating its specificity for blood coagulation activation, and it was recognized by the antilonomic serum produced in Butantan Institute. Thus, it is plausible that this protein participates in the consumption coagulopathy observed in patients.

Biochemical characterization of Losac has shown that, although its sequence did not show an equivalent among other factor X activators, Losac possess a similar mechanism of action than RVV-X, a factor X activator purified from Russell's viper venom *Daboia russelli* [28, 82, 83]. Like RVV-X, factor X activation by Losac can be accelerated in the presence of calcium and phospholipids, two important cofactor in the assembling of blood coagulation complexes [69]. In spite of this, Losac can activate factor X independently of these cofactors. Moreover, both activators require a stable conformation of factor X and the presence of the Gla-domain of factor X for an appropriated activity. Interestingly, the cleavage fragments of factor X generated by both activators were quite similar. Although there are strong functional similarities, the major difference is in the structure of both activators. Apparently, Losac activates factor X through a serine protease-like activity, while RVV-X has a typical metalloproteinase structure [20, 28, 84].

A model proposed by Morita [83] and crystallographic studies of RVV-X [85] support the hypothesis that it primarily recognizes the calcium-bound conformation of Gla-domain in factor X through an exosite formed by the light chains, followed by the catalytic conversion of factor X to factor Xa. Despite the structural differences between Losac and RVV-X, it remains possible that they share a similar mechanisms for recognition of factor X involving calcium ions, phospholipids and the Gla-domain of factor X followed by its proteolytic conversion to active factor X.

Besides its role in coagulation [22, 28], Losac is also capable of inducing proliferation and inhibiting endothelial cell death while stimulating the release of NO, a known molecule with antiapoptotic activity [86, 87], and t-PA, a component of fibrinolytic-pathway involved in matrix remodeling [88]. The authors suggest that the cell proliferation and cell viability activities elicited by Losac are probably related to the NO liberation [22], since NO was also described as an endothelial survival factor, inhibiting apoptosis [86, 87]. Moreover, it was also observed that the production/expression of some important molecules involved in inflammation and coagulation systems such as ICAM-1, PGI2, DAF, IL-8, vWF and tissue factor were not affected by Losac.

It has been show that hemolymph from some insects can increase cell longevity by inhibiting apoptosis [89, 90]. The increase of *Spodoptera frugiperda* Sf-9 cell growth in almost 3-fold was reported after supplementation with *L. obliqua* hemolymph [91]. This effect was attributed to the presence of three factors with different activities: a potential antiapoptotic factor, a growth-promoting factor, and an enzyme that hydrolyzes sucrose. Furthermore, an antiapoptotic protein of 51 kDa was purified from *L. obliqua* hemolymph [36]. This protein was able to prevent apoptosis in Sf-9 cell culture induced by nutrient deprivation and by Actinomycin D. Later reports [37, 38] described in the hemolymph a potent antiviral activity against human virus.

3.3. Molecular cloning and heterologous expression of Losac

The production of Losac in a recombinant form was important due to the disadvantages of purifying Losac from bristle extract: the use of many caterpillars to prepare the bristle extract and the low yield of native Losac (0.3%) [22]. Cloning and production scheme to obtain rLosac is shown in Figure 12 [28].

Nucleotide and deduced amino acid sequences were compared with data banks in order to identify similar genes and their products. The analysis revealed a high similarity with members of the immunoglobulin-like superfamily of cell adhesion molecules (IgCAMs), especially with neural CAMs (NCAMs) [28]. Members of this group have diverse functions but none was associated with proteolytic activities [94]. Multiple comparison of the deduced amino acid sequence revealed different degrees of identity with IgCAMs: 26% of identity with L1-NCAM from humans, 34% with the protein neuroglian from *Drosofila melanogaster*; and 47-76% with hemolins from lepidopters [95-98]. Although no structural data was reported for Losac, a tertiary structure model was built through homology modeling based on crystal structure of *Hyalophora cecropia* hemolin (HcHemolin, Protein Data Bank code 1BIH). Both proteins share 76% of sequence identity [28] and the same multi-domain structure (four Ig-like domains: D1 to D4) and conserved motifs as shown in Figures 13 and 14. Both structures are composed of β-strands, arranged in a globular shape resembling a horseshoe (Figure 14A), akin to hemolin [97], axonin [99], and the four N-terminal Ig domains of neurofascin [100]. Because Losac shares its main sequence features with hemolins, it can be perfectly classified as one of them. It was demonstrated that Losac activate factor X in a similar way than RVV-X [28]. Nevertheless, unlike Losac, no hemolins or cell adhesion molecules were associated with proteolytic activities.

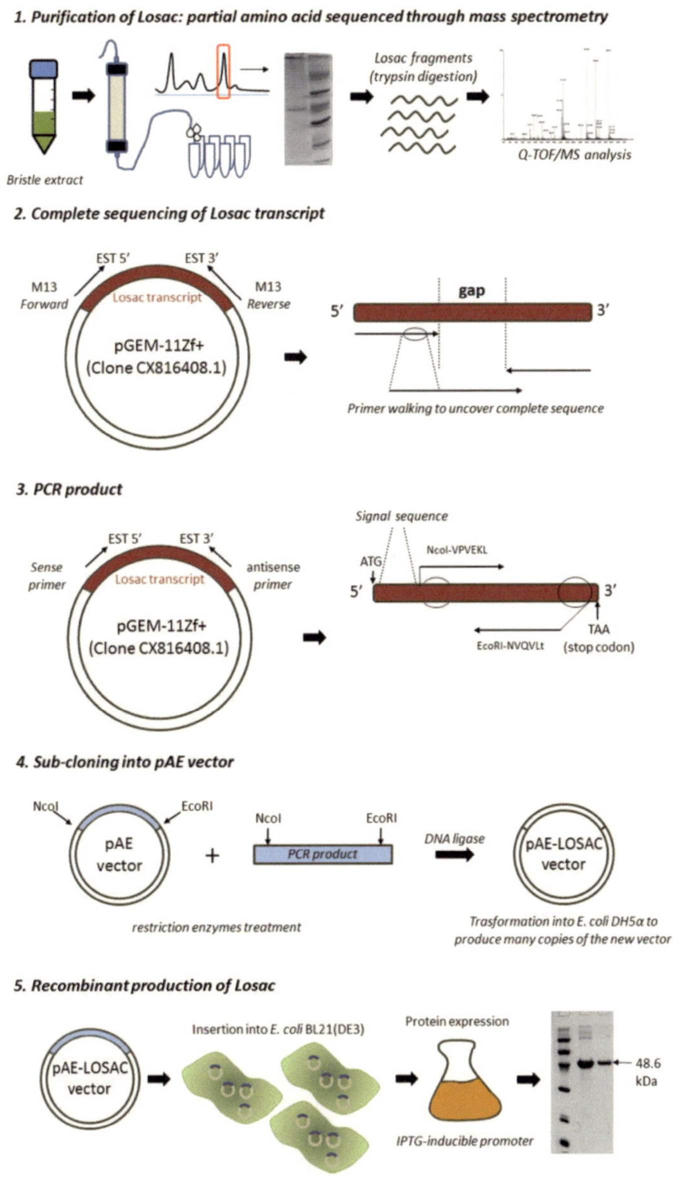

Figure 12. 1) After purification from bristle extract [22], Losac was submitted to a tryptic digestion to obtain partial amino acid sequences of internal fragments. Those sequences were obtained by mass spectrometry and used to screen the cDNA library to identify the transcript encoding the protein. The cDNA library was previously constructed with *L. obliqua* bristle mRNAs that were converted to cDNA and cloned into pGEM-11Zf+ plasmid [19, 20]. **2)** From this cDNA library, a transcript corresponding to the clone LOAH12B08 (GenBankTM accession number CX816408.1), matching the tryptic peptide sequences, was identified. However, this transcript was partially sequenced and the complete sequence was achieved through the *primer walking strategy* using a specific primer designed from an internal sequence of the transcript allowing uncover the complete sequence of Losac gene [92]. The nucleotide sequence has been deposited in GenBankTM (DQ479435), and the deduced protein has been deposited in the NCBI protein sequence database (ABF21073). **3)** The cDNA that encodes mature Losac was amplified by PCR using a sense and an

antisense primer designed according to the deduced N- and C-terminal sequences of the mature protein carrying *Nco*I or *Eco*RI restriction sites, respectively. **4)** The cDNA corresponding to mature Losac was sub-cloned into the pAE vector [93]. The PCR product and the pAE vector were restricted with *Nco*I and *Eco*RI, purified, and ligated with T4 DNA ligase and used to transform *E. coli* DH5α cells. **5)** The resulting pAE-Losac plasmid was used to transform *E. coli* BL21(DE3) cells. The recombinant protein was expressed in fusion to a minimal N-terminal His6-tag as a 48.6 kDa protein: Protein was recovered in inclusion bodies after cell lysis and subjected to refolding and purification after solubilization in urea.

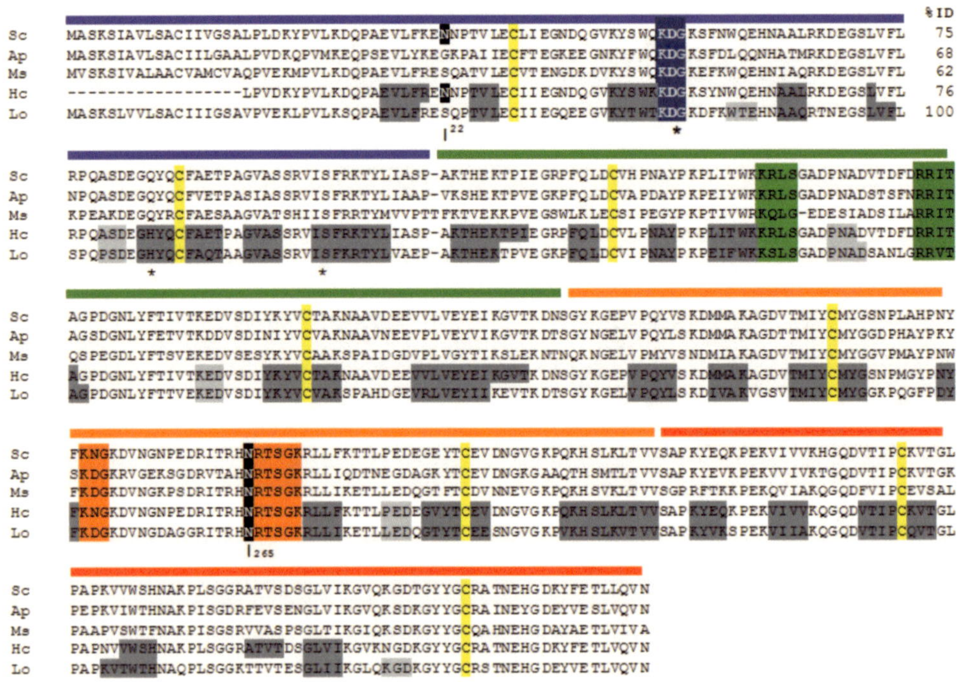

Figure 13. Multiple amino acid sequence alignment of Losac with other hemolin proteins. Sequence identity is shown for all proteins related to Losac. The structures encompass four constant-type immunoglobulin domains (cIg) (D1-D4). The bars above the sequences correspond to domains 1 (D1, blue), 2 (D2, green), 3 (D3, orange) and 4 (D4, red). Sequence identity is shown for all hemolins related to Losac (%ID). The α-helices and β-sheets observed in *Hyalophora cecropia* hemolin (Protein Data Bank code 1BIH) and Losac are shaded in light and dark gray, respectively. Previously it was predicted that hemolin contain conserved regions and motifs (28, 36). Conserved motifs are shown inside boxes according to the domain they belong. The eight cysteines (in yellow) form four intra-chain disulfide bridges. Losac conserves the well-known motifs involved in cell-adhesion mechanism (KDG motif in D1 and D3), as well as the highly conserved *N*-glycosylation site in D3 (Asn^{265}, in black). An additional *N*-glycosylation site (Asn^{22}) is found in *H. cecropia* and *S. c. ricini* hemolins (D1). The LPS-binding site (NRTS motif: Asn^{265}, Arg^{266}, Thr^{267} and Ser^{268}) in D3 (orange). In D2 are located the KRLS cAMP/cGMP-dependent protein kinase phosphorylation site and the RRIT motif (green boxes). Positions of the residues forming the putative catalytic site are evidenced with an asterisk. Hemolin sequences (with abbreviation and GenBank™ accession numbers in brackets) are from: *Samia cynthia ricini* (Sc, BAE07175), *Antheraea pernyi* (Ap, AAS99343), *Manduca sexta* (Ms, AAC46915), Losac (Lo, ABF21073) and *H. cecropia* (Hc, AAB34817).

At this stage we can only speculate about the mechanism of action of Losac. One possibility is to evaluate structural features that might contribute to the Losac-induced factor X activation. Thus, a search for serine protease active-site was undertaken based on the *Catalytic Site Atlas* (CSA) program analysis. Three possible catalytic residues, Asp(D)^{40}, His(H)^{72} and Ser(S)^{90}, were

http://dx.doi.org/10.5772/53697

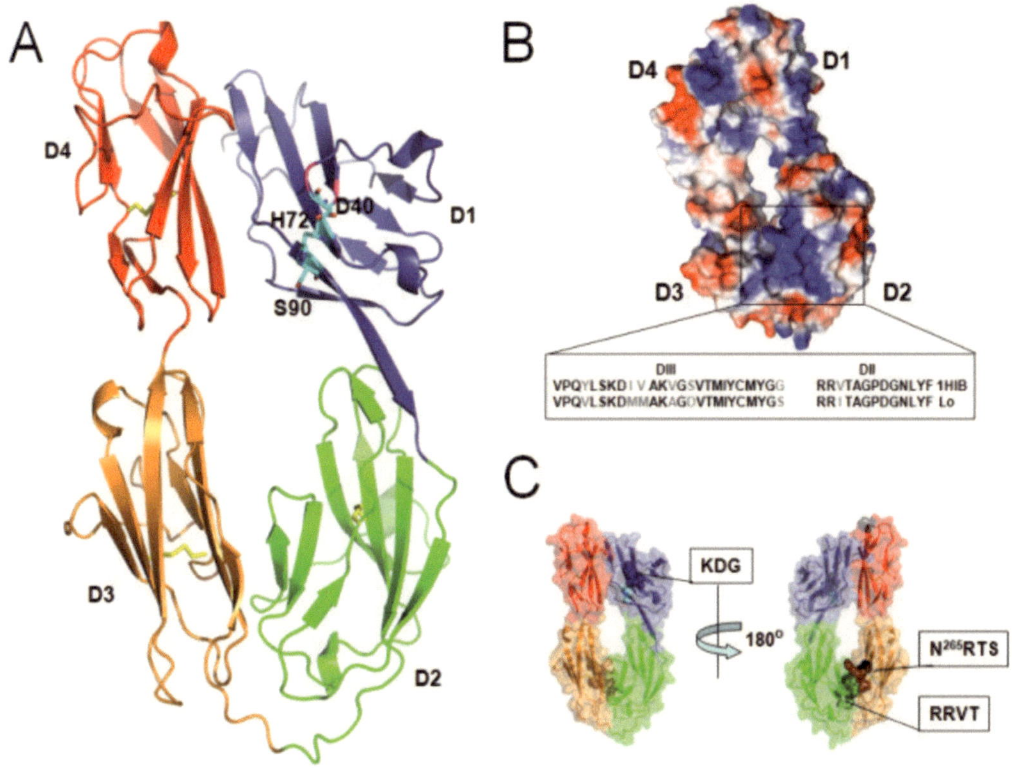

Figure 14. Three-dimensional structure model of Losac. **(A)** Cartoon view of the predicted model of Losac protein built from the structural coordinates of *H. cecropia* hemolin (PDB code 1BIH) using Modeller 9v1 [102]. Each domain (D1-D4) comprises α-helices and 7 strands arranged in 2 antiparallel β-sheets that are linked together by a disulfide bridge (shown in yellow stick). The residues of the putative catalytic triad predicted in D1 by the program *Catalytic Site Atlas* (http://www.ebi.ac.uk/thornton-srv/databases/CSA/) program, are indicated as stick cyan color by the one letter code followed by the residue number, D^{40}, H^{72}, $S^{90.}$ **(B)** Electrostatic potential surface of Losac showing inside the box the conserved phosphate-binding site at the D2-D3 interface domains, exactly as was demonstrated for HcHemolin [97]. **(C)** Surface view of Losac model evidencing the conserved adhesive motif KDG (deep blue) and the LPS-binding motif RRVT (green) and NRTS (chocolate), which contains the glycosylation site in N^{265}. All the figures were produced in Pymol v1.5 (http://www.pymol.org/).

located on D1 (Figure 13 and 14A) and could fit to such activity. Theoretical analysis (Figure 13 and 14) and observed results - total inhibition by PMSF as described in [28] - seem to suggest the presence of a serine protease-like active-site in Losac which would be responsible for the proteolytic activation of factor X [20, 28, 84]. Some molecular techniques, such as Site-directed mutagenesis [101], could be applied in an effort to understand the structural requirements for ligand binding and selectivity and identification of active site residues.

Functionally, hemolins were first associated with the insect immune system because of their over-expression after bacterial infection [103]. Due to their adhesion properties, some hemolins have been involved in the cell adhesion mechanisms. In the last two decades independent studies demonstrated that hemolins are multifunctional molecules involved in a diverse range of cell interaction [104-110]. The high identity among Losac and hemolins suggests that Losac could also assume some of these functions in *L. obliqua*. The adhesive properties of Losac probably are relevant to understanding the human umbilical vein endothelial cell responses observed in previous studies.

4. Biomedical applications

Studies on *L. obliqua* toxins with a molecular approach have applications beyond the pathophysiology and therapeutic perspectives of envenoming. As procoagulant proteins, Lopap and Losac can be useful as tools for developing clotting assays and diagnostic kits. Exogenous factor X activators, such as recombinant Losac, has also the potential to be used for detection of factor X deficiency and lupus anticoagulant [111]. In the case of Lopap, an exogenous prothrombin activator, two patents were applied to use this compound in diagnostic kits for detection of dysprothrombinemias using the native form purified from the venom as well as the recombinant form produced in bacteria. This prothrombin activator has also the potential to be used in clotting time assays, prothrombin assays, and to monitor patients anticoagulated with hirudin. A recent study suggests that exogenous procoagulant proteins could also be considered for therapeutic use to manage bleeding complications caused by anticoagulation therapy. Treatment with Lopap was able to reduce the bleeding time of rabbits anticoagulated with low molecular weight heparin, through direct prothrombin activation, bypassing factor Xa inhibition [112]. Patent information about those applications can be consulted in Table 3.

Modulation of cell responses triggered by *Lonomia* toxins can have valuable therapeutic and biotechnological applications. Promoting cell survival can be useful to improve cell culture technologies and vaccine productions, and for treatment of degenerative diseases. In addition, the effects of Lopap on extracellular matrix remodeling can be valuable to develop wound healing formulations and to regeneration issues (Table 3). For this approaches, design and synthesis of short peptides derived from Lopap amino acid sequence is an interesting task to minimize toxic and side effects and for production of this molecules for proofs of concepts, pre-clinical and clinical tests (Table 3). Isolating specific domains and sequences can also help to understand the multifunctional properties of the studied proteins and direct structure-function insights.

Unveiling the mechanisms of action and structure-function relationship of these multifunctional molecules may pointing out these molecules as promising candidates to development of new therapeutic drugs, reagents in diagnostic kits for coagulation dysfunctions, and biotechnological applications.

5. Concluding remarks

Nature has been finding ways to gift living beings with functions that are advantageous, regarding natural selection, mainly by evolutionary process. Among all the lepidopterans of

WIPO patent application	Publication date	Patent	Institutions involved
WO/2003/070746	08.28.2003	Purification and characterization of a prothrombin activator from the bristle of Lonomia obliqua: to be used in diagnosis kits for detecting plasma prothrombin in hemorrhagic state patients	Instituto Butantan (Brazil); Fapesp (Brazil) and Biolab Sanus Farmacêutica Ltda (Brazil)
WO/2006/021062	02.03.2006	Process for obtaining the recombinant prothrombin activating protease (rLopap) in monomeric form; the recombinant prothrombin activating protease (rLopap) as well as its amino acid sequence; the use of this protease as a defibrinogenase agent and the diagnosis kit for dysprothrombinemias	Instituto Butantan (Brazil); Fapesp (Brazil) and Biolab Sanus Farmacêutica Ltda (Brazil)
WO/2007/028223	03.15.2007	Lopap-based pharmaceutical compositions and uses thereof: it refers to the use of Lopap as modulators of cell death and degeneration caused by wounds, aging and external agents	Instituto Butantan (Brazil); Fapesp (Brazil) and Biolab Sanus Farmacêutica Ltda (Brazil)
WO/2009093189	07.30.2009	Peptides, compositions, and uses thereof: it refers to the uses of Lopap-derived peptides for regenerating tissues and wound repair	Instituto Butantan (Brazil); Fapesp (Brazil) and Biolab Sanus Farmacêutica Ltda (Brazil)

Table 3. International patents associated to Lopap and peptides derived from its amino acid sequence. Information was obtained from World Intellectual Property Organization (WIPO).

medical interest in the world, *Lonomia* sp. caterpillars (family: Saturniidae) is the only genus that causes dramatic damages in human blood coagulation [16, 113]. This feature is reflected in the diversity of toxins produced by the caterpillar and their unusual enzymatic properties.

Application of molecular approaches in the study of *L. obliqua* toxins has been a valuable strategy in understanding the biological means of these molecules for the source organism itself and the dynamic pathways in envenoming syndrome. On the other hand, this approach reveals these toxins as interesting tools for therapeutic and biotechnological applications. The best examples are Lopap (a prothromin activator lipocalin) and Losac (the only hemolin with proteolytic activity). If, in one hand, the molecular basis of target recognition and proteolysis of factor X and prothrombin by Losac and Lopap, respectively, needs to be further investigated, on the other hand, efforts need to be focused on understanding the pro-survival activity of both molecules.

Integrating transcriptomic, proteomic and microarray analysis will provide a wealth of valuable information about venom composition. Molecular cloning and expression of recombinant toxins from *L. obliqua* opens new perspectives in the identification and characterization of macromolecular fine structure of toxins and its implications for toxic activity as well as new action mechanisms and target cell binding that should be an area of rapid development. The next several years will likely see some very significant advances in this field and, in the future, those approaches will permit the identification of molecular mechanisms at a new level.

Acknowledgements

The authors thank the Brazilian founding agencies FAPESP and CNPq, INCTTOX program. L.C.C.-C. had a Post-Doctoral fellowship from CAT-CEPID/FAPESP.

Author details

Ana Marisa Chudzinski-Tavassi, Miryam Paola Alvarez-Flores,
Linda Christian Carrijo-Carvalho and Maria Esther Ricci-Silva

*Address all correspondence to: amchudzinski@butantan.gov.br; miryam_paolaa@hotmail.com

Laboratory of Biochemistry and Biophysics, Butantan Institute, São Paulo, Brazil

References

[1] Diaz, J.H., The evolving global epidemiology, syndromic classification, management, and prevention of caterpillar envenoming. American Journal of Tropical Medicine and Hygiene, 2005. 72(3): p. 347-357.

[2] Hossler, E.W., Caterpillars and moths: Part II. Dermatologic manifestations of encounters with Lepidoptera. J Am Acad Dermatol, 2010. 62(1): p. 13-28; quiz 29-30.

[3] Balit, C.R., et al., Prospective study of definite caterpillar exposures. Toxicon, 2003. 42(6): p. 657-662.

[4] Hossler, E.W., Caterpillars and moths. Dermatologic Therapy, 2009. 22(4): p. 353-366.

[5] Ministério-da-Saúde, Acidentes por Lepidópteros, in Manual de diagnóstico e tratamento de acidentes por animais peçonhentos, FUNASA, Editor 2001, Fundação Nacional de Saúde (FUNASA): Brasil. p. 120.

[6] Zannin, M., et al., Blood coagulation and fibrinolytic factors in 105 patients with hemorrhagic syndrome caused by accidental contact with Lonomia obliqua caterpillar in Santa Catarina, southern Brazil. Thromb Haemost, 2003. 89(2): p. 355-64.

[7] Gamborgi, G.P., E.B. Metcalf, and E.J. Barros, Acute renal failure provoked by toxin from caterpillars of the species Lonomia obliqua. Toxicon, 2006. 47(1): p. 68-74.

[8] Goncalves, L.R., et al., Efficacy of serum therapy on the treatment of rats experimentally envenomed by bristle extract of the caterpillar Lonomia obliqua: comparison with epsilon-aminocaproic acid therapy. Toxicon, 2007. 50(3): p. 349-56.

[9] Ricci-Silva, M.E., et al., Immunochemical and proteomic technologies as tools for unravelling toxins involved in envenoming by accidental contact with Lonomia obliqua caterpillars. Toxicon, 2008. 51(6): p. 1017-28.

[10] Kowacs, P.A., et al., Fatal intracerebral hemorrhage secondary to Lonomia obliqua caterpillar envenoming - Case report. Arquivos De Neuro-Psiquiatria, 2006. 64(4): p. 1030-1032.

[11] Duarte, A.C., et al., Insuficiência renal aguda por acidentes com lagartas. Journal Brasileiro de Nefrologia, 1990. 12: p. 3.

[12] Kelen, E.M.A., Z.P. Picarelli, and A.C. Duarte, Hemorrhagic syndrome induced by contact with caterpillars of the genus Lonomia (saturniidae, hemileucinae). Journal of Toxicology-Toxin Reviews, 1995. 14(3): p. 283-308.

[13] Duarte, A.C., et al., Intracerebral haemorrhage after contact with Lonomia caterpillars. Lancet, 1996. 348(9033): p. 1033-1033.

[14] Carrijo-Carvalho, L.C. and A.M. Chudzinski-Tavassi, The venom of the Lonomia caterpillar: an overview. Toxicon, 2007. 49(6): p. 741-57.

[15] Fan, H.W. and A.C. Duarte, Acidentes por Lonomia, in Animais peçonhentos no Brasil: biologia, clínica e terapêutica dos acidentes, J.L. Cardoso, et al., Editors. 2003, Sarvier: Sao Paulo. p. 224-232.

[16] Alvarez Flores, M.P., M. Zannin, and A.M. Chudzinski-Tavassi, New insight into the mechanism of Lonomia obliqua envenoming: toxin involvement and molecular approach. Pathophysiol Haemost Thromb, 2010. 37(1): p. 1-16.

[17] Chudzinski-Tavassi, A.M. and L.C. Carrijo-Carvalho, Biochemical and biological properties of Lonomia obliqua bristle extract. Journal of Venomous Animals and Toxins Including Tropical Diseases, 2006. 12(2): p. 156-171.

[18] Reis, C.V., et al., In vivo characterization of Lopap, a prothrombin activator serine protease from the Lonomia obliqua caterpillar venom. Thromb Res, 2001. 102(5): p. 437-43.

[19] Reis, C.V., et al., Lopap, a prothrombin activator from Lonomia obliqua belonging to the lipocalin family: recombinant production, biochemical characterization and structure-function insights. Biochem J, 2006. 398(2): p. 295-302.

[20] Chudzinski-Tavassi, A.M. and M.P. Alvarez Flores, Exploring new molecules and activities from Lonomia obliqua caterpillars. Pathophysiol Haemost Thromb, 2005. 34(4-5): p. 228-33.

[21] Donato, J.L., et al., Lonomia obliqua caterpillar spicules trigger human blood coagulation via activation of factor X and prothrombin. Thrombosis and Haemostasis, 1998. 79(3): p. 539-542.

[22] Alvarez Flores, M.P., et al., Losac, a factor X activator from Lonomia obliqua bristle extract: its role in the pathophysiological mechanisms and cell survival. Biochem Biophys Res Commun, 2006. 343(4): p. 1216-23.

[23] Prezoto, B.C., et al., Antithrombotic effect of Lonomia obliqua caterpillar bristle extract on experimental venous thrombosis. Braz J Med Biol Res, 2002. 35(6): p. 703-12.

[24] Reis, C.V., et al., A prothrombin activator serine protease from the Lonomia obliqua caterpillar venom (Lopap) biochemical characterization. Thromb Res, 2001. 102(5): p. 427-36.

[25] Carrijo-Carvalho, L.C., Clonagem e expressão em levedura Pichia pastoris, obtenção de um peptídeo sintético, análise estrutural e avaliação de suas potenciais aplicações. PhD Thesis, in Interunidades em Biotecnologia2009, Universidade de São Paulo.

[26] Reis, C.V., et al., A Ca++ activated serine protease (LOPAP) could be responsible for the haemorrhagic syndrome caused by the caterpillar Lonomia obliqua. L obliqua Prothrombin Activator Protease. Lancet, 1999. 353(9168): p. 1942.

[27] Lilla, S., et al., Purification and initial characterization of a novel protein with factor Xa activity from Lonomia obliqua caterpillar spicules. J Mass Spectrom, 2005. 40(3): p. 405-12.

[28] Alvarez-Flores, M.P., et al., Losac, the first hemolin that exhibits procogulant activity through selective factor X proteolytic activation. J Biol Chem, 2011. 286(9): p. 6918-28.

[29] Seibert, C.S., E.M. Shinohara, and I.S. Sano-Martins, In vitro hemolytic activity of Lonomia obliqua caterpillar bristle extract on human and Wistar rat erythrocytes. Toxicon, 2003. 41(7): p. 831-9.

[30] Seibert, C.S., et al., Intravascular hemolysis induced by Lonomia obliqua caterpillar bristle extract: an experimental model of envenomation in rats. Toxicon, 2004. 44(7): p. 793-9.

[31] Seibert, C.S., et al., Purification of a phospholipase A2 from Lonomia obliqua caterpillar bristle extract. Biochem Biophys Res Commun, 2006. 342(4): p. 1027-33.

[32] Fritzen, M., et al., Lonomia obliqua venom action on fibrinolytic system. Thromb Res, 2003. 112(1-2): p. 105-10.

[33] Veiga, A.B., A.F. Pinto, and J.A. Guimaraes, Fibrinogenolytic and procoagulant activities in the hemorrhagic syndrome caused by Lonomia obliqua caterpillars. Thromb Res, 2003. 111(1-2): p. 95-101.

[34] Pinto, A.F., et al., Lonofibrase, a novel alpha-fibrinogenase from Lonomia obliqua caterpillars. Thromb Res, 2004. 113(2): p. 147-54.

[35] Gouveia, A.I.D., et al., Identification and partial characterisation of hyaluronidases in Lonomia obliqua venom. Toxicon, 2005. 45(4): p. 403-410.

[36] Souza, A.P.B., et al., Purification and characterization of an anti-apoptotic protein isolated from Lonomia obliqua hemolymph. Biotechnology Progress, 2005. 21(1): p. 99-105.

[37] Greco, K.N., et al., Antiviral activity of the hemolymph of Lonomia obliqua (Lepidoptera: Saturniidae). Antiviral Research, 2009. 84(1): p. 84-90.

[38] Carmo, A.C., et al., Expression of an antiviral protein from Lonomia obliqua hemolymph in baculovirus/insect cell system. Antiviral Res, 2012. 94(2): p. 126-30.

[39] de Castro Bastos, L., et al., Nociceptive and edematogenic responses elicited by a crude bristle extract of Lonomia obliqua caterpillars. Toxicon, 2004. 43(3): p. 273-278.

[40] Bohrer, C.B., et al., Kallikrein-kinin system activation by Lonomia obliqua caterpillar bristles: Involvement in edema and hypotension responses to envenomation. Toxicon, 2007. 49(5): p. 663-669.

[41] Berger, M., et al., Lonomia obliqua venomous secretion induces human platelet adhesion and aggregation. Journal of Thrombosis and Thrombolysis, 2010. 30(3): p. 300-310.

[42] Berger, M., et al., Lonomia obliqua caterpillar envenomation causes platelet hypoaggregation and blood incoagulability in rats. Toxicon, 2010. 55(1): p. 33-44.

[43] Veiga, A.B., et al., A catalog for the transcripts from the venomous structures of the caterpillar Lonomia obliqua: identification of the proteins potentially involved in the coagulation disorder and hemorrhagic syndrome. Gene, 2005. 355: p. 11-27.

[44] Pinto, A.F., et al., Novel perspectives on the pathogenesis of Lonomia obliqua caterpillar envenomation based on assessment of host response by gene expression analysis. Toxicon, 2008. 51(6): p. 1119-28.

[45] Fritzen, M., et al., A prothrombin activator (Lopap) modulating inflammation, coagulation and cell survival mechanisms. Biochem Biophys Res Commun, 2005. 333(2): p. 517-23.

[46] Crick, F., Central dogma of molecular biology. Nature, 1970. 227(5258): p. 561-&.

[47] Morozova, O., M. Hirst, and M.A. Marra, Applications of New Sequencing Technologies for Transcriptome Analysis, in Annual Review of Genomics and Human Genetics2009. p. 135-151.

[48] Marra, M.A., L. Hillier, and R.H. Waterston, Expressed sequence tags--ESTablishing bridges between genomes. Trends Genet, 1998. 14(1): p. 4-7.

[49] Adams, M.D., et al., Complementary DNA sequencing: expressed sequence tags and human genome project. Science, 1991. 252(5013): p. 1651-6.

[50] Junqueira-de-Azevedo Ide, L. and P.L. Ho, A survey of gene expression and diversity in the venom glands of the pitviper snake Bothrops insularis through the generation of expressed sequence tags (ESTs). Gene, 2002. 299(1-2): p. 279-91.

[51] Yang, Y., et al., EST analysis of gene expression in the tentacle of Cyanea capillata. FEBS Lett, 2003. 538(1-3): p. 183-91.

[52] Kozlov, S., et al., A novel strategy for the identification of toxinlike structures in spider venom. Proteins, 2005. 59(1): p. 131-40.

[53] Faria, F., et al., Gene expression in the salivary complexes from Haementeria depressa leech through the generation of expressed sequence tags. Gene, 2005. 349: p. 173-85.

[54] Burke, J., D. Davison, and W. Hide, D2 cluster: A validated method for clustering EST and full-length cDNA sequences. Genome Research, 1999. 9(11): p. 1135-1142.

[55] Miller, R.T., et al., A comprehensive approach to clustering of expressed human gene sequence: The sequence tag alignment and consensus knowledge base. Genome Research, 1999. 9(11): p. 1143-1155.

[56] Vera, J.C., et al., Rapid transcriptome characterization for a nonmodel organism using 454 pyrosequencing. Molecular Ecology, 2008. 17(7): p. 1636-1647.

[57] Schena, M., et al., Quantitative monitoring of gene-expression patterns with a complementary-DNA microarray. Science, 1995. 270(5235): p. 467-470.

[58] DeRisi, J.L., V.R. Iyer, and P.O. Brown, Exploring the metabolic and genetic control of gene expression on a genomic scale. Science, 1997. 278(5338): p. 680-686.

[59] Tjalsma, H., R.M. Schaeps, and D.W. Swinkels, Immunoproteomics: From biomarker discovery to diagnostic applications. Proteomics Clin Appl, 2008. 2(2): p. 167-80.

[60] Görg, A., et al., Two-dimensional electrophoresis with immobilized pH gradients for proteome analysis: A Laboratory Manual, 2002, Amersham Biosciences.

[61] Rabilloud, T., Two-dimensional gel electrophoresis in proteomics: old, old fashioned, but it still climbs up the mountains. Proteomics, 2002. 2(1): p. 3-10.

[62] Towbin, H., T. Staehelin, and J. Gordon, Electrophoretic transfer of proteins from polyacrylamide gels to nitrocellulose sheets: procedure and some applications. Proc Natl Acad Sci U S A, 1979. 76(9): p. 4350-4.

[63] Dass, C., Principle and Practice of Biological Mass Spectrometry2000, New York: Wiley.

[64] Gutierrez, J.M., et al., Snake venomics and antivenomics: Proteomic tools in the design and control of antivenoms for the treatment of snakebite envenoming. J Proteomics, 2009. 72(2): p. 165-82.

[65] Calvete, J.J., P. Juarez, and L. Sanz, Snake venomics. Strategy and applications. J Mass Spectrom, 2007. 42(11): p. 1405-14.

[66] Petersen, J., A.W. Purcell, and J. Rossjohn, Post-translationally modified T cell epitopes: immune recognition and immunotherapy. J Mol Med (Berl), 2009. 87(11): p. 1045-51.

[67] Eyrich, B., A. Sickmann, and R.P. Zahedi, Catch me if you can: mass spectrometry-based phosphoproteomics and quantification strategies. Proteomics, 2011. 11(4): p. 554-70.

[68] Lazar, I.M., et al., Recent advances in the MS analysis of glycoproteins: Theoretical considerations. Electrophoresis, 2011. 32(1): p. 3-13.

[69] Hoffman, M. and D.M. Monroe, Coagulation 2006: A modern view of hemostasis. Hematology-Oncology Clinics of North America, 2007. 21(1): p. 1-+.

[70] Donato, J.L., et al., Lonomia obliqua caterpillar spicules trigger human blood coagulation via activation of factor X and prothrombin. Thromb Haemost, 1998. 79(3): p. 539-42.

[71] Reis, C.V., et al., Lopap, a prothrombin activator from Lonomia obliqua belonging to the lipocalin family: recombinant production, biochemical characterization and structure-function insights. Biochemical Journal, 2006. 398: p. 295-302.

[72] Flower, D.R., The lipocalin protein family: Structure and function. Biochemical Journal, 1996. 318: p. 1-14.

[73] Chudzinski-Tavassi, A.M., et al., A lipocalin sequence signature modulates cell survival. FEBS Lett, 2010. 584(13): p. 2896-900.

[74] Krishnaswamy, S., et al., Activation of human prothrombin by human prothrombinase - influence of factor Va on the reaction mechanism. Journal of Biological Chemistry, 1987. 262(7): p. 3291-3299.

[75] Kini, R.M., The intriguing world of prothrombin activators from snake venom. Toxicon, 2005. 45(8): p. 1133-1145.

[76] Reis, C.V., et al., In vivo characterization of Lopap, a prothrombin activator serine protease from the Lonomia obliqua caterpillar venom. Thrombosis Research, 2001. 102(5): p. 437-443.

[77] Chudzinski-Tavassi, A.M., et al., Effects of lopap on human endothelial cells and platelets. Haemostasis, 2001. 31(3-6): p. 257-65.

[78] Waismam, K., et al., Lopap: a non-inflammatory and cytoprotective molecule in neutrophils and endothelial cells. Toxicon, 2009. 53(6): p. 652-9.

[79] Carrijo-Carvalho, L.C., et al., A lipocalin-derived Peptide modulating fibroblasts and extracellular matrix proteins. Journal of Toxicology doi:10.1155/2012/325250, 2012.

[80] Hall, T.A., BioEdit: a user-friendly biological sequence alignment editor and analysis program for Windows 95/98/NT. Nucl Acids Symp Ser, 1999. 41: p. 95-98.

[81] Reis, C.V., Clonagem, sequenciamento, expressão e caracterização parcial da estrutura do Lopap, um ativador de protrombina da lagarta Lonomia obliqua. PhD, in Biologia Molecular2002, Universidade federal de Sao Paulo.

[82] Kisiel, W., M.A. Hermodson, and E.W. Davie, Factor-X activating enzyme from Russells viper venom - Isolation and characterization. Biochemistry, 1976. 15(22): p. 4901-4905.

[83] Morita, T., Proteases which activate factor X, in Enzymes from snake venoms, G.S. Bailey, Editor 1998, Alaken Inc.: Fort Collins, Colorado. p. 179-208.

[84] Tans, G. and J. Rosing, Snake venom activators of factor X: an overview. Haemostasis, 2001. 31(3-6): p. 225-33.

[85] Takeda, S., T. Igarashi, and H. Mori, Crystal structure of RVV-X: An example of evolutionary gain of specificity by ADAM proteinases. Febs Letters, 2007. 581(30): p. 5859-5864.

[86] Dimmeler, S., et al., Upregulation of superoxide dismutase and nitric oxide synthase mediates the apoptosis-suppressive effects of shear stress on endothelial cells. Arterioscler Thromb Vasc Biol, 1999. 19(3): p. 656-64.

[87] Rossig, L., et al., Nitric oxide inhibits caspase-3 by S-nitrosation in vivo. J Biol Chem, 1999. 274(11): p. 6823-6.

[88] Bobik, A. and V. Tkachuk, Metalloproteinases and plasminogen activators in vessel remodeling. Curr Hypertens Rep, 2003. 5(6): p. 466-72.

[89] Rhee, W.J., E.J. Kim, and T.H. Park, Kinetic effect of silkworm hemolymph on the delayed host cell death in an insect cell-baculovirus system. Biotechnol Prog, 1999. 15(6): p. 1028-32.

[90] Kim, E.J., H.J. Park, and T.H. Park, Inhibition of apoptosis by recombinant 30K protein originating from silkworm hemolymph. Biochem Biophys Res Commun, 2003. 308(3): p. 523-8.

[91] Maranga, L., et al., Enhancement of Sf-9 cell growth and longevity through supplementation of culture medium with hemolymph. Biotechnol Prog, 2003. 19(1): p. 58-63.

[92] Strauss, E.C., et al., Specific-primer-directed DNA sequencing. Analytical Biochemistry, 1986. 154(1): p. 353-360.

[93] Ramos, C.R.R., et al., r-Sm14 - pRSETA efficacy in experimental animals. Memorias Do Instituto Oswaldo Cruz, 2001. 96: p. 131-135.

[94] Shapiro, L., J. Love, and D.R. Colman, Adhesion molecules in the nervous system: Structural insights into function and diversity, in Annual Review of Neuroscience2007. p. 451-474.

[95] Haspel, J., et al., Critical and optimal Ig domains for promotion of neurite outgrowth by L1/Ng-CAM. J Neurobiol, 2000. 42(3): p. 287-302.

[96] Bieber, A.J., et al., Drosophila neuroglian: a member of the immunoglobulin superfamily with extensive homology to the vertebrate neural adhesion molecule L1. Cell, 1989. 59(3): p. 447-60.

[97] Su, X.D., et al., Crystal structure of hemolin: a horseshoe shape with implications for homophilic adhesion. Science, 1998. 281(5379): p. 991-5.

[98] Li, W., et al., Cloning, expression and phylogenetic analysis of Hemolin, from the Chinese oak silkmoth, Antheraea pernyi. Dev Comp Immunol, 2005. 29(10): p. 853-64.

[99] Freigang, J., et al., The crystal structure of the ligand binding module of axonin-1/TAG-1 suggests a zipper mechanism for neural cell adhesion. Cell, 2000. 101(4): p. 425-33.

[100] Liu, H., P.J. Focia, and X. He, Homophilic adhesion mechanism of neurofascin, a member of the L1 family of neural cell adhesion molecules. J Biol Chem, 2011. 286(1): p. 797-805.

[101] Sarkar, G. and S.S. Sommer, Double-stranded DNA segments can efficiently prime the amplification of human genomic DNA. Nucleic Acids Res, 1992. 20(18): p. 4937-8.

[102] Sali, A., Comparative protein modeling by satisfaction of spatial restraints. Mol Med Today, 1995. 1(6): p. 270-7.

[103] Faye, I. and M.R. Kanost, Function and regulation of hemolin, in Molecular Mechanism of immune Responses in insect, P.T.a.H. Brey, D., Editor 1998, Chapman and Hall: New York. p. 173-188.

[104] Ladendorff, N.E. and M.R. Kanost, Bacteria-induced protein P4 (hemolin) from Manduca sexta: a member of the immunoglobulin superfamily which can inhibit hemocyte aggregation. Arch Insect Biochem Physiol, 1991. 18(4): p. 285-300.

[105] Daffre, S. and I. Faye, Lipopolysaccharide interaction with hemolin, an insect member of the Ig-superfamily. FEBS Lett, 1997. 408(2): p. 127-30.

[106] Yu, X.Q. and M.R. Kanost, Binding of hemolin to bacterial lipopolysaccharide and lipoteichoic acid. An immunoglobulin superfamily member from insects as a pattern-recognition receptor. Eur J Biochem, 2002. 269(7): p. 1827-34.

[107] Lanz-Mendoza, H., et al., Regulation of the insect immune response: the effect of hemolin on cellular immune mechanisms. Cell Immunol, 1996. 169(1): p. 47-54.

[108] Bettencourt, R., et al., Cell adhesion properties of hemolin, an insect immune protein in the Ig superfamily. Eur J Biochem, 1997. 250(3): p. 630-7.

[109] Schmidt, O., et al., Role of adhesion in arthropod immune recognition. Annu Rev Entomol, 2010. 55: p. 485-504.

[110] Kanost, M.R., et al., Isolation and characterization of a hemocyte aggregation inhibitor from hemolymph of Manduca sexta larvae. Arch Insect Biochem Physiol, 1994. 27(2): p. 123-36.

[111] Chudzinski-Tavassi, A.M., et al., Exogenous factors affecting hemostasis: therapeutic perspectives and biotechnological approaches, in Animal toxins: State of the Art. Pesrpectives in Health and Biotachnology, M.E. De Lima, et al., Editors. 2009, UFMG: Belo Horizonte. p. 495-523.

[112] Andrade, S.A., et al., Reversal of the anticoagulant and anti-hemostatic effect of low molecular weight heparin by direct prothrombin activation. Brazilian Journal of Medical and Biological Research, 2012.

[113] Zannin, M., et al., Blood coagulation and fibrinolytic factors in 105 patients with hemorrhagic syndrome caused by accidental contact with Lonomia obliqua caterpillar in Santa Catarina, Southern Brazil. Thrombosis and Haemostasis, 2003. 89(2): p. 355-364.

Chapter 8

Molecular Pharmacology and Toxinology of Venom from Ants

A.F.C. Torres, Y.P. Quinet, A. Havt,
G. Rádis-Baptista and A.M.C. Martins

Additional information is available at the end of the chapter

http://dx.doi.org/10.5772/53539

1. Introduction

In the last decades, poisonous animals have gained notoriety since their venoms (secreted or injected) contain several of potentially useful bioactive substances (polypeptide toxins), which are mostly codified by a single gene or, in the case of venom organic compounds, by a given enzymatic route presented in a specialized tissue where the biosynthesis occur – the venom gland.

In this context, in the age of genomic sciences, sequencing the entire genome or portion of it, can be thought as the straightforward step to understand a given venom composition. Particularly because, in many cases, the venom is produced in so small quantities, requiring great challenge (natural and bureaucratic) to obtain biological material for its investigation or the necessity of sacrifice the animal to get samples for analysis by conventional biochemical methods. Genome sequencing allows us the identification of mRNAs, as well as prediction of protein structure and function. In addition, the construction of cDNA libraries is useful to clone, catalog and identify genes, and subsequently express the proteins of interest from these libraries. By this approach, we can have adequate amounts of polypeptide toxins for functional analysis and application, by which otherwise would be difficult to isolate.

According to [1], venoms' complexity in terms of peptide and protein contents, together with the number of venomous species indicate that only a small proportion (less than 1%) of the all bioactive molecules has been identified and characterized to date, and little is known about the genomic background of the venomous organisms. Consequently, if we take into account that nature, operated by evolutionary processes, is the most efficient source of new functional molecules and drug candidates, the study of all species of venomous animals, including small insects, such as those belonging to the order Hymenoptera [2] will be crucial and timely for basic and applied research.

2. Ants biology: Subfamily Ponerinae

Ants (Vespoidea: Formicidae) belong to the insect order Hymenoptera, which includes other important families like Apidae (bees) and Vespidae (wasps) [3]. The family Formicidae consists of approximately 13.000 species of ants, most of them exibiting an advanced and sophisticated social life. With colonies ranging from tens to millions of individuals, a high diversity as well as numerical and biomass dominance in almost every habitat throughout the world, ants form an important component of terrestrial biodiversity, especially in the Neotropical Region, where about 30% of all known ant species are found [4,5]. All ant species possess eusocial habits, the most conspicuous one being the reproductive division of labor, with one to many queens specialized in reproduction, while the more and less sterile, and nonreproductive workers, help the queen(s) reproduction, tending the brood and dealing with all other tasks of the colony like food collection, nest repair, nest and/territory defense [6].

With more than 1000 species distributed in 28 genera, like *Dinoponera* and *Paraponera*, the Ponerinae subfamily is a primitive group of ants mainly found in tropical habitats [4]. It is also one the four major ant groups (Myrmicinae, Formicinae, Ponerinae and Dolichoderinae), all characterized by high species diversity and widespread geographic distribution [4]. *Dinoponera* Roger, 1861 [7] is a strictly Neotropical genus with six known species [5] that are considered the largest ants of the world (3-4 cm in length): *D. australis*Emery, 1910; *D. gigantea*(Perty, 1833); *D. longipes* Emery, 1901; *D. lucida*Emery, 1901; *D. mutica*Emery, 1901; and *D. quadriceps* Santschi, 1921 (Figure 1). Like in other ponerine ants, *Dinoponera* colonies have a poor social organization, with small colonies that are queenless [9, 10]. Contrary to most ant species, all workers of the *Dinoponera* colony are potential reproductives with functional spermatheca. However, only one (sometimes more) worker mate and become the dominant worker with reproductive function that is regularly disputed by subdominant workers [9, 10]. Like most Ponerinae, *Dinoponera* are mostly predatory ants: their common prey are medium size to large arthropods (mainly insects) that they subdue with their sting [11, 12]

Like all Aculeata hymenopterans (Chrysidoidea, Apoidea, Vespoidea), *Dinoponera* ants have a sting apparatus that is located in the last portion of the gaster, and is formed by the sting itself (derived from the ovipositor of more basal hymenopteran groups) along with two associated glands: the Dufour's gland and the venom gland [4,13]. In all ants, the venom gland apparatus typically consists of paired venom secreting tubules that converge into a single convoluted gland (an elongated continuation of the secretory tubule into the venom gland reservoir), which in turn empties into a sac-like reservoir that leads into the sting (in ants with sting) [4](Figure 2). In *D. australis*, it was shown that the convoluted gland has, like the free tubules, a secretory function [14]. The free tubules and convoluted gland are responsible for toxin production [14], which seems to be composed mainly of proteins [4,15]. Furthermore, it was also shown that its morphology and ultrastructural organization presents similarity with the convoluted gland of vespine waps (Vespinae), a fact that supports the hypothesis of a phylogenetic origin of ants from wasp-like ancestors [14].

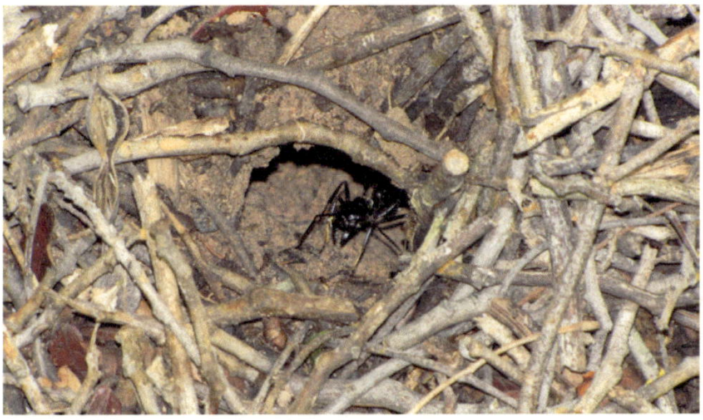

Figure 1. *Dinoponera quadriceps* (Quinet, Y.P. 2011)

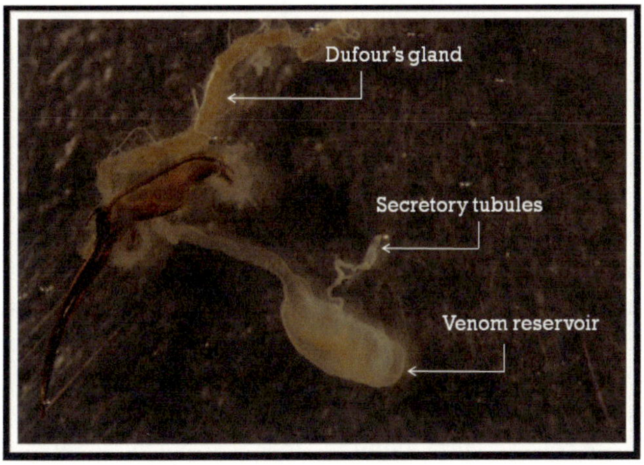

Figure 2. Secretory apparatus from *D. quadriceps* (Quinet, Y.P. 2010)

In solitary Aculeata hymenopterans, and in social bees and wasps, the venom has two main functions: prey capture and defense, respectively [13,16]. In ants, the products from the venom exhibit much higher diversity of biological roles. Particularly In stinging ants, particularly in primitive groups like Ponerinae, the primary function of venom gland products is to serve as injectable offensive or/and defensive agents (to capture prey, fight with competitors or against predators, for example) [13,16]. In more derived functions, the venom gland products are used as defensive (toxic and/or repellent) agents by non-stinging ants that topically apply them on the cuticle of enemies, as in *Crematogaster* or *Monomorium* ants for example. Venom gland products can also serve as chemical communication agents (alarm and recruitment phero- mones, for example) [16,17].

3. Clinical aspects of ants' stings

Many insect stings are associated with local pathophysiological events, characterized by pain, swelling and redness at the sting site for about 1-2 days [18]. The most severe reactions are associated with allergic disorders, presenting neutrophilic and eosinophilic infiltration and specific IgE production [19]. These manifestations are common in accidents with Hymenoptera insects. Most studies that describe the clinical aspects of ant stings reported accidents with ants of the genus *Solenopsis* (Myrmicinae), known as fire ants [20,21,22]. In most serious cases, these accidental encounter with fire ants can promote multiple body rash, seizures, heart failure, and serum sickness nephritis and, more rarely, acute renal failure [23,24].

Accidents with ants of the Ponerinae subfamily are rare or rarely reported. In fact, several concomitant or sequential stings are necessary in order to produce significant clinical symptoms of envenomation, in giant ants, multiple attacks are less probable, since workers have a solitary foraging behavior. However, some of the accidents with giants ants may have medical importance, such as the ones produced by the genus *Paraponera* and *Dinoponera*, popularly known as "true tocandira" and "false tocandira", respectively. Their stings are extremely painful and can cause potentially systemic manifestations such as fever, cold sweats, nausea, vomiting, lymphadenopathy and cardiac arrhythmias [8,25,26]. According to [27,28] the venom of these ants may be neurotoxic for other insects.

4. Venom composition and pharmacological properties

The ant's venoms have been investigated in a relatively small number of species. In the group of stinging ants, the most investigated species belong to the Myrmeciinae, Ponerinae, Pseudomyrmecinae and Myrmicinae subfamilies. They produce aqueous solutions of proteinaceous venoms containing enzymatic and non-enzymatic proteins, free amino-acids and small biologically active compounds like histamine, 5-hydroxytryptamine, acetylcholine, norepinephrine, and dopamine [16,17]. Venoms with proteinaceous components are considered as most primitive and are consequently found in other aculeate hymenopterans like wasps and bees [4,16]. A notable exception to this proteinaceous nature of the venom in ants with sting is found in ants of the genera *Solenopsis* (fire ants) and *Monomorium* (Myrmicinae) that produce alkaloid-rich venoms with few proteins. In the Formicinae ants (ex: *Camponotus*, *Formica*), the sting is no more presented, but the poison gland produces a mixtures of simple organic acids an aqueous solution. Formic acid is presented in concentrations up to 65% along with some peptides and free amino-acids [16,17].

As a member of a group of predatory ants (Ponerinae), it is expected that *Dinoponera* would produces such a kind of proteinaceous venom. However, until now few studies have been done with *Dinoponera* venoms. In two of these studies, which compared venoms of a variety of hymenopterans, the presence of proteins, some with enzyme activities (phospholipase A, hyaluronidase, and lipase), was shown for *D. grandis* (in fact, *D. gigantea*) venom [16,29]. In a more recent study, in which the peptide components from the venom of *D. australis* was investigated, over 75 unique protein components were found with a large diversity of properties ranging in size, hydrophobicity, and overall abundance [30]. The biological effects of several ants' venoms have been attributed to their protein repertoire. As showed by [31] high molecular weight proteins are present in the venom of *Dinoponera australis*. In a comparative evaluation of protein composition of hymenopteran venom reservoirs, proteins with molecular weight ranging from 24 to 75kDa were evidenced [29]. Additionaly, two peptides with less than 10 kDa, as well as proteins with molecular weight ranging from 26-90 kDa were also found in the venom of *Myrmecia pilosula* [32]. The electrophoretic profile of wasps also shows variation in the protein molecular weight, ranging from 5 to 200kDa [33,34], whereas the venoms of bees was shown to range from 2 to108 kDa [35].

5. Pharmacology and therapeutic uses of venom form ants

The first reported case about the therapeutic use of venoms from ants were to treat rheumatoid arthritis. In fact, insects might have components that justify its use in traditional medicine in countries of East Asia, Africa and South America [36]. Lately, several studies of ant venom aimed to demonstrate their beneficial intrinsic properties such as reduction of inflammation, pain relief, improved function of the immune system and liver [37,38].

As the venom from Ponerinae subfamily is composed of a complex mixtures of proteins and neurotoxins [39] we would expected to have several pharmacological properties. Small peptides isolated from *Paraponera clavata* venom, called poneratoxin (PoTx) interfere with sodium channels function and have potential use as a biological insecticide [40,41].

Several distinctive pharmacological activities were demonstrated with peptides isolated from *Pachycondyla goeldii* and *Myrmecia* sp. In one of these works, antimicrobial activity against both Gram positive and Gram negative bacteria was observed [42, 43]. In a recent study [44], it was reported that the venom from *Pachycondila sennaarensis* has a significant antitumor effect on breast cancer cells in a dose and time dependent manner without affecting the viability of non tumor cells. In addition, some studies have also shown the renal effects of Hymenoptera venoms. In fact, in more serious accidents with venoms from wasps and bees acute renal failure generally occurs [45,46, 47, 48].

6. Genomic study of ant venom composition

Since the description of DNA double helix by Francis Crick and James Watson (1953), recombinant DNA technology and genomics revolutionized numerous areas of life science. The comprehension of the biochemical and molecular basis of inheritance had been improved our knowledge about the complexity of all forms of life and the manner how genes and proteins interact to create diversity. The genomic revolution was additionally expanded with the advent of bioinformatic, the 'omic' science (transcriptomic, proteomic, peptidome, metabolomic, glycome) and, presently, system biology.

Collective efforts have been joined to annotate the gene composition of insects. The first complete sequenced genome of insect was from the fruit fly *Drosophila melanogaster*, in 2000, followed by a flurry of activities aimed at sequencing the genomes of several additional insect species. In the field of toxinology, the hymenopterans are receiving special attention due to their behavior and the ability to produce venom.

Up to now, at least 10 ant species had their genomes analyzed and published. The ants whose genomes were sequenced include: the fire ant *Solenopsis invicta* found in South America, United States, China, Taiwan, Australia [49]; the Argentine ant *Linepithema humile* [50], the leaf-cutting ant *Acromyrmex echinator* [51] and *Atta cephalote* [52] found in South America; the red harvester *Pogonomyrmex barbatus* found in North and South America [53], the florida carpenter ant *Camponotus floriandus* from United States; and, the jumper ant *Harpegnatos saltator* from India, Sri Lanka and Southeast Asia [54]. Those ant genomes have provided hundreds of new available nucleotide data.

Apart of a detailed genome analysis, the construction of cDNA libraries from ants' venom glands is an important tool in order to analyze venom composition and discover new molecules that could have biological and pharmacological properties. But an important question arises: why hymenopteran venoms? As we pointed at the beginning of this chapter, there are several reports that hymenopteran venom could have biological properties useful for medical purposes. In this scope, from traditional and modern medicine reports, description can be found not only about clinical manifestation caused by hymenopterans venom, as allergic response, but also the benefits of ant venom to treat disease like rheumatoid arthritis and pain [36].

Genomic and transcriptomic studies of hymenopteran cDNA libraries would provide useful information about their protein constituents. Some of these informations would include signal peptide sequences and the presence of post-translational modifications, which cannot be predicted by the studies of mature proteins. Ants genomic studies have shown a number of substances involved in the biology of these insects, such as: vittelogenins, gustatory and odorant receptors, molecules involved in immune response, as well as metabolic and structural proteins like cytochrome P450.

7. Molecular pharmacology and toxinology of *D. quadriceps* venom

Recently, we have initiated a research project dedicated to investigate the composition, the pharmacological properties, and the transcripts from the venom gland components of *Dinoponera quadriceps.*

Using one-dimensional (SDS-PAGE) electrophoresis (1-DE) to resolve *Dinoponera quadriceps* venom proteins, only eight major large polypeptides (ranging from 15 to 100 kDa) were visualized by Comassie Brilliant Blue (CBB) Staining. The 1-DE and the insensitive method of staining with CBB was not adequate to separate small proteins below 15 kDa and peptides (Figure 3)

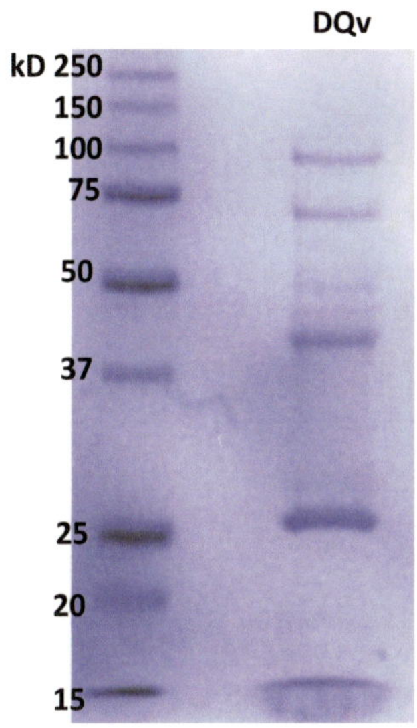

Figure 3. Electrophoretic profile of *Dinoponera quadriceps* total venom (DQv) in one-dimensional SDS-PAGE gel electrophoresis visualized with Comassie Brilliant Blue.

The peptide mass fingerprint (PMF), as well as other proteomic analysis is being conducted and a report will be published elsewhere.

Pharmacological studies have been realized with *Dinoponera quadriceps* venom, particularly, in a system of isolated perfused rat kidney. We now know that at concentrations of approximately 10μg/mL increased urinary flow, glomerular filtration rate and decreased vascular resistance and sodium tubular transport, suggesting a natriuretic and diuretic effect. Furthermore, in studies with renal tubule cells (MDCK - Madin-Darbin Canine Kidney) the same venom induced cell cytotoxicity, on MTT assay (3-(4,5-dimethylthiazol-2-yl)-2,5-diphenyltetrazolium bromide) at a dose and time dependent manner. Interestingly, greater cytotoxicity was observed in the shorter incubation periods, suggesting that the cell culture could recover after a given exposure time. Additional assays have been designed to evaluate the biological and pharmacological activity of purified component of this venom, as well as highlighting the mechanisms related to the observed effects.

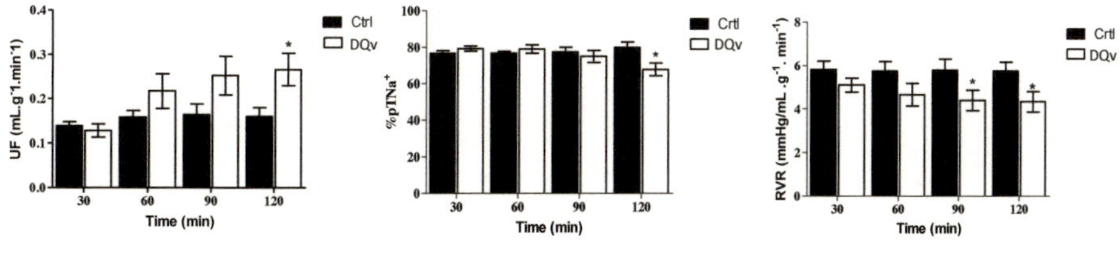

Figure 4. Effect of *D. quadriceps* total venom (DQv) on Urinary flow (UF; A), sodium tubular transport percent(%pTNa; B) and renal vascular resistence (RVR; C). Ctrl=control. Results are expressed as means ± S.E.M., *p<0.05 (ANOVA).

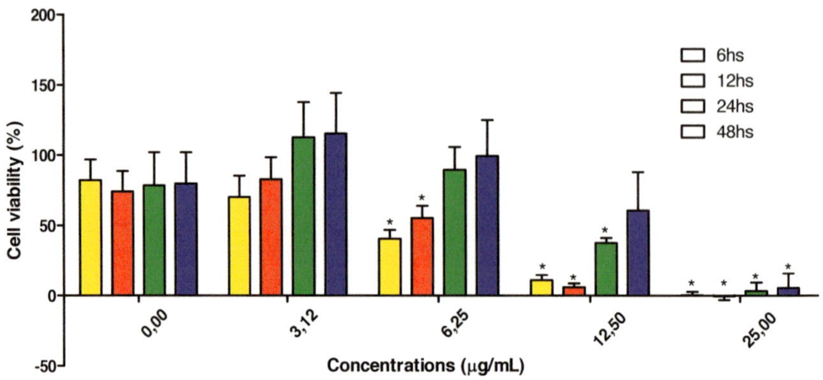

Figure 5. Citotoxicity of *D. quadriceps* total venom on MDCK (Madin-Darbin Canine Kidney) cells culture on MTT assay. Results are expressed as means ± S.E.M., *p<0,05 (ANOVA).

Recently we also demonstrated the neuroprotective activity of *D. quadriceps* venom in models of seizures induced by pentylenetetrazol (PTZ), when administered intraperitoneally. The effect was an increase in latency to first seizure and a tendency to increased latency of death, as well as reduction of lipid peroxidation in the prefrontal cortex of mice [55].

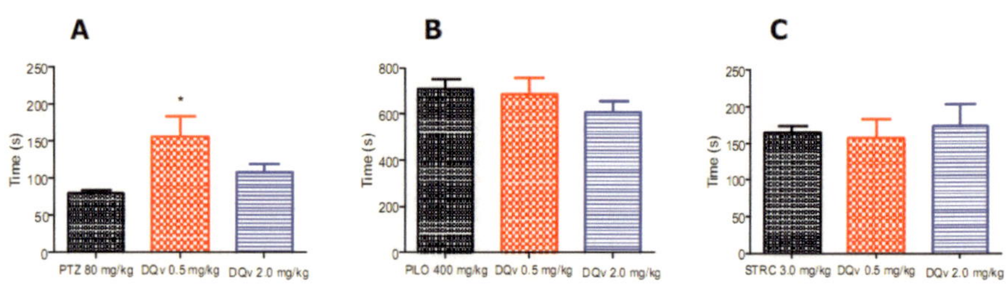

Figure 6. Effects of *D. quadriceps* venom (DQv) on latency of the first seizure in the models of seizure of pentylenetetrazol (PTZ) (A), pilocarpine (PILO) (B) and strychnine (STRC) (C). Results are expressed as means ± S.E.M., *p<0.05 (ANOVA).

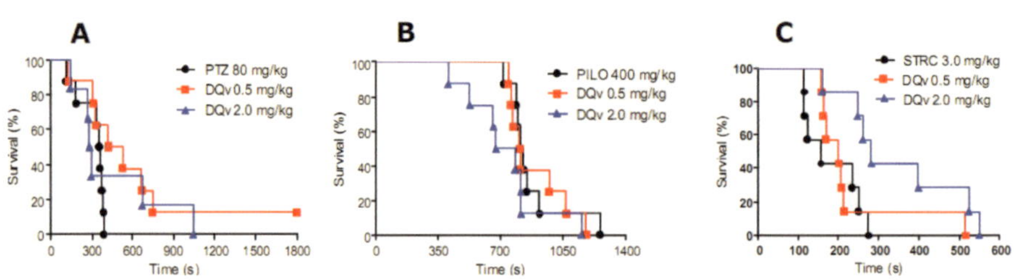

Figure 7. Effects of *D. Quadriceps* total venom (DQv) on latency of death in models of seizure of pentylenetetrazol (PTZ) (A), pilocarpine (PILO) (B) and strychnine (STRC) (C). Results are expressed as means ± S.E.M (n=8), *p<0.05.

A part of proteomic and pharmacological studies, we prepared a *D. quadriceps* venom gland cDNA library to use an EST-strategy to identify the major transcripts expressed in the giant ant venom.we successfully constructed a full-length cDNA library of approximately 20 venom glands from *D. quadriceps,* using In-Fusion SMARTer kit (Clontech, USA). We obtained an efficiency of $1x10^5$ cfu/μg of DNA, our medium insert was 700bp and the library was amplified and stored at -80°C. A total of 432 individual ESTs were sequenced by the dideoxy chain termination (Sanger) method. Of these, 125 were undergone to a preliminary analysis through BLASTx. The Tabel 1 and Figure 8(A) shows an overview of the relative abundance of the protein groups.Most of the transcripts represent proteins involved in the whole metabolism as transferases, ATP synthase, dehydrogenases, ribosomal proteins, cytocrome c. Those sequences are being annotated for deposit in DNA and protein data bank. A note of caution is that, as in most trancriptome project, a significant number of transcripts showed no similarities with well-known sequences in data bank. These ESTs presents a typical structure of true ORFs (Open Reading Frame), that is start and stop codons, in addition a poly A tail. They were classified as (1) hypothetical proteins with unknown function and (2) cDNA precursors with no hits found. However, by comparing against DNA and protein data the hypothetical proteins showed high similarities with proteins from scorpions (*Opisthacanthus cayaporum)* and others ants, as *Harpegnatos saltator, Solenopsis invicta* and *Camponotus floriandus*. The Figure 8(B) represents the percentage of three classification of hits over the total clones analyzed, were probable toxins comprises a significant percentage of ESTs, representing about 34% of messages. Other 37% represents no-significant hits, which give us a number of perspectives to analyze several novel proteins.

Class	Function	% Clones
No hit	Typical ORF with no hits	40.8
DnTx	Mast cell degranulation	28.8
Hypothetical protein	Unknown function	12.0
Antigen like	Allergenic	9.6
Cytocrome c oxidase	Metabolism	1.6
Cytocrome b	Metabolism	1.6
Transferase	Metabolism	2.4
Ionic channel blocker	Toxin	1.6
Ribossomal protein	Structural protein	1.6
Chymotripsin inhibitor	Metabolism	0.8
Dehydrogenase	Metabolism	0.8
ATP synthase	Metabolism	0.8
Phospholipase A1	Enzyme/Toxin	0.8
Bacterial ESTs	Symbionts (?)	4.0
Mitocondrial protein	Metabiolism	0.8

Table 1. Classification of ESTs from *D. quadriceps* venom gland cDNA library on their putative functions.

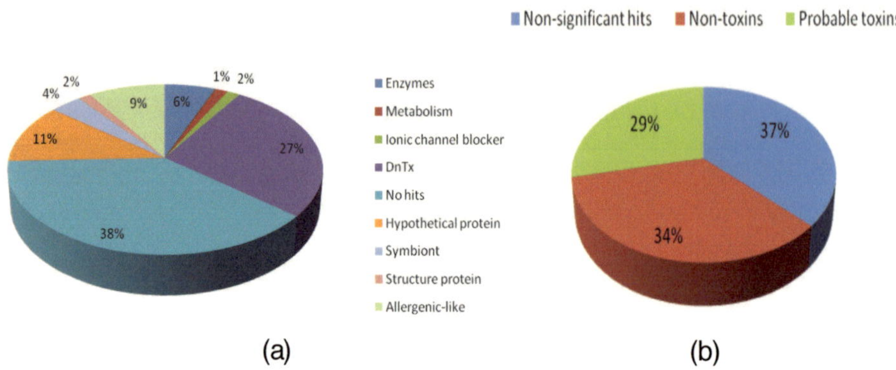

Figure 8. Classification of ESTs from *D. quadriceps* venom gland cDNA library on their putative functions (A). Relative proportion of toxin-encoding, non-toxing encoding and no significant hit ESTs (B).

As a matter of example, the most abundant toxin was dinoponera toxin (DnTx). The dinoponeratoxin whole sequence (accounting for 27% of the total clones analysed) was identified in this cDNA library. Deduced aminoacid sequences (DnTx01 and DnTx02), corresponding to two cDNA isoform precursos, from *D. quadricipes* transcriptome (this work) and three mature venom peptides (DnTx_Da-3105, DnTx_Da-3177 and TX01_DINAS - GenBank accession numbers GI:294863162, GI:294863159 and GI:294863158, respectively) from *D. australis* [30] were aligned with ClustalW software using default parameters (http://www.ebi.ac.uk). DnTx01 and DnTx02 are represented with their respective signal peptides and pro-peptides, in which putative cleavage sites are shown in green and blue, respectively, according to SignalP software (http://www.cbs.dtu.dk/services/SignalP) and proteomic data. In the alignment A is clearly observed that DnTX01 shares high similarity with DnTx_Da-3105 and DnTx_Da-3177, whereas the mature DnTx02 and TX01_DINAS are highly similar to each other (part B).

```
A

DnTx01          MKLSAFTLAFALILMMAIMYNMAEAAALADADADAEAIAGLKDWWNKHKDKIVKVVKEMG 60
DnTx_Da-3105    ---------------------------------------GLKDWWNKHKDKIIAVAKEMG 21
DnTx_Da-3177    ---------------------------------------GLKDWWNKHKDKIIDVVKEMG 21
                                                       *************: *.****

DnTx01          -KAGINAAGK 69
DnTx_Da-3105    -KAGLQAA-- 28
DnTx_Da-3177    -KAGLQAA-- 28
                 ***::**


B

DnTx02          MKLSALSIIFGMILVMTIMYTKAEAEAEAEADADADAKAEAEAFWGTLAKWALKAIPAAM 60
TX01_DINAS      -------------------------------------------FWGTLAKLALKAVPAVM 17
                                                           ******* ****:**.*

DnTx02          -GMKQNK 66
TX01_DINAS      -GMIKKE 23
                 ** :::
```

Figure 9. Alignment of dinoponeratoxin precursors and mature peptides from *D. quadricipes* and *D. australis* using ClustalW software (http://www.ebi.ac.uk).

http://dx.doi.org/10.5772/53539

8. Conclusion

Taking into account the information presented in this chapter, a second question arises and should be answered in the near future: "Is there any hymenopteran venom component that could be used as a biotechnological tool?" The majority of works done to discovery new biotechnological tools from hymenopteran venoms were performed using proteomic science analysis, probably because ants apparatus venom is so hard to identify and dissect. Nevertheless, the size of some poneromorph primitive ants may permit subdue these difficulties allowing us to construct a cDNA library and thus opening new perspectives to better understand the biology of ants as well as to analyze the properties of the venom in the search for new molecules with pharmacological and / or biotechnological potential.

Thus, its clear that further work is necessary to understand ant venom, as well venoms from hymenopteran, since several precursors comprises hypothetical and predicted toxins/polypeptides with unknown function. Moreover, a deep functional analysis in the coming period will be made to comprehend the effects presented by total venom and peptides isolated from it.

Acknowledgements

CNPq/CAPES and FUNCAP for financial support.

Author details

A.F.C. Torres[1*], Y.P. Quinet[2], A. Havt[3], G. Rádis-Baptista[4] and A.M.C. Martins[1]

*Address all correspondence to: alba.fabiola@gmail.com

1 Departament of Clinical and Toxicological Analysis, Federal University of Ceara, Fortaleza, Brazil

2 Laboratory of Entomology, State University of Ceara, Fortaleza, Brazil

3 Biomedicine Institute, Department of Physiology and Pharmacology, Federal University of Ceara, Fortaleza, Brazil

4 Marine Science Institute, Federal University of Ceara, Fortaleza, Brazil

References

[1] Ménez A, Stocklin R, Mebs D. 'Venomics' or: The venomous system genome project. Toxicon 2006; 47(3):255-9.

[2] Harvey AL, Bradley KN, Cochran SA, Rowan EG, Pratt JA, Quillfeldt JA, Jerusalinsky DA. What can toxins tell us for drug discovery? Toxicon 1998; 36(11):1635-40.

[3] Gullan PJ, Cranston PS. The insects: an outline of entomology. Wiley-Blackwell:Chichester; 2010.

[4] Holldobler B, Wilson EO. The ants. Belknap Press of Harvard University Press:Cambridge;1990.

[5] Fernández F, Ospina M. Sinopsis de las hormigas de La región Neotropical. In: Fernández F (ed.) Introduccíon a lãs Hormigas de La región Neotropical. Instituto de Investigación de Recursos Biológicos Alexander Von Humboldt: Colombia; 2003. p49-64

[6] Wilson EO. The insect societies. Belknap Press of Harvard University Press:Cambridge;1971

[7] Roger J. Die Ponera-artigen Ameisen. (Schluss.)Berliner Entomologische Zeitschrift 1861; 5:1–54.

[8] Haddad Jr V, Cardoso JLC, Moraes RHP. Description of an injury in a human caused by a false tocandira (*Dinoponera gigantea*, Perty, 1833) with a revision on folkloric, pharmacological and clinical aspects of the giant ants of the genera Paraponera and Dinoponera (sub-family ponerinae). Rev Inst Med Trop 2005; 47(4):235-38.

[9] Monnin T, Peeters C. Monogyny and regulation of worker mating in the queenless ant *Dinoponera quadriceps*. Animal Behaviour 1998; 55(2):299-306.

[10] Araújo CZD, Jaisson P. Modes de fondation dês colonies chez La fourmi sans reine *Dinoponera quadriceps* Santschi (Hymenoptera,Formicidae, Ponerinae). Actes de Colloques Insects Sociaux 1994; 9:79-88.

[11] Fourcassié V, Oliveira PS. Foraging ecology of the giant Amazonian ant *Dinoponera gigantea* (Hymenoptera, Formicidae, Ponerinae): activity schedule, diet and spatial foraging patterns. Journal of Natural History 2002; 36:2211-27.

[12] Araujo A, Rodrigues Z. Forraging behavior of the queenless ant *Dinoponera quadriceps* Santschi (Hymenoptera, Formicidae., Neotrop Entomol 2006; 35(2):159-64.

[13] Buschinger A, Maschwitz U..Defensive behavior and defensive mechanisms in ants. In: *Defensive mechanisms in social insects* (H.R. Hermann - Ed.), Praeger, New York; 1984. p95-150

[14] Schoeters E, Billen J. Morphology and ultra structure of the convoluted gland in the ant *Dinoponera australis* (Hymenoptera:Formicidae). Int J Insect Morphol Embryol 1995; 24(3):p323-32.

[15] Siquieroli ACS, Santana FA, Rodrigues RS, Vieira CU, Cardoso R, Goulart LR, Bonetti AM. Phage display in venom gland in *Dinoponera australis* (HYMENOP-

TERA:FORMICIDAE). J Venom Anim Toxins incl Trop Disc, IX Symposium of the Brazilian Society on Toxinology 2007; 13(1):p291.

[16] Schmidt JO, Blum MS, Overal WL. Comparative enzymology of venoms from stinging Hymenoptera. Toxicon1986; 24(9):p907–21.

[17] Attygalle AB. Morgan ED. Chemicals from the glands of ants. Chemical Society Review 1984;13:p245-78.

[18] Ellis AK, Day JH. Clinical reactivity to insect stings. Current Opinion in Allergy and Clinical Immunol 2005; 5(4):p349-54.

[19] Haddad Jr V. Identificação de enfermidades agudas causadas por animais e plantas em ambientes rurais e litorâneos: auxílio à prática dermatológica. An Bras Dermatol 2009;84(4):p343-8.

[20] Lee EK, Jeong KY, Lyuz DP, Lee YW, Sohn JH, Lim KJ, Hong CS, Park JW. Characterization of the major allergens of Pachycondyla chinensis in ant sting anaphylaxis patients. Clinical and Experimental Allergy 2009; 39:p602-07.

[21] Tankersley MS. The stinging impact of the imported fire ant. Current Opinion in Allergy and Clinical Immunology 2008, 8:p354–59.

[22] Chianura L, Pozzi F. Case Report: A 40-year-old man with ulcerated skin lesions caused by bites of safari ants. Am J Trop Med Hyg 2010; 83(1):p9.

[23] Koya S, Crenshaw D, Agarwal A. Rhabdomyolysis and acute renal failure after fire ant bites. Society of General Internal Medicine 2007;22:p145–47.

[24] Deshazo RD. My journey to the ants. Transactions of the american clinical and climatological association 2009; 120:p85-95.

[25] HADDAD Jr V. Acidentes por formigas. In: Manual de diagnóstico e tratamento de acidentes por animais peçonhentos. Brasília, FNS 2001.p65-66

[26] Cruz Lopez L, Morgan ED. Explanation of bitter taste of venom of ponerine ant *Pachycondyla apicalis*. J Chem Ecol 1997; 23(3):p705-12.

[27] Hermann HR, Blum MS, Wheeler JW, Overal WL, Schmidt JO, Chao J. Comparative anatomy and chemistry of the venom apparatus and mandibular glands in Dinoponera grandis (Guérin) and Paraponera clavata (F.) (Hymenoptera:Formicidae:Ponerinae). Annals of the Entomological Society of America 1984; 77(3):p272-79.

[28] Orivel J, Dejean A. Comparative effect of the venoms of ants of the genus Pachycondyla (Hymenoptera: Ponerinae). Toxicon 2001; 39(2-3):p195-201.

[29] Leluk K, Schmidt J, Jones, D. Comparative studies on the protein composition of hymenopteran venom reservois. Toxicon 1989; 27(1):p105-14.

[30] Johnson SR, Copello JA, Evans MS, Suarez AV. A biochemical characterization of the major peptides from the venom of the giant neotropical hunting ant *Dinoponera australis.* Toxicon 2010; 55(4):p702-10.

[31] Cologna CT, Barbosa DB, Santana FA, Rodovalho CM,Oliveira LA, Brandeburgo MAM. Estudo da peçonha de *Dinoponera australis* – Roger, 1861 (Hymenoptera, Ponerinae). In: V Encontro interno de Iniciação científica, Convênio CNPq/UFU, Uberlândia, 2005.

[32] Wiese MD, Chataway TK, Davies NW, Milne RW, Brown SGA, Gai WP, Heddle RJ. Proteomic analysis of *Myrmecia pilosula* (jack jumper) ant venom. Toxicon 2006; 47(2):p208-17.

[33] Rivers DB, Uckan F, Ergin E. Characterization and biochemical analyses of venom from the ectoparasitic was Nasonia vitripennis (Walker)(Hymenoptera:Pteromalidade). Arch Insect Biochem Physiol 2006; 61(1):p24-41.

[34] Parkinson N, Richards EH, Conyers C, Smith I, Edwards JP. Analysis of venom constituents from the parasitoid wasp Pimpla hypocondriaca and cloning of a cDNA encoding a venom protein.Insect Biochem Mol Biol 2002; 32(7):p729-35.

[35] Zalat S, Nabil Z, Hussein A, Rakha M. Biochemical and haematological studies of some solitary and social bee venoms. Egyptian J of Biology 1999;1:p55-71.

[36] Cherniak EP. Bugs as drugs, Part 1: Insects: the new alternative medicine for the 21st century?. Altern Med Rev 2010; 15(2):p124-35.

[37] Kou J, Ni Y, Li N, Wang J, Liu L, Jiang ZH. Analgesic and anti-inflammatory activities of total extract and individual fractions of Chinese medicinal ants *Polyrhachis lamellidens*. Biol Pharm Bull 2005; 28:p176-180.

[38] Wang CP, Wu YL. Study on mechanism underlying the treatment of rheumatoid arthritis by Keshiling, Zhongguo Zong Yao Za Zhi 2006; 31:155-158.

[39] Sousa PL, Quinet Y, Ponte EL, do Vale JF, Torres AF, Pereira MG, Asseury AM. Venom's antinociceptive property in the primitive ant *Dinoponera quadriceps*. J Ethnopharmacol 2012; 144(1):p213-216.

[40] Lima PRM, Brochetto-Braga MR. Hymenoptera venom review focusing on *Apis mellifera*. J Venomous Animals and Toxins including Tropical Diseases 2003; 9:p149-62.

[41] Duval A, Malécot CO, Pelhate M, Piek T. Poneratoxin, a new toxin from ant venom, reveals an interconversion between two gating modes of the Na channels in frog skeletal muscle fibres. Pflugers Arch 1992; 420(3-4):p239-47.

[42] Szolajska E, Poznanki J, Ferber ML, Michalik J, Gout E, Fender P, Bailly I, Dublet B, Chroboczek J. Poneratoxin, a neurotoxin from ant venom.Structure and expression in insect cells and construction of a bio-insecticide. Europ J Biochem 2004; 271(11):p2127-36.

[43] Orivell J, Redeker V, Caer JP, Krier F, Revol-Junelles A, Longeon A, Chaffotte A, Dejean A, Rossier J. Ponericins, new antibacterial and insecticidal peptides from venom of the ant *Pachycondyla goeldii*. J Biochem Chem 2001; 286(21):p17823-9.

[44] Zelezetsky I, Pag U, Antcheva N, Sahl HG, Tossi A. Identification and optimization of an antimicrobial peptide from the ant venom toxin pilosulin. Biochem Biophys 2005; 434(2):p358-64.

[45] Badr G, Garraud O, Daghestani M, Al-Khalifa MS, Richard Y. Human breast carcinoma cells are induced to apoptosis by samsum ant venom through an IGF-1-dependant pathway, PI3K/AKT and ERK signaling. Cellular Immunology 2012; 273 (1): p10-6.

[46] Daher EF, Oliveira RA, Silva LSV, Silva BEM, Morais TP. Acute renal failure following bee stings: case reports. Rev Soc Bras Med Trop 2009; 42(2):p209-12.

[47] Grisotto LS, Mendes GE, Castro I, Baptista MA, Alves VA, Yu L, Burdmann EA. Mechanisms of bee venom-induced acute renal failure.Toxicon 2006; 48(1):p44-54.

[48] Loh HH, Tan CH. Acute renal failure and posterior reversible encephalopathy syndrome following multiple waspstings: a case report. Med J Malaysia 2012; 67(1):p133-5.

[49] Rachaiah NM, Jayappagowda LA, Siddabyrappa HB, Bharath VK.Unusual case of acute renal failure following multiple wasp stings. N Am J Med Sci 2012; 4(2):p104-6.

[50] Wurm Y, Wang J, Riba-Grognuz O, Corona M, Nygaard S, Hunt BG, Ingram KK, Falquet L, Nipitwattanaphon M, Gotzek D, Dijkstra MB, Oettler J, Comtesse F, Shih CJ, Wu WJ, Yang CC, Thomas J, Beaudoing E, Pradervand S, Flegel V, Cook ED, Fabbretti R, Stockinger H, Long L, Farmerie WG, Oakey J, Boomsma JJ, Pamilo P, Yi SV, Heinze J, Goodisman MA, Farinelli L, Harshman K, Hulo N, Cerutti L, Xenarios I, Shoemaker D, Keller L. The genome of the fire ant *Solenopsisinvicta*. Proc Natl Acad Sci U S A 2011; 108(14):p5679-84.

[51] Smith CD, Zimin A, Holt C, Abouheif E, Benton R, Cash E, Croset V, Currie CR, Elhaik E, Elsik CG, Fave MJ, Fernandes V, Gadau J, Gibson JD, Graur D, Grubbs KJ, Hagen DE, Helmkampf M, Holley JA, Hu H, Viniegra AS, Johnson BR, Johnson RM, Khila A, Kim JW, Laird J, Mathis KA, Moeller JA, Muñoz-Torres MC, Murphy MC, Nakamura R, Nigam S, Overson RP, Placek JE, Rajakumar R, Reese JT, Robertson HM, Smith CR, Suarez AV, Suen G, Suhr EL, Tao S, Torres CW, van Wilgenburg E, Viljakainen L, Walden KK, Wild AL, Yandell M, Yorke JA, Tsutsui ND. Draft genome of the globally widespread and invasive Argentine ant (*Linepithema humile*). Proc Natl Acad Sci U S A 2011; 108(14):p5673-8.

[52] Nygaard S, Zhang G, Schiøtt M, Li C, Wurm Y, Hu H, Zhou J, Ji L, Qiu F, Rasmussen M, Pan H, Hauser F, Krogh A, Grimmelikhuijzen CJ, Wang J, Boomsma JJ. The genome of the leaf-cutting ant *Acromyrmex echinatior* suggests key adaptations to advanced social life and fungus farming.Genome Res 2011; 21(8):p1339-48.

[53] Suen G, Teiling C, Li L, Holt C, Abouheif E, Bornberg-Bauer E, Bouffard P, Caldera EJ, Cash E, Cavanaugh A, Denas O, Elhaik E, Favé MJ, Gadau J, Gibson JD, Graur D, Grubbs KJ, Hagen DE, Harkins TT, Helmkampf M, Hu H, Johnson BR, Kim J, Marsh SE, Moeller JA, Muñoz-Torres MC, Murphy MC, Naughton MC, Nigam S, Overson R, Rajakumar R, Reese JT, Scott JJ, Smith CR, Tao S, Tsutsui ND, Viljakainen L, Wissler L, Yandell MD, Zimmer F, Taylor J, Slater SC, Clifton SW, Warren WC, Elsik CG, Smith CD, Weinstock GM, Gerardo NM, Currie CR. The genome sequence of the leaf-cutter ant *Atta cephalotes* reveals insights into its obligate symbiotic lifestyle. PLoS Genet 2011; 7(2):e1002007.

[54] Smith CR, Smith CD, Robertson HM, Helmkampf M, Zimin A, Yandell M, Holt C, Hu H, Abouheif E, Benton R, Cash E, Croset V, Currie CR, Elhaik E, Elsik CG, Favé MJ, Fernandes V, Gibson JD, Graur D, Gronenberg W, Grubbs KJ, Hagen DE, Viniegra AS, Johnson BR, Johnson RM, Khila A, Kim JW, Mathis KA, Munoz-Torres MC, Murphy MC, Mustard JA, Nakamura R, Niehuis O, Nigam S, Overson RP, Placek JE, Rajakumar R, Reese JT, Suen G, Tao S, Torres CW, Tsutsui ND, Viljakainen L, Wolschin F, Gadau J.Draft genome of the red harvester ant *Pogonomyrmex barbatus*. Proc Natl Acad Sci U S A 2011; 108(14):p5667-72.

[55] Bonasio R, Zhang G, Ye C, Mutti NS, Fang X, Qin N, Donahue G, Yang P, Li Q, Li C, Zhang P, Huang Z, Berger SL, Reinberg D, Wang J, Liebig J. Genomic comparison of the ants *Camponotus floridanus* and *Harpegnathos saltator*.Science 2010; 329(5995):p1068-71.

[56] Lopes KS, Rios E, Dantas RT, Lima C, Linhares M, Torres AFC, Menezes R, Quinet YP, Havt A, Fonteles MM, Martins AMC. Effect of *Dinoponera quadriceps* venom on chemical-induced seizures models in mice. Rencontres en Toxinologie – Meeting on Toxinology SFET Editions 2011. http://www.sfet.asso.fr (accessed 20 August 2012).

Chapter 9

Discovering the Role of MicroRNAs in Microcystin-Induced Toxicity in Fish

Paweł Brzuzan, Maciej Woźny, Lidia Wolińska and
Michał K. Łuczyński

Additional information is available at the end of the chapter

http://dx.doi.org/10.5772/52204

1. Introduction

MicroRNAs (miRNAs) form a class of endogenously expressed small, non-coding RNAs, that play key roles in the regulation of gene expression of a broad spectrum of biological processes. However, in the field of toxinology, a science of naturally occurring toxins, the relationship between toxicity and microRNA expression is poorly understood. Microcystins (MCs) are potent cyclic peptide hepatotoxins produced by cyanobacteria, which pose a serious threat to aquatic organisms and may also affect human health through the consumption of contaminated waters or food. Although a number of cell physiologic pathways, potential targets for miRNA regulation, are implicated in the response to MCs in animals, no research so far investigated the role for miRNA genes in the mechanism of microcystin (MC)-induced toxicity in fish. The chapter aims to summarize recent achievements of our team in the field, focusing on expression profiling *in vivo* of liver microRNA levels of whitefish (*Coregonus lavaretus*) following MC-LR exposure.

2. Body

2.1. MicroRNAs in fish cells

MicroRNAs (miRNAs) form a class of endogenously expressed small, non-coding RNAs, that play key roles in the regulation of gene expression of a broad spectrum of biological processes. Figure 1 summarizes crucial steps in microRNA processing. MiRNAs are transcribed by RNA polymerases II or III as primary transcripts (pri-miRNAs), which are further processed by the nuclear RNase III enzyme Drosha to stem-loop-structured miRNA precursor molecules (pre-miRNAs). The pre-miRNAs are subsequently transported to the cytoplasm where the RNase III enzyme Dicer cleaves off the double stranded (ds) portion of the hairpin and generates a short-lived dsRNA of about 19–23 nucleotides (nt) in size. The duplex is subsequently unwound and only one strand gives rise to the mature miRNA, which is incorporated into miRNA-protein complexes (miRNPs) [1-2]. The mature miRNAs binds to partially complementary recognition sequences located in the 3'-untranslated regions (3'-UTRs) of mRNAs and target them for degradation or translational repression (reviewed in [3]).

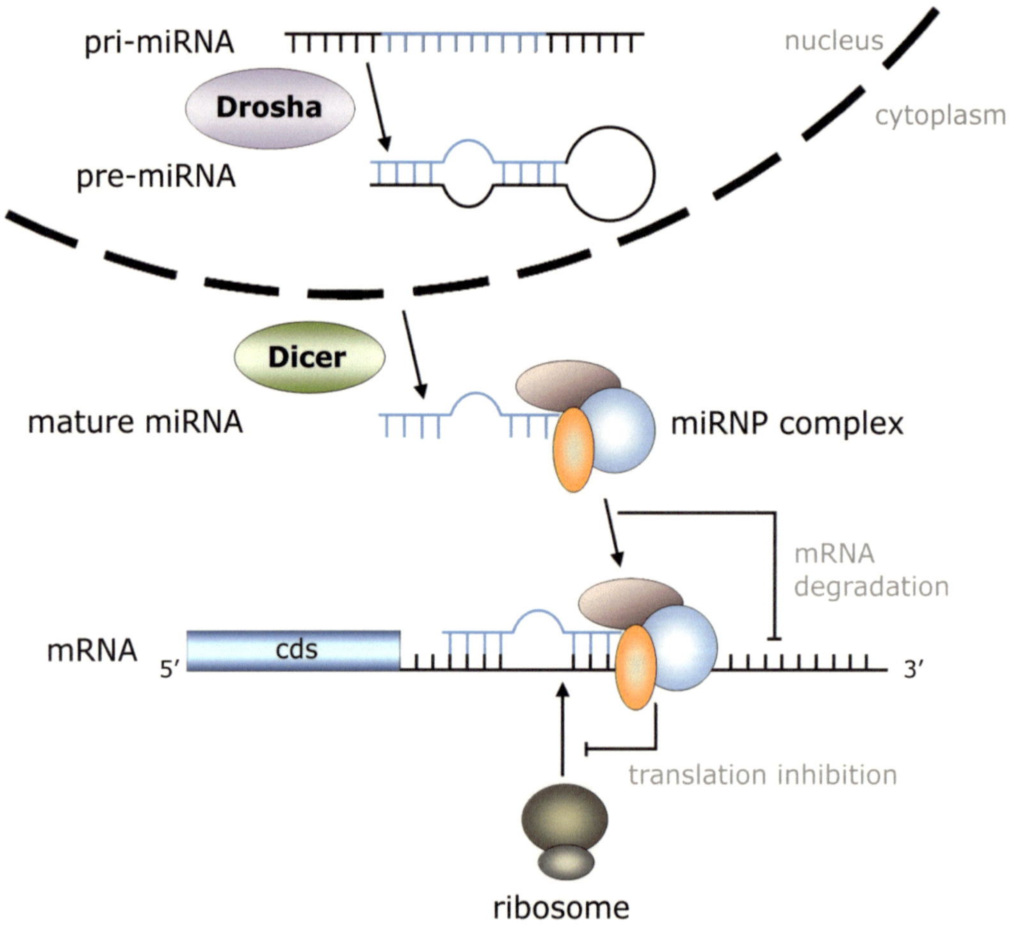

Figure 1. miRNA processing and target recognition. The pri-miRNA is processed by the Drosha enzyme to a stem-loop-structured miRNA precursor molecule (pre-miRNA). The pre-miRNAs is transported to the cytoplasm where the Dicer enzyme cleaves off the double stranded (ds) portion of the hairpin and generates the mature miRNA, which is incorporated into miRNA-protein complexes (miRNPs). The mature miRNA binds to partially complementary recognition sequences on 3'-UTRs of mRNAs and targets them for decay or translational repression.

In metazoans miRNA complementarity to their targets is far from perfect, so one miRNA can bind up to 200 targets, and each mRNA could have recognition sites for more than one miRNA. It is estimated that about 30% of the human protein-coding genes are negatively regulated by miRNA, which suggests that miRNAs are very important regulators of gene expression process [3]. Although specific functions and target mRNAs have been assigned to only a few dozen of miRNAs, much experimental evidence suggests that miRNAs participate in the regulation of a vast spectrum of biological processes. miRNAs control diverse cellular processes including animal development and growth, cell differentiation, signal transduction, cancer, neuronal disease, virus-induced immune defense, programmed cell death, insulin secretion, and metabolism (see [4] and references therein). Understanding of RNA interference (RNA*i*) has been made possible through a variety of experimental and bioinformatics approaches using different model organisms, including fish [5-6].

To discover aberrantly expressed miRNAs in fish and to determine how altered miRNA function contributes to a disease, new RNA*i* technologies may be applied (Figure 2). In toxicological studies attention is focused on the relationship between exposure to a chemical and adverse effects it produces in cells, tissues or organisms. So, when a treatment study is carried out small RNA may be collected from a tissue to generate miRNA libraries, from either control or exposed fish. That is the first important step to establish the full repertoire of miRNAs that are differentially regulated in treated fish. Then the miRNA libraries are subjected to massively parallel sequencing, a next generation sequencing technique, which is a combination of emulsion PCR and pyrosequencing [7]. In comparison to microarray analyses, this approach is not limited to previously identified miRNAs and is expected to have superior sensitivity at high sequencing depth. Such approaches have expanded the catalogue of differentially expressed miRNA genes in various fish tissues [6]. The genome-wide screen for regulated miRNAs should yield candidate miRNAs for further profiling (Real Time qPCR) and functional analyses (e.g. Renilla luciferase reporter assay).

As miRNAs regulate many different pathways and orchestrate integrated responses in cells and tissues, it is reasonable to think that they also play key roles in coordinating networks in the poisoned organs. Indeed, there are reports concluding that miRNAs may be key molecules involved in aberrant gene expression in liver cells exposed to hepatotoxic agents, other than MC-LR. For example, Fukushima and co-workers [8] have shown that two well known hepatotoxicants which induce hepatocellular injuries and necrosis, acetaminophen or carbon tetrachloride, were capable of modulating expression of two miRNAs (miR-298 and miR-370) in rats, and that those effects were accompanied by impaired liver metabolism. The observation that miRNAs levels in rat livers were changed by hepatotoxic compounds prompted our team to investigate the role of fish microRNAs in the context of liver-specific MC-LR toxicity.

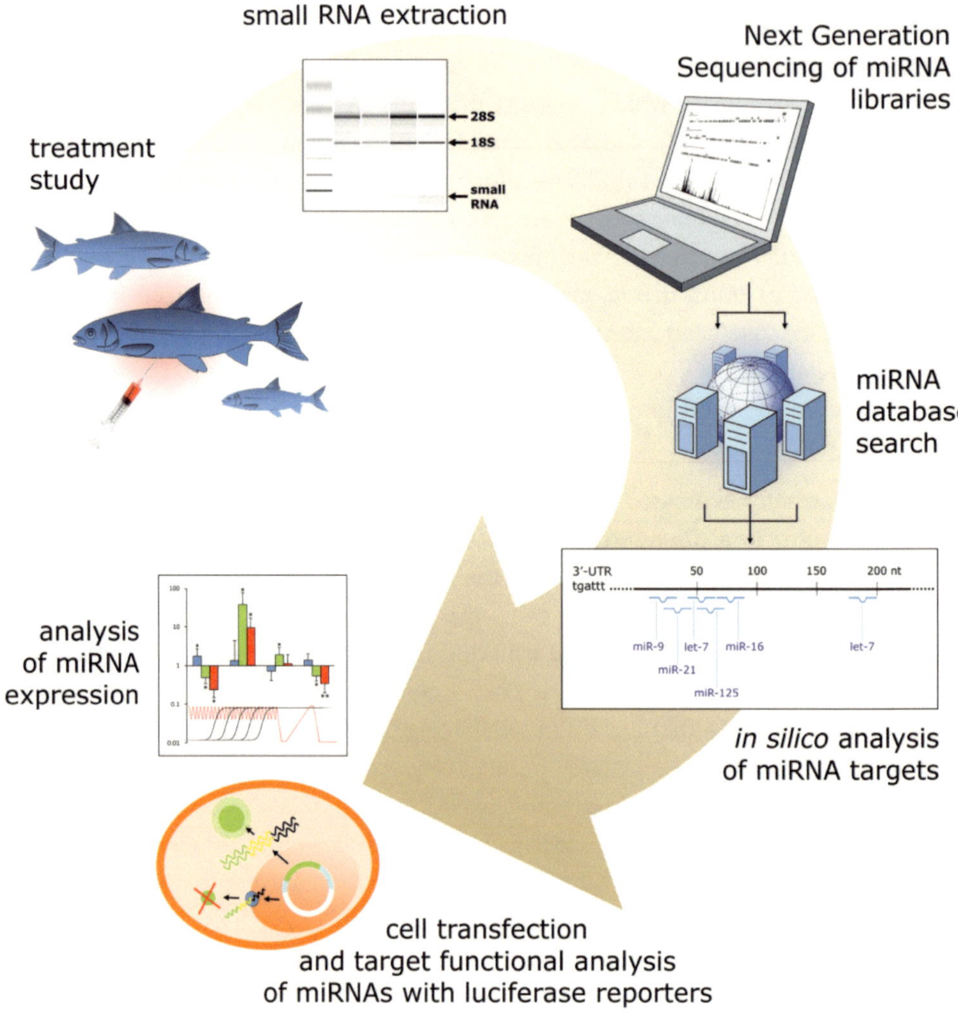

Figure 2. Studying fish miRNAs. MicroRNA discovery has been recently revolutionized by next-generation sequencing. Following ligation of specific linkers to small RNAs (which comprise miRNAs), cDNAs can be produced, which are ideally suited to sequencing using short-read platforms. Databases now offer online catalogues of known microRNAs, which may further be examined for their pathways and functions through a variety of approaches, such as target functional analysis of candidate miRNAs using luciferase reporter assays and miRNA profiling with Real Time PCR.

2.2. Microcystins as potent cyanobacterial toxins

Microcystins (MCs) are potent hepatotoxins produced by cyanobacteria of the genera *Planktothrix, Microcystis, Aphanizomenon, Nostoc,* or *Anabaena,* which have received worldwide concern in recent decades. Mass growths of cyanobacteria, leading to production of blooms, scums and mats, can occur in nutrient-enriched waterbodies (particularly with phosphorus and nitrogen), enhanced by higher temperature and pH values. MCs can be found in lakes, ponds and rivers used for recreational activities as well as in sources for drinking water preparation [9]. In surface waters, concentrations of total MCs (cell-bound and dissolved) measured with ELISA may reach high levels, of up to 1300 μg/l [9], and thus the toxins may pose a threat to aquatic organisms and humans [10]; the World Health Organization recommends 1 μg/l as the maximum acceptable level for microcystin-LR (MC-LR) in drinking water [11]. So far, more than 100 different structural analogues of MCs have been identified, among which MC-LR is one of the most common and abundant [12].

MCs have strong affinity to serine/threonine specific protein phosphatases (PP1 and PP2A), thereby acting as inhibitors of the enzymes [13]. The acute toxicity of MC can be explained by the PP inhibition, which leads to an excessive phosphorylation of cell proteins, to alterations in the cytoskeleton, and a loss of cell shape [14]. Another biochemical feature of MC toxicity is the production of reactive oxygen species (ROS). MC-related ROS generation has been reported using both *in vitro* approaches with different cell lines of fish and mammals [15-16], as well as in a number of *in vivo* studies in rodent liver, heart and reproductive system [17-19]. This process is related to mitochondrial metabolism and it may lead to cell death and to genotoxicity [20]. Oxidative stress caused by MC exposure is believed to be involved in a series of heart, liver and kidney pathologies [19, 21], neurodegenerative effects [22] and embryotoxicity [23].

In recent years, new insights on the key molecules involved in the signal-transduction and toxicity have been reported [24], which highlighted the complexity of the interaction of these toxins with animal cells (Figure 3). Key proteins involved in MC up-take, biotransformation and excretion have been identified, demonstrating the ability of aquatic animals to metabolize and excrete the toxin. After having caused damage to intestinal (or gill) cells these toxins penetrate liver cell membranes through a bile acid carrier. In liver cells MCs inhibit serine/threonine-specific protein phosphatases, PP1 and PP2A, through the binding to them, thus perturbing signaling pathway controlled by the enzymes. The consequences are induction of mitochondrial permeability and loss of mitochondrial membrane potential leading to dysfunction of the mitochondria, induction of reactive oxygen species (ROS), DNA damage (through lowered expression of DNA-PK), and cell apoptosis (through increase Ca2+ levels, CaMKII). MC activity leads to the differential expression/activity of transcriptional factors (e.g. c-myc, p53) and protein kinases (NeK2) involved in the pathways of cellular differentiation, proliferation, tumor promotion activity, and metastasis [25].

2.3. Likely silencing targets in MC-exposed fish cells

In the field of toxinology, a science of naturally occurring toxins, the relationship between toxicity and microRNA expression is poorly understood. However, based on current knowledge about genes involved in the animal cell response on the exposure to environmental stressors, putative targets for miRNA regulation emerge. Genes of transcription factors, *p53* and mapk (mitogen activated protein kinases) regulated proto-oncogenes e.g. *c-myc*, that are involved in MC-LR toxicity (Figure 3), are good candidates for tight and robust regulation by microRNAs. The nuclear phosphoprotein p53 is induced in response to cellular stress. It plays a role as a transcriptional trans-activator in DNA repair, apoptosis and tumor suppression pathways. Interestingly, the protein is a substrate of PP2A [26] and therefore its activity is likely to be regulated, in part, by MC-LR. Furthermore, p53 is a regulator of the expression of the anti- and pro-apoptotic genes including members of the BCL-2 family such as *BCL-2* and *BAX*, as well as *CDKN1A*, encoding p21^{Cip1}, which is a cyclin dependent kinase inhibitor (CDKI), an important effector that acts by inhibiting CDK activity in p53-mediated cell cycle arrest in response to various agents. Indeed, we have shown previously that intraperitoneal injection of whitefish, *Coregonus lavaretus*, with MC-LR at subacute dose of 100 μg/kg body weight induced mRNA expression of tumor suppressor p53 and cyclin dependent kinase inhibitor 1 (cdkn1a) in the liver of exposed fish [27]. Interestingly, it was proven in human cell lines that p53 is a transcription factor for some miRNAs, such as miR-34a [7]. miR-34a mediates some of the well-known effects of p53, i.e. cell cycle arrest or apoptosis, and reduced miR-34a levels can serve as a biomarker for any dysfunction along the p53 axis [28]. Yet, its role in controlling miRNA network in fish awaits investigation (Figure 3).

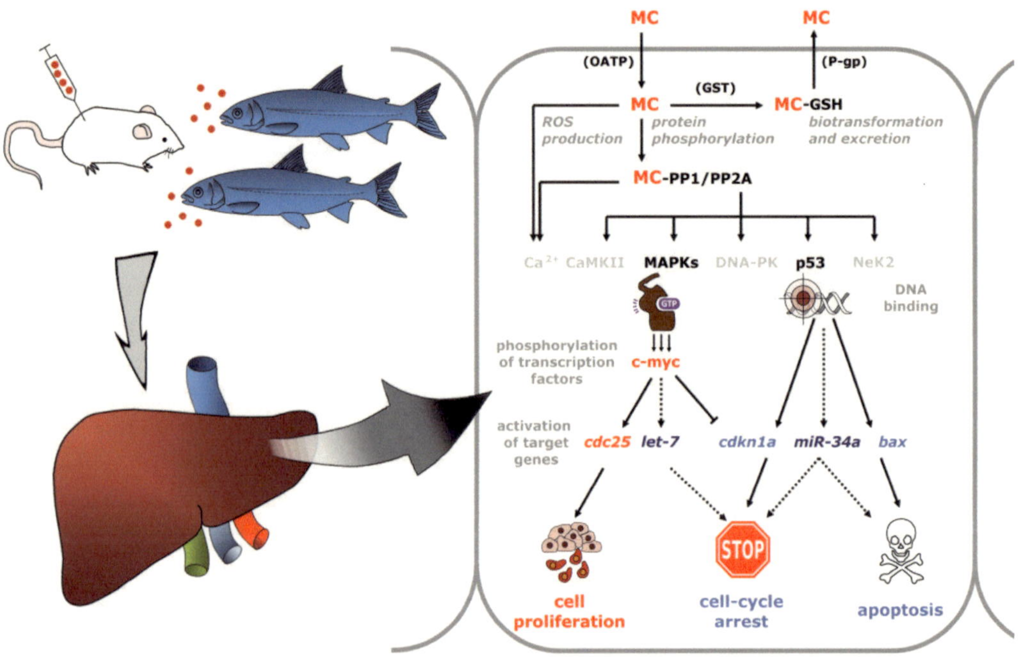

Figure 3. Suggested pathways of MC up-take, toxicity, biotransformation and excretion in vertebrates. Based on the current knowledge, microRNAs (e.g. let-7 or miR-34a) may play roles in MC-LR dependent cell proliferation, cell-cycle arrest or apoptosis.

In the other pathway (Figure 3), mitogen-activated protein kinases (MAPKs) regulate the expression of proto-oncogenes which on the other hand regulate the transcription of genes involved in the growth and differentiation [29]. Expression of MAPKs is mediated by PP2A and are likely to be regulated by MC. The expression of three proto-oncogenes c-fos, c-jun and c-myc were reported to increase in liver, kidney and testis of Wistar rats injected intravenously with MC-LR, with higher levels registered in liver [30]. Expression of these genes suggest that a possible mechanism for the tumor-promoting activity of the toxin could be controlled by MAPKs. Importantly, c-MYC controls expression of let-7 miRNA members by binding to their promoters. The levels of let-7 have been reported to decrease in models of MYC-mediated tumorigenesis, and to increase when MYC is inhibited by chemicals [31]. It is also found that MYC can repress $p21^{Cip1}$ transcription (Figure 1), thereby overriding a p21-mediated cell cycle checkpoint [32].

2.4. miRNA expression in whitefish exposed to MC-LR

In 2008, we began a study of MC-LR induced transcriptional changes in European whitefish, *Coregonus lavaretus* L., a sentinel organism frequently used for pollution monitoring in aquatic systems [27]. To obtain necessary information for the study, full-length cDNA of p53 or cdkn1a of whitefish were determined, using molecular cloning and rapid amplification of cDNA ends (RACE). The *short term* treatment study showed that MC-LR at a dose of 100 μg/kg body weight induced hepatocyte cell DNA fragmentation and up-regulated mRNA expression of p53 and cdkn1a genes in whitefish liver. Interestingly, the elevated transcript levels of both genes were observed only from 48 through the 72 h of exposure, and were accompanied by pathological signs of severe injury of the liver and loss of normal organ functions (elevated levels of blood AspAT AlaAT, and hepatosomatic index; [27]).

Whereas, the above study confirms that MC-LR exposure underlies various acute and chronic effects in fish, it is still little known about aberrant gene expression profiles and molecular pathways involved in the liver of MC-LR challenged organisms. Therefore, to improve our knowledge about adverse effects of MC-LR on hepatocyte cell responses in fish, we performed an initial microRNA study to examine the abundance of 9 selected miRNAs (omy-miR-21, omy-miR-21t, omy-miR-122, omy-miR-125a, omy-miR-125b, omy-miR-125t, omy-miR-199-5a, omy-miR-295, omy-let-7a), in liver samples of whitefish exposed for 24 or 48h to MC-LR at a dose of 100μg/kg body weight [4]. Interestingly, the study showed that MC-LR treatment affected expression levels of two miRNAs, omy-miR-125a (up-regulation) and omy-let-7a (down-regulation) [4].

Following the early demonstration that MC-LR modulates expression of let-7a and miR-125a, in our most recent work [33] we aimed at profiling expression of other 6 miRNAs and 8 mRNAs (Table 1) in the liver of challenged whitefish during the first 48 h after single intraperitoneal injection. From studies on mammals we chose miRNAs which play regulatory roles in pathways of signal transduction (let-7c, [34]; miR-9b, [35]), apoptosis and cell cycle (miR-16a, [36]; miR-21a, [37]; miR-34a, [7]) and fatty-acid metabolism (miR-122, which is a liver specific miRNA, [38]). The selection of mRNA targets (Table 1) was based on their reported aberrant tissue expression on exposure to environmental stressors, and included mRNAs involved in apoptosis and cell cycle (bax, [20]; cas6, cdkn1a, p53, [27]), signal transduction (p-ras, [39]), cellular iron homeostasis (frih, [40]), gene silencing by miRNAs (dcr, [41]), and nucleosome assembly (h2a, [4]). Together with the RNA expression, we analyzed levels of tumor suppressor protein p53 to assess its potential contribution in molecular mechanisms of liver toxicity induced by MCs in fish.

miRNA	Putative biological process*
omy-let-7c	signal transduction
omy-miR-9b	signal transduction
omy-miR-16a	apoptosis, cell cycle
omy-miR-21a	apoptosis, cell cycle
dre-miR-34**	cell cycle, signal transduction
omy-miR-122	fatty-acid metabolism, maintenance of adult liver phenotype
mRNA [gene abbreviation]	Biological process***
bcl2-associated X protein (bax)	apoptosis
caspase 6 (cas6)	apoptosis
cyclin-dependent kinase inhibitor 1a (cdkn1a)	cell cycle
dicer (dcr)	gene silencing by miRNA
ferritin heavy chain (frih)	cellular iron ion homeostasis
histone 2A (h2a)	nucleosome assembly
tumor protein 53 (p53)	apoptosis, cell cycle, signal transduction
HNK Ras –like protein (p-ras)	signal transduction

* based on literature review; see text for details.

** putative *miR-34* gene is present in *Salmo salar* genome; Contig_142190, whole genome shotgun sequence, GenBank ACC. No. AGKD01142167.1, nucleotides from 5978 through 6053.

*** in terms of Gene Ontology Annotation (http://www.ebi.ac.uk/QuickGO).

Table 1. miRNA and mRNA targets selected under study.

Quantifying miRNAs in different tissues is an important initial step in investigating their biological functions. To this end, we determined the expression levels of 6 selected miRNAs in adult whitefish liver using Real-Time qPCR. Prominent expression of miR-122 in the liver of whitefish was observed which is consistent with other data from fish [4,6] and mammals [42]. Variable expression levels of other miRNAs studied in the liver of whitefish corroborated results of previous work on normal human tissues [43], and they are also in agreement with available data on the fish miRNome isolated from rainbow trout [6] and zebrafish [44] miRNA libraries. While the actual expression values of miRNAs can vary by orders of magnitude between whitefish and humans [43], their relative abundance in a particular tissue should tend to be more conserved in evolution. Indeed, the order of individual miRNA abundances in human liver (miR-122 > let-7c ≈ miR-21 ≈ miR16 > miR-34a > miR-9; [43]) held in whitefish as well [33].

Our treatment study [33] identified miRNAs whose expression levels rose (from 2.7-fold for miR-122 to 6.8-fold for let-7c) in MC-LR treated fish, compared to the respective levels in control fish (Figure 4). The increase, which was most apparent at 24 h of the experiment, was correlated with a reduction in the expression of mRNAs: ferritin H (frih) and HNK Ras –like protein (p-ras) and an overexpression of bcl2-associated X protein (bax), cyclin dependent kinase inhibitor 1a (cdkn1a), dicer (dcr), histone 2A (h2a) and p53. Expression of the remaining caspase 6 (cas6) mRNA did not change over 48 h of the treatment. Moreover, exposure to MC-LR did not alter whitefish p53 protein levels [33].

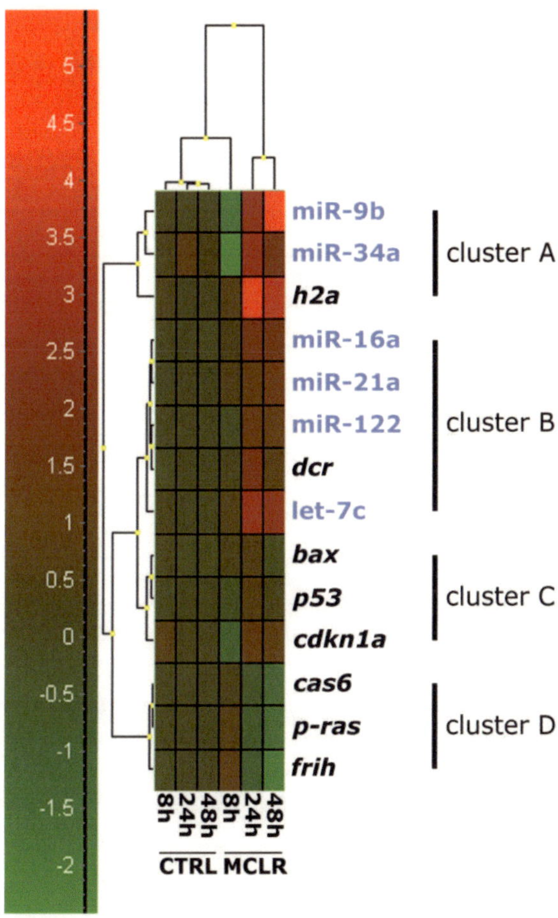

Figure 4. Heat map and hierarchical clustering of differentially expressed genes and miRNAs in MC-LR treated whitefish. Each row represents one gene/miRNA and each column represents a mean of 5 replicates/duration of exposure. Colors represent expression levels of each individual gene/miRNA: red, up-regulation; green, down-regulation. Four distinct clusters (A through D) based on the observed expression profiles could be identified by the analysis. The analysis and visualization were performed using GenEx 5 software (MultiD Analyses AB; Sweden), based on raw expression data from our recent study [33].

The experiment allows one to determine which miRNAs change expression as a group or as a cluster. Genes that function together may define regulatory networks and regulate a common set of regulated genes. Using clustering software, we divided the significantly regulated miRNAs into different groups. In Figure 4 there were four different types of expression profiles among the miRNAs and genes. Some groups showed transient changes in the expression profile (clusters B and C) while others stably increase (cluster A) or decrease (cluster D) during the treatment with MC-LR. Bearing in mind a variety of likely silencing targets for, and the onset of, the aberrant miRNAs expression (Table 2; [33]) it may be concluded that they are involved in diverse molecular pathways, such as liver cell metabolism, cell cycle regulation and apoptosis, and may contribute to the early phase of MC-LR induced hepatotoxicity. Whereas, this argues that at least some of miRNAs listed in Table 2 are good candidates to pursue in future studies, a key to further elucidation of the miRNA role in the toxicity mechanism is the generation of more complete lists of their numbers and expression changes in healthy and challenged fish.

MicroRNA*	Fold change	Reported silencing targets	Reference
let-7c	6.8	Rat sarcoma viral oncogene, RAS	[34]
		Myelocytomatosis viral related oncogene, c-MYC	[45]
miR-9b	4.4	Caudal related homebox protein, CDX2	[35]
miR-34a	4.0	B-cell lymphoma 2, BCL2	[46]
		Myelocytomatosis viral related oncogene, neuroblastoma derived (avian), MYCN	[47]
miR-16a	3.6	B-cell lymphoma 2, BCL2	[36]
miR-122	2.7	Cationic amino acid transporter, CAT-1	[48]

*Only miRNAs which were significantly up-regulated ($p<0.05$) are included in the column.

Table 2. Reported mammalian silencing targets for differentially expressed miRNAs in MC-LR treated whitefish (100μg/kg body weight) after 24 h of the challenge [33].

On the other hand, the lack of p53 stabilization observed in our study infers the presence of alternate checkpoint mechanisms for deregulated growth signals and/or DNA damage in whitefish cells and may suggest post-transcriptional regulation of *p53*. Indeed, recent work by Liu and coworkers [49] suggest that two checkpoint kinases, ATM and ATR, which act upstream of p53, are promising candidates for the role. Further studies should also reveal if the lack of p53 induction in fish liver following exposure to many compounds known to cause DNA damage and DNA replication defects [49-50], is controlled by the miRNA network, a role it is known to fulfill in other organisms. For example, miR-125b has been previously confirmed to be a negative regulator of p53 in both zebrafish and humans [51].

3. Conclusions

We are only beginning to understand the complexities of miRNA-mediated gene regulatory networks in fish cells. It should be expected that environmental contaminants that have the potential to induce oxidative stress and hypoxia in animal cells, like MCs, will also be agents deregulating miRNA expression. In our initial studies [4, 33] we observed rapid changes in liver microRNA levels of whitefish following MC-LR exposure. Bearing in mind a variety of likely silencing targets for and the onset of the aberrant miRNAs expression observed in the study, one may conclude that they are involved in various molecular pathways and may contribute to the early phase of MC-hepatotoxicity. This argues that studied miRNAs are good candidates to pursue in future studies, however, a key to further elucidation of the miRNA role in the toxicity mechanism will be the generation of more complete lists of their numbers and expression changes in healthy and challenged fish, using next generation sequencing methods (Figure 2). As miRNA field continues to evolve, the new markers should help elucidating a variety of issues intrinsic to MC toxicity. As more profiling studies are performed after MC-LR treatment, and on different model organisms, it might be possible to obtain a miRNA snapshot map, the "core of the MC-LR toxicity connectivity grid". Finally, the revealed miRNA pathways underlying hepatotoxic effects of MC-LR may provide therapeutic targets for a variety of liver diseases.

Acknowledgments

This work was supported by the Polish Ministry of Science and Higher Education (MNiSW), project UWM No. 0809-0801.

Author details

Paweł Brzuzan[1*], Maciej Woźny[1], Lidia Wolińska[1] and Michał K. Łuczyński[2]

1 Department of Environmental Biotechnology, Faculty of Environmental Sciences, University of Warmia and Mazury in Olsztyn, Olsztyn, Poland

2 Department of Chemistry, Faculty of Environmental Management and Agriculture, University of Warmia and Mazury in Olsztyn, Olsztyn, Poland

References

[1] Meister G, Tuschl T. Mechanisms of gene silencing by double-stranded RNA. Nature 2004;431(7006): 343-349.

[2] Ambros V. The functions of animal microRNAs. Nature 2004;431(7006): 350-355.

[3] Zhang B, Wang Q, Pan X. MicroRNAs and their regulatory roles in animals and plants. Journal of Cellular Physiology 2007;210(2): 279-289.

[4] Brzuzan P, Woźny M, Wolińska L, Piasecka A, Łuczyński MK. MicroRNA expression in liver of whitefish (Coregonus lavaretus) exposed to microcystin-LR. Environmental Biotechnology 2010;6(2): 53-60.

[5] Flynt AS, Thatcher EJ, Patton JG. RNA interferences and miRNAs in zebrafish. In: Gaur RK, Rossi JJ. (ed.) Regulation of gene expression by small RNAs. CRC Press; 2009. p149-172.

[6] Salem M, Xiao C, Womack J, Rexroad III CE, Yao J. MicroRNA repertoire for functional genome research in rainbow trout (Oncorhynchus mykiss). Marine Biotechnology 2010;12(4): 410-429.

[7] Tarasov V, Jung P, Verdoodt B, Lodygin D, Epanchintsev A, Menssen A, Meister G, Hermeking H. Differential regulation of microRNAs by p53 revealed by massively parallel sequencing: miR-34a is a p53 target that induces apoptosis and G1-arrest. Cell Cycle 2007;6(13): 1586-1593.

[8] Fukushima T, Hamada Y, Yamada H, Horii I. Changes of micro-RNA expression in rat liver treated by acetaminophen or carbon tetrachloride – regulating role of micro-RNA for RNA expression. Journal of Toxicological Sciences 2007;32(4): 401-409.

[9] Fromme H, Köhler A, Krause R, Führling D. Occurrence of cyanobacterial toxins-microcystins and anatoxin-a–in Berlin water bodies with implications to human health and regulations. Environmental Toxicology 2000;15(2): 120-130.

[10] Carmichael WW. Cyanobacteria secondary metabolites – the cyanotoxins. Journal of Applied Bacteriology 1992;72(6): 445-459.

[11] WHO. Guidelines for Drinking-water Quality, Volume 1. Recommendations, 3rd edition. World Health Organization Publishing 2004; Geneva, Switzerland.

[12] Dietrich D, Hoeger S. Guidance values for microcystins in water and cyanobacterial supplement products (blue-green algal supplements): a reasonable or misguided approach? Toxicology and Applied Pharmacology 2005;203(3): 273-289.

[13] Honkanen RE, Zwiller J, Moore RE, Daily SL, Khatra BS, Dukelow M, Boynton AL. Characterization of microcystin-LR, a potent inhibitor of type 1 and type 2A protein phosphatases. Journal of Biological Chemistry 1990;265(32): 19401-19404.

[14] van Apeldoorn ME, van Egmond HP, Speijers GJA, Bakker GJI. Toxins of cyanobacteria. Molecular Nutrition and Food Research 2007;51(1): 7-60.

[15] Nong Q, Komatsu M, Izumo K, Indo HP, Xu B, Aoyama K, Majima HJ, Horiuchi M, Morimoto K, Takeuchi T. Involvement of reactive oxygen species in Microcystin-LR-induced cytogenotoxicity. Free Radical Research 2007;41(12): 1326-1337.

[16] Pichardo S, Jos A, Zurita JL, Salguero M, Cameán AM, Repetto G. Acute and subacute toxic effects produced by microcystin-YR on the fish cell lines RTG-2 and PLHC-1. Toxicology In Vitro 2007;21(8): 1460-1467.

[17] Ding WX, Shen HM, Ong CN. Pivotal role of mitochondrial Ca(2+) in microcystin-induced mitochondrial permeability transition in rat hepatocytes. Biochemical and Biophysical Research Communications 2001;285(5): 1155-1161.

[18] Li Y, Sheng J, Sha J, Han X. The toxic effects of microcystin-LR on the reproductive system of male rats in vivo and in vitro. Reproductive Toxicology 2008;26(3-4): 239-245.

[19] Qiu T, Xie P, Liu Y, Li G, Xiong Q, Hao L, Li H. The profound effects of microcystin on cardiac antioxidant enzymes, mitochondrial function and cardiac toxicity in rat. Toxicology 2009;257(1-2): 86-94.

[20] Žegura B, Filipič M, Šuput D, Lah T, Sedmak B. In vitro genotoxicity of microcystin-RR on primary cultured rat hepatocites and Hep G2 cell line detected by Comet assay. Radiology and Oncology 2002;36(2): 159-161.

[21] Wei Y, Weng D, Li F, Zou X, Young DO, Ji J, Shen P. Involvement of JNK regulation in oxidative stress-mediated murine liver injury by microcystin-LR. Apoptosis 2008;13(8): 1031-1042.

[22] Feurstein D, Stemmer K, Kleinteich J, Speicher T, Dietrich DR. Microcystin congener- and concentration-dependent induction of murine neuron apoptosis and neurite degeneration. Toxicological Sciences 2011;124(2): 424-431.

[23] Zhao Y, Xiong Q, Xie P. Analysis of microRNA expression in embryonic developmental toxicity induced by MC-RR. PLoS ONE 2011;6(7): e22676.

[24] Campos A, Vasconcelos V. Molecular mechanism of microcystin toxicity in animal cells. International Journal of Molecular Sciences 2010;11(1): 268–287.

[25] Zhang XX, Zhang Z, Fu Z, Wang T, Qin W, Xu L, Cheng S, Yang L. Stimulation effect of microcystin-LR on matrix metalloproteinase-2/-9 expression in mouse liver. Toxicology Letters 2010;199(3): 377-382.

[26] Li HH, Cai X, Shouse GP, Piluso LG, Liu X. A specific PP2A regulatory subunit, B56γ, mediates DNA damage-induced dephosphorylation of p53 at Thr55. EMBO Journal 2007;26(2): 402-411.

[27] Brzuzan P, Woźny M, Ciesielski S, Łuczyński MK, Góra M, Kuźmiński H, Dobosz S. Microcystin-LR induced apoptosis and mRNA expression of p53 and cdkn1a in liver of whitefish (Coregonus lavaretus L.). Toxicon 2009;54(2): 170-183.

[28] Asslaber D, Piñón JD, Seyfried I, Desch P, Stöcher M, Tinhofer I, Egle A, Merkel O, Greil R. microRNA-34a expression correlates with MDM2 SNP309 polymorphism and treatment-free survival in chronic lymphocytic leukemia. Blood 2010;115(21): 4191-4197.

[29] Gehringer MM. Microcystin-LR and okadaic acid-induced cellular effects: a dualistic response. FEBS Letters 2004;557(1-3): 1-8.

[30] Li H, Xie P, Li G, Hao L, Xiong Q. In vivo study on the effects of microcystin extracts on the expression profiles of proto-oncogenes (c-fos, c-jun and c-myc) in liver, kidney and testis of male Wistar rats injected i.v. with toxins. Toxicon 2009;53(1): 169-175.

[31] Chang TC, Yu D, Lee YS, Wentzel EA, Arking DE, West KM, Dang CV, Thomas-Tikhonenko A, Mendell JT. Widespread microRNA repression by Myc contributes to tumorigenesis. Nature genetics. 2008;40(1): 43-50.

[32] Gartel AL, Ye X, Goufman E, Shianov P, Hay N, Najmabadi F, Tyner AL. Myc represses the p21(WAF1/CIP1) promoter and interacts with Sp1/Sp3. Proceedings of the National Academy of Sciences U.S.A. 2001;98(8): 4510-4515.

[33] Brzuzan P, Woźny M, Wolińska L, Piasecka A. Expression profiling in vivo demonstrates rapid changes in liver microRNA levels of whitefish (Coregonus lavaretus) following microcystin-LR exposure. Aquatic Toxicology 2012;122-123: 188-196.

[34] Johnson SM, Grosshans H, Shingara J, Byrom M, Jarvis R, Cheng A, Labourier E, Reinert KL, Brown D, Slack FJ. RAS is regulated by the let-7 microRNA family. Cell 2005;120(5): 635-647.

[35] Rotkrua P, Akiyama Y, Hashimoto Y, Otsubo T, Yuasa Y. MiR-9 downregulates CDX2 expression in gastric cancer cells. International Journal of Cancer 2011;129(11): 2611-2620.

[36] Cimmino A, Calin GA, Fabbri M, Iorio MV, Ferracin M, Shimizu M, Wojcik SE, Aqeilan RI, Zupo S, Dono M, Rassenti L, Alder H, Volinia S, Liu CG, Kipps TJ, Negrini M, Croce CM. miR-15 and miR-16 induce apoptosis by targeting BCL2. Proceedings of the National Academy of Sciences U.S.A. 2005;102(39): 13944-13949.

[37] Chan JA, Krichevsky AM, Kosik KS. MicroRNA-21 is an antiapoptotic factor in human glioblastoma cells. Cancer Research 2005;65(14): 6029-6033.

[38] Girard M, Jacquemin E, Munnich A, Lyonnet S, Henrion-Caude A. miR-122, a paradigm for the role of microRNAs in the liver. Journal of Hepatology 2008;48(4): 648-656.

[39] Žegura B, Zajc I, Lah TT, Filipič M. Patterns of microcystin-LR induced alteration of the expression of genes involved in response to DNA damage and apoptosis. Toxicon 2008;51(4): 615-623.

[40] Woźny M, Brzuzan P, Wolińska L, Góra M, Łuczyński MK. Differential gene expression in rainbow trout (Oncorhynchus mykiss) liver and ovary after exposure to zearalenone. Comparative Biochemistry and Physiology, Part C: Toxicology and Pharmacology 2012; doi:10.1016/j.cbpc.2012.05.005.

[41] Mishra PK, Tyagi N, Kundu S, Tyagi SC. MicroRNAs are involved in homocysteine-induced cardiac remodeling. Cell Biochemistry and Biophysics 2009;55(3): 153-162.

[42] Ason B, Darnell DK, Wittbrodt B, Berezikov E, Kloosterman WP, Wittbrodt J, Antin PB, Plasterk RH. Differences in vertebrate microRNA expression. Proceedings of the National Academy of Sciences U.S.A. 2006;103(39): 14385-14389.

[43] Liang Y, Ridzon D, Wong L, Chen C. Characterization of microRNA expression profiles in normal human tissues. BMC Genomics 2007;8: 166.

[44] Chen PY, Manninga H, Slanchev K, Chien M, Russo JJ, Ju J, Sheridan R, John B, Marks DS, Gaidatzis D, Sander C, Zavolan M, Tuschl T. The developmental miRNA profiles of zebrafish as determined by small RNA cloning. Genes and Development 2005;19(11): 1288-1293.

[45] Koscianska E, Baev V, Skreka K, Oikonomaki K, Rusinov V, Tabler M, Kalantidis K. Prediction and preliminary validation of oncogene regulation by miRNAs. BMC Molecular Biology 2007;8: 79.

[46] Ji Q, Hao X, Meng Y, Zhang M, DeSano J, Fan D, Xu L. Restoration of tumor suppressor miR-34 inhibits human p53-mutant gastric cancer tumorspheres. BMC Cancer 2008;8: 266.

[47] Wei JS, Song YK, Durinck S, Chen QR, Cheuk AT, Tsang P, Zhang Q, Thiele CJ, Slack A, Shohet J, Khan J. The MYCN oncogene is a direct target of miR-34a. Oncogene 2008;27(39): 5204-5213.

[48] Chang J, Nicolas E, Marks D, Sander C, Lerro A, Buendia MA, Xu C, Mason WS, Moloshok T, Bort R, Zaret KS, Taylor JM. miR-122, a mammalian liver-specific microRNA, is processed from hcr mRNA and may downregulate the high affinity cationic amino acid transporter CAT-1. RNA Biology 2004;1(2): 106-113.

[49] Liu M, Tee C, Zeng F, Sherry JP, Dixon B, Bols NC, Duncker BP. Characterization of p53 expression in rainbow trout. Comparative Biochemistry and Physiology, Part C: Toxicology and Pharmacology 2011;154(4): 326-332.

[50] Rau EM, Billiard SM, Di Giulio RT. Lack of p53 induction in fish cells by model chemotherapeutics. Oncogene 2006;25(14): 2004-2010.

[51] Le MTN, Teh C, Shyh-Chang N, Xie H, Zhou B, Korzh V, Lodish HF, Lim B. MicroRNA-125b is a novel negative regulator of p53. Genes and Development 2009;23(7): 862-876.

Section 2

Molecular Cloning and Genetics

Chapter 10

Identification of Key Molecules Involved in the Protection of Vultures Against Pathogens and Toxins

Lourdes Mateos-Hernández, Elena Crespo,
José de la Fuente and José M. Pérez de la Lastra

Additional information is available at the end of the chapter

http://dx.doi.org/10.5772/54191

1. Introduction

Vultures may have one of the strongest immune systems of all vertebrates (Apanius et al., 1983; Ohishi et al., 1979). Vultures are unique vertebrates able to efficiently utilize carcass from other animals as a food resource. These carrion birds are in permanent contact with numerous pathogens and toxins found in its food. In addition, vultures tend to feed in large groups, because carcasses are patchy in space and time, and feeding often incurs fighting and wounding, exposing vultures to the penetration of microorganisms present in the carrion (Houston & Cooper, 1975). When an animal dies, the carcass provides the growth conditions necessary for many pathogens to thrive and produce high levels of toxins. Vultures are able to feed upon such a carcasses with no apparent ill effects. Therefore, vultures were predicted to have evolved immune mechanisms to cope with a high risk of infection with virulent parasites.

Despite the potential interest in carrion bird immune system, little is known about the molecular mechanisms involved in the regulation of this process in vultures. The aim of this chapter was to explore the genes from the griffon vulture (*Gyps fulvus*) leukocytes, particularly to search novel receptors, such as the toll-like receptor (TLRs) and other components involved in the immune sensing of pathogens and in the mechanism by which vulture are protected against toxins. This study is, to the best of our knowledge, the first report of exploring the transcriptome in this interesting specie.

The toll-like receptor (TLR) family is an ancient pattern recognition receptor family, conserved from insects to mammals. Members of the TLR family are vital to immune function through the sensing of pathogenic agents and initiation of an appropriate immune response. The rapid identification of Toll orthologues in invertebrates and mammals suggests that these genes must be present in other vertebrates (Takeda, 2005). During the recent years, members of the multigene family of TLRs have been recognised as key players in the recognition of microbes during host defence (Hopkinsn & Sriskandan, 2005). Recognition of pathogens by immune receptors leads to activation of macrophages, dendritic cells, and lymphocytes. Signals are then communicated to enhance expression of target molecules such as cytokines and adhesion molecules, depending on activation of various inducible transcription factors, among which the family NF-kappaB transcription factors plays a critical role. The involvement of nuclear factor-kappa B (NF-κB) in the expression of numerous cytokines and adhesion molecules has supported its role as an evolutionarily conserved coordinating element in organism's response to situations of infection, stress, and injury. In many species, pathogen recognition, whether mediated via the Toll-like receptors or via the antigen-specific T- and B-cell receptors, initiates the activation of distinct signal transduction pathways that activate NF-κB (Ghosh et al., 1998). TLR-mediated NF-κB activation is also an evolutionarily conserved event that occurs in phylogenetically distinct species ranging from insects to mammals.

Botulinun toxins are the most deadly neurotoxins known to man and animals. When an animal dies from botulism or other causes, the carcass provides the growth conditions necessary for *C. botulinun* to thrive and produce high levels of toxins. Certain species of carrion-eater birds and mammals are able to feed upon such carcasses with no apparent ill effects. Turkey vultures (*Cathartes aura*), have been shown to be highly resistant to botulinun toxins (Kalmbach, 1993; Pates, 1967, cited by Oishi et al., 1979). The mechanism by which these species are protected against botulinun toxin was investigated by exploring the genes from the griffon vulture (*Gyps fulvus*) leukocytes, particularly with the identification of ORFs with homology to the Ras-related botulinun toxin substrate 2 (RAC2), ADP-ribosylation factor 1 (a GTP-binding protein that functions as an allosteric activator of the cholera toxin catalytic subunit); a ras-related protein Rabb-11-B-like, and other ORFs with homology to some chemical mediators, such as IL-8, Chemokine (C-C motif) ligand 1.

2. Exploring the genes from the griffon vulture (*Gyps fulvus*) leukocytes

Given that the vulture is protected in Spain, we have used an *ex-vivo* approach. We have generated a cDNA library from from vulture peripheral blood monuclear cells (PBMC) and screened it, either with specific probes or randomly, to search for molecules involved in the immune recognition of pathogens and in the mechanism of resistance to toxins. In order to search for molecules involved in the immune recognition of pathogens and in the mechanism of resistance to toxins, we screened the cDNA library randomly. Several clones were identified and sequenced from the screening of the cDNA library from vulture´s leukocytes. A total of 49 open reading frames (ORFs) were identified by BLAST analysis from 100 plaques approximately. The identification and function of each ORF are summarized in the Table 1.

ORF /Acs number	Function	Assignment[1]
Phosphogycerato kinase 1 PGK1 JX889400	Glycolytic enzyme, also PGK-1 may acts as a polymerase alpha cofactor protein (primer recognition protein).	CA
Activity-dependent neuroprotector homeobox (ADNP) JX889402	Potential transcription factor. May mediate some of the neuroprotective peptide VIP-associated effects involving normal growth and cancer proliferation.	RP
Serpin B5-like JX889399	Tumor suppressor. It blocks the growth, invasion, and metastatic properties of mammary tumors.	RP
40S ribosomal protein S3a JX889382	May play a role during erythropoiesis through regulation of transcription factor DDIT3.	OT
Mps one binder kinase activator-like 1B, JX889412	Activator of LATS1/2 in the Hippo signaling pathway which plays a pivotal role in organ size control and tumor suppression by restricting proliferation and promoting apoptosis.	OT
Lymphocyte antigen 86 [LY86] JX889396	May cooperate with CD180 and TLR4 to mediate the innate immune response to bacterial lipopolysaccharide (LPS) and cytokine production. Important for efficient CD180 cell surface expression.	IS
IL-8 JX889394	Chemotactic factor that attracts neutrophils, basophils, and T-cells, but not monocytes. It is also involved in neutrophil activation. It is released from several cell types in response to an inflammatory stimulus.	IS
Constitutive coactivator of PPAR-gamma-like protein 1, JX889388	May participate in mRNA transport in the cytoplasm. Critical component of the oxidative stress-induced survival signaling.	OT
Interferon regulatory factor 1 (IRF-1), JX889416	Specifically binds to the upstream regulatory region of type I IFN and IFN-inducible MHC class I genes and activates those genes. Acts as a tumor suppressor.	IS
Annexin A1 [ANXA1], JX889410	Calcium/phospholipid-binding protein which promotes membrane fusion and is involved in exocytosis. This protein regulates phospholipase A2 activity.	RP
Chemokine (C-C motif) ligand 1, JX889398	Cytokine that is chemotactic for monocytes but not for neutrophils. Binds to CCR8	IS
Ras-related C3 botulinum toxin substrate 2 (RAC2) JX889392	Enzyme regulation: Plasma membrane-associated small GTPase which cycles between an active GTP-bound and inactive GDP-bound state. In active state binds to a variety of effector proteins to regulate cellular responses, such as secretory processes, phagocytose of apoptotic cells and epithelial cell polarization. Augments the production of reactive oxygen species (ROS) by NADPH oxidase	IS
Activating transcription factor 4 (ATF4), JX889393	Transcriptional activator. Binds the cAMP response element (CRE), a sequence present in many viral and cellular promoters.	RP
Elongation factor 1-alpha 1 (EF-1-alpha-1), JX889383	This protein promotes the GTP-dependent binding of aminoacyl-tRNA to the A-site of ribosomes during protein biosynthesis	OT
Polynucleotide 5'-hydroxyl-kinase NOL9, JX889408	Polynucleotide 5'-kinase involved in rRNA processing.	RP
Sodium/potassium -transporting ATPase subunit alpha-1, JX889386	Catalytic activity: Catalytic component of the active enzyme, which catalyzes the hydrolysis of ATP coupled with the exchange of sodium and potassium ions across the plasma membrane. This action creates the electrochemical gradient of sodium and potassium ions, providing the energy for active transport of various nutrients.	CA
Tyrosyl-DNA phosphodiesterase 2 (TDP2), JX889415	DNA repair enzyme that can remove a variety of covalent adducts from DNA through hydrolysis of a 5'-phosphodiester bond, giving rise to DNA with a free 5' phosphate.	OT
Transaldolase (EC 2.2.1.2) [TALDO1] JX889384	Important for the balance of metabolites in the pentose-phosphate pathway.	CA
60S ribosomal	Binds to a specific region on the 26S rRNA	RP

protein L23a variant 1, JX889411		
2',3'-cyclic-nucleotide 3'-phosphodiesterase (EC 3.1.4.37) (CNP), JX889397	Catalytic activity: Nucleoside 2',3'-cyclic phosphate + H(2)O = nucleoside 2'-phosphate	CA
Ribosomal protein S6 (RPS6), JX889418	May play an important role in controlling cell growth and proliferation through the selective translation of particular classes of mRNA.	RP
Hippocalcin-like protein 1 (Protein Rem-1), JX889389	May be involved in the calcium-dependent regulation of rhodopsin phosphorylation	OT
Sel-1 suppressor of lin-12-like	May play a role in Notch signaling. May be involved in the endoplasmic reticulum quality control (ERQC) system also called ER-associated degradation (ERAD) involved in ubiquitin-dependent degradation of misfolded endoplasmic reticulum proteins.	IS
Arf-GAP domain and FG repeats-containing protein 1-like, JX889409	Required for vesicle docking or fusion during acrosome biogenesis. May play a role in RNA trafficking or localization. In case of infection by HIV-1, acts as a cofactor for viral ISRev and promotes movement of Rev-responsive element-containing RNAs from the nuclear periphery to the cytoplasm.	OT
TNF receptor-associated factor 6 (TRAF-6) JX889385	E3 ubiquitin ligase that, together with UBE2N and UBE2V1, mediates the synthesis of 'Lys-63'-linked-polyubiquitin chains conjugated to proteins, such as IKBKG, AKT1 and AKT2. Seems to also play a role in dendritic cells (DCs) maturation and/or activation. Represses c-Myb-mediated transactivation, in B lymphocytes. Adapter protein that seems to play a role in signal transduction initiated via TNF receptor, IL-1 receptor and IL-17 receptor.	IS
Sorting nexin-5, JX889390	May be involved in several stages of intracellular trafficking.	OT
F-box protein 34 (FBXO34), JX889403	Substrate-recognition component of the SCF (SKP1-CUL1-F-box protein)-type E3 ubiquitin ligase complex	OT
Low density lipoprotein receptor-related protein 5 (LRP5) JX889414	Component of the Wnt-Fzd-LRP5-LRP6 complex that triggers beta-catenin signaling through inducing aggregation of receptor-ligand complexes into ribosome-sized signalsomes.	IS
Coronin, actin binding protein 1C JX889404	May be involved in cytokinesis, motility, and signal transduction.	CM
tumor protein, translationally-controlled 1 (TPT1) JX889417	Involved in calcium binding and microtubule stabilization.	CM
SH3 domain binding glutamic acid-rich protein like (SH3BGRL) JX889401	Acts as a transcriptional regulator of PAX6. Acts as a transcriptional activator of PF4 in complex with PBX1 or PBX2. Required for hematopoiesis, megakaryocyte lineage development and vascular patterning.	RP
GATA-binding factor 2 (GATA-2) (Transcription factor NF-E1b) JX889387	Transcriptional activator, which regulates endothelin-1 gene expression in endothelial cells. Binds to the consensus sequence 5'-AGATAG-3'	RP
Cytochrome b5 JX889381	Membrane bound hemoprotein which function as an electron carrier for several membrane bound oxygenases, including fatty acid desaturases	OT
iron sulfur cluster assembly 1 homolog mitochondria JX889395	Acts as a co-chaperone in iron-sulfur cluster assembly in mitochondria	OT

Table 1. ORFs found from the random screening of the vulture leukocyte cDNA library. Assignment of the function of each ORF was performed based on the information shown at the Universal Protein Resource (UniProt) web page (http://www.uniprot.org/) and it was assigned as immune system (IS), Catalytic activity (CA), Cell motility (CM), Regulatory protein (RP) and Other (OT).

Interestingly, we found ORFs with homology to the Ras-related botulinun toxin substrate 2 (RAC2); the interferon regulatory factor I (IRF1), ADP-ribosylation factor 1 (a GTP-binding protein that functions as an allosteric activator of the cholera toxin catalytic subunit); a ras-related protein Rabb-11-B-like; some chemical mediators, such as IL-8, Chemokine (C-C motif) ligand 1, etc. These sequences were deposited in the Genbank under accession numbers indicated in Table 1.

The *ras* and *ras-related* genes represent a superfamily coding for low molecular weight GTPases (Bourne et al., 1991). These proteins, which share significant homology in the four regions shown for the H-ras protein to be involved in the binding and hydrolysis of GTP, regulate a diverse number of cellular processes including growth and differentiation, vesicular trafficking, and cytoskeleton organization. GTPases are in an active state when GTP is bound and are inactive when GDP is bound, and a variety of additional proteins have been identified that regulate the switch between active and inactive states. ADP-ribosylation of cellular proteins by a number of bacterial toxins (*i.e.* cholera, pertussis, pseudomonas exotoxins A., and diphtheria) is the primary mechanism for their toxicity (Eidels et al., 1983). Botulinun toxins C1 and D contain an ADP-ribosyltransferase activity that is able to ADP-ribosylate 21-26 kDa eukaryotic proteins. The ORF found with high homology to the Ras-related botulinun toxin substrate 2 (RAC2) led us to hypothesize that this ORF is candidate for such a regulatory function in the vulture and it may be involved in the protection of vultures against toxins.

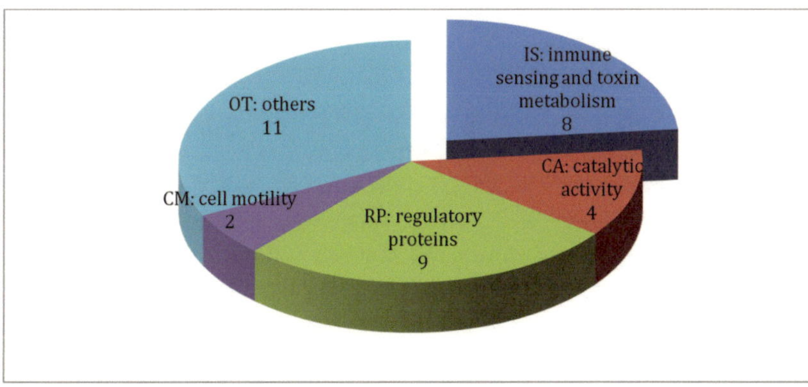

Figure 1. Pie-chart showing number of ORFs with different functions.

3. Strategy for cloning of vulture TLR1 and IκBα

In order to identify key components of the vulture system for sensing of pathogens, we screened a cDNA library from vulture peripheral blood monuclear cells (PBMC) using specific probes for TLR1 and IκBα.

Since the majority of toll-like receptors are expressed in leukocytes and lymphoid tissues in human and other vertebrates, we decided to use vulture PBMC as the source of RNA to obtain a specific probes for TLR1 and IκBα and to construct a cDNA library. Using this strategy we cloned cDNAs encoding for griffon vulture (*Gyps fulvus*) orthologues of mammalian

TLR1 (CD281) and for the alpha inhibitor of NF-κB (IκBα). The tissue and cell expression pattern of vulture TLR1 and IκBα were analyzed by real-time RT-PCR and correlated with the ability to respond to various pathogenic challenges.

3.1. Design of specific probes for vulture TLR1 and IκBα

To obtain specific probes for vulture TLR1 and IκBα, total RNA was isolated from vulture PBMC and from cells and tissues using the Ultraspec isolation reagent (Biotecx Laboratories, Houston TX, USA). Ten micrograms of total RNA was heated at 65 °C for 5 min, quenched on ice for 5 min and subjected to first strand cDNA synthesis. The RNA was reverse transcribed using an oligo dT12 primer by incubation with 200 U RNase H- reverse transcriptase (Invitrogen, Barcelona, Spain) at 25°C for 10 min, then at 42°C for 90 min in the presence of 50 mM Tris-HCl, 75 mM KCl, 3 mM MgCl2, 10 mM DTT, 30 U RNase-inhibitor and 1mM dNTPs, in a total volume of 20 μl.

For the vulture TLR probe, a partial fragment of 567 bp showing sequence similarity to human TLR-1 was amplified by PCR from vulture PBMC cDNA using two oligonucleotide primers TLR1/2Fw (5′-GAT TTC TTC CAG AGC TG–3′) and TLR1/3Rv (5′-CAA AGA TGG ACT TGT AAC TCT TCT CAA TG -3′), which were designed based on regions of high homology among the sequences of human and mouse TLR1 (GenBank, accession numbers NM_003263 and NM_030682, respectively). Cycling conditions were 94°C for 30 s, 52°C for 30 s and 72°C for 1.5 min, for 30 cycles.

For the vulture IκBα probe, a partial fragment of 336 bp showing sequence similarity to human and chicken IκBα was amplified by PCR from vulture PBMC cDNA using two oligonucleotide primers IκBα-Fw (5′-CCT GAA CTT CCA GAA CAA C-3′) and IκBα-Rv (5′-GAT GTA AAT GCT CAG GAG CCA TG-3′), which were designed based on regions of high homology among the sequences of human and chicken IκBα (GenBank, accession numbers M69043 and S55765, respectively). Cycling conditions were 94°C for 30 s, 52°C for 30 s and 72°C for 1.5 min, for 30 cycles.

The obtained PCR products were cloned into pGEM-T easy vector using a TA cloning kit (Promega, Barcelona, Spain) and sequenced bidirectionally to confirm their respective specificities. These fragments were DIG-labelled following the recommendation of the manufacturer (Roche, Barcelona, Spain) and used as probes to screen 500 000 plaque colonies of the vulture-PBMC cDNA library.

3.2. cDNA library construction and screening

Total RNA (500 μg) was extracted from PBMC (pooled from 6 birds) using the Ultraspec isolation reagent (Biotecx). mRNA (20 μg) was extracted by Dynabeads (Dynal biotech-Invitrogen, Barcelona, Spain) and used in the construction of a cDNA library in Lambda ZAP vector (Stratagene, La Jolla, CA, USA) by directional cloning into EcoRI and XhoI sites. The cDNA library was plated by standard protocols at 50 000 plaque forming units (pfu) per plate and grown on a lawn of XL1-Blue E. coli for 6-8 h. Screening of the library was performed with DIG labelled probes. Plaques were transferred onto Hybond-N+ membranes

(Amersham, Barcelona, Spain) denatured in 1.5 M NaCl/0.5M NaOH, neutralised in 1.5 M NaCl/0.5 Tris (pH 8.0) and fixed using a cross-linker oven (Stratagene). The filters were then pre-incubated with hybridisation buffer (5XSSC [1XSSC is 150 mM NaCl, 15 mM trisodium citrate, pH 7.7], 0.1% N-laurylsarcosine, 0.02% SDS and 1% blocking reagent (Roche)) at 65 °C for 1 h and then hybridised with hybridisation buffer containing the DIG-labelled probe, overnight at 65 °C. The membranes were washed at high stringency (2XSSC, 0.1% SDS; 2x5 min at ambient temperature followed by 0.5XSSC, 0.1% SDS; 2x15 min at 65 °C). DiG-labelled probes were detected using phosphatase-labelled anti-digoxygenin antibodies (Roche) according to the manufacturer's instructions. Positive plaques on membranes were identified, isolated in agar plugs, eluted in 1 ml of SM buffer (0.1M NaCl, 10 mM MgSO4, 0.01% gelatin, 50 mM Tris-Hcl, pH 7.5) for 24 h at 4°C and replated. The above screening protocol was then repeated. Individual positive plaques from the secondary screening were isolated in agar plugs and eluted in SM buffer. The cDNA inserts were recovered using the Exassist/SOLR system (Stratagene). Individual bacterial colonies containing phagemid were grown up in LB broth (1% NaCl, 1% trytone, 0.5% yeast extract, pH 7.0) containing 50 µg/ml ampicillin. Phagemid DNA was purified using a Bio-Rad plasmid mini-prep kit and sequenced.

4. Structural analysis of vulture TLR1 and IκBα sequences

Sequences were analyzed using the analysis software LaserGene (DNAstar, London, UK) and the analysis tools provided at the expasy web site (http://www.expasy.org). PEST regions are sequences rich in Pro, Glu, Asp, Ser and Thr, which have been proposed to constitute protein instability determinants. The analysis of the PEST region for the putative protein was made using the webtool PESTfind at http://www.at.embnet.org/toolbox/pestfind. The potential phosphorylation sites were calculated using the NetPhos 2.0 prediction server at http://www.cbs.dtu.dk/services/NetPhos. The prediction of the potential attachment of small ubiquitin-related modifier (SUMO) was made using the webtool SUMOplot™.

The alignment of vulture TIR domain sequences with TLR-1 from other species and of the vulture IκBα sequences with IκBα from other species was done using the program ClustalW v1.83 with Blosum62 as the scoring matrix and gap opening penalty of 1.53. Griffon vulture TLR-1 and IκBα sequences were deposited in the Genbank under accession numbers DQ480086 and EU161944, respectively.

4.1. Vulture TLR1

The screening of the vulture PBMC cDNA library for TLR1 yielded seven clones with identical open reading frame (ORF) sequences. The fact that the screening of 500,000 vulture cDNA clones resulted in 7 identical sequences suggested that this TLR receptor is broadly represented in PBMC, possibly illustrating its important role in pathogen recognition during vulture innate immune response. This result was consistent with the real time RT-PCR analysis of TLR1 transcripts in vulture cells.

```
cccagttctcagaagcatgcttcacaaatacggatcatactatgtgacttacacgcttatc     61
aggcaaaagtctctgaagtttcccataaaggatattctgaagaaagtttgaaggtactca      121
taaataatttgactgaatgccaggatataggaaggagaaagaaaattaagcacatgtgga      181
agaattgtatccttctttcacctagtccctggatattgatgaaattttgtcctaagaaga      241
aataacgacttgaaggattagaacaaaggtggacagataagagaagtattgagcatctcc      301
aaggaaacagaaaccagtatgacagaaaatatgagatctctcagaaactttttctttac       361
                  M  T  E  N  M  R  S  L  R  N  F  F  L  Y        14
aagtgtctgtttgcattaacttttggaattgtgtcagcctgtctgtggaaaatgaactc       421
 K  C  L  F  A  L  T  F  W  N  C  V  S  L  S  V  E  N  E  L       34
ttcacatctgtttctaacgaagatggttctgacaaaaaaatcaagagcctgccactcctc      481
 F  T  S  V  S  N  E  D  G  S  D  K  K  I  K  S  L  P  L  L       54
tatacaaatagtcatcagtccaaagctaatttgactgggttgtgatacaaaatactaca       541
 Y  T  N  S  H  Q  S  K  A  N  F  D  W  V  V  I  Q  N  T  T       74
gaaagcctatcgttgtcagaaatcacaaatgacaatgtaaaaaaattagtagcattatta      601
 E  S  L  S  L  S  E  I  T  N  D  N  V  K  K  L  V  A  L  L       94
tctaatttcagacaaggctccaggttacaaaatctgacactgacaaatgtgtcagttgac      661
 S  N  F  R  Q  G  S  R  L  Q  N  L  T  L  T  N  V  S  V  D       114
tggaatgctcttattgaaacttttcagactgtatggcactcacccattgaatacttcagt      721
 W  N  A  L  I  E  T  F  Q  T  V  W  H  S  P  I  E  Y  F  S       134
gttaacggtgtaacacaattgtcggacatcgaaagctatgactttgactattcaggtacg      781
 V  N  G  V  T  Q  L  S  D  I  E  S  Y  D  F  D  Y  S  G  T       154
tctatgaaagcggtcacaatgaagaaagtttaatcacagatctgtacttctcacagaat       841
 S  M  K  A  V  T  M  K  K  V  L  I  T  D  L  Y  F  S  Q  N       174
gacctatacaaaatatttgcagacatgaatattgcagccttgacaatagctgaatcagag      901
 D  L  Y  K  I  F  A  D  M  N  I  A  A  L  T  I  A  E  S  E       194
atgatacatatgctgtgtccttcgtctgacagtccctttagatacttaaatttttaaag       961
 M  I  H  M  L  C  P  S  S  D  S  P  F  R  Y  L  N  F  L  K       214
aacgatttaacagatctgcttttcaaaaatgtgacaaattaattcaactggagacatta       1021
 N  D  L  T  D  L  L  F  Q  K  C  D  K  L  I  Q  L  E  T  L       234
atcttgccgaagaataaatttgagagcctttccaaggtaagcttcatgactagccgtatg      1081
 I  L  P  K  N  K  F  E  S  L  S  K  V  S  F  M  T  S  R  M       254
aaatcactgaaatacctggacatcagcagcaacttgctgagtcacgatggagctgatgtg      1141
 K  S  L  K  Y  L  D  I  S  S  N  L  L  S  H  D  G  A  D  V       274
caatgccaatgggctgagtctctgacagagttggacctgtcctcaaatcagttgacggat      1201
 Q  C  Q  W  A  E  S  L  T  E  L  D  L  S  S  N  Q  L  T  D       294
gccgtgtttgagtgcttgccagtcaacatcagaaaactcaacctccaaaacaatcacatc      1261
 A  V  F  E  C  L  P  V  N  I  R  K  L  N  L  Q  N  N  H  I       314
accagtgtccccaagggaatggctgagctgaaatccttgaaagagctgaacctggcatcg      1321
 T  S  V  P  K  G  M  A  E  L  K  S  L  K  E  L  N  L  A  S       334
aacaggctggctgacctgccggggtgcagtggctttacgtcgctggagttcctgaacgta      1381
 N  R  L  A  D  L  P  G  C  S  G  F  T  S  L  E  F  L  N  V       354
gagatgaattcgatcctcaccccatctgccgacttcttccagagctgcccacaggtcagg      1441
 E  M  N  S  I  L  T  P  S  A  D  F  F  Q  S  C  P  Q  V  R       374
gagctgcaagccgggcacaacccattcaagtgttcctgtgaactgcaagactttatccgt      1501
 E  L  Q  A  G  H  N  P  F  K  C  S  C  E  L  Q  D  F  I  R       394
ctggcgaggcagtctgggggaagctgtttggctggccagcggcgtatgtgtgcgagtac       1561
 L  A  R  Q  S  G  G  K  L  F  G  W  P  A  A  Y  V  C  E  Y       414
ccggaagacttgcaaggaacgcagctgaaggacttccacctgactgaactggcttgcaac      1621
 P  E  D  L  Q  G  T  Q  L  K  D  F  H  L  T  E  L  A  C  N       434
acggtgctcttgctggtgacagctctgctgctgacgctggtgctggtggctgtcgtggcc      1681
 T  V  L  L  L  V  T  A  L  L  L  T  L  V  L  V  A  V  V  A       454
tttctgtgcatctacttggatgtgccgtggtacgtgcggatgacgtggcagtggacgcag      1741
 F  L  C  I  Y  L  D  V  P  W  Y  V  R  M  T  W  Q  W  T  Q       474
acaaagcggagggcttggcacagccaccccgaagagcaggagaccattctgcagtttcac      1801
 T  K  R  R  A  W  H  S  H  P  E  E  Q  E  T  I  L  Q  F  H       494
gcgttcatttcctacagcgagcgcgattcgttgtgggtgaagaacgagctgatcccgaac      1861
 A  F  I  S  Y  S  E  R  D  S  L  W  V  K  N  E  L  I  P  N       514
ctggagaagggggagggctgtgtacaactgtgccagcacgagaggaactttatccccggc      1921
 L  E  K  G  E  G  C  V  Q  L  C  Q  H  E  R  N  F  I  P  G       534
aagagcattgtggagaacatcattaactgcattgagaagagctacaggtcgatctttgtg      1981
 K  S  I  V  E  N  I  I  N  C  I  E  K  S  Y  R  S  I  F  V       554
ttgtctcccaactttgtgcagagcgagtggtgtcactatgagctgtactttgcccatcac      2041
 L  S  P  N  F  V  Q  S  E  W  C  H  Y  E  L  Y  F  A  H  H       574
aaattattcagtgagaattccaacagcttaatcctcattttactggagccgatccctccg      2101
 K  L  F  S  E  N  S  N  S  L  I  L  I  L  L  E  P  I  P  P       594
tacattatccctgccaggtatcacaagctgaaggctctcatggcaaagcgaacctacctg      2161
 Y  I  I  P  A  R  Y  H  K  L  K  A  L  M  A  K  R  T  Y  L       614
gagtggccaaaggagaggagcaagcatcccctttttctgggctaacctgagggcagctatt      2221
 E  W  P  K  E  R  S  K  H  P  L  F  W  A  N  L  R  A  A  I       634
agcattaacctgctaatggctgatggaaagaggtgtggggaaacagattaagaatctttc      2281
 S  I  N  L  L  M  A  D  G  K  R  C  G  E  T  D  *                650
taatggagtttcttccatttttttcttggtgaagcaataaatgctttatgatttccaaaaa     2341
aaaaaaaaaaaaaa
```

Figure 2. Nucleotide and deduced amino acid sequence of vulture TLR1. Complete sequence of the full-length Vulture TLR obtained from the cDNA library (GenBank accession number: DQ480086). Translated amino acid sequence is also shown under nucleotide sequence. Numbers to the right of each row refer to nucleotide or amino acid position. The cleavage site for the putative signal peptide is indicated by an arrow. LRRs domains are shaded. Potential N-glycosylation sites are circled. The predicted transmembrane segment is underlined. The initiation codon (atg) and the polyadenilation site are underlined. The translational stop site is indicated by an asterisk. The cysteines critical for the maintenance of the structure of LRR-CT are in bold.

The largest clone (2,355 bp) contained an ORF that encoded a 650 amino acid putative vulture orthologue to TLR1, flanked by 319 bp 5'UTR and a 83 bp 3'UTR that contained a potential polyadenylation signal, AATAAA, 21 bp upstream of the poly (A) tail (Fig. 2). The predicted molecular weight of the putative vulture TLR1 was of 74.6 KDa. The predicted protein sequence had a signal peptide, an extracellular portion, a short transmembrane region and a cytoplasmic segment (Fig. 2). In assigning names to the vulture TLR, we looked at the closest orthologue in chicken and followed the nomenclature that was proposed for this species (Yilmaz et al., 2005). Therefore, the discovered sequence was identified as vulture TLR1.

4.1.1. *Amino acid sequence comparison of vulture TLR1 with other species*

The comparison of the deduced amino acid sequence of vulture TLR1 with the sequence of chicken, pig, cattle, human and mouse TLR1 indicated that the deduced protein had a higher degree of similarity to chicken (64% of amino acid similarity) than to pig (51%), cattle (51%), human (51%) and mouse (48%) sequences (Fig. 3). Protein sequence similarity was different on different TLR domains (Fig. 3).

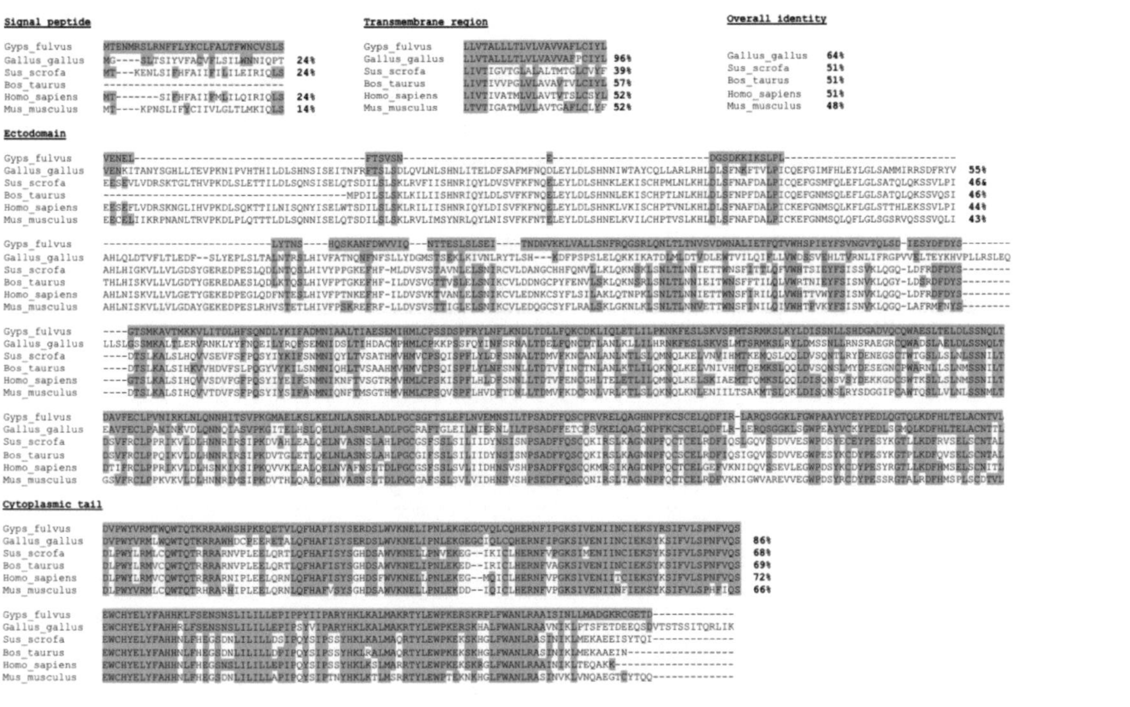

Figure 3. Alignment of amino acid sequences of TLR1 from different species.

Amino acid sequence of vulture TLR1 was aligned with the orthologous sequence of chicken (*Gallus gallus*), pig (*Sus scrofa*), cattle (*Bos taurus*), human (*Homo sapiens*) and mouse (*Mus musculus*) based on amino acid identity and structural similarity. Identical amino acid residues to vulture TLR1 from the aligned sequences are shaded. Gaps were introduced for optimal alignment of the sequences and are indicated by dashes (-). GenBank or Swiss protein accession numbers are: DQ480086, Q5WA51, Q59HI9, Q706D2, Q5FWG5 and Q6A0E8, respectively.

For the TLRs, it is assumed that the structure of the ectodomain has evolved more quickly than the structure of the TIR (Johnson et al., 2003). Similarly to other TLR receptors, the degree of homology of vulture TLR1 was higher in the transmembrane and cytoplasmic domains than in the extracellular domain.

The vulture TLR1 with 650 amino acids is probably the TLR with the shortest length and the smallest predicted MW (74.6 kDa). Recently, a chicken isoform of TLR1 (Ch-TLR1 type 2) was identified *in silico* and predicted to have a similar number of residues than vulture TLR1 (Yilmaz et al., 2005). However, this receptor also contains an additional transmembrane region in its N-terminal end, and the pattern of expression in tissues is also different from that ChTLR1 type 1 (Yilmaz et al., 2005).

Comparison of the structure obtained from the SMART analysis (at expasy web server) of the amino acid sequence from human, bovine, pig, mouse, chicken and vulture TLR1. Each diagram shows a typical structure of a member of the toll-like receptor family. Vulture TLR1 consists of an ectodomain containing five leucine rich repeats (LRRs) followed by an additional leucine rich repeat C terminal (LRR-CT) motif. The Vulture TLR has a transmembrane segment and a cytoplasmic tail which contains the TIR domain. Genbank or swiss accession number for proteins are DQ480086 (vulture), Q5WA51 (chicken), Q59HI9 (pig), Q706D2 (bovine), Q5FWG5 (human) and Q6A0E8 (mouse).

Structural feature	***G fulvus***	***G gallus***	***S scrofa***	***B taurus***	***H sapiens***	***M musculus***
Amino acid residues	650	818	796	727	786	795
Number of LRRs	5	5	5	5	4	6
N-glycosylation sites	3	5	4	6	7	8
Predicted MW(KDa)	74.60	94.46	90.94	83.04	90.29	90.67
Length of ectodomain	409	569	560	521	560	558

Table 2. Structural features of TLR1 receptor from Griffon vulture (*G. fulvus*), Chicken (*G. gallus*), pig (*S. scrofa*), cattle (*B. taurus*) human (*H. sapiens*) and mouse (*M. musculus*) amino acid sequences. The theoretical molecular weight, number of LRRs, and of glycosilation sites was calculated using the software available at the expasy web server (http://www.expasy.org). Genbank or Swiss accession number for proteins are DQ480086 (*G. fulvus*), Q5WA51 (*G. gallus*), Q59HI9 (*S. scrofa*), Q706D2 (*B. taurus*), Q5FWG5 (*H. sapiens*) and Q6A0E8 (*M. musculus*).

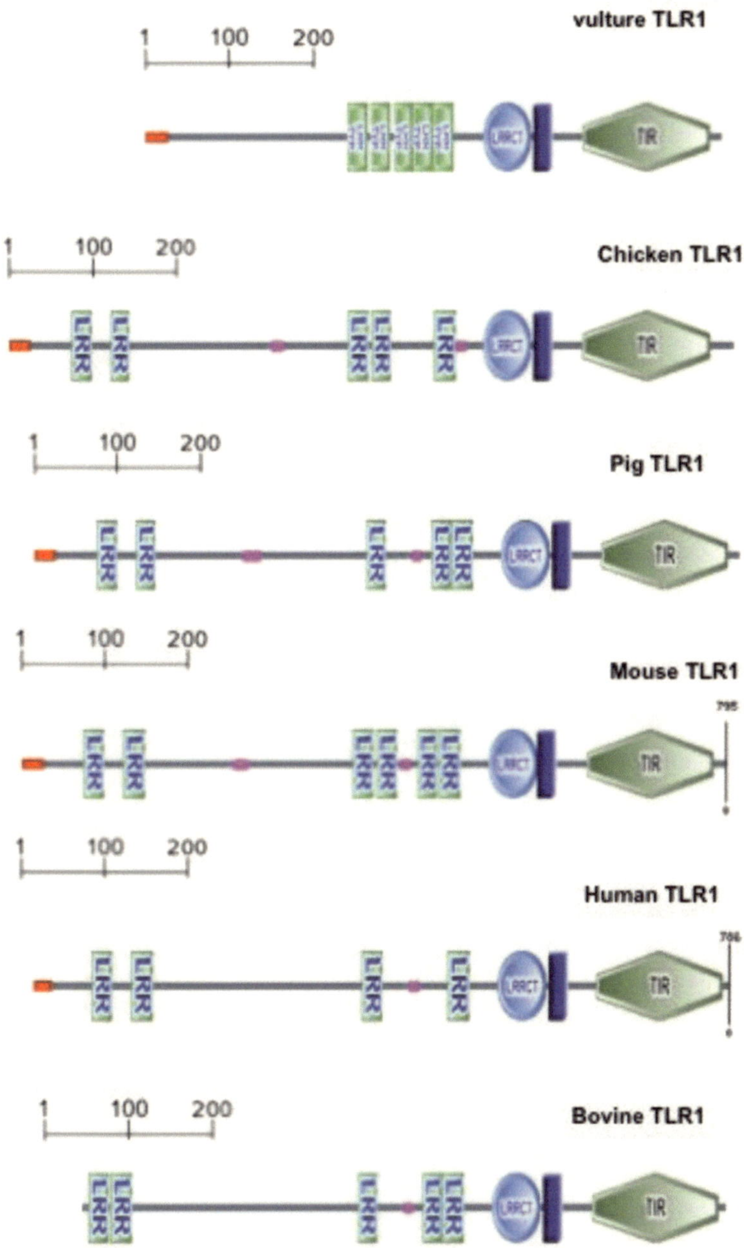

Figure 4. Schematic structure of TLR1 from various species

In general, the structure of vulture TLR1 shows similarity to chicken and mammalian TLR1 (Table 2). However, vulture TLR1 exhibits some structural features that could influence its functional role as pathogen receptor (Fig. 4). For example, it is possible that the smaller size of vulture TLR1, the lower number of N-glycosylation sites and the grouping of its LRRs in the proximal half of its ectodomain have functional implications.

The set of Toll proteins for humans and insects each contain widely divergent LRR regions, and this is viewed as providing the potential to discriminate between different ligands. Perhaps these features provide vulture TLR1 some advantages on pathogen recognition. TLR glycosylation is also likely to influence receptor surface representation, trafficking and pattern recognition (Weber et al., 2004).

4.2. Vulture IκBα

The screening of the vulture PBMC cDNA library yielded one clone that contained an ORF that encoded a 313 amino acid putative vulture orthologue to IκBα, flanked by 15 bp 5'UTR and a 596 bp 3'UTR (Fig. 5).

```
cggagccctgccgctatgatcagcgcccgccgcctcgtcgagccgccggttatggagggc   60
 M  I  S  A  R  R  L  V  E  P  P  V  M  E  G   15
tacgagcaagcgaagaaagagcgccagggcggcttcccgctcgacgaccgccacgacagc   120
 Y  E  Q  A  K  K  E  R  Q  G  G  F  P  L  D  D  R  H  D  S    35
ggcttggactccatgaaggaggaagagtaccggcagctggtgaaggagctggaggacata   180
 G  L  D  S  M  K  E  E E  Y  R  Q  L  V  K  E  L  E  D  I   55
cgcctgcagccccgcgagccgcccgcctgggcgcagcagctgacggaggacggagacact   240
 R  L  Q  P  R  E  P  P  A  W  A  Q  Q  L  T  E  D  G  D  T    75
tttctccacttggcgattattcacgaggaaaaagccctgagcctggaggtgatccggcag   300
 F  L  H  L  A  I  I  H  E  E  K  A  L  S  L  E  V  I  R  Q    95
gcggccggggaccgtgctttcctgaacttccagaacaacctcagccagactcctcttcac   360
 A  A  G  D  R  A  F  L  N  F  Q  N  N L  S  Q  T  P  L  H   115
ctggcagtgatcaccgatcagcctgaaattgccgagcatcttctgaaggccggatgcgac   420
 L  A  V  I  T  D  Q  P  E  I  A  E  H  L  L  K  A  G  C  D    135
ctggaactcagggacttccgaggaaacacccccctgcatattgcctgccagcagggctcc   480
 L  E  L  R  D  F  R  G  N  T  P  L  H  I  A  C  Q  Q  G  S    155
ctcaggagcgtcagcgtcctcacgcagtactgccagccgcaccacctcctcgctgtcctg   540
 L  R  S  V  S  V  L  T  Q  Y  C  Q  P  H  H  L L  A  V  L   175
caggcaaccaactacaacgggcatacatgtctccatttggcatctattcaaggatacctg   600
 Q  A  T  N  Y  N  G  H  T  C  L  H  L  A  S  I  Q  G  Y  L    195
cctattgtcgaatacttgctgtccttgggagcagatgtaaatgctcaggagccatgcaat   660
 A  I  V  E  Y  L  L  S  L  G  A  D  V  N  A  Q  E  P  C  N    215
ggcagaacggcactacatttggctgtcgacctgcagaattcagacctggtgtcgcttctg   720
 G  R  T  A  L  H  L  A  V  D  L  Q  N  S  D  L  V  S  L  L    235
gtgaaacatggggcggacgtgaacaaagtgacctaccaaggctattcccccctatcagctc   780
 V  K  H  G  A  D  V  N  K  V  T  Y  Q  G  Y  S  P  Y  Q  L    255
acatggggaagagacaactccagcatacaggaacagctgaagcagctgaccacagccgac   840
 T  W  G  R  D  N  S  S  I  Q  E  Q  L  K  Q  L  T  T  A  D    275
ctgcagatgttgccagaaagtgaggacgaggagagcagtgaatcggagcctgaattcaca   900
 L  Q  M  L  P  E  S  E  D  E  E  S  S  E  S  E  P  E  F  T    295
gaggatgaacttatatacgatgactgccttattggaggacgacagctggcatttaaagc   960
 E  D  E  L  I  Y  D  D  C  L  I  G  G  R  Q  L  A  F  *       313
agagctatctgtgaaaagaagtgactgtgtacatatgtatagaaaaaggactgacttcat   1020
ttaaaaagaaagtcgcaatgcaaagggaaaaaccaggagggaaatactacactgcccagc   1080
aaggagcacataattgtaacaggttctggcctgtgtttaaatacaggagtgggatgtgta   1140
acatcagtagggatctgtgattattcacaccacctgataaagagccacatagccaatctt   1200
ctcagccctacaaaggtaacagactacacatccaacctgctggttacagagagctatctt   1260
gtggtgttaagtaccacgaggaatgcgtgtcgcctcgtggcaaggcaggctcataccaac   1320
ccccccatcttctcggagactgcgtgttaatctgcgttgggctggtggtgctccctggcc   1380
ttactgaccggcctcagctgctcttggtggggtgtcccaggtggaggagtcaaaccaagg   1440
gactggtgacctcctgactgttagaagaaagtagcaataatgttaactgtgggcattgga   1500
aactgtgtgtttcacaccatgtgtgtcataattgctacacttttagcaattg            1553
```

Figure 5. Nucleotide and deduced amino acid sequence of vulture IκBα. Complete sequence of the full-length vulture IκBα obtained from the cDNA library (GenBank accession number: EU161944). Translated amino acid sequence is also shown under nucleotide sequence. Numbers to the right of each row refer to nucleotide or amino acid position. Ankyrin domains are shaded. The PEST region is underlined. The ATTTA domain is in bold. Phosphorylation sites Ser-35 and Ser-39 are circled. The translational stop site is indicated by an asterisk.

http://dx.doi.org/10.5772/54191

The predicted molecular weight of the putative vulture IκBα was of 35170 Da. Structurally, the vulture I kappa B alpha molecule could be divided into three sections: a 70-amino-acid N terminus with no known function, a 205-residue midsection composed of five ankyrin-like repeats, and a very acidic 42-amino-acid C terminus that resembles a PEST sequence. Examination of the Griffon vulture sequence revealed the features characteristic of an IκB molecule (Fig. 6) The putative vulture IκBα protein was composed of a N-terminal regulatory domain, a central ankyrin repeat domain (ARD), required for its interaction with NF-κB, and a putative PEST-like sequence in the C-terminus (Fig. 6), which is similar to IκBα proteins from other organisms (Jaffray et al., 1995). Together with the N-terminal regulatory domain and the central ARD domain, the presence of an acidic C-terminal PEST region rich in the amino acids proline (P), glutamic acid (E), serine (S) and threonine (T) is characteristic of IκBα inhibitors (Luque & Gelinas, 1998). PEST regions have been found in the C-terminus of avian IκBα (Krishnan et al., 1995) and mammalian IκBα and it was also present in the vulture IκBα sequence (Fig. 6). Particularly, the PEST sequence of IκBα seems to be critical for its calpain-dependent degradation (Shumway et al., 1999).

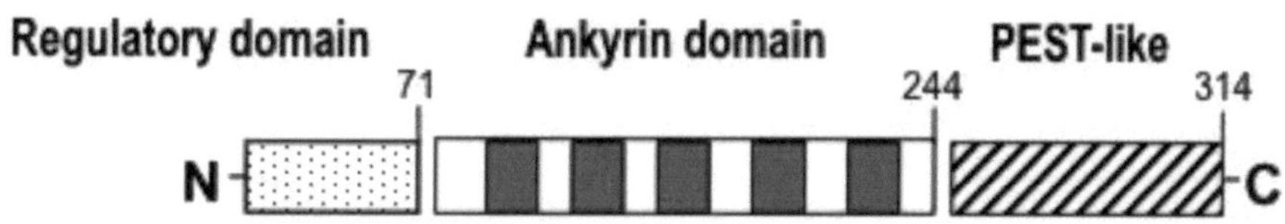

Figure 6. Schematic structure of vulture IκBα.

Structure obtained from the SMART analysis (at expasy web server) of the amino acid sequence from vulture IκBα. Each box shows a typical structure of a member of the IκBα inhibitor. Vulture IκBα consists of an N-terminus regulatory domain, a central ankyrin domain containing five ankyrin repeats followed by an additional PEST-like motif. Number shows the amino acid flanking the relevant domains.

Classical activation of NF-kappaB involves phosphorylation, polyubiquitination and subsequent degradation of IκB (Figure. Several residues are known to be important in the N-terminal regulatory domain (Luque & Gelinas, 1998, Luque et al., 2000). In nonstimulated cells, NF-kappa B dimers are maintained in the cytoplasm through interaction with inhibitory proteins, the IκBs (Fig. 7).

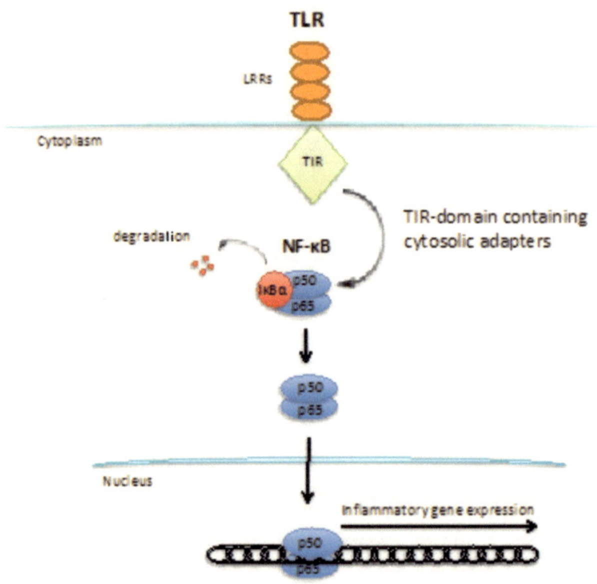

Figure 7. Activation of the NFκB pathway by TLRs. Ligand binding of TLR results in direct or indirect recruitment of a series of TIR-domain containing adapters, which in turn phosphorylates IκBs, causing degradation of the inhibitor and translocation of the transcription factor to the nucleus, where it initiates the transcription of genes encoding chemokines and pro-inflammatory cytokines.

In response to cell stimulation, mainly by proinflammatory cytokines, a multisubunit protein kinase, the I kappa B kinase (IKK), is rapidly activated and phosphorylates two critical serines in the N-terminal regulatory domain of the I kappa Bs. Phosphorylated IκBs are recognized by a specific E3 ubiquitin ligase complex on neighboring lysine residues, which targets them for rapid degradation by the 26S proteasome, which frees NFκ-B and leads to its translocation to the nucleus, where it regulates gene transcription (Karin & Ben-Neriah, 2000). It has been demonstrated that phosphorylation of the N-terminus residues Ser-32 and Ser-36 is the signal that leads to inducer-mediated degradation of IκBα in mammals (Brown et al., 1997; Good et al., 1996).

As can be observed in the alignment of Figure 8, the griffon vulture equivalent residues seem to be Ser-35 and Ser-39, which are part of the conserved sequence DSGLDS (Luque et al., 2000; Pons et al., 2007). This observation suggests that the phosphorylation of these serine residues could trigger the IκBα inducer-mediated degradation in vulture in a similar manner to that in mammals. Unlike ubiquitin modification, which requires phosphorylation of S32 and S36, the small ubiquitin-like modifier (SUMO) modification of IκBα is inhibited by phosphorylation. Thus, while ubiquitination targets proteins for rapid degradation, SUMO modification acts antagonistically to generate proteins resistant to degradation (Desterro et al., 1998; Mabb & Miyamoto, 2007). This SUMO modification occurs primarily on K21 (Mabb & Miyamoto, 2007). This residue was also conserved in the IκBα sequence from human, mouse, pig, rat and vulture, but not from chicken (Fig. 8).

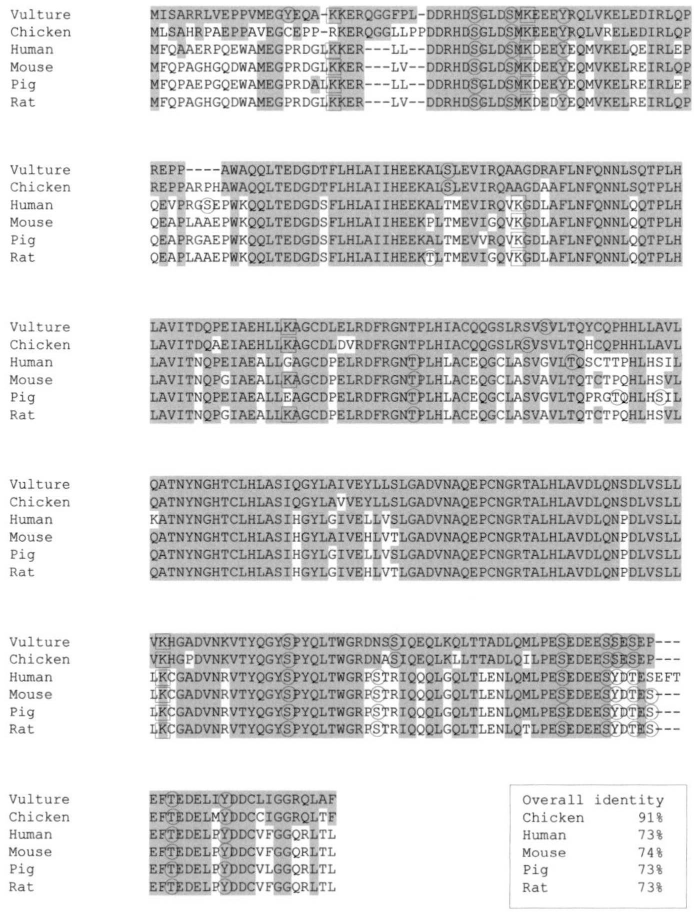

Figure 8. Alignment of amino acid sequences of IκBα from different species.

Amino acid sequence of vulture IκBα was aligned with the orthologous sequence of chicken (*Gallus gallus*), pig (*Sus scrofa*), cattle (*Bos taurus*), human (*Homo sapiens*) and mouse (*Mus musculus*) based on amino acid identity and structural similarity. Identical amino acid residues to vulture IκBα from the aligned sequences are shaded. Gaps were introduced for optimal alignment of the sequences and are indicated by dashes (-). SUMOlation sites are squared and phosphorylation sites are circled. GenBank or Swiss protein accession numbers are: DQ480086, Q5WA51, Q59HI9, Q706D2, Q5FWG5 and Q6A0E8, respectively. Griffon vulture IκBα sequence was deposited in the Genbank under accession number EU161944.

A common characteristic of the IκB proteins is the presence of ankyrin repeats, which interact with the Rel-homology domain of NF-κB (Aoki et al., 1996; Luque & Gelinas, 1998). In the vulture sequence, five ankyrin repeats were detected using the Simple Modular Architecture Research Tool (SMART) at EMBL (Table 2). Five ankyrin repeats also exist in human and other vertebrates IκBα (Jaffray et al., 1995). It is possible that individual repeats have remained conserved because of their important structural and functional roles in regulating NF-κB.

Compared with other species, vulture IκBα exhibited the lowest number of predicted SUMOlation sites (Table 3).

Structural feature	*G fulvus*	*G gallus*	*H sapiens*	*S scrofa*	*R norvegicus*	*M musculus*
Amino acid residues	313	318	317	314	314	314
Number of ankyrin repeats	5	5	5	5	5	5
Phosphorylation sites	14	13	14	15	14	13
Predicted MW(KDa)	35,17	35,40	35,61	35,23	35,02	35,02
SUMOlation sites	2	3	4	4	5	5

Table 3. Structural features of IκBα from Griffon vulture (*G. fulvus*), Chicken (*G. gallus*), human (*H. sapiens*), pig (*S. scrofa*), rat (*R. norvegicus*) and mouse (*M. musculus*) amino acid sequences. The theoretical molecular weight, number of ankyrin repeats, SUMOlation and of phosphorylation sites was calculated using the software available at the expasy web server (http://www.expasy.org). Genbank or Swiss accession number for proteins are EU161944 (*G. fulvus*), Q91974 (*G. gallus*), P25963 (*H. sapiens*), Q08353 (*S. scrofa*), Q63746 (*R. norvegicus*), and Q9Z1E3 (*M. musculus*).

4.2.1. Amino acid sequence comparison of vulture IκBα with other species

The comparison of the deduced amino acid sequence of vulture IκBα with the sequence of chicken, human, mouse, pig, and rat IκBα indicated that the deduced protein had a higher degree of similarity to chicken (91% of amino acid similarity) than to human (73%), mouse (74%), pig (73%) and rat (73%) sequences (Fig. 7). The analysis of the vulture IκBα sequence using the software NetPhos 2.0 (cita) revealed 14 potential phosphorylation sites: 10 Ser (S35, S39, S89, S160, S251, S263, S282, S287, S288, and S290), 1 Thr (T295) and 3 Tyr (Y16, Y45, and Y301). Although many of these residues were conserved in the aligned sequences from chicken, human, mouse, pig and rat IκBα, two phosphorylation sites (Y16 and S160) were distinctive to the vulture sequence (Fig.8).

5. Detection of vulture TLR1 and IκBα expression in tissues

In order to better understand the biological roles of TLR1 and IκBα, we analyzed their tissue expression pattern. The presence of transcripts encoding vulture TLR1 and IκBα in tissues was determined by real time RT-PCR. Biological samples were collected from vultures (about 8-10 months old) that were provisionally captive at the Centre for Wild Life Protection, "El Chaparrillo", Ciudad Real, Spain. Blood was obtained by puncture of the branquial vein, located in the internal face of the wing, and collected in 10 ml tubes with EDTA as anticoagulant. Blood (10 ml) was diluted 1:1 (vol:vol) with PBS (Sigma) and the mononuclear fraction containing PBMC was obtained by density gradient centrifugation on Lymphoprep (Axis-Shield, Oslo, Norway). All vulture tissues used for cDNA preparation were obtained fresh from euthanised birds that were impossible to recover.

http://dx.doi.org/10.5772/54191

RT-PCR was performed on a SmartCycler® II thermal cycler (Cepheid, Sunnyvale, CA, USA) using the QuantiTect® SYBR® Green RT-PCR Kit (Quiagen, Valencia, CA, USA), following the recommendations of the manufacturer. We used primers GfTLR-Fw (5′-GCT TGC CAG TCA ACA TCA GA-3′) and GfTLR-Rv (5′-GAA CTC CAG CGA CGT AAA GC-3′), which amplify a fragment of 158 bp of vulture TLR1 and primers IκBα -L (5′- CTG CAG GCA ACC AAC TAC AA -3′) and IκBα –R (5′- TGA ATT CTG CAG GTC GAC AG-3′), which amplify a fragment of 165 b of vulture IκBα. Cycling conditions were: 94°C for 30 sec, 60°C for 30 sec, 72°C for 1 min, for 40 cycles. As an internal control, RT-PCR was performed on the same RNAs using the primers BA-Fw (5′-CTA TCC AGG CTG TGC TGT CC-3′) and BA-Rv (5′-TGA GGT AGT CTG TCA GGT CAG G-3′), which amplify a fragment of 165 bp from the conserved housekeeping gene beta-actin. Control reactions were done using the same procedures, but without RT to control for DNA contamination in the RNA preparations, and without RNA added to control contamination of the PCR reaction. Amplification efficiencies were validated and normalized against vulture beta actin, (GenBank accession number DQ507221) using the comparative Ct method. Experiments were repeated for at least three times with similar results. Tissues used for the study were artery, liver, lung, bursa cloacalis, heart, small intestine, peripheral blood mononuclear cells (PBMC), large intestine and kidney.

The level of TLR1 mRNA was higher in kidney, small intestine and PBMC (Fig. 9).

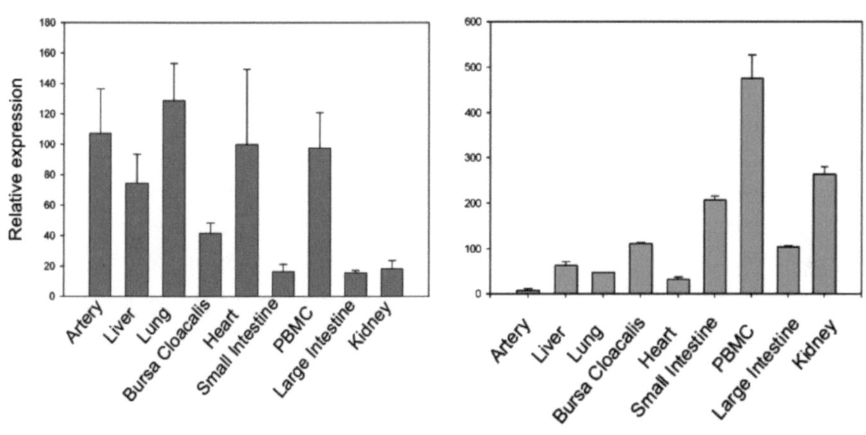

Figure 9. Relative expression of TLR1 and IκBα mRNA transcripts in vulture cells and tissues.

Real time RT-PCR was used to examine the relative amount of TLR1 (right) and IκBα (left) transcripts in vulture cells and tissues. The data were normalised using the beta-actin gene and calculated by the delta Ct method.

Moderate vulture TLR1 mRNA levels were observed in Bursa cloacalis and large intestine, whereas the lowest TLR1 mRNA levels were found in liver, heart and artery (Fig. 9). It has been reported that the patterns of TLR tissue expression are variable, even among closely related species (Zarember & Godowski 2002). Likewise, the intensity and the anatomic location of the innate immune response may vary considerably among species (Rehli, 2002). Consistent with its role in pathogen recognition and host defense, the tissue and cell expression pattern of vulture TLR1, as revealed by real time RT-PCR, correlated with vulture ability to respond to various pathogenic challenges. The expression of vulture TLR1 was higher in cells such as circulating PBMC and intestinal epithelial cells that are immediately accessible to microorganisms upon infection.

The analysis of the relative expression of IκBα mRNA transcripts, using real-time RT-PCR, demonstrated that vulture IκBα mRNAs were higher in lung, artery, heart, and in PBMC cells (Fig. 9), which was consistent with its role in numerous physiological processes. Interestingly, the expression of vulture IκBα mRNA was observed in tissues at which the lowest expression of vulture Toll-like receptor was found. This is consistent with the role of IκBα as inhibitor of the TLR-signalling pathway.

6. Analysis of the evolutionary relationship of vulture TLR and IκBα

The dendrogram of sequences was calculated based on the distance matrix that was generated from the pairwise scores and the phylogenetic trees were constructed based on the multiple alignment of the sequences using the PHYLIP (Phylogeny Inference Package) available at the expasy.org web page. All ClustalW phylogenetic calculations were based around the neighbor-joining method of Saitou and Nei (Saitou & Nei, 1987).

For the analysis of the evolutionary relationship of vulture and other vertebrate TLR and IκBα, a phylogenetic tree was constructed with the TIR-domain sequences of human, macaque, bovine, pig, mouse, Japanese pufferfish and chicken TLR1. GenBank or swiss protein accessions numbers Q5WA51, Q706D2, Q6A0E8, Q59HI9, Q5H727 and Q5FWG5, respectively. The phylogenetic analysis of the TIR domain of vulture TLR1 revealed separate clustering of TLR1 from birds, fish, mouse and other mammals (Fig. 10B)

For the TLRs, it is assumed that the structure of the ectodomain has evolved more quickly than the structure of the TIR (Johnson, 2003). Similarly to other TLR receptors, the degree of homology of vulture TLR1 was higher in the transmembrane and cytoplasmic domains than in the extracellular domain. As expected, phylogenetic analysis of the TIR domains revealed separate clustering of TLR1 from birds, fish and mammals (Fig. 9B), suggesting independent evolution of the Toll family of proteins and of innate immunity (Beutler & Rehli, 2002; Roach et al., 2005).

The unrooted trees were constructed by neighbor-joining analysis of an alignment of the ankirin repeats of IκBα sequences from vulture and other species (A) or the alignment of the TIR domains of TLR1 from vulture and other species (B). The branch lengths are proportional to the number of amino acid differences. GenBank or swiss protein accessions numbers of chicken (*Gallus gallus*), human (*Homo sapiens*), mouse (*Mus musculus*), rat (*Rattus norvegicus*), African frog (*Xenopus laevis*), cattle (*Bos taurus*), zebrafish (*Danio rerio*), Mongolian gerbil (*Meriones unguiculatus*), Rainbow trout (*Oncorhynchus mykiss*) and pig (*Sus scrofa*) sequences

http://dx.doi.org/10.5772/54191

used for the phylogenetic tree were Q91974, P25963, Q08353, Q63746, Q1ET75, Q6DCW3, Q8WNW7, Q6K196, Q1ET75, Q8QFQ0 and Q9Z1E3, respectively.

For the analysis of the evolutionary relationship of vulture and other vertebrate IκBα, a phylogenetic tree was constructed with the sequences of chicken, human, mouse, rat, African frog, cattle, zebrafish, Mongolian gerbil, Rainbow trout and pig IκBα. The phylogenetic analysis of the ankyrin domain of vulture IκBα revealed separate clustering of IκBα from rodents, fish and other species and the sequence of vulture IκBα clustered together with that of chicken IκBα (Fig 10A). The IκB family includes IκBα, IκBβ, IκBγ, IκBε, IκBζ, Bcl-3, the precursors of NFκB1 (p105), and NF-κB2 (p100), and the Drosophila protein Cactus (Hayden et al., 2006; Karin & Ben-Neriah, 2000; Totzke et al., 2006; Gilmore, 2006). Why multiple IκB proteins now exist in vertebrates has been a subject of great interest, and much effort has been expended on establishing the roles of individual members of this protein family in the regulation of NF-κB. The recent identification of a novel member of IκB family (IκBζ) indicates that there might exist species-specific differences in the regulation of NF-κB (Totzke et al., 2006).

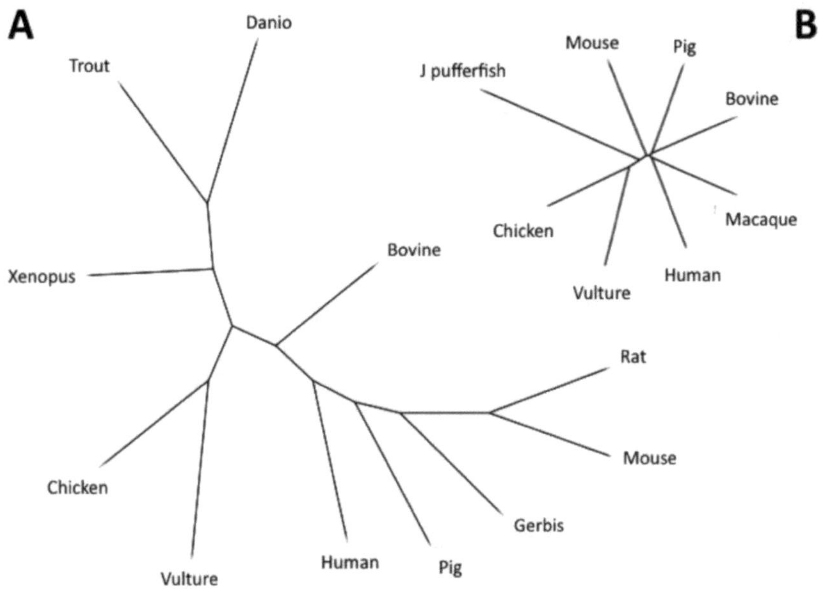

Figure 10. Phylogenetic trees illustrating the relationship between TLR and IκBα sequences from vulture and other species.

Evolutionarily, the IκB protein family is quite old, as members have been found in insects, birds and mammals (Ghosh & Kopp, 1998). However, the finding that individual ankyrin repeats within each IκB molecule are more similar to corresponding ankyrin repeats in other IκB family members, rather than to other ankyrin repeats within the same IκB, suggests that all IκB family members evolved from an ancestral IκB molecule (Huguet, et al., 1997).

Consistent with the hypothesis that all these factors evolved from a common ancestral RHD-ankyrin structure within a unique superfamily, explaining the specificities of interaction between the different Rel/NF-kappa B dimers and the various I kappa B inhibitors (Huguet, et al., 1997).

Recently, the presence of two IkappaB-like genes in Nematostella encoded by loci distinct from nf-kb suggested that a gene fusion event created the nfkb genes in insects and vertebrates (Sullivan et al., 2007). This is consistent with the hypothesis that interactions between transcription factors of the Rel members and members of the IκB gene family evolved to regulate genes mainly involved in immune inflammatory responses (Bonizzi & Karin, 2004).

NF-kappaB represents an ancient, generalized signaling system that has been co-opted for immune system roles independently in vertebrate and insect lineages (Friedman & Hughes, 2002). Therefore, while these proteins share a basic three-dimensional structure as predicted by their shared ankyrin repeat pattern and sequence, a possible evolutionary scenario based on this phylogenetic tree could be that subtle differences in the amino acid substitutions in the ankyrin repeats and flanking sequences occurred throughout evolution, which contributed to their specificity of interaction with various members of the Rel family.

7. Summary

The ORFs reported herein identified and characterized the vulture orthologues to TLR1 (CD281) and to IκBα, the first NF-κB pathway element from the griffon vulture *G. fulvus*. In addition, we have also identified sequences that may be involved in the protection of vultures against toxins. These results have implications for the understanding of the evolution of pathogen-host interactions. Particularly, these studies help to highlight a potentially important regulatory pathway for the study of the related functions in vulture immune system (Perez de la Lastra & de la Fuente, 2007; 2008). Despite the overall structure of vulture TLR1 and expression pattern was similar to that of chicken, pig, cattle, human and mouse TLR, vulture TLR1 had differences in the length of the ectodomain, number and position of LRRs and N-glycosylation sites that makes vulture TLR1 structurally unique with possible functional implications.

Strong selective pressure for recognition of and response to pathogen-associated molecular patterns (PAMPs) has probably maintained a largely unchanged TLR signalling pathways in all vertebrates. The IκBα gene reported here expands our understanding of the immune regulatory pathways present in carrion birds that are in permanent contact with pathogens. Current investigations should focus on the cloning and characterization of other members of NF-κB signalling cascade and genes controlled by this signalling pathway. At this point it is difficult to understand the implications of the structural differences between vulture TLR1, chicken TLR1 and TLR1 in different mammalian species. A greater understanding of the functional capacity of non-mammalian TLRs and, particularly in carrion birds that are in permanent contact with pathogens, has implications for the understanding of the evolutionary pressures that defined the TLR repertoires in present day animals. The discovery of molecules that neutralize toxins found in the genetic and phenotypic background of an organism (like vulture) is extremely adequate for bio compatible drugs and antidote development.

8. Biotechnological applications of molecules involved in the recognition of pathogens

Our growing understanding of host-pathogen interactions and mechanisms of protective immunity have allowed for an increasingly rational approach to the design of immune based therapeutics. One posible biomedical application of the discovery of efficient pathogen receptors could be the generation of "immunoadhesins" (Perez de la Lastra et al., 2009). Because of the versatility of immunoadhesins, immunoadhesin-based therapies could, in theory, be developed against any existing pathogen. Some advantages of immunoadhesin-based therapies include versatility, low toxicity, pathogen specificity, enhancement of immune function, and favorable pharmacokinetics; the disadvantages include high cost, limited usefulness against mixed infections and the need for early and precise microbiologic diagnosis.

The patent by Visintin *et al.* (cited in Perez de la Lastra et al., 2009) discloses anti-pathogen immunoadhesins (APIs), a subset of which is "tollbodies", which have a pathogen recognition module derived from the binding domain of a toll-like receptor (TLR). A schematic illustration of an exemplary API is shown in Fig. 11.

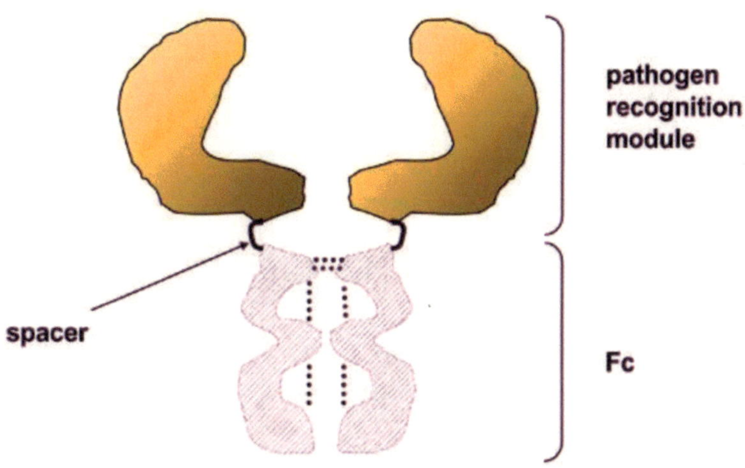

Figure 11. Schematic structure of an anti-pathogen immunoadhesin (API). Gray undashed area, pathogen recognition module; dashed, Fc portion. Disulfide bridges are represented by dashed line, which include intrachain bridges (that stabilize the Ig domains) and the interchain bridges (that covalently link two immunoadhesin molecules).

APIs can be used as therapeutics, e.g., for treating pathogen-associated disorders, e.g., infections and inflammatory conditions (e.g. inflammatory conditions associated with a pathogen- associated infection) and other disorders in which it is desirable to inhibit signaling pathways associated with the pathogen recognition protein from which the extracellular domain of the API is derived. These APIs are particularly useful therapeutics because pathogens generally cannot mutate the PAMPs (e.g., LPS) that are recognized by the pathogen recognition proteins. Thus, APIs can be used as antipathogenic agents to whom the targeted pathogen cannot develop resistance. The APIs can thus be used both *in vivo* and *in vitro/ex vivo*, e.g. to remove pathogens from blood or a water supply, or other liquids to be consumed, e.g., beverages, or even in the air, e.g. to combat a weapon of biological warfare. It is envisaged that these immunotechnological advances will increase the available antiinfective armamentarium and that immunoadhesin-therapy is poised to play an important part in modern anti-infective drugs.

Acknowledgements

This work was supported by the Junta de Comunidades de Castilla-La Mancha (JCCM), project PII1I09-0243-4350.

Author details

Lourdes Mateos-Hernández[1], Elena Crespo[1], José de la Fuente[1,2] and José M. Pérez de la Lastra[1]

1 Instituto de Investigación en Recursos Cinegéticos (UCLM-CSIC-JCCLM), Ronda Toledo s/n, Ciudad Real, Spain

2 Department of Veterinary Pathobiology, Center for Veterinary Health Sciences, Oklahoma State University, Stillwater, OK, USA

References

[1] Aoki, T., et al., The ankyrin repeats but not the PEST-like sequences are required for signal-dependent degradation of IkappaBalpha. Oncogene, 1996. 12(5): p. 1159-64.

[2] Apanius, V., S.A. Temple, and M. Bale, Serum proteins of wild turkey vultures (Cathartes aura). Comp Biochem Physiol B, 1983. 76(4): p. 907-13.

[3] Beutler, B. and M. Rehli, Evolution of the TIR, tolls and TLRs: functional inferences from computational biology. Curr Top Microbiol Immunol, 2002. 270: p. 1-21.

[4] Bonizzi, G. and M. Karin, The two NF-kappaB activation pathways and their role in innate and adaptive immunity. Trends Immunol, 2004. 25(6): p. 280-8.

[5] Bourne, H.R., D.A. Sanders and F. McCornick, The GTPase superfamily: conserved structure and molecular mechanism. Nature, 1991. 349: p. 117-126.

[6] Brown, K., et al., The signal response of IkappaB alpha is regulated by transferable N- and C-terminal domains. Mol Cell Biol, 1997. 17(6): p. 3021-7.

[7] Desterro, J.M., M.S. Rodriguez, and R.T. Hay, SUMO-1 modification of IkappaBalpha inhibits NF-kappaB activation. Mol Cell, 1998. 2(2): p. 233-9.

[8] Eidels, L., R.L. Proia and D.A. Hart, Membrane receptors for bacterial toxins. Microbiol Rev, 1983. 47: p. 596-620.

[9] Friedman, R. and A.L. Hughes, Molecular evolution of the NF-kappaB signaling system. Immunogenetics, 2002. 53(10-11): p. 964-74.

[10] Ghosh, S., M.J. May, and E.B. Kopp, NF-kappa B and Rel proteins: evolutionarily conserved mediators of immune responses. Annu Rev Immunol, 1998. 16: p. 225-60.

[11] Gilmore, T.D., Introduction to NF-kappaB: players, pathways, perspectives. Oncogene, 2006. 25(51): p. 6680-4.

[12] Hayden, M.S., A.P. West, and S. Ghosh, NF-kappaB and the immune response. Oncogene, 2006. 25(51): p. 6758-80.

[13] Hopkins, P.A. and S. Sriskandan, Mammalian Toll-like receptors: to immunity and beyond. Clin Exp Immunol, 2005. 140(3): p. 395-407.

[14] Houston, D.C. and J.E. Cooper, The digestive tract of the whiteback griffon vulture and its role in disease transmission among wild ungulates. J Wildl Dis, 1975. 11(3): p. 306-13.

[15] Huguet, C., P. Crepieux, and V. Laudet, Rel/NF-kappa B transcription factors and I kappa B inhibitors: evolution from a unique common ancestor. Oncogene, 1997. 15(24): p. 2965-74.

[16] Jaffray, E., K.M. Wood, and R.T. Hay, Domain organization of I kappa B alpha and sites of interaction with NF-kappa B p65. Mol Cell Biol, 1995. 15(4): p. 2166-72.

[17] Johnson, G.B., et al., Evolutionary clues to the functions of the Toll-like family as surveillance receptors. Trends Immunol, 2003. 24(1): p. 19-24.

[18] Karin, M. and Y. Ben-Neriah, Phosphorylation meets ubiquitination: the control of NF-[kappa]B activity. Annu Rev Immunol, 2000. 18: p. 621-63.

[19] Krishnan, V.A., et al., Structure and regulation of the gene encoding avian inhibitor of nuclear factor kappa B-alpha. Gene, 1995. 166(2): p. 261-6.

[20] Luque, I. and C. Gelinas, Distinct domains of IkappaBalpha regulate c-Rel in the cytoplasm and in the nucleus. Mol Cell Biol, 1998. 18(3): p. 1213-24.

[21] Luque, I., et al., N-terminal determinants of I kappa B alpha necessary for the cytoplasmic regulation of c-Rel. Oncogene, 2000. 19(9): p. 1239-44.

[22] Mabb, A.M. and S. Miyamoto, SUMO and NF-kappaB ties. Cell Mol Life Sci, 2007. 64(15): p. 1979-96.

[23] Ohishi, I., et al., Antibodies to Clostridium botulinum toxins in free-living birds and mammals. J Wildl Dis, 1979. 15(1): p. 3-9.

[24] Perez de la Lastra, J.M. and J. de la Fuente, Molecular cloning and characterisation of the griffon vulture (Gyps fulvus) toll-like receptor 1. Dev Comp Immunol, 2007. 31(5): p. 511-9.

[25] Perez de la Lastra, J.M. and J. de la Fuente, Molecular cloning and characterisation of a homologue of the alpha inhibitor of NF-kB in the griffon vulture (Gyps fulvus). Vet Immunol Immunopathol, 2008. 122: p. 318-25

[26] Perez de la Lastra, J.M., L. Kremer and J. De la Fuente, Recent advances in the development of immunoadhesins for immune therapy and as anti-infective agents. Recent Patents on Anti-Infective Drug Discovery, 2009, 4: p. 183-189.

[27] Pons, J., et al., Structural studies on 24P-IkappaBalpha peptide derived from a human IkappaB-alpha protein related to the inhibition of the activity of the transcription factor NF-kappaB. Biochemistry, 2007. 46(11): p. 2958-72.

[28] Roach, J.C., et al., The evolution of vertebrate Toll-like receptors. Proc Natl Acad Sci U S A, 2005. 102(27): p. 9577-82.

[29] Saitou, N. and M. Nei, The neighbor-joining method: a new method for reconstructing phylogenetic trees. Mol Biol Evol, 1987. 4(4): p. 406-25.

[30] Shumway, S.D., M. Maki, and S. Miyamoto, The PEST domain of IkappaBalpha is necessary and sufficient for in vitro degradation by mu-calpain. J Biol Chem, 1999. 274(43): p. 30874-81.

[31] Sullivan, J.C., et al., Rel homology domain-containing transcription factors in the cnidarian Nematostella vectensis. Dev Genes Evol, 2007. 217(1): p. 63-72.

[32] Takeda, K. and S. Akira, Toll-like receptors in innate immunity. Int Immunol, 2005. 17(1): p. 1-14.

[33] Takeda, K., Evolution and integration of innate immune recognition systems: the Toll-like receptors. J Endotoxin Res, 2005. 11(1): p. 51-5.

[34] Totzke, G., et al., A novel member of the IkappaB family, human IkappaB-zeta, inhibits transactivation of p65 and its DNA binding. J Biol Chem, 2006. 281(18): p. 12645-54.

http://dx.doi.org/10.5772/54191

[35] Weber, A.N., M.A. Morse, and N.J. Gay, Four N-linked glycosylation sites in human toll-like receptor 2 cooperate to direct efficient biosynthesis and secretion. J Biol Chem, 2004. 279(33): p. 34589-94.

Chapter 11

Glutathione *S*-Transferase Genes from Ticks

Yasser Shahein, Amira Abouelella and
Ragaa Hamed

Additional information is available at the end of the chapter

http://dx.doi.org/10.5772/52482

1. Introduction

For a long time before the discovery of glutathione S–transferases (GSTs; EC 2.5.1.18), it was a well known fact that some orally administered electrophilic compounds ultimately become excreted in the urines as a conjugates of N- acetyl cysteine, the so called mercapturic acids. Glutathione was then identified by [1] to be the source of cysteine used for biosynthesis of the mercapturic acids. As a consequence, the GSTs were discovered as enzymes catalyzing the first step in the formation of mercapturic acids. The first paper on GSTs was presented by [2], who described the partial purification and some properties of cytosolic rat liver enzymes capable of catalyzing the formation of GSH conjugation with halogenated aromatic compounds. GSTs form a group of ubiquitous enzymes that catalyze the conjugation between glutathione and several molecules, and play the most important role in the cellular detoxification pathway of endogenous and xenobiotic compounds [3].

GST family classified based on primary structure, substrate specificity and immunological properties. Presently, seven classes of GSTs are recognized in mammals, namely the specific Alpha, Mu, Pi and the common Sigma, Theta, Zeta and Omega. The classification of GSTs into different classes is also reflected in the chromosomal location of the genes. In human, each class is encoded by genes organized into clusters on different chromosomes. For example, the genes of all known class Mu GSTs are clustered on chromosome l, the genes of the class Alpha, Pi and Theta are clustered on chromosomes 6, 11, 22, respectively [4]. Polymorphisms have been identified in the GSTM1, GSTT1 and GSTPl genes coding for enzymes in the μ, θ, and π classes, respectively. The GSTM1 and the GSTT1 genes are polymorphic in humans, and the phenotypic absence of enzyme activity is due to a homozygous inherited deletion of the gene [5-7].

Ticks are blood sucking ectoparasites that infest a wide array of species. They are vectors of diseases in humans and other animals. The southern cattle tick, *Rhipicephalus microplus*, transmits the cattle fever pathogen (*Babesia spp.*) and is one of the most important cattle pests. Chemical pesticides continue to be the primary means of control for ectoparasites on livestock. Intensive use of these materials has led to the development of resistance in Rhipicephalus ticks to all currently used organophosphates [8], synthetic pyrethroids and amidines [9]. Despite previous studies that suggested increased detoxification [10] and target site insensitivity may contribute to the increased tolerance to acaricides, the mechanisms conferring resistance on ticks are poorly understood.

In the past years, significant advancement has been made to determine the potential role of GSTs in toxicology. Besides the well established role of GSTs in detoxification of xenobiotic compounds, it has been observed that GSTs have other intracellular substrates including the metabolites released from cellular molecules. In ticks, GSTs have attracted attention because of their involvement in the defense towards insecticides mainly organophosphates, organochlorines and cyclodienes. This chapter will give highlight on some of the cloned GST genes in ticks and will discuss and review the folding and unfolding states of a GST mu class from the cattle tick *Rhipicephalus annulatus* distributed in Egypt.

2. Glutathione S-transferase genes in ticks

Ticks are blood feeding external parasites of mammals, birds, and reptiles throughout the world. Tick infestations of animals and especially farm ones like cattle and camels, economically impact food industry by reducing weight gain and milk production, and by transmitting pathogens that cause babesiosis (*Babesia bovis* and *Babesia bigemina*) and anaplasmosis (*Anaplasma marginale*). The most important and widely distributed ticks include American dog tick (*Dermacentor variabilis*) is the most commonly identified species responsible for transmitting *Rickettsia rickettsii*, which causes Rocky Mountain spotted fever in humans, *R. microplus* and *R. annulatus* which infest cattle and distributed in Asia, Latin America, and Africa, *Hyalomma dromedarii* which infest camels (Asia and Africa), and the blacklegged tick (*Ixodes scapularis*), commonly known as "deer tick" and can transmit the organisms responsible for anaplasmosis, babesiosis, and Lyme disease and is widely distributed in the northeastern and upper midwestern United States.

Acaricide application constitutes a major component of integrated tick control strategies [11]. However, use of acaricides has had limited efficacy in reducing tick infestations and is often accompanied by serious drawbacks, including the selection of acaricide-resistant ticks, environmental contamination, and contamination of milk and meat products with drug residues.

GST enzymes are one of the important supergene families that are involved in protecting the organism from oxidative stress and xenobiotics including the acaricides. Different studies have been carried out to explore the role of the different GST families in detoxification in ticks. The methods applied in these studies used biochemical approaches, direct cloning using consensus sequences or using the available information from whole genome sequence information. Niranjan Reddy et al. [12] studied the GST superfamily organization in *Ixodes scapularis* using the whole genome sequence information (IscaW1.1, December' 2008) by applying different phylogenetic and bioinformatic tools. They identified all the three broad GST classes, the canonical, mitochondrial, and microsomal forms. A total of 35 GST genes belong to five different canonical GST classes, namely Delta (7 genes), Epsilon (5), Mu (14), Omega (3), and Zeta (3 genes) GST classes, and two mitochondrial Kappa class GST genes, and a single microsomal GST gene were found. The analysis of these sequences identified members of the Delta- and Epsilon-classes which are thought to be specific to the Insecta. Surprisingly, Ixodes has lost two of the functionally important gene families, Theta-and Sigma-GSTs.

GSTs had been reported to play a major role in the organophosphate resistance pathway of the *Musca domestica* (Corrnell-HR strain) [13]. On the contrary, Li et al. [14] reported that GSTs play only a minor role against organophosphate toxicity in *R. microplus*. Several GST coding frames had been cloned from *R. microplus* as done by [15] (accession number AAL99403), and [16] described that the activity of this protein is enhanced by organophosphate and coumaphos.

Some GST genes were cloned from different tick species and are of the mu class. The conservation score is represented in figure 1, and three state secondary structure is in figure 2. However, several attempts were carried out to explore the distribution of the different GST classes in ticks. The most widely distributed and economically important; the cattle tick *R. microplus* was used to initiate a study of the genome using an expressed sequence tag (EST) approach [17]. They reported the construction of a gene index named BmiGI from 20417 ESTs derived from a normalized cDNA library. The BmiGI was used to identify genes which might be involved in the acaricide resistance including GSTs.

Gurrero et al. [17] reported 15 possible GST coding genes identified from the BmiGI. One of these sequences was reported to be similar to the human GST class Omega 1, and the other clone was similar to mouse GST of Zeta 1 class. The total 15 clones are listed in table 1.

3. Unfolding/refolding of *Rhipicephalus annulatus* GST mu class

GSTs are dimeric proteins composed of identical or structurally related subunits. Each subunit has a molecular weight of about 25 kDa and is built of two domains and contains a complete active site consisting of a highly conserved G-site (GSH binding site) and a divergent H-site (Hydrophobic substrate binding site). The functional soluble enzymatic forms are found in dimers and only subunits within the same class can form heterodimers as found in alpha subunits, but this would not happen with either pi or mu subunits.

The nature of protein folding mechanisms and the manner in which the compact native state is achieved are still not well understood. From a wide range of experiments, it is now evident that specific pathways of folding are involved, at least for many proteins. At equilibrium, most monomeric and many oligomeric proteins display essentially a two-state pathway upon folding/unfolding, for which thermodynamically stable folding intermediates do not exist. Other mechanisms result in the formation of stable intermediates. These monomeric intermediates sometimes have preserved tertiary structure or appear as molten globules [18-20]. For proteins composed of subunits, the intermediates are either partially folded oligomeric states or monomeric states.

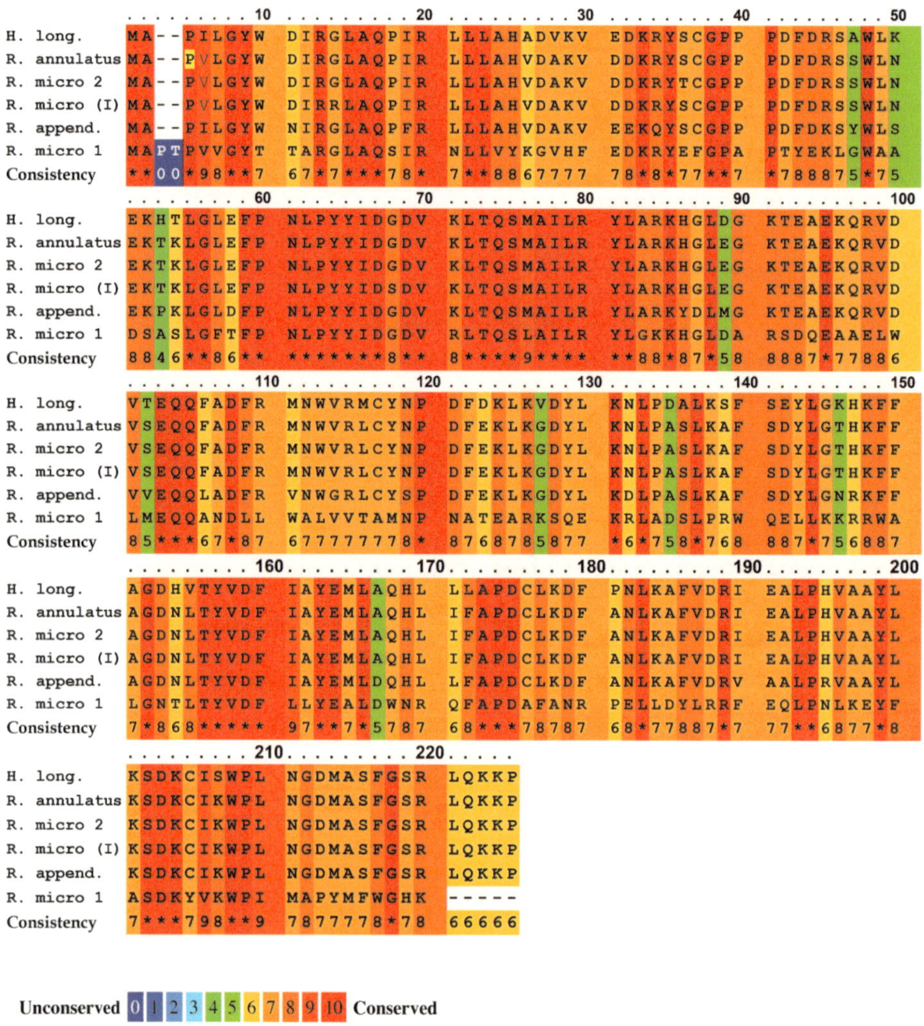

Figure 1. Amino acid conservation of Glutathione S-transferase mu class of different tick species. H. long. refers to *Haemaphysalis longicornis* GST (AAQ74441), R. annulatus is the *Rhipicephalus annulatus* GST (ABR24785), R. micro 2 refers to *Rhipicephalus microplus* GST (AAD15991), R. micro I is *Rhipicephalus microplus* Indian strain GST (ADQ01064),

http://dx.doi.org/10.5772/52482

R. micro 1 refers to *Rhipicephalus microplus* GST (AF366931_1), and R. append. refers to *Rhipicephalus appendiculatus* GST (AAQ74442). The conservation scoring was performed by PRALINE software (http://zeus.few.vu.nl). The scoring scheme works from 0 for the least conserved alignment position, up to 10 for the most conserved alignment position.

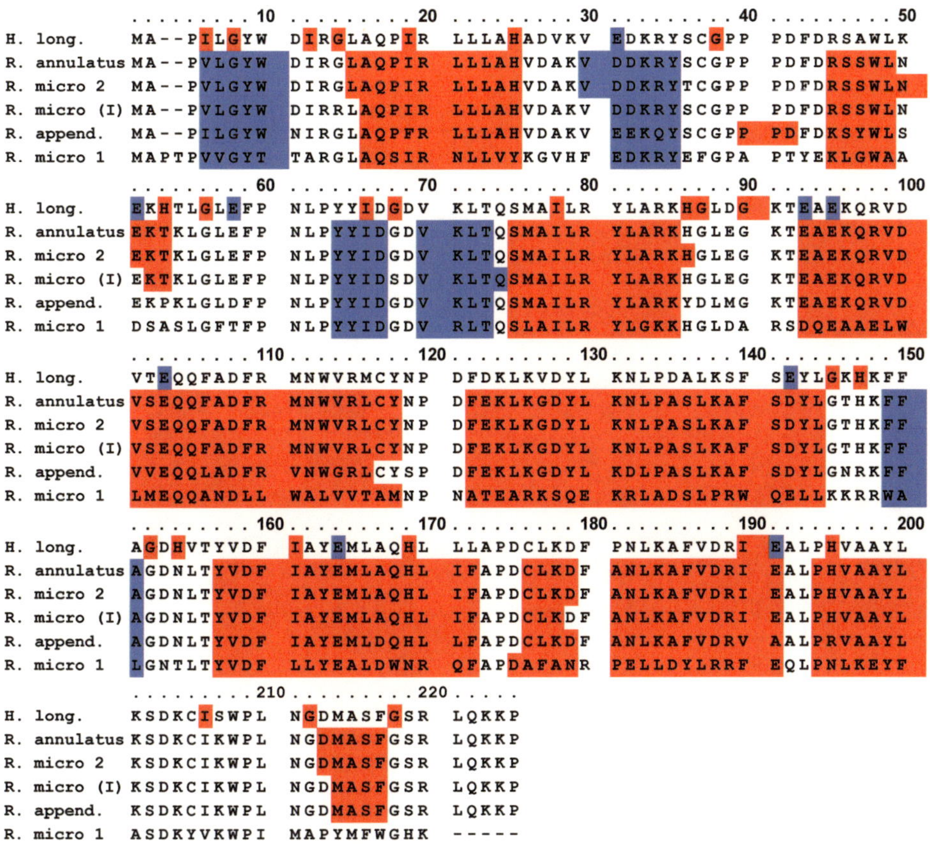

Figure 2. Three state (H, E C) secondary structure of Glutathione S-transferase mu class sequences from different tick species. H. long. refers to *Haemaphysalis longicornis* GST (AAQ74441), R. annulatus is *Rhipicephalus annulatus* GST (ABR24785), R. micro 2 refers to *Rhipicephalus microplus* GST (AAD15991), R. micro I is *Rhipicephalus microplus* Indian strain GST (ADQ01064), R. micro 1 refers to *Rhipicephalus microplus* GST (AF366931_1), and R. append. refers to *Rhipicephalus appendiculatus* GST (AAQ74442). The Helix (H) structure is in red and the Strand (E) is in blue. The sequence in the alignment has no color assigned for the coil (C) because there is no DSSP information available, or that no prediction was possible for that sequence.

Eftink et al. [18] proposed three models for proteins unfolding; the first is the two-state model. This model assumes that the protein exists only as a native dimer, D, and unfolded monomers, U, [D←→ 2U]. The second is three-state model (Folded monomers model). Unlike the first model, this one assumes that there is a two-step (three-state) unfolding process, with the formation of a folded monomeric intermediate, N. "folded" means that the intermediate can be further unfolded, in a cooperative manner, by addition of denaturant. However, it is not known to what extent the intermediate's structure actually resembles the subunits of the native dimer [D←→2N←→2U]. The third model is also three-state model and also considers the existence of an intermediate in the unfolding process but the intermediate is a partially unfolded dimeric state, D', which can then be further unfolded to unfolded monomers [D←→ D'←→2U].

Clone	Length (bp)	Top Blastx Hit e value cutoff=0.001	(TC)-GST Class subfamily*	Accession number of the Hit
TC 213	861	*Galleria mellonella*	Delta or Epsilon	AAK64362
TC2718	808			
TC 298	908	*Homo sapiens* Omega 1	Omega 1	NP004823
TC 614	756	*Dermacentor variabilis*	Delta or Epsilon	AAO92279
TC3165	855			
TC 762	1061			
TC3881	831			
TC4914	718			
TC1038	742	*R. microplus*	Mu	AAL99403
TC2910	813			
TC3317	984			
TC3737	825	*R. microplus*	Mu	AAD15991
TC1082	1236	*Mus musculus* Zeta 1	Zeta	Q9WVL0
TC 811	859	*Anopheles gambiae*	Zeta	AAM61889
TC2689	1007	*Xenopus laevis*	Mu	CAD01094

Table 1. Glutathione S-transferase sequences identified in *Boophilus microplus* Gene Index (BmiGI). The asterisk means that there is no practical evidence of the subfamily. The assigned class is based on prediction similarity.

Full understanding of the protein folding process requires the identification and characterization of all intermediate steps, which are often very transient and detected by kinetic studies only. In these cases, some properties of the intermediates can be inferred, but little structural information can be derived from this approach. It is known that mild denaturing conditions, such as moderately high temperature or low pH, promote partially unfolded states that are similar to those observed at moderate concentrations of guanidinium chloride [19]. Therefore a large number of studies have been performed on these partially folded states [21]. Some of these more or less stable intermediates, called "molten globules"are characterized by a largely conserved secondary structure but loss of tertiary structure and, due to the presence of a loosely packed hydrophobic core, binding of ANS is often observed

[22, 23]. Clear evidence of acidic pH induced stable folding intermediates has been obtained with some lipocalins, such as β-lactoglobulin [24, 25], retinol binding protein [26] and hGSTP1-1 [27].

Electrostatic interactions between charged residues on the surface of a protein play an important role in conferring stability to its folded structure. Change of pH alters the ionization state of these residues, causing intramolecular charge repulsion and possible disruption of salt bridges that can lead to destabilization of the native protein conformation [28]. pH is an important factor determining protein structure and function. Most proteins are stable and active at physiological pH and show varying degrees of denaturation in acid medium. However, as the acid concentration increases, a number of these proteins revert back to a compact conformation containing substantial secondary structure that resemble the folding intermediates known as molten globules [29, 30]. Study of the structural stability of a protein as a function of pH thus helps understand the thermodynamic or kinetic intermediates in its folding pathway and identifies the electrostatic interactions important for the stability of its folded state [31, 32].

In ticks, no data is available about the unfolding pathway of GST classes except for the *Rhipicephalus* (*Boophilus*) *annulatus* (*R. annulatus*) recombinant GST mu class (BaGSTM) [33]. Because of the non-identity of the different transitions monitored, the acid denaturation of BaGSTM does not appear to be a simple two-step transition, rather a multi-step process during which several intermediates coexist in equilibrium.

Shahein et al. [34] cloned the GST mu class from λZAP cDNA library of *R. annulatus*. The GST protein (Figure 3) contains four tryptophan residues (Try 7, Try 45, Try 110 and Try 214) and ten tyrosine residues [34]. Comparison of BaGST with the protein databank for GST sequences revealed the presence of the SMAILRYL motif that may play an important structural role in GSH binding site and the interface domain The authors showed that the *E. coli* expressed recombinant protein (BaGSTM) exhibited peroxidatic activity on cumene hydroperoxide sharing this property with GSTs belonging to the GST α class. The inhibition studies using cibacron blue and bromosulfophthalein showed that the *R. annuatus* GST shares this property with thc mammalian GST mu class.

In its native state, the BaGSTM enzyme exhibits an emission spectrum with a maximum at 329 nm (excitation 280 nm). This feature characteristic of tryptophan residues partially buried in the protein matrix (Figure 4 a). The addition of increasing concentrations of GdmCl at equilibrium caused a red shift of λmax of the emission spectra from 329 nm to 352 nm. As shown in figure 4, compared with the native dimer, the fluorescence intensity increased with a slight red shift of λmax as the GdmCl concentration was increased. The intensity reached a maximum at approximately 1.45 M (partially unfolded dimer or nonnative dimeric intermediate). At GdmCl concentration between 1.5 M and 1.9 M there was no change in the fluorescence intensity or in λmax. The nonnative dimeric intermediate undergoes dissociation into monomeric intermediate at these GdmCl concentrations. Increasing the GdmCl concentration leads to another increase in the fluorescence intensity with a red shift of λmax and the intensity reached a maximum at approximately 2.4 M. This might be due to the formation of a partially unfolded monomer. After this concentration the intensity started to decrease with a red shift of λmax and at 4.0 M GdmCl, a λmax of 352 nm occurred, indicating the complete exposure of the tryptophan residues to the aqueous solvent which is consistence with the complete unfolding of the protein (unfolded monomer). From these results, at least two transition states between the native dimer and unfolded monomer could be identified for BaGSTM.

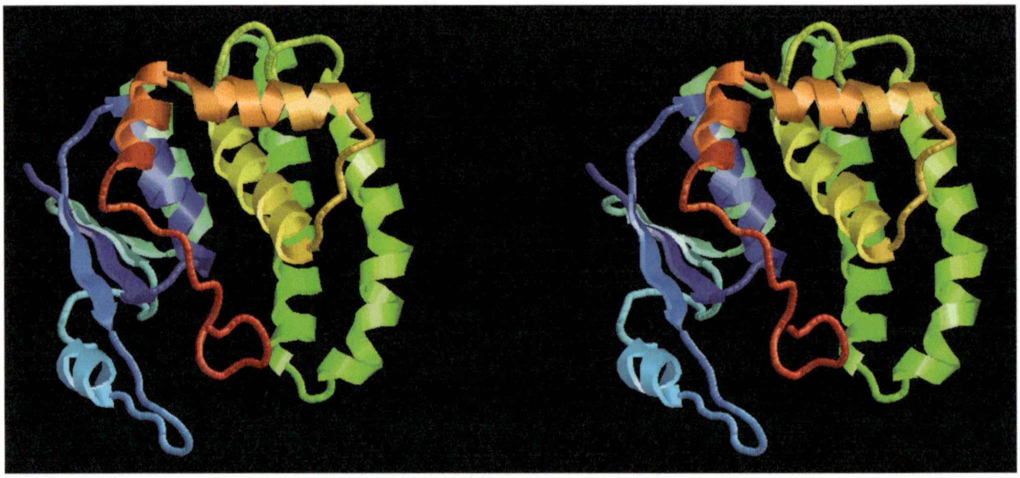

Figure 3. Theoretical model of *R. annulatus* GST mu class (ABR24785) built with M4T server. The numbers of groups are 218, atoms 1765, and bonds 1813 [35, 36].

As shown in the figure 5, at the concentration of urea between 0 and 1.75 M, there was an increase in the fluorescence intensity, as the concentration of urea increased, without any detectable shift of λmax. The intensity of fluorescence was increased by 50% at 1.75 M urea concentration compared with the native state of the protein indicating a partial exposure of the fluorophore (first phase). Increasing the concentration of urea, between 2.0 M and 3.0 M, resulted in a slight red shift (by 3 nm) of the emission maximum (second phase). Whereas, the increase in fluorescence intensity decreased as the concentration of urea was increased. The fluorescence intensity at the end of the first phase was higher than that at the end of the second phase. This indicates the movement of the fluorophore back into a more hydrophobic environment. At higher urea concentration, (between 3.25 and 4.5 M) the fluorescence intensity started to increase again with a shift of λmax (10 nm red shift). The fluorescence intensity was increased by three fold at 4.5 M urea compared to that of the native protein (third phase) [33].

Addition of higher concentrations of urea (5.0-7.0 M) did not change the intensity of the fluorescence significantly compared to that at 4.5 M urea but progressively shifted the λmax to 347 nm. At 8.0 M urea, the fluorescence intensity was decreased again with a shift of λmax to 352 nm indicating the complete unfolding of the protein. The present results indicate that three intermediates could be identified between the native dimer and unfolded monomer during the unfolding of BaGSTM.

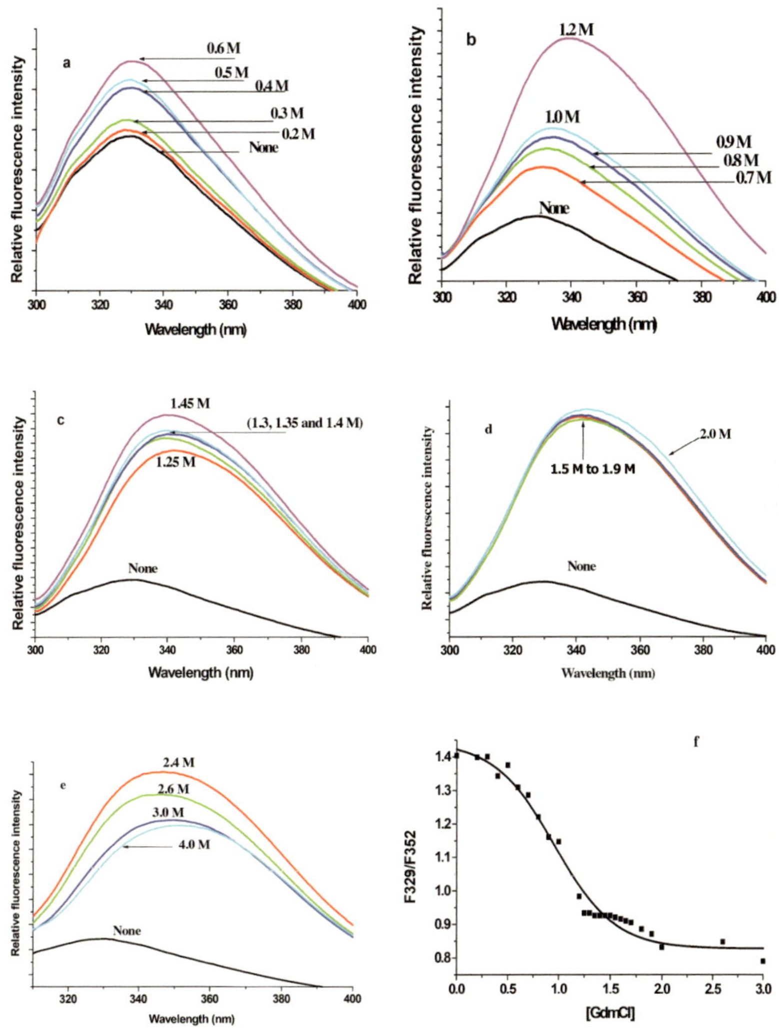

Figure 4. Fluorescence–emission spectra of BaGSTM (20 µg/ml) equilibrated in buffer A (20 mM potassium phosphate buffer, pH 7.0 containing 1 mM EDTA/1 mM dithiothreitol) at different GdmCl concentrations ranging from 0 to 4.0 M at room temperature. Excitation was done at 280 nm and fluorescence was recorded from 300 to 400 nm (a to e). Unfolding was expressed as the ratio of fluorescence at 329 nm to the fluorescence at 352 nm (f).

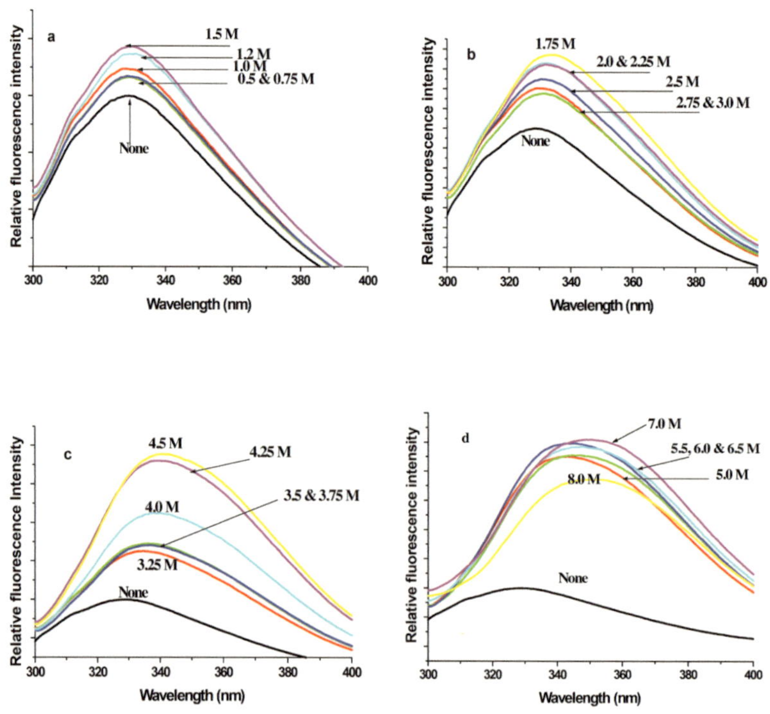

Figure 5. Urea-induced equilibrium unfolding for BaGSTM monitored by fluorescence. The protein (20µg/ml) was equilibrated in buffer A in the presence of the indicated concentration of urea at room temperature. Excitation was done at 280 nm and fluorescence was recorded from 300 to 400 nm.

In particular, the pH-dependent fluorescence transition of BaGSTM is clearly characterized by many distinct steps. The behavior of the protein in an acidic environment was investigated and analyses of fluorescence emission spectra of BaGSTM in solutions at different pH values were performed. The position of the emission maximum of a protein's fluorescence spectrum, upon excitation at 280 nm, was highly sensitive to the environment around its tryptophanyl and tyrosyl residues. As shown in figure 6, the acid denaturation of BaGSTM, as followed by the intrinsic fluorescence changes, was characterized by the presence of at least three transition states [33].

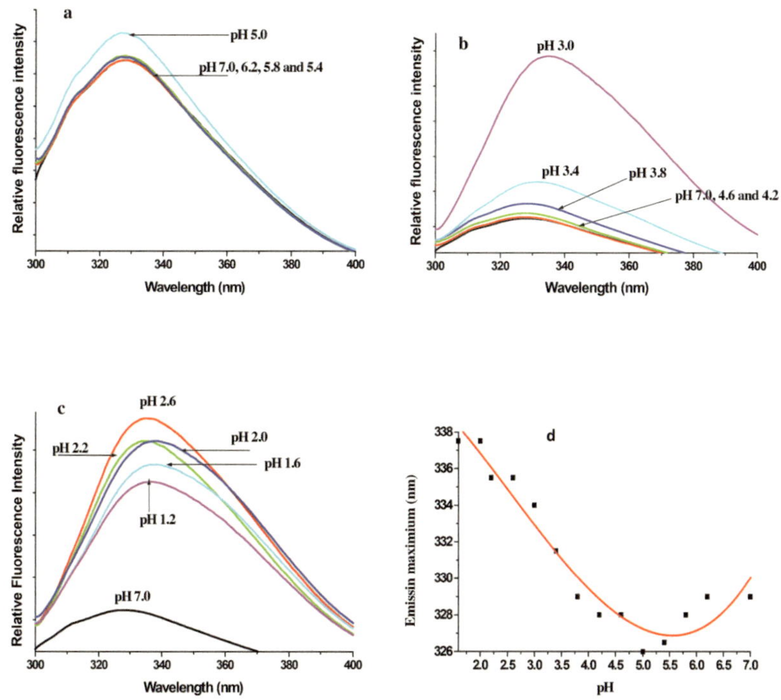

Figure 6. pH-induced equilibrium unfolding for BaGSTM monitored by fluorescence. The protein (20µg/ml) was equilibrated at room temperature in 0.02 M citrate-phosphate buffer at pH from 7.0 to 1.2 for 1 h before measurement. Excitation was done at 280 nm and fluorescence was recorded from 300 to 400 nm (a-c). Emission maxima were determined using the same excitation wavelength (d).

However, between pH 5.0 and 3.5, an initial red shift, from 338 to 342 nm of the maximum fluorescence emission, indicates a partial exposure of one or more tryptophanyl residues to the solvent. From pH 3.5 to pH 2.0 a second fluorescence transition occurs, characterized by a blue shift of λmax to 337 nm. This indicates the formation of a new type of structure in which the environment of the tryptophanyl residues is more hydrophobic. It has been proposed that the molten globule represents a common intermediate of the acid denaturation of many monomeric proteins.

GSTs are crystallized as dimers, but in solution class mu GST from rat its Asp97 mutant enzymes undergo reversible association and dissociation, the extent of which depends on protein concentration. Addition of 3 M potassium bromide to buffer solutions containing the wild-type rGSTM1-1 has generated monomers (GSTM1) [37]. A monomeric species of a human GSTpi has been constructed by introducing 10 site specific mutations. This drastically changed enzyme was structurally stable, but retained no activity [38].

The nonsubstrate ligand 8-anilino-1-naphthalene sulfonate (ANS) is a negatively charged hydrophobic fluorescent molecule, largely used to check the presence of compact partially folded intermediates. In fact, its very low fluorescence quantum yield in polar environment is strongly increased in non polar solvents [39]. Therefore, the binding of this molecule to partially folded proteins, containing clusters of hydrophobic side chains accessible to solvent, is often observed in the presence of molten globules [23].

Unbound ANS emission spectra showed a maximum at 530 nm that was blue shifted upon binding of the dye to the protein. Binding of ANS to BaGSTM as a function of GdmCl concentration showed one peak centered at 1.5 M and one peak as a function of urea concentrations centred at 3.5 M (Figures 7 a and b). ANS binding fluorescence of BaGSTM as a function of pH did not show any transition peak. However, the fluorescence intensity was increased as the pH decreased. The fluorescence intensity about 2000 fold higher at pH 2.0 compared with that at neutral pH (Figure 7 c). At the neutral pH, the fluorescence of ANS in the presence of BaGSTM is perfectly super imposable to that of ANS alone. At less than pH 3.8, ANS binds to BaGSTM showed a blue shift displacement with an enhancement of fluorescence intensity. Binding of the dye occurs at the dimer interface and unfolded GST does not bind ANS. This makes ANS an excellent probe to monitor changes at the packing of hydrophobic cores in protein which undergoes structural changes and has been broadly used to study the presence of monomeric intermediates at the urea/GdmCl unfolding of several GSTs [38, 40-42]. ANS was also used to detect the presence of folding intermediates with hydrophobic patches such as the molten globule in penicillin G acylase [43] and apomyoglobin [44].

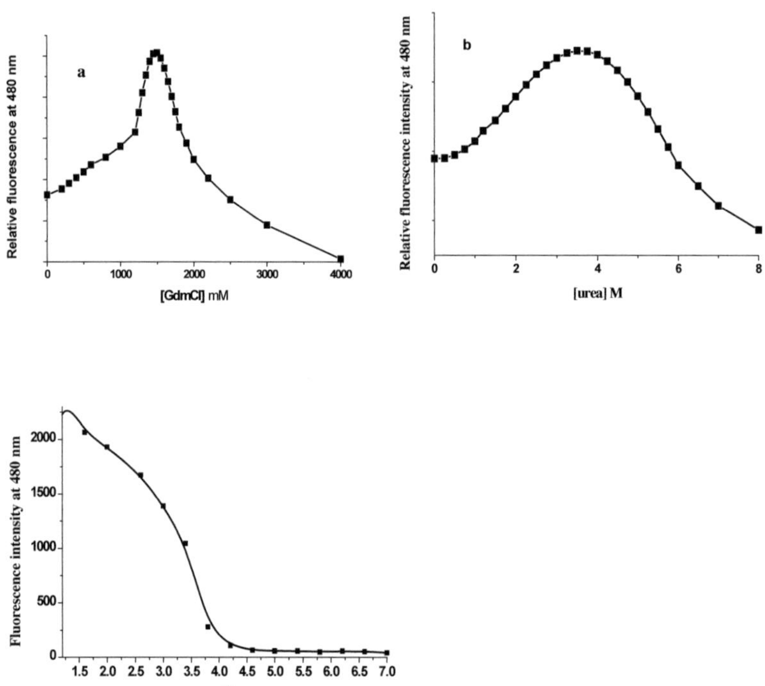

Figure 7. Variation of ANS binding fluorescence at 480 nm as a function of GdmCl concentrations (a) or urea (b) or as a function of pH (c). The proteins (20 µg/ml) were equilibrated in buffer A at room temperature in the presence of the indicated concentration of denaturant or pH. 100 µM ANS was added to the solution. Excitation was done at 380 nm and emission at 480 nm.

The unfolding results of the *R. (Boophilus) annulatus* (BaGSTM) demonstrate that the probes used (intrinsic fluorescence, excitation of tryptophan and tyrosine and ANS binding fluorescence) are differentially sensitive to various conformational states of BaGSTM. The presence of multiple nonsuperimposable transitions for this enzyme indicates that the two states unfolding mechanism is not applicable, and it is highly suggestion of the existence of at least two well-populated stable intermediates. Similar data were reported demonstrating the existence of stable intermediates at the unfolding of GSTs [42, 45-48]. However, only one transition intermediate was detected using ANS binding fluorescence for BaGSTM in presence of different concentrations of GdmCl or urea. This result is similar to that observed for sigma class GST in the presence of urea [46].

4. GST and immune system

Tick control is considered crucial all over the world to minimize the major drawbacks of tick infestations. The control strategies were adopted to use the acaricides which become less efficient. Seixas et al. [49] has stated the alternative approaches used in tick control and are classified into four groups: (i) biological control by tick pathogens or predators [50]; (ii) habitat alterations by planting tick-killing or repelling vegetation [51]; (iii) immunological control [52]; and (iv) development of tick-resistant breeds. They stated that although these methods have been proved to be theoretically valuable, most of them have been forsaken, since they did not afford acceptable cost/benefit ratios under field conditions, except for vaccines.

Many types of chemical tick control were started since 1893 including the application of arsenic acaricides, gamma BHC (organochlorine acaricide) and DDT. However, resistance to DDT was reported within 5 years of field application [53]. The toxicity plus the environmental awareness and other factors led to the removal of the previously mentioned acaricides from the tick control market.

In early 1960's, Diazinon and other organophosphate acaricides were applied and in 1970's, Triatix was the first amidine to be registered for tick control. In the 1980's, pyrethroids (Flumethrin and Permethrin) were also registered for tick control. The following table 2 shows the different acaricides used in tick control.

Along with the application of these chemicals with acaricidal properties as the predominant method of tick control throughout the world, resistance to the majority of the groups of chemicals had been evolved. Generally, the resistance may arise through several mechanisms including target sites, metabolic mechanism or reduced penetration. The target site resistance occurs when an allele of the gene coding for the target molecule is attacked by the acaricide. The penetration resistance occurs when an acaricide fails to penetrate the target individual. This type of resistance has not been reported in ticks. The third type of resistance mechanisms is the metabolic pathway which occurs through changes in the abilities of acaricide detoxification by an organism [17]. Three enzyme families including cytochrome P450s

(115 individual members), esterases (81 individual members), and GSTs (39 individual members), are involved in the metabolic resistance mechanism.

Type of Acaricide	Examples	Mode of Action
Arsenical Compounds	Arsenic Trioxide	Arsenite may bind to intracellular thiols, such as glutathione, and hence disrupting the ratio of reduced to oxidized glutathione leading to inhibition of cell division [54]
Chlorinated Hydrocarbons (Organochlorines)	DDT Gamma BHC Lindane Toxaphene	Interfere with the nerve conduction of ticks by affecting the ion channels, especially the voltage gated Na^+ channels [55]
Organophosphates	Diazinon Dichlorphos	Suppress the enzyme acetyl-cholinesterase [56]. This group of acaricides is used in the form of phosphorothionates which are converted by the ticks into an active more toxic ingredient named "phosphate" or the "Oxon".
Carbamates	Propoxure	Very similar to organophosphates
Amidines	Amitraz Cymiazol	They inhibit the monoamine oxidase enzyme which is responsible for the metabolism of neurotransmitter amines in tick nervous system. They probably interact with octopamine receptors causing an increase in nervous activity causing detaching of ticks from the animal [57]
Pyrethroides	Cypermethrin Flumethrin Cyhalothrin Alphamethrin	They interfere with nerve conduction [58]
Macrocyclic lactones (eg. Avermectin group)	Ivermectin	It affects neural transmission. In ticks, ivermectin inhibits female engorgement by reduction of body weight [59]

Table 2. Different acaricide groups used in tick control.

Anti-tick vaccine development is focused on the identification, molecular cloning and in vitro production of proteins playing key putative roles in tick physiology, such as cell signaling, modulation of host immune response, pathogen transmission, embryogenesis, digestion, and intermediary metabolism [60]. Of the different antigens used as an anti-tick vaccine was the GST molecule. GST was of special interest to stimulate cattle immune system and their critical role in the metabolic resistance of acaricides. The immunological bases of using GSTs as vaccines may be derived from the hypothesis that parasites can survive within their hosts for a period of time despite the complex immune environment surrounding them possibly accomplish this by adopting various immunomodulatory strategies, which include release of GSTs that counteract the oxidative reactive oxygen species (ROS) produced by the host activated cells and attach parasite cell membrane [61].

Since GSTs produced by parasites appear to be critical for the survival of parasites in the host, several studies evaluated the potential of parasite GSTs as vaccine candidates especially against schistosomiasis, fascioliasis and filarial parasites. However, several immunological studies were carried out to identify potential vaccines against helminth parasites including *Schistosoma mansoni* where the successful Sm28GST vaccine was developed by Capron et al. [62] and is in Phase II clinical trials. The injection of Sm28GST antigen elicited the production of immunoglobulins (especially IgE) and activation of eosinophils which could interfere with the function of parasitic GST [62]. Interestingly, the injection of Sm28GST in toxicity studies performed in dogs, rabbits and rats showed no system or local toxicity and no cross reactivity with rat or human GST [62]. Bushara et al. [63] and Morrison et al. [64] suggested that GST of *Schisotosoma spp*. and *Fasciola spp*. improved host immunity against these parasites. In this respect, GSTs were found to be up-regulated in response to rickettsial infection of *D. variabilis* ovaries [65]. They found that there is 0.25 fold increase in the mRNA expression of the GST gene.

Previous studies correlated the role of GSTs in insect innate immunity with increased GST expression in response to infection-induced oxidative stress [66-70]. Increasing numbers of insect GSTs are being characterized due to their roles in insecticide detoxification. Dreher-Lesnick et al. [71] had cloned two GST variants and sequenced from the American dog tick; *D. variabilis* tick. Their structural analysis revealed that one of them belongs to the theta class (Figure 8) but no data is available about their biological activities. The secondary structure prediction using the DSSP prediction is shown in figure 9. Comparison of these two GST molecules with those of other species indicates that GST1 is related to the mammalian class theta and insect class delta GSTs, while GST2 does not seem to fall in the same family. Northern blotting analyses revealed differential expression patterns, where GST1 and GST2 transcripts are found in the tick gut, with GST2 transcripts also present in the ovaries. Both *D. variabilis* GST transcripts are up-regulated upon tick feeding. The up-regulation of GST in this state is probably due to the stresses incurred during blood feeding. The authors could not rule out the possibility that up-regulation of GST in ticks may serve other purposes including cell protection from oxidative stress caused by infection with the intracellular bacterium Rickettsia.

D. variabilis serves as a host for an obligate intracellular cattle pathogen belongs to the genus Anaplasma; *Anaplasma marginale*. The developmental cycle of this pathogen begins in the gut cells of the host and the transmission to cattle occurs from the salivary glands during a second tick feeding. The *A. marginale* parasite has two stages occur within parasitophorous vacuole in the tick cell cytoplasm; the reticulated form (RF) which will transform to the infective dense form (DF). Kocan et al. [72] studied the characterization of the silencing effects of 4 different *D. variabilis* genes (separately) including the GST (DQ224235) on the development and infection levels of the *A. marginale*. They used the RNAi technology to silence these genes in male ticks and they showed that the *A. marginale* infection was inhibited both in tick guts after acquisition feeding and salivary glands after transmission feeding. *D. variabilis* ticks injected with GST dsRNA showed significant lower density of dense forms in guts after acquisition feeding. In general, the results of GST silencing demonstrate that GST is required for pathogen infection of *D. variabilis* guts and salivary glands and IDE8 cells. It would suggest that GST may reduce the harmful effects of the metabolites, produced by the cellular oxidative stress, which may affect the development of the pathogen. Surprisingly, Kocan et al. [72] noticed that *A. marginale* infection was increased in the fat body cells in the GST silenced ticks.

Vaccination studies using tick proteins like GST from *Haemaphysalis longicornis* (Hl-GST) demonstrated the immunogenicity and antigenicity of this protein in bovines. Ultimately, immunization with GST protein triggered a partial immune response against *R. microplus* infestation in cattle, manifested mainly as a reduction of 7.9% in egg fertility, 53% in the number of fully engorged ticks and 57% overall efficacy ratio [73]. These data suggest that GST proteins have potential to be used as antigens in an anti-tick vaccine.

In conclusion, the phylogenetic analysis of the different cloned GST genes from different tick species indicates that numerous GSTs are present in the tick genome, which may or may not belong to different classes. These sequences are distributed in different tick organs including ovaries, gut and salivary glands. However, it is clear that protective immunity against tick infestation can be achieved; demonstrating that vaccination is a realistic unconventional approach for tick control and GST would be a candidate.

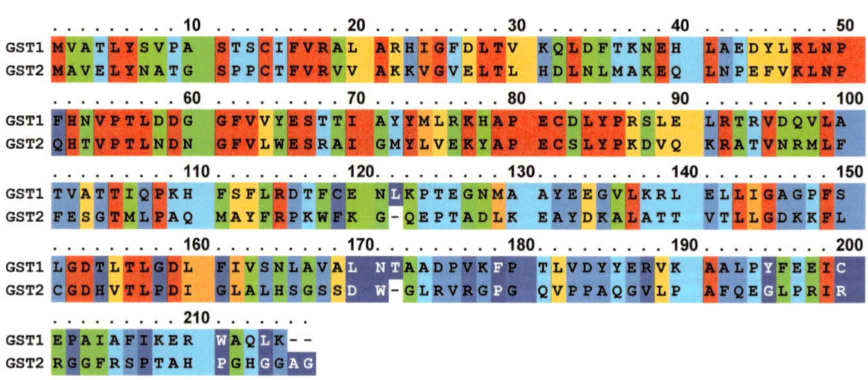

Figure 8. *Dermacentor variabilis* Glutathione S-transferase GST1 and GST2 (DQ224235 and AY241958, respectively) amino acid conservation. The conservation scoring is performed by PRALINE software (http://zeus.few.vu.nl). The scoring scheme works from 0 for the least conserved alignment position, up to 10 for the most conserved alignment position. The color assignments are as in figure 1.

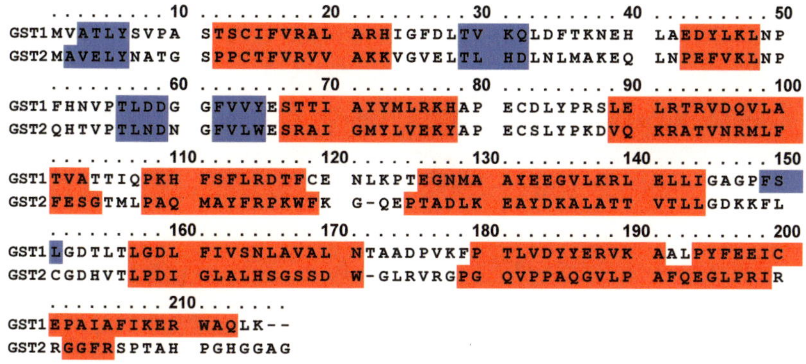

Figure 9. *Dermacentor variabilis* theta Glutathione S-transferase GST1 and GST2 (DQ224235 and AY241958, respectively) 3-state (H, E C) secondary structure. The Helix (H) structure is in red and the Strand (E) is in blue. The sequence in the alignment has no color assigned for the coil (C) because there is no DSSP information available, or that no prediction was possible for that sequence. The conservation scoring was performed by PRALINE software (http://zeus.few.vu.nl).

Author details

Yasser Shahein[1], Amira Abouelella[2] and Ragaa Hamed[1]

1 Department of Molecular Biology, National Research Centre, Egypt

2 Department of Radiation Biology, National Centre for Radiation Research and Technology, Egypt

References

[1] Barnes M. M., James S. P., Wood P. B. The formation of mercapturic acids. 1. Formation of mercapturic acid and the levels of glutathione in tissues. Biochemical Journal 1959; 71 680-690.

[2] Booth J., Boyland E., Sims P. An enzyme from rat liver catalyzing conjugations with glutathione. Biochemical Journal 1961; 79 516-524.

[3] Freitas D.R., Rosa R.M., Moraes J., Campos E., Logullo C., Da Silva Vaz I. Jr., Masuda A. Relationship between glutathione S-transferase, catalase, oxygen consumption, lipid peroxidation and oxidative stress in eggs and larvae of *Boophilus microplus* (Acarina: Ixodidae). Comparative Biochemistry and Physiology. Part A Molecular Integrative Physiology 2007; 146(4) 688-694.

[4] Pearson W.R., Vorachek W.R., Xu S.J., Berger R., Hart I., Vannais D., Patterson D. Identification of class-mu glutathione transferase genes GSTM1–GSTM5 on human chromosome 1p13. American Journal of Human Genetics 1993; 53 (1) 220-233.

[5] Davies S.M., Robison L.L., Buckley J.D., Tjoa T., Woods W.G., Radloff G.A., Ross J.A., Perentesis J.P. Glutathione S-transferases polymorphisms and outcome of chemotherapy in childhood acute myeloid leukemia. Journal of Clinical Oncology 2001; 19(5) 1279-1287.

[6] Davies S.M., Bhatia S., Ross J.A., Kiffmeyer W.R., Gaynon P.S., Radloff G.A., Robison L.L., Perentesis J.P. Glutathione S-transferases genotypes, genetic susceptibility, and outcome of therapy in childhood acute lymphoblastic leukemia. Blood 2002; 100(1) 67-71.

[7] Mannervik B. Novel polymorphisms in the glutathione transferase superfamily. Pharmacogenetics 2003; 13 127-128.

[8] Baxter G.D., Green P., Stuttgen M., Baker S.C. Detecting resistance to organophosphates and carbamates in the cattle tick *Boophilus microplus,* with a propoxur-based biochemical test. Experimental and Applied Acarology 1999; 23 (11) 907-914.

[9] Martinez M.L., Machado M.A., Nascimento C.S., Silva M.V., Teodoro R.L., Furlong J., Prata M.C., Campos A.L., Guimaraes M.F., Azevedo A.L., Pires M.F., Verneque R.S. Association of BoLA-DRB3.2 alleles with tick (*Boophilus microplus*) resistance in cattle. Genetics and Molecular Research 2006; 5 (3) 513-524.

[10] [10] De La Fuente J., Kocan K.M. Strategies for development of vaccines for control of ixodid tick species. Parasite Immunology 2006; 28 275-283.

[11] Graf J.-F., Gogolewski R., Leach-Bing N., Sabatini G. A., Molento M. B., Bordin E. L., Arantes G. J. Tick control: an industry point of view. Parasitology 2004; 129 S427-S442.

[12] Niranjan Reddy B.P., Prasad G.B., Raghavendra K. In silico analysis of glutathione S-transferase supergene family revealed hitherto unreported insect specific δ- and ε-GSTs and mammalian specific μ-GSTs in *Ixodes scapularis* (Acari: Ixodidae).Computational Biology and Chemistry 2011; 35 114–120

[13] Wei S.H., Clark A.G., Syvanen M. Identification and cloning of a key insecticide-metabolizing glutathione S-transferase (MdGST-6A) from a hyper insecticide-resistant strain of the housefly *Musca domestica*. Insect Biochemistry and Molecular Biology 2001; 31 1145-1153.

[14] Li A., Davey R.B., Miller R.J., George J.E. Resistance to coumaphos and diazinon in *Boophilus microplus* (Acari: Ixodidae) and evidence for the involvement of an oxidative detoxification mechanism. Journal of Medical Entomology 2003; 40 482-490.

[15] He H., Chen A.C., Davey R.B., Ivie G.W., George J.E. Characterization and molecular cloning of glutathione S-transferase gene from the tick, *Boophilus microplus* (Acari; Ixodidae). Insect Biochemistry and Molecular Biology 1999; 29 737-743.

[16] Da Silva Vaz I., Torino Lermen T., Michelon A., Sanchez Ferreira C.A., Joaquim de Freitas D.R., Termignoni C., Masuda A. Effect of acaricides on the activity of a *Boophilus microplus* glutathione S-transferase. Veterinary Parasitology 2004; 119 (2/3) 237-245.

[17] Guerrero F. D., Lovis L., Martins J. R. Acaricide resistance mechanisms in *Rhipicephalus (Boophilus) microplus*. Revista Brasileira de Parasitologia Veterinária, Jaboticabal 2012; 21(1) 1-6.

[18] Eftink M. R., Helton K. J., Beavers A., Ramsay G. D. The unfolding of trp aporepressor as a function of pH: Evidence for an unfolding intermediate. Biochemistry 1994; 33(34) 10220-10228.

[19] Ptitsyn O. B. Molten globule and protein folding. Advances in Protein Chemistry 1995; 47 83-229.

[20] Ptitsyn, O. B. Structures of folding intermediates. Current Opinion in Structural Biology 1995; 5(1) 74-78.

[21] Ausili A., Scire A., Damiani E., Zolese G., Bertoli E., Tanfani F. Temperature-induced molten globule-like state in human alpha1-acid glycoprotein: An infrared spectroscopic study. Biochemistry 2005; 44(49) 15997-16006.

[22] Kuwajima K. The molten globule state as a clue for understanding the folding and cooperativity of globular-protein structure. Proteins 1989; 6(2) 87-103.

[23] Arai M., Kuwajima K. Role of the molten globule state in protein folding. Advances in Protein Chemistry 2000; 53 209-282.

[24] D'Alfonso L., Collini M., Baldini G. Does betalactoglobulin denaturation occur via an intermediate state? Biochemistry 2002; 41(1) 326-333.

[25] Ikeguchi M., Kato S., Shimizu A., Sugai S. Molten globule state of equine beta-lactoglobulin. Proteins 1997; 27(4) 567-575.

[26] Bychkova V. E., Dujsekina A. E., Fantuzzi A., Ptitsyn O.B., Rossi G. Release of retinol and denaturation of its plasma carrier, retinol binding protein. Folding and Design 1998; 3(4) 285-291.

[27] Dragani B., Cocco R., Principe D.R., Cicconetti M., Aceto A. Structural characterization of acid-induced intermediates of human glutathione transferase P1-1. International Journal of Biochemistry and Cell Biology 2000; 32(7) 725-736.

[28] Goto Y., Calciano L. J., Fink A. L. Acid-induced folding of proteins. Proceedings of the National Academy of Sciences USA 1990; 87(2) 573-577.

[29] Goto Y., Takahashi N., Fink A. L. Mechanism of acid induced folding of proteins. Biochemistry 1990; 29(14) 3480-3488.

[30] Fink A. L. Molten globules. Methods in Molecular Biology 1995; 40 343-360.

[31] Pace C. N., Alston R. W., Shaw K. L. Charge-charge interactions influence the denatured state ensemble and contribute to protein stability. Protein Science 2000; 9(7) 1395-1398.

[32] Sheinerman F. B., Honig B. On the role of electrostatic interactions in the design of protein-protein interfaces. Journal of Molecular Biology 2002; 318(1) 161-177.

[33] Abdalla A., Shahein Y., Hamdy Y. M., El-Hakim A. E., Hamed R. Chemical and Acidic Denaturation of a Homodimeric Glutathione Transferase mu Class from *Rhipicephalus (Boophilus) annulatus*. Journal of Genetic Engineering and Biotechnology 2008; 6(1) 67-76.

[34] Shahein Y. E., EL-Hakim A. E. S., Abouelella A.M., Hamed R.R., Allam S.A., Farid N.M. Molecular cloning, expression and characterization of a functional GSTmu class from the cattle tick *Boophilus annulatus*. Veterinary Parasitology 2008; 152(12) 116-126.

[35] Fernandez-Fuentes N., Rai B.K., Madrid-Aliste C.J., Fajardo J.E., Fiser A. Comparative protein structure modeling by combining multiple templates and optimizing sequence-to-structure alignments. Bioinformatics 2007; 23(19) 2558-2565.

[36] Rykunov D., Steinberger E., Madrid-Aliste C.J., Fiser A. Improved scoring function for comparative modeling using the M4T method. Journal of Structural and Functional Genomics 2009; 10(1) 95-99.

[37] Hearne J.L., Colman R.F. Catalytically active monomer of class mu glutathione transferase from rat. Biochemistry 2006; 45(19) 5974-5984.

[38] Abdalla A. M., Bruns C. M., Tainer J. A., Mannervik B., Stenberg G. Design of a monomeric human glutathione transferase GSTP1, a structurally stable but catalytically inactive protein. Protein Engineering 2002; 15(10) 827-834.

[39] Turner D. C., Brand L. Quantitative estimation of protein binding site polarity. Fluorescence of N-arylaminonaphthalenesulfonates. Biochemistry 1968; 7(10) 3381-3390.

[40] Bico P., Erhardt J., Kaplan W., Dirr H. Porcine class pi glutathione S-transferase: Anionic ligand binding and conformational analysis. Biochimica et Biophysica Acta 1995; 1247(2) 225-230.

[41] Erhardt J., Dirr H. Native dimer stabilizes the subunit tertiary structure of porcine class pi glutathione S-transferase. European Journal of Biochemistry 1995; 230(2) 614-620.

[42] Andujar-Sanchez M., Clemente-Jimenez J. M., Rodriguez-Vico F., Las Heras-Vazquez F.J., Jara-Pérez V., Cámara-Artigas A. A monomer form of the glutathione S-transferase Y7F mutant from *Schistosoma japonicum* at acidic pH. Biochemical and Biophysical Research Communications 2004; 314(1) 6-10.

[43] Lindsay C. D., Pain R. H. The folding and solution conformation of penicillin G acylase. European Journal of Biochemistry 1990; 192(1) 133-141.

[44] De Young L. R., Dill K. A., Fink, A. L. Aggregation and denaturation of apomyoglobin in aqueous urea solutions. Biochemistry 1993; 32(15) 3877-3886.

[45] Aceto A., Caccuri A. M., Sacchetta P., Bucciarelli T., Dragani B., Rosato N., Federici G., Di Ilio C. Dissociation and unfolding of Pi-class glutathione transferase. Evidence for a monomeric inactive intermediate. The Biochemical Journal 1992; 285(1) 241-245.

[46] Stevens J. M., Hornby J. A., Armstrong R. N., Dirr, H. W. Class sigma glutathione transferase unfolds via a dimeric and a monomeric intermediate: Impact of subunit interface on conformational stability in the superfamily. Biochemistry 1998; 37(44) 15534-15541.

[47] Sacchetta P., Pennelli A., Bucciarelli T., Cornelio L., Amicarelli F., Miranda M., Di Ilio C. Multiple unfolded states of glutathione transferase bbGSTP1-1 by guanidinium chloride. Archives of Biochemistry and Biophysics 1999; 369(1) 100-106.

[48] Abdalla A. M., Hamed, R. R. Multiple unfolding states of glutathione transferase from *Physa acuta* (Gastropoda [correction of Gastropada]: Physidae). Biochemical and Biophysical Research Communications 2006; 340(2) 625-632.

[49] Seixas A., Oliveira P., Termignoni C., Logullo C., Masuda A., da Silva Vaz I Jr. *Rhipicephalus (Boophilus) microplus* embryo proteins as target for tick vaccine. Veterinary Immunology and Immunopathology 2011; doi:10.1016/j.vetimm.2011.05.011

[50] Samish M., Glazer I. Entomopathogenic nematodes for the biocontrol of ticks. Trends in Parasitology 2001; 17 368-371

[51] Sutherst R.W., Jones R.J., Schnitzerling H.J. Tropical legumes of the genus Stylosanthes immobilize and kill cattle ticks. Nature 1982; 295 320-321.

[52] Willadsen P. Anti-tick vaccines. Parasitology 2004; 129 S367-S387.

[53] Whitehead G. DDT resistance in the blue tick, *B. decoloratus* (Koch). Journal of the South African Veterinary Medical Association 1956; 27 117-120.

[54] Levy J., Stauber J., Adams M., Maher W., Kirby J., Jolley D. Toxicity, biotransformation, and mode of action of arsenic in two freshwater microalgae (*Chlorella sp.* and *Monoraphidium arcuatum*). Environmental Toxicology and Chemistry 2005; 24 2630-2639.

[55] Adams H.R. Veterinary pharmacology and therapeutic. 7th Ed. Iowa State University Press, United States of America.

[56] Wharton R.H., Roulston W.J. Resistance of ticks to chemicals. Annual Review of Entomology 1970; 15 381-404.

[57] Thullner F., Kemp D.H., Mckenna R.V., Willadsen P. Dispersal test for the diagnosis of amitraz resistance in tick larvae (*Boophilus microplus*). Proceedings of the 3rd International Conference "Ticks and Tick-borne pathogens: Into the 21st Century". Eds. M. Kazimirova, M. Labuda and P.A. Nuttall. Institute of Zoology, Slovak Academy of Sciences, Bratislava, Slovakia. 2000; 205-208.

[58] Solomon K.R. Acaricide resistance in ticks. Advances in Veterinary Science and Comparative Medicine 1983; 27 273-296.

[59] Wilkins C.A., Conroy J.B., Ho P., O'shanny W.J., Capizzi T., The effect of ivermectin on the live mass period of attachment and percent control of ticks. In Whitehead, G.B. and Gibson, J.D. (Eds) Tick Biology and Control. Proceedings of International Conference, Tick Research Unit, Rhodes University, Grahamstown, South Africa 1981; 137-142.

[60] Parizi L.F., Pohl P.C., Masuda A., Da Silva Vaz I. New approaches toward anti-*Rhipicephalus (Boophilus) microplus* tick vaccine. Brazilian Journal of Veterinary Parasitology 2009; 18 1–7.

[61] Veerapathran A., Dakshinamoorthy G., Gnanasekar M., Reddy M.V.R., Kalyanasundaram R. Evaluation of *Wuchereria bancrofti* GST as a vaccine candidate for lymphatic filariasis. PLOS Neglected Tropical Diseases 2009; 3(6) e457-e468.

[62] Capron A., Capron M., Riveau G. Vaccine development against schistosomiasis from concepts to clinical trials. British Medical Bulletin 2002; 62 139-148.

[63] Bushara H.O., Bashir M.E.N., Malik K.H.E., Mukhtar M.M., Trottein F., Capron A., Taylor M.G. Suppression of *Schistosoma bovis* egg-production in cattle by vaccination with either glutathione-S- transferase or keyhole limpet hemocyanin. Parasite Immunolology 1993; 15 383-390.

[64] Morrison C.A., Colin T., Sexton J.L., Bowen F., Wicker J., Friedel T., Spithill T.W. Protection of cattle against *Fasciola hepatica* infection by vaccination with glutathione S-transferase. Vaccine 1996; 14 1603-1612.

[65] Mulenga A., Macaluso K. R., Simser J. A., Azad A. F. Dynamics of Rickettsia–tick interactions: identification and characterization of differentially expressed mRNAs in uninfected and infected *Dermacentor variabilis*. Insect Molecular Biology (2003); 12 (2) 185-193.

[66] Lehane M.J., Aksoy S., Gibson W., Kerhornou A., Berriman M., Hamilton J., Soares M.B., Bonaldo M.F., Lehane S., Hall N. Adult midgut expressed sequence tags from the tsetse fly *Glossina morsitans morsitans* and expression analysis of putative immune response genes. Genome Biology 2003; 4 R63 1-10.

[67] Loseva O., Engstrom, Y. Analysis of signal-dependent changes in the proteome of Drosophila blood cells during an immune response. Molecular and Cellular Proteomics 2004; 3 796-808.

[68] Vierstraete E., Verleyen P., Baggerman G., D'Hertog W., Van den Bergh G., Arckens L., De Loof A., Schoofs L. A proteomic approach for the analysis of instantly released wound and immune proteins in *Drosophila melanogaster* hemolymph. Proceedings of the National Academy of Sciences USA 2004; 101 470-475.

[69] De Morais Guedes S., Vitorino R., Domingues R., Tomer K., Correia A.J., Amado F., Domingues, P. Proteomics of immune-challenged *Drosophila melanogaster* larvae hemolymph. Biochemical and Biophysical Research Communications 2005; 328 106-115.

[70] Rudenko N., Golovchenko M., Edwards M.J., Grubhoffer L. Differential expression of *Ixodes ricinus* tick genes induced by blood feeding or *Borrelia burgdorferi* infection. Journal of Medical Entomology 2005; 42 36-41.

[71] Dreher-Lesnick S.M., Mulenga A., Simser J.A., Azad A.F. Differential expression of two glutathione S-transferases identified from the American dog tick, *Dermacentor variabilis*. Insect Molecular Biology 2006; 15 445-453.

[72] Kocan K. M., Zivkovic Z., Blouin E. F., Naranjo V., Almazán C., Mitra R., de la Fuente J. Silencing of genes involved in *Anaplasma marginale*-tick interactions affects the pathogen developmental cycle in *Dermacentor variabilis*. BMC Developmental Biology 2009; 9 42-52.

[73] Parizi L.F., Utiumi K.U., Imamura S., Onuma M., Ohashi K., Masuda A., Da Silva Vaz I. Cross immunity with *Haemaphysalis longicornis* glutathione S-transferase reduces an experimental *Rhipicephalus (Boophilus) microplus* infestation. Experimental Parasitology 2011; 127 113–118.

Chapter 12

From Molecular Cloning to Vaccine Development for Allergic Diseases

José Cantillo and Leonardo Puerta

Additional information is available at the end of the chapter

http://dx.doi.org/10.5772/52821

1. Introduction

Allergic diseases are manifested in susceptible individual by exposure to proteins named allergens that induce an immune response mediated by IgE antibody. Numerous allergens from different sources such as plants, insects, mites and mammals have been obtained as recombinant molecules by molecular cloning. These types of molecules have shown molecular, functional and immunological properties similar to the corresponding natural allergens and, therefore, could be used for in vitro and in vivo diagnosis test of allergy. An important step was done with the development of variants of allergens with reduced allergenicity and preserved immunogenicity, which paved the way toward its rational use in allergen specific immunotherapy to treat allergies. Few of the allergens cloned have been developed to a stage at which they are suitable for use in clinical studies. However, today the academic and scientific communities note a broad and important activity to offer in the near future preparations with enhanced clinical efficacy and safety. In this work, basic aspects and experimental and clinical results of this process are presented.

2. Progress in the molecular cloning and production of allergens

The molecular cloning has provided a practical and efficient way to obtain highly purified molecules for different purposes; in the biomedical sciences this is evident by the increasing amount of biological products, obtained by recombinant DNA technology, which are commercially available for diagnosis and treatment of different diseases, as well as the wide variety of reagents for basic research. The era of molecular cloning of allergen molecules was initiated in 1988 with the report of a cDNA clone coding for the allergen Der p 1 isolated from a cDNA library of the house dust mite *Dermatophagoides pteronyssinus,* screened with rabbit anti -Der p 1 antiserum [1, 2]. Latter, Tovey, E.R *et al.* [3], using sera from allergic individuals for screening a mite cDNA library also isolated a clone of Der p 1. This strategy was useful to explore the whole spectrum of IgE binding proteins in a natural source and to isolate positive clones to express the molecules [4, 5]. The development and optimization of technology based on the polymerase chain reaction (PCR), have given an important impulse to cloning and identification of new allergens. PCR can be applied to screen cDNA library and amplify specific clones, or to obtain by RT- PCR the nucleotide sequence coding for specific allergens and then cloning in an appropriate vector for expression [6-10]. The numerous nucleotide sequences of allergens reported in data bank have facilitated the isolation of new allergens from RNA material using PCR technology, avoiding the construction of cDNA library and the use of sera from allergic subjects for screening, which is time consuming [11-14]. An expressed sequence tagging (EST) approach was applied to obtaining a large sampling and overview of expressed genomes of several mite species [15], the EST approach involved the partial sequencing of random clones selected from cDNA libraries, allowing the identification of allergens with homology to genes from more distantly related species or even across taxonomic kingdoms.

The bacteria *E. coli* is the preferred expression system used for the production of recombinant allergens, most of the house dust mite allergens have been expressed in this system with success, allowing the molecular characterization [4, 5, 9, 10, 16-18]. The use of *E. coli* may result in non-functional products expressed in inclusion bodies, and without the post-translational modifications necessaries for their appropriate folding and biologic functions [19]. However, by genetic engineering modified strains of this bacteria and novel expression vectors have been obtained, which allow expression of heterologous protein in soluble form with functional properties and high yield; Origami, Rosetta or BL21(DE3)-CodonPlus-pRIL and Rosetta-gami are strains commercially available for obtain recombinants with some pos-translational modifications [20]. In these *E. coli* strains the expression of allergens from the pollen *Artemisia vulgaris* (Art v 3), the peanut (Ara h 2) and the beta-lactoglobulin from bovine have been obtained in higher yield and solubility, and with structural and immunological properties comparable to native allergens [21-23]. The GST tag used in the expression of the first recombinant allergens have been replace for His x6 tag, which is shorter, the recombinant can be analyzed without removing the tag due to the negligible effect on the properties of the molecule, and several efficient purification systems are commercially available.

The eukaryotic expression system have the capacity of performing many of the post-translational modifications including signal sequences, disulfide bond formation, and addition of lipid and carbohydrates. A variety of eukaryotic expression systems like yeast, insect cells, mammalian cells and plants are available. The yeast *P. pastoris* is easy to manipulate and frequently used to express recombinant molecules with all the characteristics of their natural counterparts, with a yield about 10 to 100 times higher than *E. coli* [24, 25]. Several recombinant allergens have been obtained by expression in this yeast and their biologic properties demonstrated by different methods, this system have resulted especially practical when post-translational modifications or biochemical activity exist [26-29]. The human cells have been used to obtain the *Phleum pretense* allergen, Phl p 5, as a secreted or membrane-anchored protein and showed to be biologically active, with capacity to bind human IgE, to induce mediator release from basophiles and to stimulate T cell proliferation [30]. A large percentage of allergens are from plants, thus the plant-based expression systems are ideal for the production of certain recombinant allergens, which could have problems such as incorrect processing, incorrect folding and insolubility when expressed in bacteria or other non-plant systems. Thaumatin or thaumatin-like proteins, only when expressed in *Nicotiana benthamiana* result in fully IgE-reactive proteins [31]. Interesting, expression in plants offers the opportunity for oral delivery of recombinant allergens of non- plant origin as a therapeutic approach for mucosal immunization for treating allergic diseases. Oral treatment of mice with squash extracts containing virus-expressed Der p 5 allergen caused inhibition of both allergen-specific IgE synthesis and airway inflammation [32], this plant-based edible vaccines is very promising.

3. Current vaccines for allergic diseases

Allergies are inflammatory diseases characterized by a Th2 biased response induced in atopic individuals for exposure to allergens. The Th2 response is also induced by helminthes, which occur in an environment characterized by the presence of IL-4, IL-5 and IL-13. Nuocytes [33, 34], basophiles [35] and type 2 multi-potent progenitor cells [36] seem to be an important source of this cytokines and necessary for the development of allergic response. Allergen-specific IgE antibodies produced by B cells bind to Fc epsilon receptor 1 (FcεRI) on basophiles or mast cells, sensitizing them. After consecutive exposure, allergen binds to IgE on these cells leading to the release of inflammatory mediators of immediate-type symptoms of allergic diseases and paves the way for late-phase inflammatory responses caused by basophiles, eosinophils and T cells. Allergen specific Th1, Th9, Th17 and Treg cells are also produced in this process [37, 38].

Allergen-specific immunotherapy (SIT) is the only curative and specific approach for treatment of allergies [39, 40]. The current SIT consists of gradual administration of increasing amounts of allergenic extract with the aim to avoid allergic symptoms associated to the exposition. The induction of allergen tolerance is the essential immunological mechanisms of SIT, and involve allergen-specific memory T and B-cell that lead to immune tolerance characterized by a specific noninflammatory reactivity to a given allergen and prevention of new sensitizations and progression of allergic disease. During the immunotherapy, different regulatory and effectors components of the immune system are involved (Figure 1). Allergen tolerance is characterized by the generation of two subgroups of Treg cells: FOXP3$^+$ CD4$^+$ CD25$^+$ Treg cells and inducible Treg cells [41]. T-regulatory type 1 (Tr1) cells have shown to play a major role in allergen tolerance induced by SIT [42, 43]. The immunosuppressor mechanism of Treg cells is mediated by the production of high level of anti-inflammatory cytokines IL-10 and TGF-β, although IFN-γ could also be produced [44-46]. The expression of different subtypes of antibodies during SIT is mediated by the activity of regulatory cytokines secreted by Treg cells; IL-10 is a potent suppressor of allergen-specific IgE and simultaneously increases IgG4 production [42]. SIT increase 10 to 100 folds the serum levels of allergen-specific IgG1 and IgG4 [43, 47]. The IgG4 seems to act as a blocking antibody that interacts with the allergen, avoiding interaction of allergen with the IgE [48].

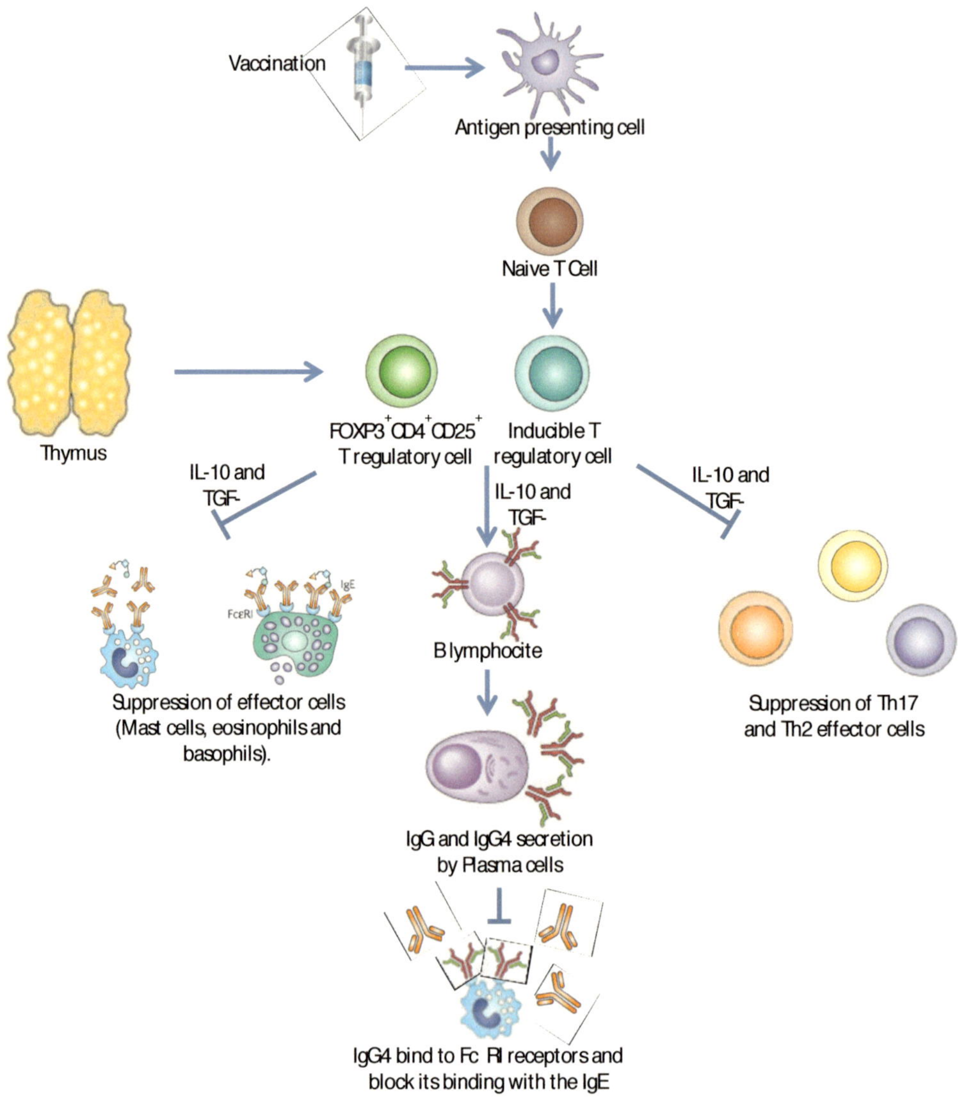

Figure 1. Mechanism of allergen-specific immunotherapy. After vaccination, allergen is taken up by antigen presenting cells leading to the differentiation of naïve T cells to inducible T regulatory cells. These cells with the thymus-derived FOXP3+CD4+CD25+ T regulatory cells, suppress allergic response by the following mechanisms. 1. Suppression of mast cells, eosinophils and basophils. 2. Induction of IgG4 antibodies production from B cells that block the binding of allergen with the IgE. 3. Suppression of effector T cells.

Vaccines composed of whole allergenic extract are complex mixtures of known and unknown material, prepared directly from the allergen source, thus containing allergenic and non-allergenic material and being difficult to standardize [49-51]. Some non-allergenic components have been shown to prime a Th2 response [52], which offset the efficacy of this type of vaccines. SIT with allergenic extract induce a variety of side effects ranging from local to systemic which in some case may be life-threatening [53]. Moreover, in some preparations the important allergens are not well represented or they exhibit poor immunogenicity [51]. Administration of whole allergenic extracts can induce new IgE specificities against allergens present which were not recognized by the patient before treatment [54]. All these facts decrease the efficacy and safety of the current allergen SIT [50]. Therefore, among new approaches to provide a better treatment for allergic diseases is to develop vaccines based on preparations with a well-defined composition, suitable for a good standardization and very low risk of anaphylaxis, here the recombinant allergens or modification of these represent a good option, they show characteristics that could allow to replace advantageously the whole allergenic extracts [55], (Table 1).

Disadvantages of natural allergen extracts
Contain undefined components, some of which may promote allergic responses
Lack or contain low amounts of important allergens
Can be contaminated with unwanted materials or allergens from other sources
Cannot be tailored to the patient's sensitization profile
May induce new sensitizations
Do not suit the international quality standards for vaccines
Cannot be compared between different products or batches
Do not allow the precise monitoring and investigation of mechanisms underlying treatment
Advantages of recombinant allergens
Represent molecules with defined physicochemical and immunologic properties that can be modified to foster advantageous characteristics
Amounts can be easily controlled on the basis of mass units
Potencies and ratios can be exactly adjusted for each molecule
Represents pure molecules
Vaccines can be exactly tailored according to the patient's sensitization profile
Fit the international quality standards for vaccines
Can be precisely compared to give consistent and reproducible products or batches
Allow the precise monitoring and investigation of mechanisms underlying treatment
Can be reproducible modified to suit different treatment strategies

Table 1. Advantages of recombinant allergens over traditional allergen extracts

4. Recombinant allergens for diagnosis and allergen-specific immunotherapy

Recombinant allergens may be obtained with the same structural and immunological properties of its natural equivalent, therefore, the usefulness for diagnosis or immunotherapy is guarantee. These can be expressed in large amounts in *E. coli* or eukaryotic systems at low cost and without contaminants, and manipulating the nucleotide sequence of allergens followed by molecular cloning and protein expression, modified version of allergens that preserve the specific T cell recognition of the natural offending molecule but reduced allergenicity, can be obtained providing a good material for allergen vaccine development.

4.1. Diagnosis of allergy

A more appropriate diagnostic of allergic diseases would be obtained by identification of the particular molecules involved in allergic response, which could be done using purified wild type or recombinant allergens in order to define the sensitization profile of each allergic subject, the concept "Component-resolved diagnosis" was applied to this kind of diagnosis [56], that would allow a "component-resolved immunotherapy", in which only the allergens involved in the sensitization are applied to an allergic subject, avoiding new sensitizations. There are some illustrative examples of the goodness of this future practice: in skin tests with three recombinant cherry allergens, rPru av 1, rPru av 3 and rPru av 4, the diagnosis of allergic population could be obtained with sensitivity similar to that obtained with the allergenic extract [57]. The population allergic to peanut was identified using three recombinant peanut allergens (rAra h 1, rAra h 2 and rAra h 3) [58], in this study and another with celery allergens was demonstrated that recombinant allergens improve the sensitivity of diagnosis compared to allergenic extracts [58, 59]. In allergies with a high compromise of cross-reactivity such as the pollen-related food allergy the power of *in vitro* testing using allergenic extracts is very low [60]. Component resolved diagnosis with recombinant allergens result in excellent sensitivity, when applied to allergy to hazelnut that shows cross-reactivity with pollen allergy. Vespid allergy is characterized by cross-reactivity between hymenoptera species, and it has been established that the true source of sensitization must be defined to ensure the efficacy of venom immunotherapy [61]. Monsalve, *et al.* [62], found that in the Mediterranean regions, a component-resolved diagnosis for wasp allergy could be accurately defined using a mixture of the allergens Ves v 1 and Ves v 5 from Vespula spp, and Pol d 1 and Pol d 5 from *Polistes dominilus*. A combination of these four allergens is enough to differentiate the real causative venom in at least 69% of the population. In allergy with a wide spectrum of sensitization profile as the induced by *Phleum pretense* pollens, the use of recombinants is useful to establish a tailor made immunotherapy approach [63]. A hybrid molecule composed of several segments of a grass pollen allergen showed in skin tests on 32 allergic individuals that with only this molecule all the allergic patients can be identified [64].

The technology of microarrays can be applied to target protein interactions and the serological immune response to antigens [65]. Microarrays are highly useful for detecting all antibodies isotypes and are a powerful tool for component-resolved diagnosis. The primary advantage of microarrays is that specific IgE to thousands allergens can be assayed in parallel with small amounts of serum, at the same time, much less amount of allergen is required. The advantages of protein microarrays to detect specific-antibodies against multiple targets have been taken to develop component-based diagnosis tools. A microarray based test developed by VBC Genomic and Phadia market as "ISAC" that uses a combination of 103 purified natural and recombinant allergens from 47 species, is available in Europe, however, in the United States it has not yet been approved for use by the US Food and Drug Administration and is available only as a research tool (Available at: http://www.pirllab.com/). One of its potentials lies in the recognition of individual patterns of IgE reactivity to protein families with homologues across plant or animal species [66, 67]. When microarray test for diagnosis of birch and timothy allergy were compared with other *in vitro* tests (Phadia CAP-FEIA and in-house ELISA), a correlation greater than 0.9, with high sensitivity and specificity was obtained [68]. Latex allergy diagnosis is well known to be confounded by a high rate of false positive results when using conventional testing, and positive specific IgE results does not always mirror the clinical situation. A combination of recombinant latex allergens (Hev b 1, Hev b 3, Hev b 5 and Hev b 6.02) on a microarray, was enough to detect individuals allergic to latex with a sensitivity of 80%, and allows discrimination between genuine allergy and sensitization [69]. Recently, a library of 419 overlapping peptides corresponding to the aminoacid sequence of peanut allergens Ara h 1, Ara h 2 and Ara h 3, printed onto glass slides to asses IgE reactivity, was evaluated as a diagnostic tool that could replace the traditional used double-blind, placebo controlled food challenge, that is time consuming, expensive, stressful for the patient and have the risk for potentially life-threatening anaphylactic reaction [70, 71]. Based on the number or peptides that bind IgE and the intensity of the reaction, was possible to distinguish peanut allergic and peanut tolerant individuals with approximately 90% sensitivity and 95% specificity [71].

To evaluate the clinical significance and allergenicity of several recombinant allergens from *B. tropicalis* and *D. pteronyssinus* in asthmatic patients from a tropical environment, IgE level were determined in sera from 90 asthmatic patients and 10 healthy controls. In addition, SPT was performed in a selected group of these patients [72]. Three recombinant allergens Der p 1, Der p 2, and Der p 10 were able to detect 93% of *D. pteronyssinus* allergic subjects. No adverse reactions were observed in the allergic or control subjects who were skin tested. We can conclude that recombinant allergens from *B. tropicalis* and *D. pteronyssinus* are useful for *in vitro* and *in vivo* diagnostic tests of mite allergy diseases.

4.2. Allergen-specific immunotherapy

Allergen SIT with recombinant allergens was proposed when it was demonstrated that these molecules have similar or the same biological properties of their natural counterparts [73, 74], and the necessity of highly purified and well standardized allergens were required for overcome the problems related to difficult standardization and management of the doses observed with the whole allergenic extracts. A study with the recombinant pollen allergen Bet v 1 (rBet v 1) demonstrated that immunotherapy with a single allergen is effective for the specific treatment of allergy [75]. In a multicenter, double-blind, placebo-controlled clinical trial, patients with history of birch pollen–related rhinoconjunctivitis were divided in four groups and treated for two years with rBet v 1, natural birch pollen extract, natural Bet v 1 (nBet v 1) or placebo, to compare the efficacy of each preparation for allergen-specific immunotherapy. Treatment with rBet v 1 reduced symptoms of rhinoconjunctivitis and skin reactivity induced by birch pollen, and showed to be safety without serious adverse events. In contrast, one adverse event appears in the group treated with nBet v 1. Clinical improvement and reduction of sensitivity were accompanied with marked increase in Bet v 1-specific IgG1, IgG2 and IgG4 levels, which were higher in the rBet v 1-treated group than in nBet v 1-treated group. Importantly, new IgE specificities were induced in 3 patients treated with birch pollen extract, but in none of rBet v 1 or nBet v 1 treated patients.

In a placebo controlled immunotherapy study, a mixture of equimolar concentration of five *Phleum pretense* allergens (Phl p 1, Phl p 2, Phl p 5a, Phl p 5b and Phl p 6) was administered via subcutaneous for 18 months in patients with grass pollen–induced allergic rhinitis, to determining efficacy and safety [43]. The immunotherapy showed a 36.5% lower median average symptom score for active treatment compared with placebo and reduction in the need for medication. By the first and second pollen season, improvement in quality of life scores was present in the patients receiving active treatment. Active treatment induced IgG1 concentrations approximately 60-fold, peaking during the rusty 12 months of the study and IgG4 levels showed a 4000 fold increase by the end of treatment. In contrast, after immunotherapy IgE levels in the active treated group were significantly lower than placebo group. Only about 1% of recombinant grass allergen injections led to systemic reactions. This was the first clinical study of immunotherapy with a cocktail of 5 recombinant grass pollen allergens that showed its clinical efficacy, good tolerance and strong induction of allergen specific IgG antibody response.

5. Approaches for an immunotherapy of allergy based on modified recombinant allergens

Several *in vitro* and *in vivo* assays indicate that allergy vaccines based on recombinant allergens might have provide a safe and efficacious immunotherapy. However, recombinants with the same amino acid sequence and similar allergenic activity as the natural allergens can elicit IgE-mediated side effects, which are a major risk during allergen-specific immunotherapy. To overcome this problem different approach have been designed to obtain molecules without or reduced IgE reactivity [76]. Recombinant DNA technology has allowed the rational design and production of well-defined modified allergens for this purpose. Hypo-allergens are molecules derived from wild type allergen which exhibits reduced capacity to react with IgE antibodies and low ability to induce IgE-mediated mast cells or basophile degranulation. They are designed to reduce the risk of anaphylaxis during the course of immunotherapy, are molecules with conserved T-cell epitopes that could be recognized by specific T lymphocytes to induce a protective response against wild-type allergen.

Some allergens are present in the nature as a mix of several isoforms with high structural homology but different IgE reactivity. The production by molecular cloning of natural isoforms with low IgE reactivity has been used to propose anti-allergy vaccines. Bet v 1.0401 and Bet v 1.1001 are isoforms that have lower IgE reactivity compared to the Bet v 1.0101 [77, 78]. Antibody response against Bet v 1.0401 is IgG4-specific and has low capacity to induce basophile degranulation [79].

Hypo-allergens obtained by site-directed mutagenesis

The availability of multiple clones of recombinant allergens has facilitated the implementation of site directed mutagenesis to obtain modified allergens for a better immunotherapy. There are several examples of this approach that illustrate the potential use for the development of new vaccines. Mouse allergic individuals are sensitized mainly against the major allergen Mus m 1 a urinary protein belonging to the lipocalin superfamily which have typicall β-barrel fold, that can be modified by mutation in the Tyr 120 residue, [80, 81]. Two hypo-allergenic variants of this allergen; mutants 1Y120A, and Mus m 1-Y120F were expressed in *P. pastoris* with a modified fold [82]. The mutants showed low capacity to react with IgE from allergic individuals and induced lower basophil degranulation than those induced by Mus m 1. In lymphoproliferation assays, using cells from mouse allergic individuals the mutants induced similar lymphoproliferation to that induced by Mus m 1. In other study three variants of an allergen from Artemisia (Art v 1), C22S, C47S and C49S [83], showed low IgE reactivity and mediator release from RBL cells. In addition, the variants C49S and C22S induced significantly higher T cell proliferative response in Artemisia allergic patients compared to the obtained with rArt v 1, suggesting a potential utility for the immunotherapy of population allergic to Artemisia. Using a different approach; mutations in residues involved in IgE binding but maintaining the 3D structure of the natural allergen, Spangforth et al. showed that mutants Gln45-Ser and Pro108-Gly of allergen Bet v 1 displayed lower IgE reactivity and induced synthesis of IgG antibodies that block the IgE reactivity against the natural Bet v1 [84]. Unlike the above mentioned studies. The x-ray crystallography structures of the mutants were similar to the natural allergen, indicating that the reduced IgE reactivity is not mediated by an inadequate folding.

Hybrid proteins

Hybrid proteins are structures composed by two or more allergens or short portions of them in only one molecule, in this way new interaction and bonds are generated, which may alter the 3D structure and B epitopes characteristic of natural allergens. Decreasing the capacity of IgE binding and mast cell degranulation. However, if these proteins conserve the T cell epitopes, they could induce a protective response after allergen challenge. A single molecule composed by different allergen polypeptides might reduce the number of molecules to be included in the vaccine. Furthermore, hybrid molecules consisting of several copies of homologous allergens or immunologically unrelated allergens could be used for the allergy treatment in the patients who are sensitized to several allergens.

T. P. King, who constructed a molecule composed by two allergens from insect and demonstrated *in vitro* and mice models studies its anti-allergenic properties [85], pioneered the design of hybrid proteins for allergen immunotherapy. Gonzales-Rioja *et al.* [86] obtained by PCR-based engineering a molecule composed by two allergens from the pollen *Parietaria judaica*

(Par j 1 and Par j 2) and demonstrated an important reduction of the IgE binding capacity by skin prick test. Linhart *et al.* [87], constructed by PCR-based recombination, a nucleotide sequence coding for principal allergens of timothy grass, Phl p 1, Phl p 2, Phl p 5 and Phl p 6. The hybrid protein induced T cell proliferation similar to the equimolar mix of individual allergens, the lymphocytes secreted regulatory and Th1 cytokines, IL-10 and IFN-γ, showing capacity to induce immune deviation to a protective profile. In an allergic mouse model, exposure to hybrid molecule induced the production of IgG that blocked mast degranulation. However, this molecule was also capable to bind IgE from allergic individuals, and to induce basophile degranulation, and high percentage of individuals allergic to timothy grass were identified using this molecule, suggesting a potential as a diagnosis reagent.

The utility of hybrid proteins for the immunotherapy of house dust mite allergy have been studied by Asturias, *et al.* [88], who designed two hybrid proteins composed by *D. pteronyssinus* allergens Der p 1 and Der p 2. The QM1 structure was composed of almost the whole sequence of both allergens; a Der p 2-fragment from residues 5 to 123 at the N-terminus, introducing point mutations on cysteine 8 and 119 to serine to avoid the formation of a disulphide bridge, and a Der p 1-fragment from residues 4 to 222 at the C-terminus were joined. The QM2 structure, was composed with the residues 1 to 73 and 74 to 129 of Der p 2, linked to residues 5 to 222 of Der p 1. Western-blot assays with a serum pool from house dust mite allergic patients showed decrease IgE reactivity of QM1, while QM2 showed no detectable IgE binding capacity. The hypoallergenic properties of both hybrids were demonstrated by skin tests. In vitro test with sample from allergic patients QM2 induced similar lymphoproliferation that the induced by natural Der p 1 and Der p 2, whereas, QM1 induced higher proliferation. It was demonstrated that antisera raised by immunization of mice with QM1 or QM2 lead to the production of specific antibodies capable of blocking the binding of IgE reactivity to natural allergens.

Recently, a hybrid protein composed of three allergens of *Chenopodium album* pollen, in the order Che a 3-Che a 1-Che a 2, was constructed by using overlapping extension polymerase chain reaction, expressed in *E. coli* BL21-CodonPlus(DE3)-RIL, to obtain a 46 kDa protein. Sera from allergic patients showed lower IgE binding affinity to the hybrid molecule than the mixture of recombinant allergens and the *C. album* pollen extract. Most of the allergic patients showed positive skin test to a mixture of the three allergens, however, when tested with the hybrid molecule allergic patients showed negative test or highly reduced weal area compared to the mixture or to the pollen extract [89].

Mosaic proteins

Mosaic proteins are constituted by different segments of the same allergen, in different order as they are present in the native molecule, such re-arrange generate new intra-molecular interactions that alter B cell epitopes. A mosaic protein called P1m constructed with four segments of the pollen allergen Phl p 1, showed lower IgE reactivity compared to the natural allergen and was unable to induce histamine release from basophiles of allergic individuals. However, this molecule conserved capacity to induce the proliferation of PBMCs. Immunized rabbits expressed IgG antibodies that blocked the binding of Phl p 1 to the IgE and inhibit histamine release from basophiles obtained from allergic individuals [90]. Other mosaic protein constructed with segments derived from Phl p 2 reassembled in altered order and expressed as a trimer showed absence of IgE reactivity with sera from allergic patients. Basophile activation and skin prick tests, showed reduction of the allergenicity of this molecule compared to recombinant Phl p 2. Furthermore, IgG antibodies produced by immunized mice were able to inhibit the binding of recombinant Phl p 2 to the IgE from allergic subjects [91]. Mosaic proteins have been studied as a potential vaccine for immunotherapy of birch allergy [92] and house dust mite allergy [93]. A mosaic protein composed of reorganized segments of Bet v 1 preserved the specific T cell epitopes and showed approximately 100-fold reduced allergenic activity compared with recombinant Bet v 1 [94, 95] and induced specific IgG antibodies inhibitors of IgE reactivity to Bet v1 of sera from patients with pollen allergy [96]. The mosaic protein exhibited none IgE reactivity and lower basophile activation. Furthermore, immunization with Bet v 1 derivatives induced IgG antibodies that recognized Bet v 1 and inhibited IgE binding to Bet v 1 [92].

Fragments of allergens or modification of these, might be poorly immunogenic because they don′t have enough T cell epitopes capable to stimulate a protective immune response. An increase of immunogenicity can be obtained when proteins are made as oligomers which enhance the number of T cell epitopes in the molecule. It has been observed that immunogenicity of Bet v1 increase when obtained as oligomer [97, 98]. By dot-blot analysis and lymphoproliferative responses in PBMCs from birch pollen allergic patients, trimers of re-organized segments of Bet v1 had lower capacity to bind IgE and enhanced capacity to stimulate lymphoproliferation. The CD203c expression analysis showed reduced allergenicity of these oligomers, and when administrated to mice in an immunization scheme, induced the production of high titer of IgG1 antibody, that inhibited human IgE binding to wild type Bet v 1 [99].

5.1. Molecules to target specific compartments or receptors

Targeting allergens to endoplasmic reticulum

It has been suggested that administration of higher allergen doses enhances the efficacy of immunotherapy [100]. However, administration of high doses increases the risk of anaphylaxis. One approach to overcome this problem is to deliver high doses of allergen to B and T cells directly, thus providing higher effective doses to stimulate a protective response, and avoiding the interaction of allergen with IgE antibodies [101]. An allergen vaccine for cat allergy composed of the major cat allergen Fel d 1 fused to the HIV-derived translocation peptide TAT was designed to mediate cytoplasmic uptake of extracellular proteins [102, 103]. Un modified version of this approach, denominated Modular Antigen Translocation (MAT) technology have been developed [104, 105], which consists of allergen fused to a peptide, to direct them to the cytosol, and a truncated human invariant chain (Ii), to target the protein to MHC class II heterodimers assembled in the endoplasmic reticulum and thus circumventing phagosomal uptake and degradation. The allergens Asp f 1, Der p 1, Bet v 1, PLA2 and Fel d 1 fused to MAT, induced lymphoproliferation of PBMCs stimulated *ex vivo* with low allergen doses, induced the secretion of Th1 type cytokines and IL-10, and inhibit the production of Th2 cytokines [105]. The cat allergen Fel d 1 fused to MAT (MAT- Fel d 1) when administered directly to the inguinal lymph nodes of allergic mice, showed capacity to stimulate the production of high levels of IFN-γ and reduced levels of IL-4, compared to unmodified Fel d 1. Immunized mice expressed higher levels of IgG2a and showed protection against the challenge of high doses of allergenic extract. Furthermore, MAT-Fel d 1 produced 100-fold less degranulation and histamine release from basophiles compared to unmodified Fel d 1 [106].

Targeting allergens to receptors on dendritic cells

Dendritic cells (DCs) play an important role in the initiation and maintenance of T cell response to allergens. Its role in the type of T cell response generated can be influenced by the maturation state, while mature DCs induce effector T cell responses characterized by Th1 or Th2 response [107], immature or semi-mature DCs are tolerogenic and have the ability to induce Tregs [108]. DCs express an array of Fc receptors which have the capacity to enhance allergen uptake through internalization of allergen/antibody receptors complexes. When stimulated with allergen, DCs express FcεRI, and activated a signal-transducing cascade involving immunoreceptor tyrosine-based activation motif (ITAM), which result in increased production of proinflammatory cytokines and chemokines, the induction of robust proliferation of allergen-specific T cells and the development of allergic symptoms [109]. DCs also express the receptor FcγRIIb that contains immunoreceptor tyrosine-based inhibition motif (ITIM) which induces inhibitory signaling events. This receptor can co-aggregate with FcεRI that activating a signaling cascade that culminates in inhibition of FcεRI signaling. Under these assumptions, Zhu, D. *et al.* [110] designed a fusion molecule called GFD composed by a human IgG Fc fragment linked to the allergen Fel d 1 by a flexible linker, with the aim to crosslink FcγRIIb and FcεRI-bounded to the cat specific-IgE. In transgenic mice expressing human FcγRIIb and FcεRI, sensitized with high doses of Fel d 1 specific-IgE and treated with several doses of GFD, the challenge with Fel d 1 didn´t cause mast cell degranulation. A scheme of immunotherapy with high doses of GFD resulted in the inhibition of allergic response against Fel d 1, pulmonary inflammation and skin reactivity in sensitized animals. Treated mice expressed IgG1 antibodies that blocked the binding of IgE to Fel d 1. When applied to mice sensitized to Fel d 1 in a scheme of rush immunotherapy, GFD blocked acute systemic allergic reaction, mast cell degranulation, bronquial hyper-reactivity and pulmonary inflammation [111]. Recently, a fusion protein composed of Fcγ chain and the *Dermatophagoides farina*e allergen, Der f 2, was obtained and tested in a Der f 2 allergic murine model [112]. After treatment with the fusion molecule, the levels of specific IgE to Der f 2, histamine and pro-inflammatory cytokines were lowered in the Fcγ-Der f 2 treated allergic mice, compared to saline-treated allergic mice. These results suggest that specific targeting of allergens to Fcγ receptors could be used as a strategy in the development of antigen-specific immunotherapy for human allergic diseases.

A different molecular design was applied to target allergens to CD64 receptor on antigen presenting cells; a fusion protein (H22-Fel d 1) composed by Fel d 1 linked to the variable region of a monoclonal antibody anti-CD64 was designed to stimulate receptor internalization [113]. Flow cytometry analysis showed that H22-Fel d 1 binds to CD64 and reacted with IgE and IgG with similar affinity compared to native allergen. *In vitro* assays demonstrated that the fusion molecule stimulates the proliferation of T lymphocytes derived from allergic individuals and the secretion of IL-5, IL-10 and IFN-γ [114]. Although H22-Fel d 1 is responsible of a positive effect that could result in a protective response against allergen challenge, it also stimulated

Th2 cytokines, in a mechanism in which the thymic stromal lymphopoietin (TSLP) cytokine seems to be involved. This cytokine was shown to maintain and polarize circulating Th2 central memory cells, including allergen-specific T cells [115]. Therefore, the usefulness of this kind of preparation for allergy immunotherapy deserves further evaluation.

6. Insect sting allergy

Insect sting allergy are frequently caused by insect stings of the Apidae family (honeybees and bumblebees), those from the Vespidae family (Vespula, Dolichovespula, Vespa and Polistes genera) and, in some regions, also of the Formicidae family (ants). The sting can induce local or systemic IgE-mediated hypersensitivity reactions that can be fatal [116]. Prevalence of systemic reactions caused by insect stings are reported from 0,3% to 7,5% in the United States and Europe [117, 118]. Up to one fifth of these subjects will eventually experience severe life-threatening reactions. Hymenoptera venoms contain protein allergens, as well as non-allergenic components, including toxins, vasoactive amines, acetylcholine, and kinins. Among the multiple allergens in Hymenoptera venoms, two allergens are importan, the phospholipase A2 from of honey bee (*Apis mellifera*) (Api m 1), and of the vespid venoms antigen 5 from *Vespula vulgaris* (common wasp) denominated Ves v 5.

Several studies have demonstrated that immunotherapy for vespid allergy with venom extracts is clinically effective and improve the quality of life and allergic symptoms. This improvement is correlated to a significant decrease of total IgE levels, and increase in specific IgG and IgG4 levels [119]. However, severe and life-threatening anaphylactic side effects may be induced after the administration of crude allergen extracts [120].

One of the first attempts to obtain safer methods for immunotherapy of insect allergies was made with allergen-derived peptides, containing T-cell epitopes. Peptides derived from the bee allergen Api m 1, were applied to allergic individuals in different immunotherapy schemes. *In* vitro and clinical phase trials showed that T cells from such patients showed marked responsiveness to Api m 1 after long term treatment, a shift in the pattern of cytokine secretion form a Th0 to a Th1 profile and increase in specific IgG4 levels [121-123].

The use of recombinant venom allergens for allergen specific immunotherapy has been analyzed in animal models. Intranasal administration of the recombinant allergen from wasp venom, rVes v 5, to mice prior to sensitization with natural allergens lead to a significant reduction of the allergic reaction, reduction of specific IgE and IgG2a levels, increase of mRNA levels of IL-10 and TGF-β. Pretreatment with the whole venom was less effective and caused toxic side reactions, suggesting a favorable use of the recombinant protein [124]. Hybrid proteins composed by allergens from bee venom have shown anti-allergenic properties in *in vitro* and animal models [85]. A fusion protein composed of the two major bee venom allergens Api m 1 and Api m 2 called Api m [1/2], showed reduced IgE reactivity of Api m [1/2] compared with native allergens [125]. By the other hand, basophil degranulation and skin tests showed that this fusion protein have hypo-allergenic properties. When applied subcutaneously, mice showed reduced specific IgE, IgG and IgG2 serum levels; demonstrating that such protein represents a potential candidate for specific immunotherapy.

Naturally occurring variants of insect allergens could be also useful for specific immunotherapy. For example, the sting of *Polybia scutellaris*, a South American wasp, does not cause allergic symptoms, however it has been proven that its venom contain Antigen 5 (Poly s 5), an analogue of the allergen Pol s 5 [126, 127]. In mice, Poly s 5 induced IgG antibodies that cross react with Pol a 5, but induced only minimal amounts of IgE and was poor inducer of basophil-mediator release. Moreover, Poly s 5-specific serum showed a specific protective activity and was able to inhibit Pol a 5-induced basophil degranulation [128].

Despite the promising results observed with recombinant and modified allergens in *in vitro* and *in vivo* studies, more clinical phase studies need to be performed to demonstrate their applicability for the allergen specific immunotherapy of insect allergy.

7. Recombinant allergy vaccines in clinical phase trials

Clinical trials with recombinant wild type allergens, and modified allergens have been performed (Table 2). The first studies of allergen SIT with purified molecules were done with peptides containing T cell epitopes either from the cat allergen Fel d 1 or from bee-venom-derived phospholipase, administered without adjuvant [122, 123, 129-135]. Such peptides were characterized by its low or none IgE binding capacity. However, they induced late phase systemic side effects in different grades depending in the dose and route of administration [129, 132, 134, 135]. Therapy with T cell peptides does not seem to influence IgE-mediated allergic reactions, in fact, the majority of studies didn't find evidence of changes in IgE levels or IgE-mediated allergic inflammation furthermore, no induction of IgG response was noted.

Allergic patients under immunotherapy with hypoallergenic preparations of the major birch pollen allergen Bet v 1 adsorbed to aluminum hydroxide as a pre-seasonal treatment for birch pollen allergy in a clinical trial, expressed high levels of IgG1, IgG2 and IgG4 antibodies directed against Bet v 1. These IgG antibodies blocked allergen-induced basophile degranulation and were associated with the ability of patients to tolerate higher allergen concentrations in nasal provocation tests [136]. Immunotherapy with wild-type recombinant Bet v 1 has also been examined for tablet-based sublingual immunotherapy in a phase II, multicenter, double-blind, placebo-controlled, however, this study is still on course and only have been reported good tolerability of the preparation with no serious adverse events and most side effects observed locally [137].

In a clinical trial, a group of patients with grass pollen allergy was treated with a combination of the major grass pollen allergens (Phl p 1, Phl p 2, Phl p 5a, Phl p 5b and Phl p 6) or with placebo for subcutaneous immunotherapy [43]. Patients treated with the recombinants improve their symptom medication score and had high IgG antibodies levels against natural grass pollen allergens. Several studies of immunotherapy with these mixed allergens have been performed and registered in the National Institutes of Health Clinical trial database (Table

http://dx.doi.org/10.5772/52821

2). Recently, the immunomodulatory properties of MAT-Fel d 1 was studied in a phase I/IIa clinical study [138]. In a randomized double blind trial, intralymphatic immunotherapy (ILIT) with MAT-Fel d 1 in alum was compared with placebo, consisting in 3 injections of each preparation for two months. MAT-Fel d 1 caused reduced skin reactions compared to equimolar concentration of nFel d 1 by intradermal injection, which proved practically painless and reduced drug-related adverse effects compared to placebo group. The IgG4 serum levels in MAT-Fel d 1 treated group increased by a factor of 5.66, while IgG1 and IgE levels didn′t change. After treatment, PBMCs from allergic individuals secreted higher levels of IL-10 when challenged with rFel d 1. Immunotherapy with MAT-Fel d 1 showed to be successful because patients increased their tolerance to nasal challenge, skin prick and dermal test, with cat dander extract. Improvement of quality of life of patients treated with MAT-Fel d 1 was maintained 300 days after immunotherapy.

Allergen	Allergen-based vaccine	Rout of administration/Trials	Year	NIH Registration number / Reference
Bet v 1 (Birch pollen allergen)	Bet v 1 trimer	SCIT, DBPC, Phase II	2000	[125]
	Bet v 1 fragments	SCIT, DBPC, Phase II	2000	[125]
	Bet v 1 folding variant	SCIT, OC, Phase II	2002	NCT00266526
		SCIT, DBPC, Phase III	2004	NCT00309062
		SCIT, DBPC, Phase III	2007	NCT00554983
		SCIT, Immunological and histological evaluation	2009	NCT00841516
	Recombinant Bet v 1	SCIT, DBPC, Phase II	2002	NCT00410930
		SLIT, Phase I	2006	NCT00396149
		SLIT, Phase I	2007	NCT00889460
		SLIT, DBPC, Phase II	2008	NCT00901914
Birch pollen and apple allergens	Bet v 1 / Mal d 1	SCIT, DBPC, Phase II	2011	NCT01449786
Phleum pratense allergens	Mix: Phl p 1, Phl p 2, Phl p 5a, Phl p 5b and Phl p 6	SCIT, DBPC, Phase II	2002	
		SCIT, DBPC, Phase III	2004	NCT00309036
		SCIT, DBPC, Phase II	2008	NCT0671268
		SCIT, DBPC, Phase III	2009	NCT01353755
	Phleum pratense peptide fused to carries protein	SCIT, Phase II	2011	NCT01445002
		SCIT, DBPC, Phase IIb	2012 (Initiating)	NCT01538979
Peanut allergens	Modified Ara h 1, Ara h 2, Ara h 3	Rectal	2009	NCT00850668

NCT numbers identify the trials that are registered in the National Institutes of Health Clinical trial database.

DBPC, Double-blind, placebo-controlled; OC, open controlled; SCIT, subcutaneous immunotherapy; SLIT, sublingual immunotherapy.

Table 2. Currently ongoing recombinant molecules development for allergen specific immunotherapy.

The National Institutes of Health's clinical trial database contain information about a study that intends to use the recombinant modified peanut allergens Ara h 1, Ara h 2 and Ara h 3 encapsulated in heat/phenol-killed *E.coli*. This phase I study should recruit healthy volunteers to receive four scaling doses of the peanut preparation rectally at weekly intervals. The major allergen of ragweed pollen *Ambrosia artemisifolia,* Amb a 1, was conjugated to CpG oligonucleotides to reduce the allergenic activity of Am b a 1 and to shift the specific Th2 response to a Th1 response, mediated by the binding of CpG with toll-like receptor 9. Allergic individuals treated with the conjugated vaccine showed reduction in eosinophilia and the number of IL-4-producing cells, and increased numbers of IFN-γ-producing cells compared to placebo-treated patients [139]. Furthermore, increase of regulatory T cells infiltration in the nasal mucosa was found after the course of immunotherapy [140].

8. Some considerations for a recombinant based mite allergy vaccine

The prevalence and severity of allergic diseases such as asthma and rhinitis have increased in recent decades [141], and house dust mite allergy is one of the most common allergies worldwide which affect more than 50% of allergic patients [142]. Several house dust mites species co-exist in tropical and subtropical regions, however in these places the species *B. tropicalis* and *D. pteronyssinus* are the most prevalent and a high percentage of allergic population is sensitized to allergens from these two species [143, 144], [72, 145]. Analysis if house dust mite extracts have shown that over 20 different proteins can induce IgE antibodies in allergic populations and several of them show cross-reactivity with allergens from other mite species. Most of them have been obtained and characterized by molecular cloning and its IgE reactivity analyzed [4]. However, it has been suggested that the majority of mite-allergic subjects elicit an IgE response to around five components of allergenic extracts [146, 147], and some of them may be cross-reactive. Therefore, and admixture of few allergens, including those species-specific and cross-reactive, could replace the crude allergenic extract for diagnostic and therapeutic purpose. Several studies indicate that a combination of allergens from group 1 and 2 bind to more than 50% of specific-IgE from allergic population, groups 5 and 7 are next in importance [148-150]. It has been reported from Middle Europe that more than 95% of mite allergic patients were mainly sensitized to Der p 1 and Der p 2, and that diagnostic test containing these allergens plus the highly cross-reactive allergen Der p 10 may improve the diagnostic selection of patients for immunotherapy with *D. pteronyssinus* extracts [151]. Other allergens are important given their cross-reactivity and the role that they play in tropical populations, as the case of group 10 and 12 [16, 152]. Results from our research group suggested that a combination of these allergens from D. pteronyssinus might be sufficient to identify almost all our mite allergic population [72] (Figure 2).

Recent studies with hybrid proteins composed by the most important pollen allergens, have suggested that preparations based on molecules containing the B-epitope spectrum of allergenic extracts could be useful for the diagnosis and allergen-specific immunotherapy [64, 86, 87]. We have engineered several fusion proteins composed by segments of different allergens of *B. tropicalis* and *D. pteronyssinus* with the aim to obtain preparations useful for the diagnosis and immunotherapy of allergies caused by house dust mites. The coding sequences of each molecule was cloned into expression vectors and then expressed in *E. coli* fused to 6xHis tag for further purification by affinity chromatography. One of these proteins denominated DPx4, consistent of different segments of allergens from *D. pteronyssinus* (Der p 1, Der p 2, Der p 7 and Der p 10), showed a 41% frequency of IgE reactivity in sera from mite allergic patients sensitized to *D. pteronyssinus* and the specific IgE levels against the recombinant were significantly lower than those against the whole allergenic extract from mites. Basophil activation test showed that DPx4 has lower capacity to induce basophile degranulation compared to the allergenic extract. These results suggest that the fusion protein have a hypoallergenic profile, and that is a good candidate for develop a vaccine with potential use for allergen specific immunotherapy of mite allergy [153]. Further *in vitro* studies as well as experiment with animal models are in progress to support this application.

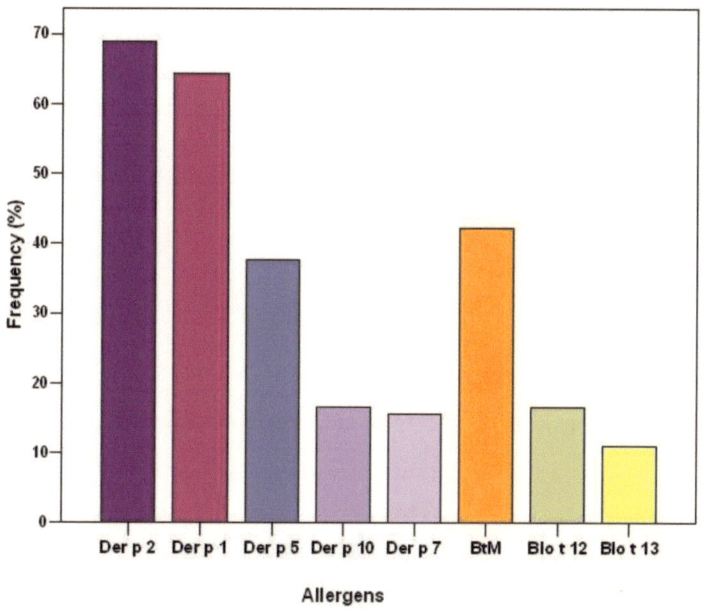

Figure 2. Frequency of IgE reactivity to allergens from *B. tropicalis and D. pteronyssinus* in asthmatic patients (From Ref 72).

9. Conclusions

For several years the allergen-specific immunotherapy has been successfully done with natural allergenic extracts. However, they are complex mixtures difficult to standardize that might cause local or systemic reactions, compromising the patient's life. In the last decades, the molecular cloning applied to the study of allergens has allowed obtaining several recombinant allergens from different sources, and their biological and molecular properties elucidated.

Component based diagnosis and immunotherapy is now possible by the availability of several recombinant allergens, which represents the best approach to achieve the most efficacious diagnosis and treatment of allergies, based on the sensitization profile and of each patient. Vaccines for allergic diseases based on recombinant allergens or modification of these, that could modulate the immune response against natural allergens toward a protective response, have been proposed. Hypoallergenic molecules obtained by molecular cloning, in different versions like hybrid molecules, oligomers, mosaic proteins or variants obtained by site-directed mutagenesis have been developed and studied by in vitro test, animal model and clinical trial in humans, indicating potential beneficial use in the near future. Recombinant allergens coupled to carriers for directing the molecule to specific cells or intracellular compartments, preventing unwanted side effects and increasing the specificity of the immune response have been explored.

The promising results showed by *in vitro* and animal models studies have encouraged the design of clinical phase trials where recombinant allergens have demonstrated their good potential to provide a more efficacious and safe diagnosis and allergen-specific immunotherapy. In the last years, the number of clinical phase trials designed and registered in the National Institutes of Health Clinical trial database is increasing. This tendency suggests that in few years several vaccines based on recombinant allergens could be commercially available in replacement of the traditional allergenic extract.

Acknowledgements

Supported by the Colciencias and University of Cartagena, Colombia. Grant No. 385-2009.

Author details

José Cantillo and Leonardo Puerta*

*Address all correspondence to: lpuertall@yahoo.com

Institute for Immunological Research, University of Cartagena, Colombia

References

[1] Thomas WR, Stewart GA, Simpson RJ, Chua KY, Plozza TM, Dilworth RJ, et al. Cloning and expression of DNA coding for the major house dust mite allergen Der p 1 in Escherichia coli. Int Arch Allergy Appl Immunol 1988;85(1):127-9.

[2] Chua KY, Stewart GA, Thomas WR, Simpson RJ, Dilworth RJ, Plozza TM, et al. Sequence analysis of cDNA coding for a major house dust mite allergen, Der p 1. Homology with cysteine proteases. J Exp Med 1988 Jan 1;167(1):175-82.

[3] Tovey ER, Johnson MC, Roche AL, Cobon GS, Baldo BA. Cloning and sequencing of cDNA expressing a recombinant house dust mite protein that binds human IgE and correspond to an important low molecular weight allergen. J Exp Med 1989;170:1457-62.

[4] Thomas WR, Smith WA, Hales BJ, Mills KL, O'Brien MR. Characterization and immunobiology of house dust mite allergens. Int Arch Allergy Immunol 2002;129:1-18.

[5] Puerta L, Caraballo L, Fernandez-Caldas E, Avjioglu A, Marsh DG, Lockey RF, et al. Nucleotide sequence analysis of a complementary DNA coding for a Blomia tropicalis allergen. J Allergy Clin Immunol 1996 Nov;98(5 Pt 1):932-7.

[6] Cui Y, Zhou Y, Shi W, Ma G, Yang L, Wang Y, et al. Molecular cloning, expression, sequence analyses of dust mite allergen Der f 6 and its IgE-binding reactivity with mite allergic asthma patients in southeast China. Mol Biol Rep 2012 Feb;39(2):961-8.

[7] An S, Chen L, Wei JF, Yang X, Ma D, Xu X, et al. Purification and characterization of two new allergens from the venom of Vespa magnifica. PLoS One 2011;7(2):e31920.

[8] An S, Ma D, Wei JF, Yang X, Yang HW, Yang H, et al. A novel allergen Tab y 1 with inhibitory activity of platelet aggregation from salivary glands of horseflies. Allergy 2011 Nov;66(11):1420-7.

[9] Caraballo L, Avjioglu A, Marrugo J, Puerta L, Marsh D. Cloning and expression of complementary DNA coding for an allergen with common antibody-binding specificities with three allergens of the house dust mite Blomia tropicalis. J Allergy Clin Immunol 1996 Sep;98(3):573-9.

[10] Caraballo L, Puerta L, Jimenez S, Martinez B, Mercado D, Avjiouglu A, et al. Cloning and IgE binding of a recombinant allergen from the mite Blomia tropicalis, homologous with fatty acid-binding proteins. Int Arch Allergy Immunol 1997 Apr;112(4): 341-7.

[11] Acevedo N, Sanchez J, Erler A, Mercado D, Briza P, Kennedy M, et al. IgE cross-reactivity between Ascaris and domestic mite allergens: the role of tropomyosin and the nematode polyprotein ABA-1. Allergy 2009 Nov;64(11):1635-43.

[12] An S, Chen L, Wei JF, Yang X, Ma D, Xu X, et al. Purification and characterization of two new allergens from the venom of Vespa magnifica. PLoS One 2012;7(2):e31920.

[13] Ayuso R, Grishina D, Bardina L, Carrillo T, Blanco C, Dolores Ibáñez M, et al. Myosin light chain is a novel shrimp allergen, Lit v 3. J Allergy Clin Immunol 2008;122:795-802.

[14] Garcia-Orozco KD, Aispuro-Hernandez E, Yepiz-Plascencia G, Calderon-de-la-Barca AM, Sotelo-Mundo RR. Molecular characterization of arginine kinase, an allergen from the shrimp Litopenaeus vannamei. Int Arch Allergy Immunol 2007;144(1):23-8.

[15] Angus A, Ong S, Chew FT. Sequence Tag catalog of Dust mite-expressed genomes. Am J Pharmacogenomics 2004;4:357-69.

[16] Yi FC, Cheong N, Shek PC, Wang DY, Chua KY, Lee BW. Identification of shared and unique immunoglobulin E epitopes of the highly conserved tropomyosins in Blomia tropicalis and Dermatophagoides pteronyssinus. Clin Exp Allergy 2002 Aug; 32(8):1203-10.

[17] Mora C, Flores I, Montealegre F, Diaz A. Cloning and expression of Blo t 1, a novel allergen from de dust mite Blomia tropicalis, homologous to the cysteine proteases. Clin Exp Allergye 2003;33:28-34.

[18] Puerta L. Obtención y caracterización de un novel alergeno mediante la tecnologia del ADN recombinante Rev Acad Colomb Cienc 2001;25(94):77-87.

[19] Villaverde A, Carrio MM. Protein aggregation in recombinant bacteria: biological role of inclusion bodies. Biotechnol Lett 2003 Sep;25(17):1385-95.

[20] Cassland P, Larsson S, Nilvebrant NO, Jonsson LJ. Heterologous expression of barley and wheat oxalate oxidase in an E. coli trxB gor double mutant. J Biotechnol 2004 Apr 8;109(1-2):53-62.

[21] Lehmann K, Hoffmann S, Neudecker P, Suhr M, Becker WM, Rosch P. High-yield expression in Escherichia coli, purification, and characterization of properly folded major peanut allergen Ara h 2. Protein Expr Purif 2003 Oct;31(2):250-9.

[22] Ponniah K, Loo TS, Edwards PJ, Pascal SM, Jameson GB, Norris GE. The production of soluble and correctly folded recombinant bovine beta-lactoglobulin variants A and B in Escherichia coli for NMR studies. Protein Expr Purif 2010 Apr;70(2):283-9.

[23] Gadermaier G, Harrer A, Girbl T, Palazzo P, Himly M, Vogel L, et al. Isoform identification and characterization of Art v 3, the lipid-transfer protein of mugwort pollen. Mol Immunol 2009 Jun;46(10):1919-24.

[24] Jia D, Li J, Liu L, Zhang D, Yang Y, Du G, et al. High-level expression, purification, and enzymatic characterization of truncated poly(vinyl alcohol) dehydrogenase in methylotrophic yeast Pichia pastoris. Appl Microbiol Biotechnol 2012 Mar 10.

[25] Vu TT, Quyen DT, Dao TT, Nguyen Sle T. Cloning, High-Level Expression, Purification, and Properties of a Novel Endo-beta-1,4-Mannanase from Bacillus subtilis G1 in Pichia pastoris. J Microbiol Biotechnol 2012 Mar;22(3):331-8.

[26] Yi MH, Jeong KY, Kim CR, Yong TS. IgE-binding reactivity of peptide fragments of Bla g 1.02, a major German cockroach allergen. Asian Pac J Allergy Immunol 2009 Jun-Sep;27(2-3):121-9.

[27] Salamanca G, Rodriguez R, Quiralte J, Moreno C, Pascual CY, Barber D, et al. Pectin methylesterases of pollen tissue, a major allergen in olive tree. FEBS J 2010 Jul; 277(13):2729-39.

[28] Goh L-T, Kuo I-C, Luo S, Chua K.Y, White M. Production and purification of recombinant Blomia tropicalis group 5 allergen from Pichia pastoris culture Biotechnology Letters 2001;23(9):661-5.

[29] Labrada M, Uyema K, Sewer M, Labrada A, Gonzalez M, Caraballo L, et al. Monoclonal antibodies against Blo t 13, a recombinant allergen from Blomia tropicalis. Int Arch Allergy Immunol 2002 Nov;129(3):212-8.

[30] Baranyi U, Gattringer M, Boehm A, Marth K, Focke-Tejkl M, Bohle B, et al. Expression of a Major Plant Allergen as Membrane-Anchored and Secreted Protein in Human Cells with Preserved T Cell and B Cell Epitopes. Int Arch Allergy Immunol 2011;156:259-66.

[31] Wagner B, Fuchs H, Adhami F, Ma Y, Scheiner O, Breiteneder H. Plant virus expression systems for transient production of recombinant allergens in Nicotiana benthamiana. Methods 2004;32:227-34.

[32] Hsu CH, Lin SS, Liu FL, Su WC, Yeh SD. Oral administration of a mite allergen expressed by zucchini yellow mosaic virus in cucurbit species downregulates allergen-induced airway inflammation and IgE synthesis. J Allergy Clin Immunol 2004;113:1079-85.

[33] Neill DR, Wong SH, Bellosi A, Flynn RJ, Daly M, Langford TK, et al. Nuocytes represent a new innate effector leukocyte that mediates type-2 immunity. Nature 2010 Apr 29;464(7293):1367-70.

[34] Barlow JL, Bellosi A, Hardman CS, Drynan LF, Wong SH, Cruickshank JP, et al. Innate IL-13-producing nuocytes arise during allergic lung inflammation and contribute to airways hyperreactivity. J Allergy Clin Immunol 2012 Jan;129(1):191-8 e1-4.

[35] Sokol CL, Barton GM, Farr AG, Medzhitov R. A mechanism for the initiation of allergen-induced T helper type 2 responses. Nat Immunol 2008 Mar;9(3):310-8.

[36] Saenz SA, Siracusa MC, Perrigoue JG, Spencer SP, Urban JF, Jr., Tocker JE, et al. IL25 elicits a multipotent progenitor cell population that promotes T(H)2 cytokine responses. Nature 2010 Apr 29;464(7293):1362-6.

[37] Veldhoen M, Uyttenhove C, van Snick J, Helmby H, Westendorf A, Buer J, et al. Transforming growth factor-beta 'reprograms' the differentiation of T helper 2 cells and promotes an interleukin 9-producing subset. Nat Immunol 2008 Dec;9(12): 1341-6.

[38] Zhao Y, Yang J, Gao YD, Guo W. Th17 immunity in patients with allergic asthma. Int Arch Allergy Immunol 2010;151(4):297-307.

[39] Durham SR, Walker SM, Varga EM, Jacobson MR, O'Brien F, Noble W, et al. Long-term clinical efficacy of grass-pollen immunotherapy. N Engl J Med 1999 Aug 12;341(7):468-75.

[40] Frew AJ, Powell RJ, Corrigan CJ, SR D. Efficacy and safety of specific immunotherapy with SQ allergen extract in treatment-resistant seasonal allergic rhinoconjunctivitis. J Allergy Clin Immunol 2006;117:319–25.

[41] Akdis M, Blaser K, Akdis CA. T regulatory cells in allergy: novel concepts in the pathogenesis, prevention, and treatment of allergic diseases. J Allergy Clin Immunol 2005 Nov;116(5):961-8; quiz 9.

[42] Jutel M, Akdis M, Budak F, Aebischer-Casaulta C, Wrzyszcz M, Blaser K, et al. IL-10 and TGF-beta cooperate in the regulatory T cell response to mucosal allergens in normal immunity and specific immunotherapy. Eur J Immunol 2003 May;33(5):1205-14.

[43] Jutel M, Jaeger L, Suck R, Meyer H, Fiebig H, Cromwell O. Allergen-specific immunotherapy with recombinant grass pollen allergens. J Allergy Clin Immunol 2005 Sep;116(3):608-13.

[44] Sakaguchi S, Yamaguchi T, Nomura T, Ono M. Regulatory T cells and immune tolerance. Cell 2008 May 30;133(5):775-87.

[45] Izcue A, Hue S, Buonocore S, Arancibia-Carcamo CV, Ahern PP, Iwakura Y, et al. Interleukin-23 restrains regulatory T cell activity to drive T cell-dependent colitis. Immunity 2008 Apr;28(4):559-70.

[46] Akdis CA, Kussebi F, Pulendran B, Akdis M, Lauener RP, Schmidt-Weber CB, et al. Inhibition of T helper 2-type responses, IgE production and eosinophilia by synthetic lipopeptides. Eur J Immunol 2003 Oct;33(10):2717-26.

[47] Reisinger J, Horak F, Pauli G, van Hage M, Cromwell O, Konig F, et al. Allergen-specific nasal IgG antibodies induced by vaccination with genetically modified allergens are associated with reduced nasal allergen sensitivity. J Allergy Clin Immunol 2005 Aug;116(2):347-54.

[48] Strait RT, Morris SC, Finkelman FD. IgG-blocking antibodies inhibit IgE-mediated anaphylaxis in vivo through both antigen interception and Fc gamma RIIb cross-linking. J Clin Invest 2006 Mar;116(3):833-41.

[49] Finkelman MA, Lempitski SJ, Slater JE. beta-Glucans in standardized allergen extracts. J Endotoxin Res 2006;12(4):241-5.

[50] Focke M, Marth K, Valenta R. Molecular composition and biological activity of commercial birch pollen allergen extracts. Eur J Clin Invest 2009 May;39(5):429-36.

[51] Focke M, Marth K, Flicker S, Valenta R. Heterogeneity of commercial timothy grass pollen extracts. Clin Exp Allergy 2008 Aug;38(8):1400-8.

[52] Trivedi B, Valerio C, Slater JE. Endotoxin content of standardized allergen vaccines. J Allergy Clin Immunol 2003 Apr;111(4):777-83.

[53] Traidl-Hoffmann C, Mariani V, Hochrein H, Karg K, Wagner H, Ring J, et al. Pollen-associated phytoprostanes inhibit dendritic cell interleukin-12 production and augment T helper type 2 cell polarization. J Exp Med 2005 Feb 21;201(4):627-36.

[54] Moverare R, Elfman L, Vesterinen E, Metso T, Haahtela T. Development of new IgE specificities to allergenic components in birch pollen extract during specific immunotherapy studied with immunoblotting and Pharmacia CAP System. Allergy 2002 May;57(5):423-30.

[55] Cromwell O, Hafner D, Nandy A. Recombinant allergens for specific immunotherapy. J Allergy Clin Immunol 2011 Apr;127(4):865-72.

[56] Valenta R, Lidholm J, Niederberger V, Hayek B, Kraft D, Gronlund H. The recombinant allergen-based concept of component-resolved diagnostics and immunotherapy (CRD and CRIT). Clin Exp Allergy 1999 Jul;29(7):896-904.

[57] Ballmer-Weber BK, Scheurer S, Fritsche P, Enrique E, Cistero-Bahima A, Haase T, et al. Component-resolved diagnosis with recombinant allergens in patients with cherry allergy. J Allergy Clin Immunol 2002 Jul;110(1):167-73.

[58] Astier C, Morisset M, Roitel O, Codreanu F, Jacquenet S, Franck P, et al. Predictive value of skin prick tests using recombinant allergens for diagnosis of peanut allergy. J Allergy Clin Immunol 2006 Jul;118(1):250-6.

[59] Bauermeister K, Ballmer-Weber BK, Bublin M, Fritsche P, Hanschmann KM, Hoffmann-Sommergruber K, et al. Assessment of component-resolved in vitro diagnosis of celeriac allergy. J Allergy Clin Immunol 2009 Dec;124(6):1273-81 e2.

[60] Akkerdaas JH, Wensing M, Knulst AC, Krebitz M, Breiteneder H, de Vries S, et al. How accurate and safe is the diagnosis of hazelnut allergy by means of commercial skin prick test reagents? Int Arch Allergy Immunol 2003 Oct;132(2):132-40.

[61] Dalmau Duch G, Gazquez Garcia V, Gaig Jane P, Galan Nieto A, Monsalve Clemente RI. Importance of controlled sting challenge and component-resolved diagnosis in the success of venom immunotherapy. J Investig Allergol Clin Immunol 2012;22(2): 135-6.

[62] Monsalve RI, Vega A, Marques L, Miranda A, Fernandez J, Soriano V, et al. Component-resolved diagnosis of vespid venom-allergic individuals: phospholipases and antigen 5s are necessary to identify Vespula or Polistes sensitization. Allergy 2012 Apr;67(4):528-36.

[63] Tripodi S, Frediani T, Lucarelli S, Macri F, Pingitore G, Di Rienzo Businco A, et al. Molecular profiles of IgE to Phleum pratense in children with grass pollen allergy: implications for specific immunotherapy. J Allergy Clin Immunol 2012 Mar;129(3): 834-9 e8.

[64] Metz-Favre C, Linhart B, Focke-Tejkl M, Purohit A, de Blay F, Valenta R, et al. Skin test diagnosis of grass pollen allergy with a recombinant hybrid molecule. J Allergy Clin Immunol 2007 Aug;120(2):315-21.

[65] Hueber W, Utz PJ, Robinson WH. Autoantibodies in early arthritis: advances in diagnosis and prognostication. Clin Exp Rheumatol 2003 Sep-Oct;21(5 Suppl 31):S59-64.

[66] Gadermaier G, Wopfner N, Wallner M, Egger M, Didierlaurent A, Regl G, et al. Array-based profiling of ragweed and mugwort pollen allergens. Allergy 2008 Nov; 63(11):1543-9.

[67] Ott H, Folster-Holst R, Merk HF, Baron JM. Allergen microarrays: a novel tool for high-resolution IgE profiling in adults with atopic dermatitis. Eur J Dermatol 2010 Jan-Feb;20(1):54-61.

[68] Jahn-Schmid B, Harwanegg C, Hiller R, Bohle B, Ebner C, Scheiner O, et al. Allergen microarray: comparison of microarray using recombinant allergens with conventional diagnostic methods to detect allergen-specific serum immunoglobulin E Clin Exp Allergy 2003;33.

[69] Ebo DG, Hagendorens MM, De Knop KJ, Verweij MM, Bridts CH, De Clerck LS, et al. Component-resolved diagnosis from latex allergy by microarray. Clin Exp Allergy 2010 Feb;40(2):348-58.

[70] Perry TT, Matsui EC, Conover-Walker MK, Wood RA. Risk of oral food challenges. J Allergy Clin Immunol 2004 Nov;114(5):1164-8.

[71] Lin J, Bruni FM, Fu Z, Maloney J, Bardina L, Boner AL, et al. A bioinformatics approach to identify patients with symptomatic peanut allergy using peptide microarray immunoassay. J Allergy Clin Immunol 2012 May;129(5):1321-8 e5.

[72] Jimenez S, Puerta L, Mendoza D, K.W.Chua, Mercado D, Caraballo L. IgE Antibody Responses to Recobinant Allergens of Blomia tropicalis and Dermatophagoides pteronyssinus in a Tropical Enviroment. Allergy Clin Immunol Int - J World Allergy Org 2007;19:233-8.

[73] Pauli G, Oster JP, Deviller P, Heiss S, Bessot JC, Susani M, et al. Skin testing with recombinant allergens rBet v 1 and birch profilin, rBet v 2: diagnostic value for birch pollen and associated allergies. J Allergy Clin Immunol 1996 May;97(5):1100-9.

[74] Godnic-Cvar J, Susani M, Breiteneder H, Berger A, Havelec L, Waldhor T, et al. Recombinant Bet v 1, the major birch pollen allergen, induces hypersensitivity reactions equal to those induced by natural Bet v 1 in the airways of patients allergic to tree pollen. J Allergy Clin Immunol 1997 Mar;99(3):354-9.

[75] Pauli G, Larsen TH, Rak S, Horak F, Pastorello E, Valenta R, et al. Efficacy of recombinant birch pollen vaccine for the treatment of birch-allergic rhinoconjunctivitis. J Allergy Clin Immunol 2008 Nov;122(5):951-60.

[76] Focke M, Swoboda I, Marth K, Valenta R. Developments in allergen-specific immunotherapy: from allergen extracts to allergy vaccines bypassing allergen-specific immunoglobulin E and T cell reactivity. Clin Exp Allergy 2010 Mar;40(3):385-97.

[77] Ferreira F, Hirtenlehner K, Jilek A, Godnik-Cvar J, Breiteneder H, Grimm R, et al. Dissection of immunoglobulin E and T lymphocyte reactivity of isoforms of the major birch pollen allergen Bet v 1: potential use of hypoallergenic isoforms for immunotherapy. J Exp Med 1996 Feb 1;183(2):599-609.

[78] Arquint O, Helbling A, Crameri R, Ferreira F, Breitenbach M, Pichler WJ. Reduced in vivo allergenicity of Bet v 1d isoform, a natural component of birch pollen. J Allergy Clin Immunol 1999 Dec;104(6):1239-43.

[79] Wagner S, Radauer C, Bublin M, Hoffmann-Sommergruber K, Kopp T, Greusenegger EK, et al. Naturally ocurring hypoallergenic Bet v 1 isoforms fail to induce IgE responses in individuals with birch pollen allergy. J Allergy Clin Immunol 2008;121:246-52.

[80] Chapman MD, Smith AM, Vailes LD, Arruda LK, Dhanaraj V, Pomes A. Recombinant allergens for diagnosis and therapy of allergic disease. J Allergy Clin Immunol 2000 Sep;106(3):409-18.

[81] Sharrow SD, Edmonds KA, Goodman MA, Novotny MV, Stone MJ. Thermodynamic consequences of disrupting a water-mediated hydrogen bond network in a protein:pheromone complex. Protein Sci 2005 Jan;14(1):249-56.

[82] Ferrari E, Breda D, Longhi R, Vangelista L, Nakaie CR, Elviri L, et al. In search of a vaccine for mouse allergy: significant reduction of Mus m 1 allergenicity by structure-guided single-point mutations. Int Arch Allergy Immunol 2012;157(3):226-37.

[83] Gadermaier G, Jahn-Schmid B, Vogel L, Egger M, Himly M, Briza P, et al. Targeting the cysteine-stabilized fold of Art v 1 for immunotherapy of Artemisia pollen allergy. Mol Immunol 2010 Mar;47(6):1292-8.

[84] Spangfort MD, Mirza O, Ipsen H, Van Neerven RJ, Gajhede M, Larsen JN. Dominating IgE-binding epitope of Bet v 1, the major allergen of birch pollen, characterized by X-ray crystallography and site-directed mutagenesis. J Immunol 2003 Sep 15;171(6):3084-90.

[85] King TP, Jim SY, Monsalve RI, Kagey-Sobotka A, Lichtenstein LM, Spangfort MD. Recombinant allergens with reduced allergenicity but retaining immunogenicity of the natural allergens: hybrids of yellow jacket and paper wasp venom allergen antigen 5s. J Immunol 2001 May 15;166(10):6057-65.

[86] Gonzalez-Rioja R, Ibarrola I, Arilla MC, Ferrer A, Mir A, Andreu C, et al. Genetically engineered hybrid proteins from Parietaria judaica pollen for allergen-specific immunotherapy. J Allergy Clin Immunol 2007 Sep;120(3):602-9.

[87] Linhart B, Hartl A, Jahn-Schmid B, Verdino P, Keller W, Krauth MT, et al. A hybrid molecule resembling the epitope spectrum of grass pollen for allergy vaccination. J Allergy Clin Immunol 2005 May;115(5):1010-6.

[88] Asturias JA, Ibarrola I, Arilla MC, Vidal C, Ferrer A, Gamboa PM, et al. Engineering of major house dust mite allergens Der p 1 and Der p 2 for allergen-specific immunotherapy. Clin Exp Allergy 2009 Jul;39(7):1088-98.

[89] Nouri HR, Varasteh A, Vahedi F, Chamani J, Afsharzadeh D, Sankian M. Constructing a hybrid molecule with low capacity of IgE binding from Chenopodium album pollen allergens. Immunol Lett 2012 May 30;144(1-2):67-77.

[90] Ball T, Linhart B, Sonneck K, Blatt K, Herrmann H, Valent P, et al. Reducing allergenicity by altering allergen fold: a mosaic protein of Phl p 1 for allergy vaccination. Allergy 2009 Apr;64(4):569-80.

[91] Mothes-Luksch N, Stumvoll S, Linhart B, Focke M, Krauth MT, Hauswirth A, et al. Disruption of allergenic activity of the major grass pollen allergen Phl p 2 by reassembly as a mosaic protein. J Immunol 2008 Oct 1;181(7):4864-73.

[92] Campana R, Vrtala S, Maderegger B, Jertschin P, Stegfellner G, Swoboda I, et al. Hypoallergenic derivatives of the major birch pollen allergen Bet v 1 obtained by rational sequence reassembly. J Allergy Clin Immunol 2010 Nov;126(5):1024-31, 31 e1-8.

[93] Chen KW, Fuchs G, Sonneck K, Gieras A, Swoboda I, Douladiris N, et al. Reduction of the in vivo allergenicity of Der p 2, the major house-dust mite allergen, by genetic engineering. Mol Immunol 2008 May;45(9):2486-98.

[94] Vrtala S, Akdis CA, Budak F, Akdis M, Blaser K, Kraft D, et al. T cell epitope-containing hypoallergenic recombinant fragments of the major birch pollen allergen, Bet v 1, induce blocking antibodies. J Immunol 2000 Dec 1;165(11):6653-9.

[95] Pauli G, Purohit A, Oster JP, De Blay F, Vrtala S, Niederberger V, et al. Comparison of genetically engineered hypoallergenic rBet v 1 derivatives with rBet v 1 wild-type by skin prick and intradermal testing: results obtained in a French population. Clin Exp Allergy 2000 Aug;30(8):1076-84.

[96] Focke M, Linhart B, Hartl A, Wiedermann U, Sperr WR, Valent P, et al. Non-anaphylactic surface-exposed peptides of the major birch pollen allergen, Bet v 1, for preventive vaccination. Clin Exp Allergy 2004 Oct;34(10):1525-33.

[97] Vrtala S, Hirtenlehner K, Susani M, Akdis M, Kussebi F, Akdis CA, et al. Genetic engineering of a hypoallergenic trimer of the major birch pollen allergen Bet v 1. FASEB J 2001 Sep;15(11):2045-7.

[98] Johansson J, Hellman L. Modifications increasing the efficacy of recombinant vaccines; marked increase in antibody titers with moderately repetitive variants of a therapeutic allergy vaccine. Vaccine 2007 Feb 19;25(9):1676-82.

[99] Vrtala S, Fohr M, Campana R, Baumgartner C, Valent P, Valenta R. Genetic engineering of trimers of hypoallergenic fragments of the major birch pollen allergen, Bet v 1, for allergy vaccination. Vaccine 2011 Mar 3;29(11):2140-8.

[100] Calderon MA, Larenas D, Kleine-Tebbe J, Jacobsen L, Passalacqua G, Eng PA, et al. European Academy of Allergy and Clinical Immunology task force report on 'dose-response relationship in allergen-specific immunotherapy'. Allergy 2011 Oct;66(10): 1345-59.

[101] Blaser K. Allergen dose dependent cytokine production regulates specific IgE and IgG antibody production. Adv Exp Med Biol 1996;409:295-303.

[102] Fittipaldi A, Giacca M. Transcellular protein transduction using the Tat protein of HIV-1. Adv Drug Deliv Rev 2005 Feb 28;57(4):597-608.

[103] Herce HD, Garcia AE. Molecular dynamics simulations suggest a mechanism for translocation of the HIV-1 TAT peptide across lipid membranes. Proc Natl Acad Sci U S A 2007 Dec 26;104(52):20805-10.

[104] Rhyner C, Kundig T, Akdis CA, Crameri R. Targeting the MHC II presentation pathway in allergy vaccine development. Biochem Soc Trans 2007 Aug;35(Pt 4):833-4.

[105] Crameri R, Fluckiger S, Daigle I, Kundig T, Rhyner C. Design, engineering and in vitro evaluation of MHC class-II targeting allergy vaccines. Allergy 2007 Feb;62(2): 197-206.

[106] Martinez-Gomez JM, Johansen P, Rose H, Steiner M, Senti G, Rhyner C, et al. Targeting the MHC class II pathway of antigen presentation enhances immunogenicity and safety of allergen immunotherapy. Allergy 2009 Jan;64(1):172-8.

[107] Lutz MB, Schuler G. Immature, semi-mature and fully mature dendritic cells: which signals induce tolerance or immunity? Trends Immunol 2002 Sep;23(9):445-9.

[108] Rutella S, Danese S, Leone G. Tolerogenic dendritic cells: cytokine modulation comes of age. Blood 2006 Sep 1;108(5):1435-40.

[109] Novak N, Valenta R, Bohle B, Laffer S, Haberstok J, Kraft S, et al. FcepsilonRI engagement of Langerhans cell-like dendritic cells and inflammatory dendritic epidermal cell-like dendritic cells induces chemotactic signals and different T-cell phenotypes in vitro. J Allergy Clin Immunol 2004 May;113(5):949-57.

[110] Zhu D, Kepley CL, Zhang K, Terada T, Yamada T, Saxon A. A chimeric human-cat fusion protein blocks cat-induced allergy. Nat Med 2005 Apr;11(4):446-9.

[111] Terada T, Zhang K, Belperio J, Londhe V, Saxon A. A chimeric human-cat Fcgamma-Fel d1 fusion protein inhibits systemic, pulmonary, and cutaneous allergic reactivity to intratracheal challenge in mice sensitized to Fel d1, the major cat allergen. Clin Immunol 2006 Jul;120(1):45-56.

[112] Lin LH, Zheng P, Yuen JW, Wang J, Zhou J, Kong CQ, et al. Prevention and treatment of allergic inflammation by an Fcgamma-Der f2 fusion protein in a murine model of dust mite-induced asthma. Immunol Res 2012 Jun;52(3):276-83.

[113] Vailes LD, Sun AW, Ichikawa K, Wu Z, Sulahian TH, Chapman MD, et al. High-level expression of immunoreactive recombinant cat allergen (Fel d 1): Targeting to antigen-presenting cells. J Allergy Clin Immunol 2002 Nov;110(5):757-62.

[114] Hulse KE, Reefer AJ, Engelhard VH, Satinover SM, Patrie JT, Chapman MD, et al. Targeting Fel d 1 to FcgammaRI induces a novel variation of the T(H)2 response in subjects with cat allergy. J Allergy Clin Immunol 2008 Mar;121(3):756-62 e4.

[115] Hulse KE, Reefer AJ, Engelhard VH, Patrie JT, Ziegler SF, Chapman MD, et al. Targeting allergen to FcgammaRI reveals a novel T(H)2 regulatory pathway linked to thymic stromal lymphopoietin receptor. J Allergy Clin Immunol 2010 Jan;125(1): 247-56 e1-8.

[116] Muller U, Golden DB, Lockey RF, Shin B. Immunotherapy for hymenoptera venom hypersensitivity. Clin Allergy Immunol 2008;21:377-92.

[117] Bilo BM, Bonifazi F. Epidemiology of insect-venom anaphylaxis. Curr Opin Allergy Clin Immunol 2008 Aug;8(4):330-7.

[118] Graft DF. Insect sting allergy. Med Clin North Am 2006 Jan;90(1):211-32.

[119] Brasch J, Maidusch T. Immunotherapy with wasp venom is accompanied by wide-ranging immune responses that need further exploration. Acta Derm Venereol 2009;89(5):466-9.

[120] Mosbech H, Muller U. Side-effects of insect venom immunotherapy: results from an EAACI multicenter study. European Academy of Allergology and Clinical Immunology. Allergy 2000 Nov;55(11):1005-10.

[121] Kammerer R, Chvatchko Y, Kettner A, Dufour N, Corradin G, Spertini F. Modulation of T-cell response to phospholipase A2 and phospholipase A2-derived peptides by conventional bee venom immunotherapy. J Allergy Clin Immunol 1997 Jul;100(1): 96-103.

[122] Muller U, Akdis CA, Fricker M, Akdis M, Blesken T, Bettens F, et al. Successful immunotherapy with T-cell epitope peptides of bee venom phospholipase A2 induces specific T-cell anergy in patients allergic to bee venom. J Allergy Clin Immunol 1998 Jun;101(6 Pt 1):747-54.

[123] Fellrath JM, Kettner A, Dufour N, Frigerio C, Schneeberger D, Leimgruber A, et al. Allergen-specific T-cell tolerance induction with allergen-derived long synthetic peptides: results of a phase I trial. J Allergy Clin Immunol 2003 Apr;111(4):854-61.

[124] Winkler B, Bolwig C, Seppala U, Spangfort MD, Ebner C, Wiedermann U. Allergen-specific immunosuppression by mucosal treatment with recombinant Ves v 5, a ma-

jor allergen of Vespula vulgaris venom, in a murine model of wasp venom allergy. Immunology 2003 Nov;110(3):376-85.

[125] Kussebi F, Karamloo F, Rhyner C, Schmid-Grendelmeier P, Salagianni M, Mannhart C, et al. A major allergen gene-fusion protein for potential usage in allergen-specific immunotherapy. J Allergy Clin Immunol 2005 Feb;115(2):323-9.

[126] Cascone O, Amaral V, Ferrara P, Vita N, Guillemot JC, Diaz LE. Purification and characterization of two forms of antigen 5 from polybia scutellaris venom. Toxicon 1995 May;33(5):659-65.

[127] Pirpignani ML, Rivera E, Hellman U, Biscoglio de Jimenez Bonino M. Structural and immunological aspects of Polybia scutellaris Antigen 5. Arch Biochem Biophys 2002 Nov 15;407(2):224-30.

[128] Vinzon SE, Marino-Buslje C, Rivera E, Biscoglio de Jimenez Bonino M. A Naturally Occurring Hypoallergenic Variant of Vespid Antigen 5 from Polybia scutellaris Venom as a Candidate for Allergen-Specific Immunotherapy. PLoS One 2012;7(7):e41351.

[129] Haselden BM, Kay AB, Larche M. Immunoglobulin E-independent major histocompatibility complex-restricted T cell peptide epitope-induced late asthmatic reactions. J Exp Med 189 1999;189:1885-94.

[130] Norman PS, Ohman JL, Jr., Long AA, Creticos PS, Gefter MA, Shaked Z, et al. Treatment of cat allergy with T-cell reactive peptides. Am J Respir Crit Care Med 1996 Dec;154(6 Pt 1):1623-8.

[131] Simons FE, Imada M, Li Y, Watson WT, HayGlass KT. Fel d 1 peptides: effect on skin tests and cytokine synthesis in cat-allergic human subjects. Int Immunol 1996 Dec; 8(12):1937-45.

[132] Maguire P, Nicodemus C, Robinson D, Aaronson D, Umetsu DT. The safety and efficacy of ALLERVAX CAT in cat allergic patients. Clin Immunol 1999 Dec;93(3):222-31.

[133] Haselden BM, Larche M, Meng Q, Shirley K, Dworski R, Kaplan AP, et al. Late asthmatic reactions provoked by intradermal injection of T-cell peptide epitopes are not associated with bronchial mucosal infiltration of eosinophils or T(H)2-type cells or with elevated concentrations of histamine or eicosanoids in bronchoalveolar fluid. J Allergy Clin Immunol 2001 Sep;108(3):394-401.

[134] Oldfield WL, Kay AB, Larche M. Allergen-derived T cell peptide-induced late asthmatic reactions precede the induction of antigen-specific hyporesponsiveness in atopic allergic asthmatic subjects. J Immunol 2001 Aug 1;167(3):1734-9.

[135] Ali FR, Oldfield WL, Higashi N, Larche M, Kay AB. Late asthmatic reactions induced by inhalation of allergen-derived T cell peptides. Am J Respir Crit Care Med 2004 Jan 1;169(1):20-6.

[136] Niederberger V, Horak F, Vrtala S, Spitzauer S, Krauth MT, Valent P, et al. Vaccination with genetically engineered allergens prevents progression of allergic disease. Proc Natl Acad Sci U S A 2004;101(suppl 2):14677-82.

[137] Winther L, Poulsen LK, Robin B, Mélac M, Malling H. Safety and Tolerability of Recombinant Bet v 1 (rBet v 1) tablets in sublingual immunotherapy (SLIT). J Allergy Clin Immunol 2009;123(suppl):S215.

[138] Senti G, Crameri R, Kuster D, Johansen P, Martinez-Gomez JM, Graf N, et al. Intralymphatic immunotherapy for cat allergy induces tolerance after only 3 injections. J Allergy Clin Immunol 2012 May;129(5):1290-6.

[139] Tulic MK, Fiset PO, Christodoulopoulos P, Vaillancourt P, Desrosiers M, Lavigne F, et al. Amb a 1-immunostimulatory oligodeoxynucleotide conjugate immunotherapy decreases the nasal inflammatory response. J Allergy Clin Immunol 2004 Feb;113(2): 235-41.

[140] Asai K, Foley SC, Sumi Y, Yamauchi Y, Takeda N, Desrosiers M, et al. Amb a 1-immunostimulatory oligodeoxynucleotide conjugate immunotherapy increases CD4+CD25+ T cells in the nasal mucosa of subjects with allergic rhinitis. Allergol Int 2008 Dec;57(4):377-81.

[141] Linneberg A, Gislum M, Johansen N, Husemoen LL, Jorgensen T. Temporal trends of aeroallergen sensitization over twenty-five years. Clin Exp Allergy 2007 Aug;37(8): 1137-42.

[142] Boulet LP, Turcotte H, Laprise C, Lavertu C, Bedard PM, Lavoie A, et al. Comparative degree and type of sensitization to common indoor and outdoor allergens in subjects with allergic rhinitis and/or asthma. Clin Exp Allergy 1997 Jan;27(1):52-9.

[143] Tsai JJ, Wu HH, Shen HD, Hsu EL, Wang SR. Sensitization to Blomia tropicalis among asthmatic patients in Taiwan. Int Arch Allergy Immunol 1998 Feb;115(2): 144-9.

[144] Fernandez-Caldas E, Baena-Cagnani CE, Lopez M, Patino C, Neffen HE, Sanchez-Medina M, et al. Cutaneous sensitivity to six mite species in asthmatic patients from five Latin American countries. J Investig Allergol Clin Immunol 1993 Sep-Oct;3(5): 245-9.

[145] Puerta L, Fernandez-Caldas E, Lockey RF, Caraballo LR. Mite allergy in the tropics: sensitization to six domestic mite species in Cartagena, Colombia. J Investig Allergol Clin Immunol 1993 Jul-Aug;3(4):198-204.

[146] Shen HD, Chua KY, Lin KL, Shich KH, Thomas WR. Molecular cloning of house dust mite allergens with common antibody binding-specificities with multiple components in mite extracts. Int Arch Allergy Immunol 1993;23:934-40.

[147] Puerta L, Lagares A, Mercado D, Fernandez-Caldas E, Caraballo L. Allergenic composition of the mite Suidasia medanensis and cross-reactivity with Blomia tropicalis. Allergy 2005 Jan;60(1):41-7.

[148] Weghofer M, Thomas WR, Kronqvist M, Mari A, Purohit A, Pauli G, et al. Variability of IgE reactivity profiles among European mite allergic patients. Eur J Clin Invest 2008 Dec;38(12):959-65.

[149] Lynch NR, Thomas WR, Garcia NM, Di Prisco MC, Puccio FA, L'Opez R I, et al. Biological activity of recombinant Der p 2, Der p 5 and Der p 7 allergens of the house-dust mite Dermatophagoides pteronyssinus. Int Arch Allergy Immunol 1997 Sep; 114(1):59-67.

[150] Thomas WR, Hales BJ, Smith WA. Structural biology of allergens. Curr Allergy Asthma Rep 2005 Sep;5(5):388-93.

[151] Pittner G, Vrtala S, Thomas WR, Weghofer M, Kundi M, Horak F, et al. Component-resolved diagnosis of house-dust mite allergy with purified natural and recombinant mite allergens. Clin Exp Allergy 2004 Apr;34(4):597-603.

[152] Zakzuk J, Jimenez S, Cheong N, Puerta L, Lee BW, Chua KY, et al. Immunlogical characterization of Blo t 12 isoallergen: identification of immunoglobulin E epitopes. Clin Exp Allergy 2009;39:608-16.

[153] Puerta L, Martinez D, Munera M, Cantillo J, Caraballo L. Recombinant protein assembling epitopes from different allergens of Dermatophagoides pteronyssinus. Presented at: European Academy of Allergy and Clinical Immunology Congress. June 16-20, 2012. Geneve, Switzerland.

Chapter 13

Current Advances in Seaweed Transformation

Koji Mikami

Additional information is available at the end of the chapter

http://dx.doi.org/10.5772/52978

1. Introduction

Frederick Griffith reported the discovery of transformation in 1928 [1]. Since a harmless strain of *Streptococcus pneumoniae* was altered to a virulent one by exposure to heat-killed virulent strains in mice, Griffice hypothesized that there was a transforming principle in the heat-killed strain. It took sixteen years to indentify the nature of the transforming principle as a DNA fragment released from virulent strains and integrated into the genome of a harmless strain [2]. Such an uptake and incorporation of DNA by bacteria was named transformation. Remarkably, an epoch-making technology in the form of artificial transformation protocol for the model bacterium *Escherichia coli* was established by Mandel and Higa in 1970 [3], which stimulated the development of artificial genetic transformation systems in yeasts, animals and plants. In plants, genetic transformation is a powerful tool for elucidating the functions and regulatory mechanisms of genes involved in various physiological events, and special attention has been paid to plant improvements affecting food security, human health, the environment and conservation of biodiversity. For instance, researchers have focused on the creation of organisms that efficiently produce biofuels and medically functional materials or carry stress tolerance in the face of uncertain environmental conditions [4-6].

Although the first success in the creation of transgenic mouse was carried out by injecting the rat growth hormone gene into a mouse embryo in 1982 [7], the protocol for artificial genetic transformation in plants was established earlier than that in animals. Following the discovery of the soil plant pathogen *Agrobacterium tumefaciens*, which is responsible for producing plant tumors, in 1907 [8], it was found that the tumor-inducing agent is the Ti plasmid containing T-DNA, a particular DNA segment containing tumor-producing genes that are transferred into the nuclear genome of infected cells [9]. By replacing tumor-producing genes by a gene of interest within the T-DNA region, infection of *A. tumefaciens* carrying a modified Ti plasmid results in insertion of a DNA fragment containing the desired genes into the genomes of plants by genetic recombination. Since the report of this protocol in the early 1980s [10,11], transformation mediated by *A. tumefaciens* has become the most commonly used method to transmit DNA fragment into higher plants [12].

Since not all plant cells are susceptible to infection by *A. tumefaciens*, other methods were developed and are available in plants. Particle bombardment [13], which is also referred to as microprojectile bombardment, particle gun or biolistics, makes use of DNA-coated gold particles, which enables the transient and stable transformation of almost any type of cell, regardless of rigidity of the cell wall, and is thus extensively used for land plants. For protoplasts, electroporation is well employed, for which a high-voltage electrical pulse temporarily disturbs the phospholipid bilayer of the plasma membrane, allowing cells to take up plasmid DNAs [14,15]. In addition, the polyethylene glycol (PEG)-mediated transformation system is also thought to affect the plasma membrane and induce the uptake of DNAs into cells [15,16] and is almost exclusively applied with the moss *Physcomitrella patens* and liverwort *Marchantia polymorpha* [17,18]. Therefore, several kinds of genetic transformation methods are now available in land green plants.

Seaweeds are photosynthetic macroalgae, the majority of which live in the sea, and are usually divided into green, red and brown algae. Traditionally, all classes of seaweeds are known as human foods especially in Asian countries; for instance, red algae are known as Nori and brown algae are called Konbu and Wakame in Japan. In addition, red and brown algae are utilized as the sources of industrially and medically valuable compounds such as phycoerythrin, n-3 polyunsaturated fatty acids, porphyran, ager and carrageenan from red algae, and fucoxantine, fucoidan and alginate from brown algae [19-22]. Thus, to make new strains carrying advantageous characteristics benefiting industry and medicine, researchers have worked hard since the early 1990s to establish methods of genetic transformation in seaweeds [20,23,24]. However, the process is very difficult, and most of the early studies were reported in conference abstracts without the accompanying manuscript publication [25-28]. This situation has hampered us from gaining an understanding of gene functions in various physiological regulations and also a utilization of seaweeds in biotechnological applications.

Transformation can be divided into genetic (stable) and transient transformations under the control of the genes introduced into cells. In genetic transformation, genes introduced by genetic recombination are maintained in the genome through generations of cells, whereas in transient transformation, rapid loss of introduced foreign genes is usually observed. Establishing the genetic transformation system requires four basal techniques: an efficient gene transfer system, an efficient expression system for foreign genes, an integration and targeting system to deliver the foreign gene into the genome, and a selection system for transformed cells. It is notable that the transient transformation system is completed by the first two of the four required systems. In this respect, the development of an efficient and reproducible transient transformation system is the most critical step to establishing a genetic transformation system in seaweeds.

The current progress in establishing of both transient and genetic transformation systems in macroalgae is reviewed here. Although high-quality review articles for algal transformation have been published previously [20,23,24], I believe addressing the recent activity in seaweed transformation provides valuable information for seaweed molecular biologists and breeding scientists. Since considerable technical improvement was recently made in red seaweeds

[29,30], I focus here on the current progress in red algal transient transformation with summarizing pioneer and recent studies related to seaweed genetic transformation.

2. Transformation in red seaweeds

2.1. Pioneer studies for transient transformation

As far as I know, Donald P. Cheney is the pioneer in researching red algal transformation. He and his colleague performed transient transformation of the red alga *Kappaphycus alvarezii* using particle bombardment [25], which was the first report about the transient transformation of seaweeds (Table 1). In this case, the *Escherichia coli uidA* gene encoding β-glucuronidase (GUS) was expressed as a reporter under direction of the cauliflower mosaic virus (CaMV) 35S promoter (*CaMV 35S-GUS* gene). Since the GUS expression can be visualized as a blue color following treatment with X-gluc (5-bromo-4-chloro-3-indolyl-β-D-glucuronide) and also be quantified by fluorometric analysis [31,32], this reporter gene is widely used in land green plants having no background of the GUS activity [33,34]. In addition, the *CaMV 35S* promoter is heterologously used in land green plants as a strong constitutive and non-tissue-specific transcriptional regulator [35,36]. Therefore, it is a natural choice for the selection of the *CaMV35S-GUS* gene by pioneers for initial trials of seaweed transformation.

To date, studies have been mainly focused on *Porphyra* species because of their economical values. As shown in Table 1, expression of the *CaMV 35S-GUS* gene was previously observed in *P. miniata, P. tenera* and *P. yezoensis* [37-42], all of which were performed by electoroporation using protoplasts. Kuang et al. [38] also tested the particle bombardment of the *CaMV 35S-GUS* gene in *P. yezoensis* and got positive results. Moreover, the availability of mammalian-type simian virus 40 (*SV40*) promoter was reported to express the *E. coli lacZ* reporter gene, encoding β-galactosidase cleaving colorless substrate X-gal (5-bromo-4-chloro-3-indolyl-β-galactopyranoside) to produce a blue insoluble product [43], in *P. haitanensis, Gracilaria chagii* and *K. alvarezii* by electroporation or particle bombardment [44,45].

2.2. Recent improvement of the transient transformation system in *Porphyra*

As noted above, pioneer experiments of red algal transient transformation were performed using plant viral *CaMV 35S RNA* and animal viral *SV40* promoters in combination with *GUS* and *lacZ* reporter genes (Table 1). The *CaMV 35S* and *SV40* promoters are typical eukaryotic class II promoters with a TATA box and thus are generally employed to drive transgenes in dicot plant and animal cells, respectively [46,47]. However, we have found that the TATA box is not usually found in the core promoters of *P. yezoensis* genes (unpublished observation), and we thus proposed that there were differences in the promoter structure and transcriptional regulation of protein-coding genes between red algae and dicot plants. Indeed, we recently observed quite low activity of the *CaMV 35S* promoter and the *GUS* reporter gene in *P. yezoensis* gametophytec cells [29,30,48]. These observations are completely opposite from the results in previous reports using the *CaMV 35S* promoter [25,37-41]. As a result, the transient transformation system in red seaweeds has recently been improved by resolving this problem.

Species	Status of expression	Gene transfer method	Promoter	Marker or Reporter	Ref.
Kappaphycus alvarezii	transient	particle bombardment	CaMV 35S	GUS	[25]
Porphyra miniata	transient	electroporation	CaMV 35S	GUS	[37]
Porphyra yezoensis	transient	Electroporation particle bombardment	CaMV 35S	GUS	[38]
Porphyra tenera	transient	electroporation	CaMV 35S	GUS	[39]
Porphyra yezoensis	transient	electroporation	rbcS	GUS	[40]
Porphyra yezoensis	transient	electroporation	CaMV 35S	GUS	[41]
Porphyra yezoensis	transient	electroporation	CaMV 35S β-tubulin	GUS	[42]
Gracilaria changii	transient	particle bombardment	SV40	lacZ	[44]
Porphyra haitanensis	transient		SV40	CAT	[128]
Porphyra yezoensis	transient	electriporation	SV40	CAT, GUS	[129]
Porphyra yezoensis	transient	electroporation	Rubisco	GUS, sGFP(S65T)	[130]
Porphyra yezoensis	transient	particle bombardment	CaMV 35S PyGAPDH	PyGUS	[48]
Porphyra yezoensis	transient	particle bombardment	PyAct1	PyGUS	[66]
Porphyra yezoensis	transient	particle bombardment	PyAct1	AmCFP	[70]
Porphyra yezoensis	transient	particle bombardment	PyAct1	AmCFP, ZsGFP, ZsYFP, sGFP(S65T)	[71]
Porphyra tenera Porphyra yezoensis	transient	particle bombardment	PtHSP70 PyGAPDH	PyGUS	[85]
Porphyra species* Bangia fuscopurpurea	transient	particle bombardment	PyAct1	PyGUS sGFP(S65T)	[86]
Porphyra species* Bangia fuscopurpurea	transient	particle bombardment	PtHSP70	PyGUS	[87]
Porphyra yezoensis	stable	*Agrobacterium*-mediated gene transfer	CaMV 35S	GUS	[26]
Porphyra leucostica	stable	ekectroporation	CaMV 35S	lacZ	[27]
Porphyra yezoensis	stable	*Agrobacterium*-mediated gene transfer	(unknown)	(unknown)	[28]
Kappaphycus alvarezii	stable	particle bombardment	SV40	lacZ	[45]
Porphyra haitanensis	stable	glass bead agitation	SV40	lacZ EGFP	[131]
Gracilaria changii	stable	particle bombardment	SV40	lacZ	[91]
Gracilaria gracilis	stable	particle bombardment	SV40	lacZ	[92]

**Porphyra species* used are *P. yezoensis, P. tenera, P. okamurae, P. onoi, P. variegate* and *P. pseudolinearis.*

Table 1. Transformation in red seaweeds.

http://dx.doi.org/10.5772/52978

2.2.1. *Optimization of codon usage in the reporter gene*

Inefficient expression of foreign genes in the green alga *Chlamydomonas reinhardtii* is often due to the incompatibility of the codon usage in the gene's coding regions [49-51]. Expressed sequence tag (EST) analysis of *P. yezoensis* reveals that the codons in *P. yezoensis* nuclear genes frequently contain G and C residues especially in their third letters, by which means the GC content reaches a high of 65.2% [52]. Since bacterial *GUS* and *lacZ* reporter genes have AT-rich codons, the incompatibility of codon usage, which generally inhibits the effective use of transfer RNA by rarely used codons in the host cells, thus decreasing the efficiency of the translation [53], might be responsible for the poor translation efficiency of foreign genes in *P. yezoensis* cells. It is therefore possible that modification of codon usage in the *GUS* gene would enable the efficient expression of this gene in *P. yezoensis* cells.

Accordingly, the codon usage of the *GUS* reporter gene was adjusted to that in the nuclear genes of *P. yezoensis* by introducing silent mutations [48], by which unfavorable or rare codons in the *GUS* reporter gene were exchanged for favorable ones without affecting amino acid sequences. The resultant artificially codon-optimized *GUS* gene was designated *PyGUS*, and its GC content was increased from 52.3% to 66.6% [48]. When the *PyGUS* gene directed by the *CaMV 35S* promoter was introduced into *P. yezoensis* gametophytic cells by particle bombardment, low but significant expression of the *PyGUS* gene was observed by histochemical detection and GUS activity test, indicating enhancement of the expression level of the *GUS* reporter gene [29,30,48]. Optimization of the codon usage of the reporter gene is therefore one of the important factors for successful expression in *P. yezoensis* cells [29,30,48].

2.2.2. *Employment of endogenous strong promoters*

The *CaMV 35S* promoter has very low activity in cells of green microalgae such as *Dunaliella salina* [54], *Chlorella kessleri* [55] and *Chlorella vulgaris* [56] and no activity in *C. reinhardtii* cells [57-59]. Thus, a low level of *PyGUS* expression under the direction of the *CaMV 35S* promoter is likely to be caused by the low activity of this promoter in *P. yezoensis* cells. A hint to overcoming this problem was that employment of strong endogenous promoters such as the *β-Tub*, *RbcS2* and *Hsp70* promoters results in the efficient expression of foreign genes in microalgae [60-65]. Therefore, it is likely that efficient expression of the *PyGUS* reporter gene in *P. yezoensis* cells is caused by the recruitment of endogenous strong promoters.

By comparison with steady-state expression levels by reverse transcription-polymerase chain reaction (PCR), we found two genes strongly expressed in *P. yezoensis*: genes encoding glyceraldehyde-3-phosphate dehydrogenase (PyGAPDH) and actin 1 (PyAct1) [29]. When the *PyGUS* gene fused with the 5′ upstream regions of these genes were introduced into gametophytic cells by particle bombardment, cells expressing the reporter gene and GUS enzymatic activity were dramatically increased [48,66]. These results indicate that employment of endogenous strong promoters is another important factor necessary for high-level expression of the reporter gene in *P. yezoensis* cells. In addition, the original *GUS* gene was not activated by *PyGAPDH* or *PyAct1* promoter [29,30,48], demonstrating that the *PyGUS* gene and endogenous strong promoter have a synergistic effect on the efficiency of the expression in *P. yezoensis* cells (Figure 1A). Therefore, the combination of endogenous strong promoters with codon optimized reporter genes is critical for successful transient transformation in *Porphyra* species [29,30]. The established procedure of transient transformation is schematically represented in Figure 2.

2.2.3. Application of the transient transformation for using fluorescent proteins

The *GUS* reporter gene is usually used to monitor gene expression *in planta*; however, visualization of the reporter products requires cell killing. Reporters that function in living cells have also been established to date with fluorescent proteins used most commonly. The green fluorescent protein (GFP) has the advantage over other reporters for monitoring subcellular localization of proteins in living cells, because its fluorescence can be visualized without additional substrates or cofactors [67]. At present, there are GFP variants with non-overlapping emission spectra such as cyan fluorescent protein (CFP), yellow fluorescent protein (YFP) and red fluorescent protein, which allows multicolor imaging in cells [68,69].

Until recently, there was no report about the successful expression of fluorescent proteins in seaweeds. However, based on an efficient transient transformation system in *P. yezoensis*, fluorescent reporter systems have recently been established in *P. yezoensis* [29,30,70,71]. The humanized fluorescent protein genes, AmCFP, ZsGFP, and ZsYFP (Clontech) and the plant-adapted GFP(S65T) [72], the GC contents of which are as high as 63.7%, 62.8%, 61.9% and 61.4%, respectively, were strongly expressed in gametophytic cells under the direction of the *PyAct1* promoter using the particle bombardment method [71] (see Figure 1B).

The analysis of subcellular localization of cellular molecules was available using humanized and plant-adapted fluorescent reporters. The first successful attempt at achieving this process was to monitor the plasma membrane localization of phosphoinositides in *P. yezoensis* [70]. Phosphoinositides (PIs), whose inositol ring has hydroxyl groups at positions D3, D4 and D5 for phosphorylation, constitute a family of structurally related lipids, PtdIns-monophosphates [PtdIns3P, PtdIns4P and PtdIns5P], PtdIns-bisphosphates [PtdIns(3,4)P_2, PtdIns(3,5)P_2 and PtdIns(4,5)P_2] and PtdIns-trisphosphate [PtdIns(3,4,5)P_3], all of which are detectable in plants except for PtdIns(3,4,5)P_3 [73,74]. Although the PIs are a minority among membrane phospholipids, they play important roles in regulating multiple processes of development and cell responses to environmental stimuli in land plants and green algae [74,75]. Recently, Li et al. [76,77] demonstrated that PIs are involved in the establishment of cell polarity in *P. yezoensis* monospores. The Pleckstrin homology (PH) domain, a PI-binding module, each part of which has individual substrate specificity, is usually used to monitor PIs *in vivo* by fusion with a fluorescent protein [78-80]. For instance, the PH domains from human phospholipase Cδ1 (PLCδ1) are employed for the detection of PtdIns(4,5)P_2 [81], whereas that from the v-akt murine thymoma viral oncogene homolog 1 (Akt1) has dual specificity in the detection of both PtdIns(3,4)P_2 and PtdIns(3,4,5)P_3 [82]. Because of this substrate specificity, we were able to visualize PtdIns(3,4)P_2 and PtdIns(4,5)P_2 at the plasma membrane with humanized AmCFP and ZsGFP fused to the PH domains from PLCδ1 and Akt1 via the direction of the *PyAct1* promoter [70].

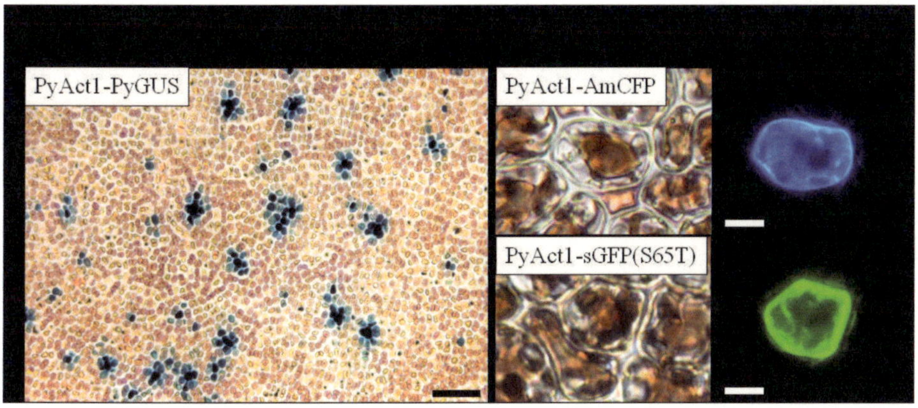

Figure 1. Efficient expression of PyGUS and fluorescent proteins by the transeint transformation with circular expression plasmids in *P. yezoensis* gametophytic cells. (A) Expression of the codon-optimized *PyGUS* reporter gene under the direction of the actin 1 (*PyAct1*) promoter. Blue histochemically stained cells are PyGUS expression cells. Scale bar corresponds to 100 µm. (B) Expression of humanized AmCFP and plant-adapted sGFP(S65T). Gametophytic cells transiently transformed with expression plasminds containng *AmCFP* or *sGFP(S65T)* gene under the control of the *PyAct1* promoter. Left and right panels show bright field and fluorescence images, respectively. Scale bar corresponds to 5 µm.

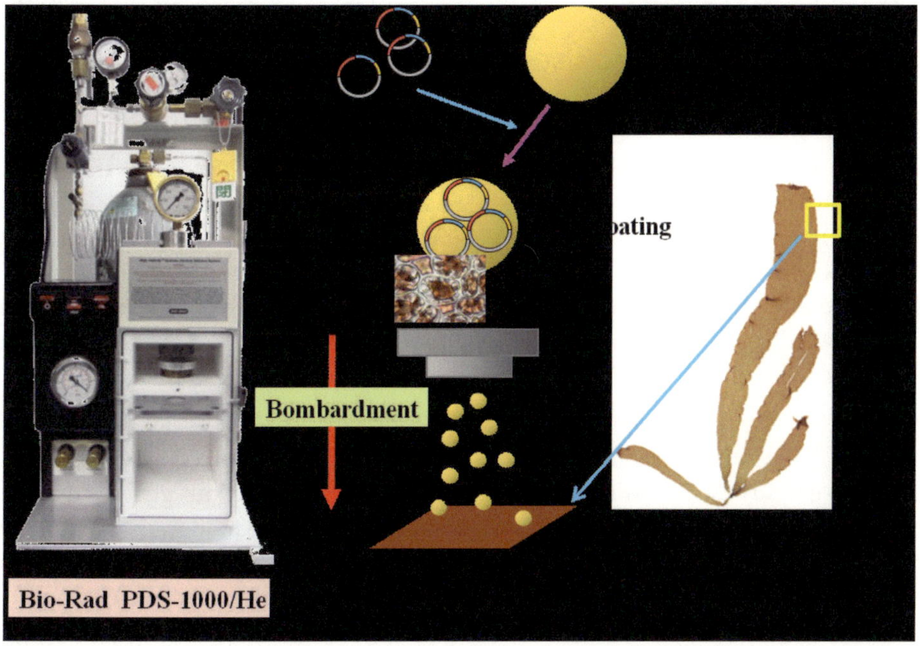

Figure 2. The established procedure of transeient transformation in *P. yezoensis.* A circular expression plasmid is bombarded into *P. yezoensis* gametophytic cells using the Bio-Rad PDS-1000/He after coating of gold particles with the plasmid. Expression of the reporter gene is observed after cultivation of the bombareded gametophyte under dark for two days; for *PyGUS* reporter gene, histochemical staining with X-gluc solution and fluorometric analysis of enzymatic activity are performed; for fluorescent reporter genes, bombarded sanples are examined with fluorescent microscopy.

Moreover, subcellular localization of transcription factors was also visualized in *P. yezoensis*. When complete open reading frames (ORFs) of transcription elongation factor 1 (PyElf1) and multiprotein bridging factor 1 (PyMBF1) from *P. yezoensis* were fused to AmCFP or ZsGFP, nuclear localization of these fusion proteins was observed in gametophytic cells, which was confirmed by overlapping of fluorescent signals with SYBR Gold staining of the nucleus [71]

With the successfull visualization of subcellular localization of cellular molecules, the transient transformation system developed in *P. yezoensis* appearst to be powerful tool to analyze functions of genes and cellular components [29,30].

2.2.4. Applicability of the P. yezoensis transient transformation system in other red seaweeds

As described above, both the adjustment of codon usage of the reporter gene according to algal preference and the employment of the strong endogenous promoters are important for providing highly efficient and reproducible expression of the reporter gene in *P. yezoensis*. In addition to Bangiophyceae like *Porphyra* species, Florideophyceae are also known, including a number of industrially important species such as *Gracilaria* and *Gelidium* as sources of agar and *Chondrus* and *Kappaphycus* as sources of carrageenan. Thus, the establishment of a genetic manipulation system for both Bangiophyceae and Florideophyceae other than *P. yezoensis* is awaited. EST analysis of *P. haitanensis* revealed that the GC content of the ORFs in this alga was as high as that in *P. yezoensis*, and analysis of the *GAPDH* gene from a Florideophycean alga *Chondrus crispus* showed a high GC content (approximately 60%) in the coding region [83,84], which is consistent with the codon preference in *P. yezoensis*. Since efficient expression of the *GAPDH-PyGUS* gene has recently been confirmed in *P. tenera* [85], the applicability of the *P. yezoensis* transient gene expression system in other red seaweeds is expected. Indeed, using the *PyGUS* and *sGFP(S65T)* reporter genes under the direction of the *PyAct1* promoter, efficient expression of *PyGUS* and *sGFP(S65T)* genes was observed in Bangiophyceae including *P. tenera, P. okamurae, P. psedolinearis* and *Bangia fuscopurpurea,* although the expression efficiency varied among species [86]. Thus, the transient transformation system developed in *P. yezoensis* is widely applicable in Bangiophycean red algae [29,30,86].

No expression of the reporter genes was seen in Florideophyceae [29,30,86]. Since the availability of the *P. yezoensis* promoter is responsible for this deficiency in gene expression, it is important to employ the 5′ upstream region of the suitable endogenous gene from Florideophycean algae. Alternatively, it is possible that the efficiency of plasmid transfer by bombardment parameters is reduced by the cell wall and thus the size of the gold particles, target distance, acceleration pressure and/or amount of DNA per bombardment should be adjusted.

Taken together, *PyGUS* and *sGFP(S65T)* genes act synergistically with the *PyAct1* promoter as a heterologous promoter for transient transformation in Bangiophycean algae. Recently, the same synergistic effect was found in *P. tenera*; that is, Son et al. [85] clearly indicated that the heat shock protein 70 (*PtHSP70*) promoter from *P. tenera* can activate the *PyGUS* gene in gametophytic cells of this alga. Moreover, the *PtHSP70-PyGUS* gene was expressed in *P. yezoensis, P. okamurae, P. psedolinearis* and *B. fuscopurpurea* [85,87]. These findings are consistent with the importance of two critical factors for transient transformation in red seaweeds, adjustment of the codon usage in reporter genes and employment of a strong endogenous promoter.

The other important message gleaned from this experimental data is the efficient heterologous activation of *PyGAPDH* and *PtHSP70* promoters in *P. tenera* and *P. yezoensis*, respectively [85, 87]. For the genetic transformation, the target site for recombination is usually determined by the DNA sequence of genes desired for disruption or modification. Thus, it is better to exclude a possibility of homologous recombination at the DNA region corresponding to the promoter sequence used for expression of the reporter gene that is usually sandwiched between two different DNA sequences from the objective gene or its flanking regions. To avoid incorrect recombination at the promoter region, it is critical to employ heterologous promoters, whose sequence has low homology to the genome sequence of the host, to direct the expression of reporter genes. It is therefore possible that *PyGAPDH* and *PtHSP70* promoters are useful for genetic transformation in *P. tenera* and *P. yezoensis*, respectively. The number of promoters acting for heterologous reporter gene expression in red algae must be increased to develop a sophisticated system for red algal genetic transformation.

2.3. Towards genetic transformation in red seaweeds

The successful genetic transformation in red alga has been established only in unicellular algae [20,88]. The first report described chloroplast transformation in the unicellular red alga *Porphyridium* sp. through integration of the gene encoding AHAS(W492S) into the chloroplast genome by homologous recombination, resulting in sulfometuron methyl (SMM) resistance at a high frequency in SMM-resistant colonies [89]. The next report was of stable nuclear transformation in the unicellular red alga *Cyanidioschyzon merolae*, for which the uracil auxotrophic mutant lacking the *URA5.3* gene was used for the genetic background to isolate mutants with uracil prototrophic by employing the wild-type *URA5.3* gene fragment as a selection maker [90].

Table 1 shows preliminary experiments with red seaweeds. The first was by Cheney et al. [26], who introduced the *CaMV 35S-GUS* and *CaMV 35S-GFP* genes in *P. yezoensis* genome via an *Agrobacterium*-mediated transformation system. In addition, they transformed *P. yezoensis* with a bacterial nitroreductase gene via an *Agrobacterium*-mediated method [28] and *P. leucosticte* monospores with an unknown gene by electroporation [27]. However, these reports appeared on conference abstracts and thus details of experimental procedures are unknown. In related work, the genetic transformation of *Gracilaria* species was recently reported [91,92], in which integration of the *SV40-lacZ* gene was checked by PCR using genomic DNAs prepared from particle-bombarded seaweeds; however, selection of transformed cells was not performed. Taken together, these preliminary experiments are not enough to conclude the establishment of genetic transformation in red seaweeds, meaning that the genetic transformation system has not yet been fully established in red macroalgae.

As mentioned above, procedures of integration and targeting of foreign genes into the genome and selection of transformed cells must be developed for establishing the genetic transformation system, although other requirements such as an efficient gene transfer system and an efficient expression system for foreign genes have been resolved by developing the transient transformation system in Bangiophyceae [29,30]. Regarding the unresolved points, knowledge about the selection of transformed cells is now accumulating. Selection marker genes are required to distinguish between transformed cells and non-transformed cells, since successful integration of a foreign gene into the host genome usually occur in only a small percentage of transfected cells. These genes confer new traits to any transformed target strain of a certain species, thus enabling the transformed cells to survive on medium containing the selective agent, where non-transformed cells die. Genes with resistance to the aminoglycoside antibiotics, which bind to ribosomal subunits and inhibit protein synthesis in bacteria, eukaryotic plastids and mitochondria [93], are generally used as selection markers. For example, the antibiotics hygromycin and geneticin (G418) are frequently used as selection agents with the hygromycin phosphotransferase (*hptII*) gene to inactivate hygromycin via an ATP-dependent phosphorylation [94] and the neomycin phosphotransferase II (*nptII*) gene to detoxify neomycin, G418 and paromomycin [93], respectively. In the green alga *Chlamydomonas reinhardtii,* the hygromycin phosphotransferase (*aph7″*) gene from *Streptomyces hygroscopicus* and the aminoglycoside phosphotransferase *aphVIII* (*aphH*) gene from *S. rimosus* had been reported as selectable marker genes for hygromycin and paromomycin, respectively, with similarity in the codon usage [95-97]. The *aphH* gene from *S. rimosus* is also applicable to the multicellular green alga *Volvox carteri* as a paromomycin-resistance gene [97,98]. In the diatom *Phaeodactylum tricornutum,* the expressed chloramphenicol acetyltransferase gene (*CAT*) detoxifies chloramphenicol [99], and the *nptII* gene confers resistance to the aminoglycoside antibiotic G418 [64]. Likewise, the *nptII* gene gives resistance to the antibiotic G418 in the diatoms *Navicula saprophila* and *Cyclotella cryptica* [100]. However, it is unknown what kinds of antibiotics-based selection marker genes are available for red seaweeds, since red algae usually have strong resistance to antibiotics.

Recently, the sensitivity of *P. yezoensis* gametophytes to ampicillin, kanamycin, hygromycin, geneticin (G418), chloramphenicol and paromomycin was investigated, and lethal effects of these antibiotics on gametophytes were observed at more than 2.0 mg mL^{-1} of hygromycin, chloramphenicol and paromomycin and 1.0 mg mL^{-1} of G418, whereas *P. yezoensis* gametophytes were highly resistant to ampicillin and kanamycin [101]. Although these concentrations are in fact very high in comparison with the cases for the red alga *Griffithsia japonica* and the green alga *C. reinhardtii* that were highly sensitive to 50 μg mL^{-1} and 1.0 μg mL^{-1} of hygromycin [96,102], these four antibiotics and corresponding resistance genes are suitable for the selection of genetically transformed cells from *P. yezoensis* gametophytes. According to these findings, it is necessary to confirm whether *P. yezoensis* gametophytes will obtain antibiotic tolerance by introducing plasmid constructs containing the antibiotic-resistance genes mentioned above. In this case, optimization of codon usage and the employment of strong endogenous promoter are expected for functional expression of the antibiotic resistance genes, according to the knowledge from the transient transformation system [29,30]. Such efforts could effectively contribute to the establishment of the genetic transformation system in red seaweeds in the near future.

http://dx.doi.org/10.5772/52978

3. Transformation in brown seaweeds

According to Qin et al. [103], trials of genetic engineering in brown seaweeds have been started by transient expression of the *GUS* reporter gene under direction of the *CaMV 35S* promoter by particle bombardment in *Laminaria japonica* and *Undaria pinnatifida*, which were first performed in 1994 by them. Descriptions of related experiments were published later [104,105]. Qin et al. then focused on the establishment of genetic transformation in brown seaweeds and provided successful reports of genetic transformation in *L. japonica* [103,106]. Genetic transformation was performed by particle bombardment only and expression of a reporter gene was driven by the *SV40* promoter that is usually used for gene expression in mammalian cells (Table 2). This promoter represented non-tissue and -cell specificity for expression of the *E. coli lacZ* reporter gene [105]. Promoters from maize ubiquitin, algal adenine-methyl transfer enzyme and diatom fucoxanthin chlorophyll a/c-binding protein (*FCP*) genes are also useful for transient expression of the *GUS* gene, and the *FCP* promoter is also employable for the genetic transformation [107]. Interestingly, there has been no successful genetic transformation using the *CaMV 35S* promoter, although this promoter is active in the transient transformation [103].

Despite the reports of successful genetic transformation, there was no experiment using antibiotics-based selection of transformants in brown seaweeds. Although the susceptibility of brown seaweeds to antibiotics has not been well studied, it was reported that *L. japonica* was sensitive to chloramphenicol and hygromycin, but not to ampicillin, streptomycin, kanamycin, neomycin or G418 [103,106]. Since hygromycin is more effective than chloramphenicol [103,106], it is necessary to confirm the utility of the *SV40-hptII* gene for the selection of transformants to fully establish the genetic transformation system in kelp.

Species	Status of expression	Gene transfer method	Promoter	Marker or Reporter	Ref.
Laminaria japonica	transient	particle bombardment	CaMV 35S	GUS	[103]
Laminaria japonica	stable	particle bombardment	SV40	GUS	[105]
Laminaria japonica	transient	particle bombardment	CaMV 35S, UBI, AMT	GUS	[107]
Laminaria japonica	stable	particle bombardment	FCP	GUS	[107]
Laminaria japonica	stable	particle bombardment	SV40	HBsAg	[113]
Laminaria japonica	stable	particle bombardment	SV40	Rt-PA	[114]
Laminaria japonica	stable	particle bombardment	SV40	bar	[114]
Undaria pinnatifida	transient	particle bombardment	CaMV 35S	GUS	[103]
Undaria pinnatifida	transient	particle bombardment	SV40	GUS	[104]

Table 2. Transformation in brown seaweeds.

To date, stably transformed microalgae have been employed to produce recombinant antibodies, vaccines or bio-hydrogen as well as to analyze the gene functions targeted for engineering [108-111]. Based on the success in genetic transformation, *L. japonica* is now proposed as a marine bioreactor in combination with the *SV40* promoter [112]. Indeed, the integration of human hepatitis B surface antigen (HBsAg) and recombinant human tissue-type plasminogen (*rt-PA*) genes into the *L. japonica* genome resulted in the efficient expression of these genes under the direction of the *SV40* promoter [113,114]. Therefore, *L. japonica* promises to be useful as the bioreactor for vaccine and other medical agents, although it is necessary to continually check the safety and value of its use by oral application.

There is no competitor against the Chinease group in the field of using brown algal genetic transformation at present [103,106,115], meaning there is currently no way to confirm the replicability of the experiments. It is necessary to re-examine the effective use of the non-plant *SV40* promoter and bacterial *lacZ* gene in brown algal genetic transformation, which is also important for the evaluation of genetic transformation in red seaweeds *Gracilaria* species, for which the *SV40-lacZ* gene was used such as transgene, as described above [91,92].

4. Transformation in green seaweeds

The first successfull genetic transformation in green algae was reported in the unicellular green alga *Chlamydomonas reinhardtii* for which the particle bombardment and glass-bead abrasion techniques were employed [116,117]. The availability of electoroporation was then confirmed in *C. reinhardtii* and *Chlorella saccharophila* [118,119]. These methods produce physical cellular damage, allowing DNA to be introduced into the cells. Moreover, particle bombardment was confirmed to be useful for a diverse range of species, including transient transformation in the unicellular *Haematococcus pluvialis* [120] and genetic transformation in the multicellular *Volvox carteri* and *Gonium pectoral* [97,120-122]. *Agrobacterium*-mediated transformation was also reported in *H. pluvialis* [123]. Thus, all methods employed in land green plants are applicable for green microalgae [88] (see Table 3).

In contrast, there is no report about genetic transformation in green seaweeds (Table 3). To date, only two examples of transient transformation have been reported in green seaweeds, *Ulva lactura* by electroporation and *U. pertusa* by particle bombardment [124,125]. As shown in Table 3, some of the experiments with micro- and macro-green algae used the promoter of the *CaMV 35S* gene and the coding region of the *E. coli GUS* gene. Although functionality of the *CaMV 35S* promoter and bacterial *GUS* coding region is the same in land green plants, the expression of the *GUS* reporter gene seems to be very low in the green seaweed *U. lactuca* [124]. In fact, codon-optimization is critical for the expression of reporters like the *GFP* gene and antibiotic-resistance genes in *C. reinhardtii* [47,90,115,126]. Moreover, the *HSP70A* promoter was employed to increase the expression level of the reporter genes [47,115]. Therefore, it is possible that changes in codon usage in the reporter gene and promoter region could result in increased reporter gene expression in transient transformation of green seaweeds. Recently, the Rubisco small subunit (*rbsS*) promoter was used for expression of the *EGFP* reporter gene in transient transformation of *U. pertusa* by particle bombardment [125]; however, it is still unclear whether the *rbsS* promoters and the *EGFP* gene work well in cells in comparison with the *CaMV 35S* promoter and codon-optimized *EGFP* gene.

Species	Status of expression	Gene transfer method	Promoter	Marker or Reporter	Ref.
Microalga					
Chlamidominas reinhardtii	stable	particle bombardment			[116]
Chlamidominas reinhardtii	stable	glass bead agitation	Nitrate reductase	Nitrate reductase	[117]
Chlamidominas reinhardtii	stable	electroporation	CaMV 35S	CAT	[118]
Chlamidominas reinhardtii	stable	glass bead agitation	rbcS2	aphVIII	[95]
Chlamidominas reinhardtii	stable	glass bead agitation	β2-tubulin	Aph7"	[96]
Chlorella saccharophila	transient	electroporation	CaMV 35S	GUS	[119]
Haematococcus pluvialis	transient	particle bombardment	SV40	lacZ	[120]
Haematococcus pluvialis	stable	*Agrobacterium*-mediated gene transfer	CaMV 35S	GUS,GFP, hptII	[123]
Volvox Carteri	stable	particle bombardment	β2-tubulin	arylsulfatase	[121]
Volvox Carteri	stable	particle bombardment glass bead agitation	Hsp70A-rbcS2 fusion	aphVIII	[98]
Volvox Carteri	stable	particle bombardment	β-tubulin, Hsp70A	aphH	[97]
Gonium pectoral	stable	particle bombardment	VcHsp70A	aphVIII	[122]
Seaweed					
Ulva lactuca	transient	electroporation	CaMV 35S	GUS	[124]
Ulva pertusa	transient	particle bombardment	UprbcS	EGFP	[125]

Table 3. Transformation in green algae.

If the *rbsS-EGFP* gene is useful as a reporter gene for genetic transformation in green seaweeds, the remaining problems to be settled are methods for foreign gene integration into the genome and selection of transformed cells, which is the same as the situation with red seaweeds. Reddy et al. [24] commented on the antibiotic sensitivity of green seaweeds, indicating the considerable resistance of protoplast from *Ulva* and *Monostroma* to hygromycin and kanamycin.

Insensitivity to hygromycin is inconsistent with the case for red and brown seaweeds [101-103,106]. It is therefore necessary to check the sensitivity of green seaweed cells to other antibiotics to identify the genes employable for selection of transformed cells, which could stimulate the development of the genetic transformation system in green seaweeds.

5. Conclusion

It is nearly 20 years since the first transient transformation of a red seaweed with a circular expression plasmid [25], and many efforts have been made to develop a system for transient and stable expression of foreign genes in many kinds of seaweeds; however, a seaweed transformation system has still not been developed. The main problem is the employment of the *CaMV 35S-GUS* gene in the pioneer attempts at system development as shown in Tables 1, 2 and 3. This problem was recently resolved through the development of an efficient transient transformation system in *P. yezoensis* [29,30]. It is clear that the *CaMV 35S* promoter and the *GUS* gene are not active in seaweed cells [48], which is supported by knowledge from green microalgae [54-65]. These findings strongly indicate that defects in the transfer and expression of foreign genes were resolved by knowledge about two critical factors required for reproducibility and efficiency of transient gene expression, namely, the optimization of codon usage of coding regions and the employment of endogenous strong promoters [29,30]. However, these significant improvements are not enough to allow the establishment of a genetic transformation system in seaweeds.

At present, genetic transformation is reported in red and brown seaweeds using the *SV40* promoter (Tables 1 and 2) [91,92,103,105-107,113,114]; however, isolation of transgenic clone lines produced from distinct single transformed cells, which is the final goal of the genetic transformation of seaweeds as a tool, has not been reported, and seaweed genetic transformation is thus not fully developed. Therefore, the next step is to develop the gene targeting system via integration of a foreign gene into the genome and the system for selection of transformed cells. Since candidates of antibiotic agents for selection of transformed algal cells were mentioned recently [101-103,106], it is necessary to confirm the possibility of stable integration of a plasmid or a DNA fragment containing the selection maker gene into the seaweed genome. Once a positive result is obtained, it could lead us to establish the gene targeting method via the homologous recombination using an appropriate antibiotics resistance gene, if possible, with the heterologous promoter. To this end, we must reevaluate the availability of the methods for gene transfer such as electroporation and *Agrobacteriumu* infection.

Due to the problems with efficient genetic transformation systems, the molecular biological studies of seaweeds are currently progressing more slowly than are the studies of land green plants. Since a genetic transformation system would allow us to perform genetic analysis of gene function via inactivation and knock-down of gene expression by RNAi and antisense RNA supression, its establishment will enhance both our biological understanding and genetical engineering for the sustainable production of seaweeds and also for the use of seaweeds as bioreactors.

http://dx.doi.org/10.5772/52978

Author details

Koji Mikami*

Address all correspondence to: komikami@fish.hokudai.ac.jp

Faculty of Fisheries Sciences, Hokkaido University, 3-1-1 Minato, Hakodate, Japan

References

[1] Griffith, F. The significance of pneumococcal types. Journal of Hygiene 1928;27(2) 113–159.

[2] Avery OT, MacLeod CM, MaCarty M. Studies on the chemical nature of the substance inducing transformation of Pneumococcal types: induction of transformation by a desoxyribonucleic acid fraction isolated from *Pneumococcus* Type III. Journal of Experimental Medicine 1944;79(2) 137–158.

[3] Mandel M, Higa A. Calcium-dependent bacteriophage DNA infection. Journal of Molecular Biology 1970;53(1) 159–162.

[4] Griesbeck C, Kobl I, Heitzer M. *Chlamydomonas reinhardtii*. A protein expression system for pharmaceutical and biotechnological proteins. Molecular Biotechnology 2006;34(2) 213-223.

[5] Torney F, Moeller L, Scarpa A, Wang K. Genetic engineering approaches to improve bioethanol production from maize. Current Opinion in Biotechnology 2007;18(3) 193-199.

[6] Bhatnagar-Mathur P, Vadez V, Sharma KK. Transgenic approaches for abiotic stress tolerance in plants: retrospect and prospects. Plant Cell Reports 2008;27(3) 411-424.

[7] Doehmer J, Barinaga M, Vale W, Rosenfeld MG, Verma IM, Evans RM. Introduction of rat growth hormone gene into mouse fibroblasts via a retroviral DNA vector: expression and regulation. Proceedings of the National Academy of Sciences of the United States of America 1982;79(7) 2268-7222.

[8] Smith EF, Townsend CO. A plant tumor of bacterial origin. Science 1907;25(643) 671-673.

[9] Chilton MD, Drummond MH, Merio DJ, Sciaky D, Montoya AL, Gordon MP, Nester EW. Stable incorporation of plasmid DNA into higher plant cells: the molecular basis of crown gall tumorigenesis. Cell 1977;11(2) 263-271.

[10] Zambryski P, Joos H, Genetello C, Leemans J, Van Montagu M, Schell J. Ti plasmid vector for the introduction of DNA into plant cells without alteration of their normal regeneration capacity. EMBO Journal 1983;2(12) 2143–2150.

[11] Bevan M. Binary *Agrobacterium* vectors for plant transformation. Nucleic Acids Research 1984;12(22) 8711-8721.

[12] Guo M, Bian X, Wu X, Wu M. *Agrobacterium*-mediated genetic transformation: history and progress. In: Alvarrez MA (ed.) Genetic Transformation. Rijeka: InTech; 2011. p5-28.

[13] Klein TM, Wolf ED, Wu R, Sanford JC. High-velocity microprojectiles for delivery of nucleic acids into living cells. Nature 1987;327(6117) 70-73.

[14] Fromm ME, Taylor LP, Walbot V. Expression of genes transferred into monocot and dicot plant cells by electroporation. Proceedings of the National Academy of Sciences of the United States of America 1985;82(17) 5824-5828.

[15] Newell CA. Plant transformation technology: developments and applications. Molecular Biotechnology 2000;16(1) 53-65.

[16] Radchuk VV, Ryschka U, Schumann G, Klocke E. Genetic transformation of cauliflower (*Brassica oleracea* var. botrytis) by direct DNA uptake into mesophyll protoplasts. Physiologia Plantarum 2002;114(3) 429-438.

[17] Cove D. The moss *Physcomitrella patens*. Annual Review of Genetics 2005;39 339-358.

[18] Takenaka M, Yamaoka S, Hanajiri T, Shimizu-Ueda Y, Yamato KT, Fukuzawa H, Ohyama K. Direct transformation and plant regeneration of the haploid liverwort *Marchantia polymorpha* L. Transgenic Research 2000;9(3) 179-185.

[19] D'Orazio N, Gemello E, Bammoue MA, de Girolamo M, Ficoneri C, Riccioni G.: A treasure from the sea. Marine Drugs 2012;10(3) 604-616.

[20] Hallmann A. Algal transgenics and biotechnology. Transgenic Plant Journal 2007;1(1) 81-98.

[21] Smit AJ. Medicinal and pharmaceutical uses of seaweed natural products: a review. Journal of Applied Phycology 2004;16(4) 245-262.

[22] van Ginneken VJTH, Helsper JPEG, de Visser W, van Keulen H, Brandenburg WA. Polyunsaturated fatty acids in various macroalgal species from north Atlantic and tropical seas. Lipids in Health and Disease 2011;10 104. (doi: 10.1186/1476-511X-10-104) http://www.lipidworld.com/content/10/1/104 (accessed 22 June 2011).

[23] Walker TL, Collet C, Purton S. Algal transgenics in the genomic era. Journal of Phycology 2005;41(6) 1077-1093.

[24] Reddy CRK, Gupta MK, Mantri VA, Jha B. Seaweed protoplasts: status, biotechnological perspectives and needs. Journal of Applied Phycology 2008;20(5) 619-632.

[25] Kurtzman AM, Cheney DP. Direct gene transfer and transient expression in a marine red alga using the biolistic method. Journal of Phycology 1991;27(Supplement) 42.

[26] Cheney DP, Metz B, Stiller J. *Agrobacterium*-mediated genetic transformation in the macroscopic marine red alga *Porphyra yezoensis*. Journal of Phycology 2001;37(Supplement) 11–12.

[27] Lin CM, Larsen J, Yarish C, Chen T. A novel gene transfer in *Porphyra*. Journal of Phycology 2001;37(Supplement) 31.

[28] Bernasconi P, Cruz-Uribe T, Rorrer G, Bruce N, Cheney DP. Development of a TNT-detoxifying strain of the seaweed *Porphyra yezoensis* through genetic engineering. Journal of Phycology 2004;40(Supplement) 31.

[29] Mikami K, Hirata R, Takahashi M, Uji T, Saga N. Transient transformation of red algal cells: Breakthrough toward genetic transformation of marine crop *Porphyra* species. In: Alvarez MA. (ed.) Genetic Transformation. Rijeka: InTech; 2011. p241-258.

[30] Mikami K, Uji T. Transient gene expression systems in *Porphyra yezoensis*: Establishment, application and limitation. In: Mikami K. (ed.) *Porphyra yezoensis*: Frontiers in Physiological and Molecular Biological Research. New York: Nova Science Publishers; 2012. p93-117.

[31] Basu C, Kausch AP, Chandlee JM. Use of β-glucuronidase reporter gene for gene expression analysis in turfgrasses. Biochemical and Biophysical Research Communications 2004;320(1) 7-10.

[32] Sun P, Tian QY, Chen J, Zhang WH. Aluminium-induced inhibition of root elongation in *Arabidopsis* is mediated by ethylene and auxin. Journal of Experimantal Botany 2010;61(2) 347-356.

[33] Jefferson RA. The GUS reporter gene system. Nature 1989;342(6251) 837-838.

[34] Cervera M. Histochemical and fluorometric assays for uidA (GUS) gene detection. Methods in Moecular Biology 2004;286(4) 203-213.

[35] Louis J, Lorenc-Kukula K, Singh V, Reese J, Jander G, Shah J. Antibiosis against the green peach aphid requires the *Arabidopsis thaliana MYZUS PERSICAEINDUCED LIPASE1* gene. Plant Journal 2010;64(5) 800-811.

[36] Wally O, Punja ZK. Enhanced disease resistance in transgenic carrot (*Daucus carota* L.) plants over-expressing a rice cationic peroxidase. Planta 2010;232(5) 1229-1239.

[37] Kübler JE, Minocha SC, Mathieson AC. Transient expression of the GUS reporter gene in protoplasts of *Porphyra miniata* (Rhodophyta). Journal of Marine Biotechnology 1994;1 165–169.

[38] Kuang M, Wang SJ, Li Y, Shen DL, Zeng CK. Transient expression of exogenous GUS gene in *Porphyra yezoensis* (Rhodophyta). Chinese Journal of Oceanology and Limnology 1998;16(1) 56–61.

[39] Okauchi M, Mizukami Y. Transient β-Glucuronidase (GUS) gene expression under control of *CaMV 35S* promoter in *Porphyra tenera* (Rhodophyta). Bulletin of National Research Institute of Aquaculture 1999;Supplement 4 13-18.

[40] Hado M, Okauchhi M, Murase N, Mizukami Y. Transient expression of GUS gene using Rubisco gene promoter in the protoplasts of *Porphyra yezoensis*. Suisan Zoushoku 2003;51(3) 355-360.

[41] Liu HQ, Yu WG, Dai JX, Gong QH, Yang KF, Zhang YP. Increasing the transient expression of *GUS* gene in *Porphyra yezoensis* by 18S rDNA targeted homologous recombination. Journal of Applied Phycology 2003;15(5) 371-377.

[42] Gong Q, Yu W, Dai J, Liu H, Xu R, Guan H, Pan K. Efficient *gusA* transient expression in *Porphyra yezoensis* protoplasts mediated by endogenous beta-tubulin flanking sequences. Journal of Ocean University of China 2005;6(1) 21-25.

[43] Bell P, Limberis M, Gao GP, Wu D, Bove MS, Sanmiguel JC, Wilson JM. An optimized protocol for detection of *E. coli* beta-galactosidase in lung tissue following gene transfer. Histochemistry and Cell Biology 2005;124(1) 77-85.

[44] Gan SY, Qin S, Othman RY, Yu D, Phang SM. Transient expression of *lacZ* in particle bombarded *Gracilaria changii* (Gracilariales, Rhodophyta). Journal of Applied Phycology 2003;15(4) 351–353.

[45] Wang J, Jiang P, Cui Y, Deng X, Li F, Liu J, Qin S. Genetic transformation in *Kappaphycus alvarezii* using micro-particle bombardment: a potential strategy for germplasm improvement. Aquaculture International 2010;18(6) 1027-1034.

[46] Kang HG, An GH. Morphological alterations by ectopic expression of the rice *OsMADS4* gene in tobacco plants. Plant Cell Reports 2005;24(2) 120-126.

[47] Funabashi H, Takatsu M, Saito M, Matsuoka H. Sox2 regulatory region 2 sequence works as a DNA nuclear targeting sequence enhancing the efficiency of an exogenous gene expression in ES cells. Biochemical and Biophysical Research Communications 2010;400(4) 554-558.

[48] Fukuda S, Mikami K, Uji T, Park EJ, Ohba T, Asada K, Kitade Y, Endo H, Kato I, Saga N. Factors influencing efficiency of transient gene expression in the red macrophyte *Porphyra yezoensis*. Plant Science 2008;174(3) 329-339.

[49] Fuhrmann M, Hausherr A, Ferbitz L, Schödl T, Heitzer M, Hegemann P. Monitoring dynamic expression of nuclear genes in *Chlamydomonas reinhardtii* by using a synthetic luciferase reporter gene. Plant Molecular Biology 2004;55(6) 869-881.

[50] Ruecker O, Zillner K, Groebner-Ferreira R, Heitzer M. Gaussia-luciferase as asensitive reporter gene for monitoring promoter activity in the nucleus of the green alga *Chlamydomonas reinhardtii*. Molecular Genetics and Genomics 2008;280(2) 153-162.

[51] Shao N, Bock R. A codon-optimized luciferase from *Gaussia princeps*facilitates the in vivo monitoring of gene expression in the model alga *Chlamydomonas reinhardtii*. Current Genetics 2008;53(6) 381-388.

[52] Nikaido I, Asamizu E, Nakajima M, Nakamura Y, Saga N, Tabata S. Generation of 10,154 expressed sequence tags from a leafy gametophyte of a marine red alga, *Porphyra yezoensis*. DNA Research 2000;7(3) 223-227.

[53] Mayfield SP, Kindle KL. Stable nuclear transformation of *Chlamydomonas reinhardtii* by using a *C. reinhardtii* gene as the selectable marker. Proceedings of the National Academy of Sciences of the United States of America 1990;87(6) 2087-2091.

[54] Tan D, Qin S, Zhang Q, Jiang P, Zhao F. Establishment of a micro-particle bombardment transformation system for *Dunaliella salina*. Journal of Microbiology 2005;43(4) 361-365.

[55] El-Sheekh MM. Stable transformation of the intact cells of *Chlorella kessleri* with high velocity microprojectiles. Biologia Plantarum 1999;42(2) 209-216.

[56] Chow KC, Tung WL. Electrotransformation of *Chlorella vulgaris*. Plant Cell Reports 1999;18(9) 778-780.

[57] Day A, Debuchy R, Dillewijn J, Purton S, Rochaix JD. Studies on the maintenance and expression of cloned DNA fragments in the nuclear genome of the green alga *Chlamydomonas reinhardtii*. Physiologia Plantarum 1990;78(2) 254-260.

[58] Blankenship JE, Kindle K. Expression of chimeric genes by the light-regulated *cabII-1* promoter in *Chlamydomonas reinhardtii*: a *cabII-1/nit1* gene functions as a dominant selectable marker in a *nit1- nit2*-strain. Molecular and Cellular Biology 1992;12(11) 5268-5279.

[59] Lumbreras V, Stevens DR, Purton S. Efficient foreign gene expression in *Chlamydomonas reinhardtii* mediated by an endogenous intron. Plant Journal 1998;14(4) 441-447.

[60] Davies JP, Weeks DP, Grossman AR. Expression of the arylsulfatase gene from the beta 2-tubulin promoter in *Chlamydomonas reinhardtii*. Nucleic Acids Res 1992;20(12) 2959-2965.

[61] Stevens DR, Rochaix JD, Purton S. The bacterial phleomycin resistance gene *ble* as a dominant selectable marker in *Chlamydomonas*. Molecular and General Genetics 1996;251(1) 23-30.

[62] Schroda M, Blocker D, Beck CF. The HSP70A promoter as a tool for the improved expression of transgenes in *Chlamydomonas*. Plant Journal 2000;21(2) 121-131.

[63] Walker TL, Becker DK, Collet CC. Characterisation of the *Dunaliella tertiolecta RbcS* genes and their promoter activity in *Chlamydomonas reinhardtii*. Plant Cell Reports 2004;23(10-11) 727-735.

[64] Zaslavskaia LA, Lippmeier JC, Kroth PG, Grossman AR, Apt KE. Transformation of the diatom *Phaeodactylum tricornutum* (Bacillariophyceae) with a variety of selectable marker and reporter genes. Journanl of Phycology 2000;36(2) 379-386.

[65] Hirakawa Y, Kofuji R, Ishida K. Transient transformation of achlorarachniophyte alga, *Lotharella amoebiformis* (Chlorarachniophyceae), with *uidA* and *egfp* reporter genes. Jounal of Phycology 2008;44(3) 814-820.

[66] Takahashi M, Uji T, Saga N, Mikami K. Isolation and regeneration of transiently transformed protoplasts from gametophytic blades of the marine red alga *Porphyra yezoensis*. Electronic Journal of Biotechnology 2010;13(2) (doi:10.2225/vol13-issue2-fulltext-7) http://www.ejbiotechnology.cl/content/vol13/issue2/full/7/index.html (accessed 15 March 2010).

[67] Ehrhardt D. GFP technology for live cell imaging. Current Opinion in Plant Biology 2003;6(6) 622-628.

[68] Lin ZF, Arciga-Reyes L, Zhong SL, Alexander L, Hackett R, Wilson I, Grierson D. SlTPR1, a tomato tetratricopeptide repeat protein, interacts with the ethylene receptors NR and LeETR1, modulating ethylene and auxin responses and development. Journal of Experimental Botany 2008;59(15) 4271-4287.

[69] Martin K, Kopperud K, Chakrabarty R, Banerjee R, Brooks R, Goodin MM. Transient expression in *Nicotiana benthamiana* fluorescent marker lines provides enhanced definition of protein localization, movement and interactions in planta. Plant Journal 2009;59(1) 150-162.

[70] Mikami K, Uji T, Li L, Takahashi M, Yasui H, Saga N. Visualization of phosphoinositides via the development of the transient expression system of a cyan fluorescent protein in the red alga *Porphyra yezoensis*. Marine Biotechnology 2009;11(5) 563-569.

[71] Uji T, Takahashi M, Saga N, Mikami K. Visualization of nuclear localization of transcription factors with cyan and green fluorescent proteins in the red alga *Porphyra yezoensis*. Marine Biotechnology 2010;12(2) 150-159.

[72] Niwa Y, Hirano T, Yoshimoto K, Shimizu M, Kobayashi H. Non-invasive quantitative detection and applications of non-toxic, S65T-type green fluorescent protein in living plants. Plant Journal 1999;18(4) 455-463.

[73] Xue HW, Chen X, Me Y. Function and regulation of phospholipid signaling in plants. Biochemical Journal 2009;421(Part 2) 145-156.

[74] Heilmann I. Using genetic tools to understand plant phosphoinositide signalling. Trends in Plant Science 2009;14(3) 171-179.

[75] Williams ME, Torabinejad J, Cohick E, Parker K, Drake EJ, Thompson JE, Hortter M, DeWald DB. Mutations in the Arabidopsis phosphoinositide phosphatase gene SAC9 lead to over accumulation of PtdIns(4,5)P_2 and constitutive expression of the stress-response pathway. Plant Physiology 2005;138(2) 686-700.

[76] Li L, Saga N, Mikami K. Phosphatidylinositol 3-kinase activity and asymmetrical accumulation of F-actin are necessary for establishment of cell polarity in the early development of monospores from the marine red alga *Porphyra yezoensis*. Journal of Experimental Botany 2008;59(13) 3575-3586.

[77] Li L, Saga N, Mikami K. Ca^{2+} influx and phosphoinositide signalling are essential for the establishment and maintenance of cell polarity in monospores from the red alga *Porphyra yezoensis*. Journal of Experimental Botany 2009;60(12) 3477-3489.

[78] Vermeer JEM, Thole JM, Goedhart J, Nielsen E, Munnik T, Gadella TW. Imaging phosphatidylinositol 4-phosphate dynamics in living plant cells. Plant Journal 2009;57(2) 356-372.

[79] Szentpetery Z, Balla A, Kim YJ, Lemmon MA, Balla T. Live cell imaging with protein domains capable of recognizing phosphatidylinositol 4,5-bisphosphate; a comparative study. BMC Cell Biology 2009;10 67. (doi:10.1186/1471-2121-10-67) http://www.biomedcentral.com/1471-2121/10/67 (accessed 21 September 2009).

[80] Loovers HM, Postma M, Keizer-Gunnink I, Huang YE, Devreotes PN, van Haastert PJ. Distinct roles of PI(3,4,5)P_3 during chemoattractant signaling in *Dictyostelium*: a quantitative in vivo analysis by inhibition of PI3-kinase. Molecular Biology of the Cell 2006;17(4) 1503-1513.

[81] Lee Y, Kim YW, Jeon BW, Park KY, Suh SJ, Seo J, Kwak JM, Martinoia E, Hwang I. Phosphatidylinositol 4,5-bisphosphate is important for stomatal opening. Plant Journal 2007;52(5) 803-816.

[82] Nishio M, Watanabe KI, Sasaki J, Taya C, Takasuga S, Iizuka R, Balla T, Yamazaki M, Watanabe H, Itoh R, Kuroda S, Horie Y, Forster I, Mak TW, Yonekawa H, Penninger JM, Kanaho Y, Suzuki A, Sasaki T. Control of cell polarity and motility by the PtdIns(3,4,5)P-3 phosphatase SHIP1. Nature Cell Biology 2007;9(1) 36-44.

[83] Fan XL, Fang YJ, Hu SN, Wang GC. Generation and analysis of 5318 expressed sequence tags from the filamentous sporophyte of *Porphyra haitanensis* (Rhodophyta). Journal of Phycology 2007;43(6) 1287–1294.

[84] Liaud MF, Valentin C, Brandt U, Bouget FY, Kloareg B, Cerff R. (1993). The GAPDH gene system of the red alga *Chondrus crispus*: promoter structures, intron/exon organization, genomic complexity and differential expression of genes. Plant Molecular Biology 1993;23(5) 981–994.

[85] Son SH, Ahn J-W, Uji T, Choi D-W, Park E-J, Hwang MS, Liu JR, Choi D, Mikami K, Jeong W-J. Development of a transient gene expression system in the red macroalga, *Porphyra tenera*. Journal of Applied Phycology 2012;24(1) 79-87.

[86] Hirata R, Takahashi M, Saga N, Mikami K. Transient gene expression system established in *Porphyra yezoensis* is widely applicable in Bangiophycean algae. Marine Biotechnology 2011;13(5) 1038-1047.

[87] Hirata R, Jeong W-J, Saga N, Mikami K. Heterologous activation of the *Porphyra tenera HSP70* promoter in Bangiophycean algal cells. Bioengineered Bugs 2011;2(5) 272-274.

[88] Coll JM. Methodologies for transferring DNA into eukaryotic microalgae. Spanish Journal of Agricultural Research 2006;4(4) 316-330.

[89] Lapidot M, Raveh D, Sivan A, Arad S, Shapira M. Stable Chloroplast transformation of the unicellular red alga *Porphyridium* species. Plant Physiology 2002;129(1) 7-12.

[90] Minoda A, Sakagami R, Yagisawa F, Kuroiwa T, Tanaka K. Improvement of culture conditions and evidence for nuclear transformation by homologous recombination in a red alga, *Cyanidioschyzon merolae* 10D. Plant and Cell Physiology 2004;45(6) 667-671.

[91] Gan SY, Qin S, Othman RY, Yu D, Phang SM. Development of a transformation system for *Gracilaria changii* (Gracilariales, Rhodophyta), a Malaysian red alga via microparticle bombardment. The 4 th Annual Seminar of National Science Fellowship 2004, 2004;BIO08, 45-48.

[92] Haddy SM, Meyers AE, Coyne VE. Transformation of *lacZ* using different promoters in the commercially important red alga, *Gracilaria gracilis*. Afreican Journal of Biotechnology 2012;11(8) 1879-1885.

[93] Miki B, McHugh S. Selectable marker genes in transgenic plants: applications, alternatives and biosafety. Journal of Biotechnology 2004;107(3) 193-232.

[94] Tian LN, Charest PJ, Seguin A, Rutledge RG. Hygromycin resistance is an effective selectable marker for biolistic transformation of *Black spruce* (Picea mariana). Plant Cell Reports 2000;19(4) 358-362.

[95] Sizova I, Fuhrmann M, Hegemann P. A *Streptomyces rimosus aphVIII* gene coding for a new type phosphotransferase provides stable antibiotic resistance to *Chlamydomonas reinhardtii*. Gene 2001;277(1-2) 221-229.

[96] Berthold P, Schmitt R, Mages W. An engineered *Streptomyces hygroscopicus aph 7"* gene mediates dominant resistance against hygromycin B in *Chlamydomonas reinhardtii*. Protist 2002;153(4) 401-412.

[97] Jakobiak T, Mages W, Scharf B, Babinger P, Stark K, Schmitt R. The bacterial paromomycin resistance gene, *aphH*, as a dominant selectable marker in *Volvox carteri*. Protest 2004;155(4) 381-393.

[98] Hallmann A, Wodnniok S. Swapped green algal promoters: *aphVIII*-based gene constructs with *Chlamydomonas* flanking sequences work as dominant selectable makers in *Volvox* and vice versa. Plant Cell Reports 2006;25(6) 582-591.

[99] Apt KE, Kroth-Pancic PG, Grossman AR. Stable nuclear transformation of the diatom *Phaeodactylum tricornutum*. Molecular and General Genetics 1996;252(5) 572-579.

[100] Dunahay TG, Jarvis EE, Roessler PG. Genetic transformation of the diatom *Cyclotella cryptic* and *Navicula saprophila*. Journal of Phycology 1995;31(6) 1004-1012.

[101] Takahashi M, Mikami K, Mizuta H, Saga N. Identification and efficient utilization of antibiotics for the development of a stable transformation system in Porphyra yezoensis (Bangiales, Rhodophyta). Journal of Aquaculture Research and Development 2011;2 118, (doi:10.4172/2155-9546.1000118). http://www.omicsonline.org/2155-9546/2155-9546-2-118.php (accessed 23 December 2011)

[102] Lee YK, An G, Lee IK. Antibiotics resistance of a red alga, *Griffithsia japonica*. Journal of Plant Biology 2000;43(2) 179-182.

[103] Qin S, Jiang P, Li X, Wang X, Zeng C. A transformation model for *Laminaria japonica* (Phaeophyta, Laminariales). Chinese Journal of Oceanology and Limnology 1998;16(Supplement 1) 50-55.

[104] Yu D, Qin S, Sun G, Chengkui Z. Transient expression of *lacZ* in the economic seaweed *Undaria pinnatifida*. High Technology Letters 2002;12(8) 93-95.

[105] Jiang P, Qin S, Tseng CK. Expression of the *lacZ* reporter gene in sporophytes of the seaweed *Laminaria japonica* (Phaeophyceae) by gametophyte-targeted transformation. Plant Cell Reports 2003;21(12) 1211-1216.

[106] Qin S, Sun GQ, Jiang P, Zou LH, Wu Y, Tseng C. Review of genetic engineering of *Laminaria japonica* (Laminariales, Phaepophyta) in China. Hydrobiologia 1999;398/399(0) 469-472.

[107] Li F, Qin S, Jiang P, Wu Y, Zhang W. The integrative expression of GUS gene driven by FCP promoter in the seaweed *Laminaria japonica* (Phaeophyta). Journal of Applied Phycology 2009;21(3) 287-293.

[108] Sun M, Qian KX, Su N, Chang HY, Liu JX, Chen GF. Foot-and-mouth disease virus VP1 protein fused with cholera toxin B subunit expressed in *Chlamydomonas reinhardtii* chloroplast. Biotechnology Letters 2003;25(13) 1087-1092.

[109] Zorin B, Lu YH, Sizova I, Hegemann P. Nuclear gene targeting in *Chlamydomonas* as exemplified by disruption of the *PHOT* gene. Gene 2009;432(1-2) 91-96.

[110] Specht E, Miyake-Stoner S, Mayfesqaxeld S. Micro-algae come of age as a platform for recombinant protein production. Biotechnology Letters 2010;32(10) 1373-1383.

[111] Wu S, Huang R, Xu LL, Yan GY, Wang QX. Improved hydrogen production with expression of *hemH* and *lba* genes in chloroplast of *Chlamydomonas reinhardtii*. Journal of Biotechnology 2010;146(3) 120-125.

[112] Qin S, Jiang P, Tseng CK. Transforming kelp into a marine bioreactor. Trends in Biotechnology 2005;23(5) 264-268.

[113] Jiang P, Qin S, Tseng CK. Expression of hepatitis B surface antigen gene (*HBsAg*) in *Laminaria japonica* (Laminariales, Phaeophyta). Chinese Science Bulletin 2002;47(17) 1438-1440.

[114] Zhang YC, Jiang P, Gao JT, Liao JM, Sun SJ, Shen ZL, Qin S. Recombinant expression of *rt-PA* gene (encoding Reteplase) in gametophytes of the seaweed *Laminaria japonica* (Laminariales, Phaeophyta). Science in China-Series C, Life sciences 2008;51(12) 1116-1120.

[115] Qin S, Jiang P, Tseng CK. Molecular biotechnology of marine algae in Chaina. Hydrobiologia 2004;512(1-3) 21-26.

[116] Kindle KL, Schnell RA, Fernandez E, Lefebvre PA. Stable nuclear transformation of *Chlamydomonas* using the *Chlamydomonas* gene for nitrate reductase. Journal of Cell Biology 1989;109(6 Part1) 2589–2601.

[117] Kindle KL. High-frequency nuclear transformation of *Chlamydomonas reinhardtii*. Proceedings of the National Academy of Sciences of the United States of America 1990;87(3) 1228-1232.

[118] Brown LE, Sprecher SL, Keller LR. Introduction of exogenous DNA into *Chlamidomonas reinhardtii* by electroporation. Molecular and Cellular Biology 1991;11(4) 2328-2332.

[119] Maruyama M, Horákova I, Honda H, Xing X, Shiragami N, Unno H. Introduction of foreign DNA into *Chlorella saccharophila* by electroporation. Biotechnology Techniques 1994;8(11) 821-826.

[120] Teng C, Qin S, Liu J, Yu D, Liang C, Tseng C. Transient expression of *lacZ* in bombarded unicellular green alga *Haematococcua pluvialis*. Journal of Applied Phycology 2002;14(6) 495-500.

[121] Hallmann A, Rappel A, Sumper M. Gene replacement by homologous recombination in the multicellular green alga *Volvox carteri*. Proceedings of the National Academy of Sciences of the United States of America 1997;94(14) 7469-7474.

[122] Lerche K, Hallmann A. Stable nuclear transformation of *Gonium pectoral*. BMC Biotechnol 2009;9 64. (doi:10.1186/1472-6750-9-64) http://www.biomedcentral.com/1472-6750/9/64 (accessed 10 July 2009).

[123] Kathiresan S, Chandrashekar A, Ravishankar GA, Sarada R. *Agrobacterium*-mediated transformation in the green alga *Haematococcus pluvialis* (Chlorophyceae, Volvocales). Journal of Phycology 2009;45(3) 642-649.

[124] Huang, X, Weber JC, Hinson TK, Mathieson AC, Minocha SC. Transient expression of the GUS reporter gene in the protoplasts and partially digested cells of *Ulva lactuca* L (Chlorophyta). Botanica Marina 1996;39(1-6) 467-474.

[125] Kakinuma M, Ikeda M, Coury DA, Tominaga H, Kobayashi I, Amano H. Isolation and characterization of the *rbcS* genes from a sterile mutant of *Ulva pertusa* (Ulvales, Chlorophytea) and transient gene expression using the *rbcS* gene promoter. Fisheries Science 2009;75(4) 1015-1028.

[126] Franklin S, Ngo B, Efuet E, Mayfield SP. Development of a GFP reporter gene for *Chlamydomonas reinhardtii* chloroplast. Plant Journal 2002;30(6) 733-744.

[127] Ohnuma M, Yokoyama T, Inouye T, Sekine Y, Tanaka K. Polyethylene glycol (PEG)-mediated transient gene expression in a red alga, Cyanidioschyzon merolae 10D. Plant and Cell Physiology 2008;49(1) 117-120.

[128] Zuo Z, Li B, Wang C, Cai J, Chen Y. Increasing transient expression of *CAT* gene in *Porphyra haitanensis* by matrix attachment regions and 18S rDNA targeted homologous recombination. Aquaculture Research 2007;38(7) 681-688.

[129] He P, Yao Q, Chen Q , Guo M, Xiong A, Wu W, Ma J. Transferring and expression of glucose oxidase gene in *Porphyra yezoensis*. Journal of Phycology 2001;37(Supplement) 23.

[130] Mizukami Y, Hado M, Kito H, Kunimoto M, Murase N. Reporter gene introduction and transient expression in protoplasts of *Porphyra yezoensis*. Journal of Applied Phycology 2004;16(1) 23-29.

[131] Wang J, Jiang P, Cui Y, Guan X, Qin S. Gene transfer into conchospores of *Porphyra haitanensis* (Bangiales, Rhodophyta) by glass bead agitation. Phycologia 2010;49(4) 355-360.

Chapter 14

Genetic Diversity and Population Structure of the Hotoke Loach, *Lefua echigonia*, a Japanese Endangered Loach

Noriyuki Koizumi, Masakazu Mizutani, Keiji Watabe,
Atsushi Mori, Kazuya Nishida and Takeshi Takemura

Additional information is available at the end of the chapter

http://dx.doi.org/10.5772/53022

1. Introduction

In Japan, conservation and regeneration projects have been actively conducted for large-sized birds such as the Japanese crested ibis, *Nipponia Nippon*, the oriental white stork, *Ciconia boyciana* and the intermediate egret, *Ardea intermedia* (Photo 1) that inhabit rural areas [1, 2]. Many people are highly interested in these projects and a lot of information about growth and breeding for large-sized birds is broadcasted through television, radio and internet media. In such a situation, a conspicuous topic has been found in recent months, that is, 2 individuals of the Japanese crested ibis displayed beriberi symptom along with human being, because of overeating great favorite food that is the Dojo loach, *Misgurnus anguillicaudatus*. Their beriberi symptom appeared to be caused by eating the Dojo loach raw. The 2 individuals were diagnosed as follows; this beriberi symptom occurred as vitamin B1 in the individual bodies was destroyed by tiaminase enzyme contained in the Dojo loach. At present the two individuals may have completely recovered from the beriberi symptom through vitamin B1 supplementation by injection.

By the way, the presence of 10 or more loach species including the Dojo loach has been observed around paddy fields in rural areas, Japan. Most loach species appear to become food attractive for large-sized birds (Photo 1) [3] and one of the reasons is that the loach species cannot move as rapidly as swimming species such as the Japanese dace, *Tribolodon hakonensis* and the Ayu, *Plecoglossus altivelis altivelis*; hence large-sized birds are able to easily catch them. In addition, only the Dojo loach has been investigated, but nutrition contained in this loach was superior to other fish species; for instance, amount of calcium in the Dojo was 9 times that of the Japanese ell, *Anguilla japonica,* and also the Dojo had the most amount of vitamin B2 in all fish [4, 5]. Actually these precise nutrient components may somewhat differ among the loach species, but their nutrient components could have to be fundamentally similar.

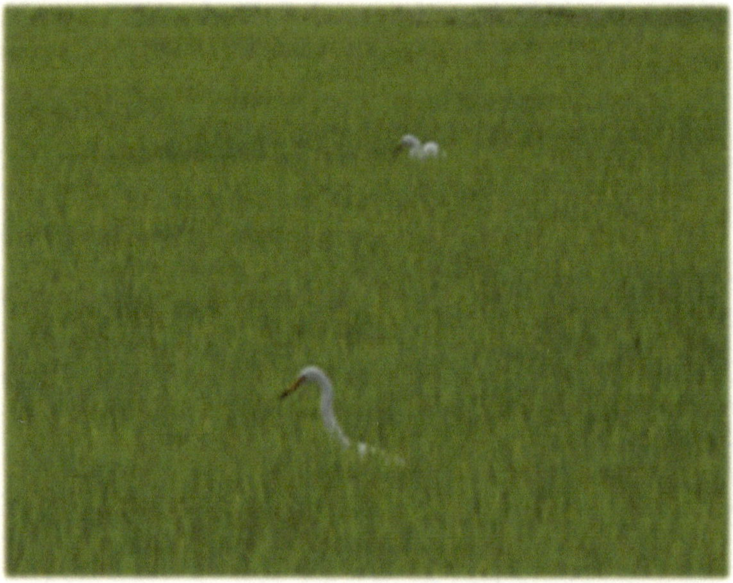

Photo 1. 2 individuals of the intermediate egret, *Ardea intermedia* that are finding individuals of many loach species as their food in paddy field (unpublished photo)

However, some of the loach species have confronted a kind of serious concerns, especially a decrease in their population size. In Japan, we have conducted many land consolidation projects for rising rice production and easing agricultural works in rural area since 1960s. In land consolidation projects, concrete canals, drops, diversion weirs, etc. have been installed around paddy fields as agricultural infrastructures; therefore not only fish populations and their habitats but also all of ecosystem and biodiversity in rural area have been extremely damaged [6-9].

The Hotoke loach, *Lefua echigonia* endemic to Japan (the above in Photo 2) has been well known as a representative loach species has been adversely impacted on its habitat due to land consolidation projects. Since populations of this loach have rapidly declined in some rural areas, consequently the Hotoke loach has been designated as an endangered species on the Red List of Japan [10]. Ecology of the loach is briefed as follows; this species is widely distributed across the Honshu Island from the Tohoku region to the Kinki region. They usually inhabits earth canals and ditches around paddy fields into which ground water flows (the bottom in Photo 2) [11, 12]. The Hotoke loach often coexists with the Dojo loach in the habitat and geographic variations for this loach based on morphological characteristics is obscure [13, 14].

http://dx.doi.org/10.5772/53022

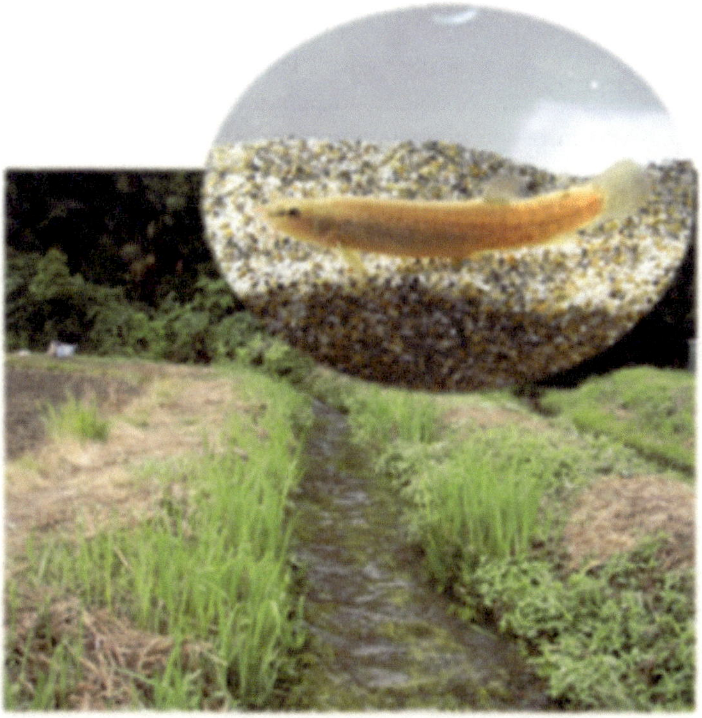

Photo 2. An adult of the Hotoke loach, *Lefua echigonia* (the above) with approximately 60 mm in body length and typical earth ditch (the bottom) where the loach inhabits around paddy field (unpublished photo)

In recent years, because importance of ecosystem and biodiversity in rural areas has been deeply realized, various research activities have been carried out for conserving and recovering populations of the Hotoke loach. Distribution pattern and habitat characteristics of this loach were elucidated in some rural areas [15-18], manners of habitat utilization and migration routes for the species were investigated [11, 12, 19, 20] and techniques of artificial propagation were developed with human chorionic gonadotropin [21-23]. Further, molecular analyses of phylogeography of the Hotoke loach using DNA sequences of mitochondrial genes revealed that populations of the species were evolutionally separated into a total of 7 genetic clades in Japan [24-29].

Unfortunately, there is also another serious concern left in populations of the Hotoke loach. That is, as this loach has experienced, diminishment of population size may often cause to improve not only fragmentation among populations but also inbreeding among individuals. Such populations tend to have distinctly poor genetic diversity, occasionally threatened with extinction [30-33]. Usually, to evaluate genetic diversity including genetic population structure for such populations, polymorphism analysis has been performed using microsatellite loci in nuclear genome [33-35]. Only preliminary investigations, however, were implemented for populations the Hotoke loach [36-38], although microsatellite analyses have been carried out for populations of several endangered species.

Genetic properties of microsatellite loci are briefed as follows (Fig. 1). These loci are repeating sequences of 2 to 6 base pairs of DNA, for instance CACA..., CTCTCT... and CATCAT... Microsatellites that are typically neutral and co-dominant are used as molecular markers in genetics for kinship, population and other studies, because of often presenting high levels of inter- and intra-specific polymorphism [33-35]. Especially, CA nucleotide repeats appear to be very frequent in human and other genomes and present every few 10,000 to 100,000 base pairs. A repeat size in a locus is treated as an allele and a pair of repeat sizes which are inherited from both of parents is used as genotypes at a locus for a diploid organism. Heterozygous describes a genotype consisting of two different sizes (alleles), while homozygous does it consisting of two identical ones (Fig. 1).

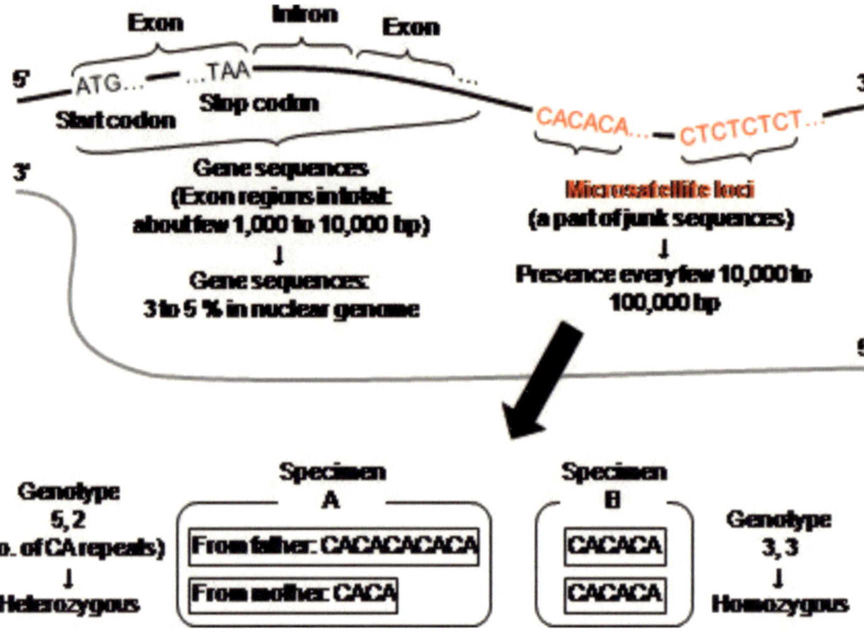

Figure 1. Scheme of microsatellite loci in nuclear genome DNA (unpublished figure)

In this chapter, to detect the existence of the above serious genetic issues, we carried out a series of analysis for genetic diversity and population structure in population of the Hotoke loach (Fig. 2). Novel microsatellite loci applied in this loach were developed and characterized in Section 2. Using these developed loci, genetic diversity and population structure were investigated for populations in the upper Kokai River along with adjacent rivers, the southeast part of Tochigi Prefecture as a case study in Section 3. Technical terms related to population and conservation genetics are often used in the sections; thus, details of meanings of these terms are able to be known by references cited in the end of this chapter.

http://dx.doi.org/10.5772/53022

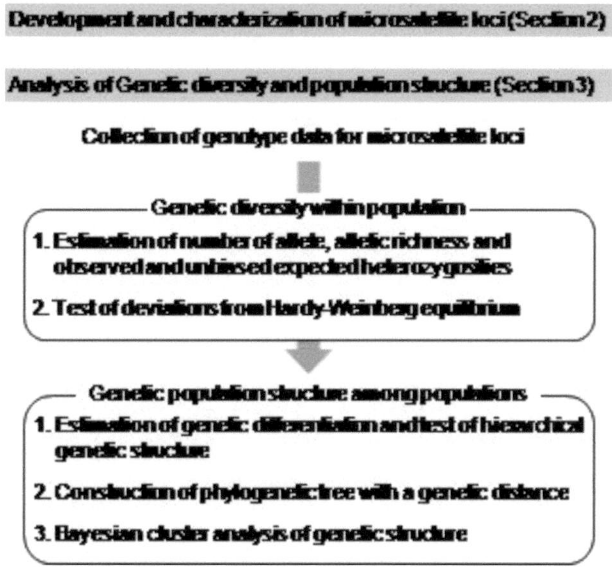

Figure 2. Analysis flow chart of microsatellite loci in this chapter (unpublished figure)

2. Development and characterization of microsatellite loci

2.1. Development of microsatellite loci

In Section 2, a total of 19 novel microsatellite loci for the Hotoke loach were isolated with an individual obtained in the Shitada R., Chiba Pref. and characterized using 32 individuals collected from the Koise R., Ibaraki Pref. The following development procedure [36] is partially improved based on the latest studies [39, 40].

A sample of this loach was collected from an agricultural canal in the Shitada R., Chiba Pref. in 2005 and preserved in 99% EtOH, and then stored at -30 °C. Genomic DNA was extracted from single caudal fin clip, approximately 5 mm × 5 mm, using a standard phenol-chloroform procedure [41]. Microsatellite enriched libraries were developed following the previous study [42] with some modifications. Briefly extracted DNA was digested with RsaI (New England Biolabs) and then ligated to SuperSNX linkers (SuperSNX24 Forward: 5′-GTT TAA GGC CTA GCT AGC AGA ATC-3′ and SuperSNX24+4P Reverse: 5′-phosphate-GAT TCT GCT AGC TAG GCC TTA AAC AAA A-3′). Linker-ligated DNA was enriched for microsatellites using streptavidin-coated magnetic beads (Dynal) treated with a blocking step [43] and using the pooled biotinylated probes $(CA)_{12}$ and $(CT)_{12}$.

Recovered DNA was amplified by the polymerase chain reaction (PCR) and PCR products were cloned using a TOPO-TA Cloning Kit (Invitrogen) following the manufacture's protocol. A total of 192 positive clones were sequenced on a 3130*xl* Genetic Analyzer (Applied Biosystems; ABI) using BigDye Terminator kit version 3.1 (ABI) and resultant sequences were proofread for repeat regions using the software DNA BASER version 3.2 (Heracle BioSoft). Oligonucleotide primers (Table 1) were designed in flanking regions of the 19 targeted microsatellite loci using the software DNASIS PRO version 3.0 (Hitachi Software Engineering).

Locus	Primer sequence (5'-3')[a]	Repeat motif	Dye	GenBank accession no.
Lec01	F: M13-ATC CCT CCC TTC ACC GTC TG R: TCC GAA ACC AGC AGC ACC AC	$(CA)_{13}$	6-FAM	AB286032
Lec02	F: M13-TGT GCT GTA GGA TTG CTT GAG C R: ATG TCA GAG GCT GAT GG GAT AC	$(CA)_{30}AA(CA)_{5}$	VIC	AB286033
Lec03	F: M13-CGT CCA CCA GCC TTA CGA AC R: TGA CGC TCA GTA GTC GGA CC	$(CA)_{14}CG(CA)_{3}$	6-FAM	AB286034
Lec04	F: M13-GCA CTG CTG ATG ACA ATC ATT G R: GCT TTG GGT TAG AAC ATC AGT G	$(GA)_{29}$	6-FAM	AB286035
Lec05	F: M13-TGT CTG CTG TGA TGA TGA CAT C R: CTC ACA GCA CTA TTC ACT GAT G	$(GT)_{13}$	NED	AB286036
Lec06	F: M13-CCG TGT CTG TTT TGC TTT CTC R: CTC CCT TCA CAA AGT AAC TGG	$(CT)_{10}$	PET	AB286037
Lec07	F: M13-TGT GAA GAA ACC TGA ACA CGC R: ATT CTG TGT CCC TGA ACA CAC	$(CT)_{7}(GT)_{11}$	NED	AB286038
Lec08	F: M13-GAC GCA ACA ATC TCA GGG TC R: ACA GGA CCA AGT GGA CTC TC	$(GA)_{5}AA(GA)_{8}$ $AA(GA)_{17}$	6-FAM	AB286039
Lec09	F: M13-GGG GAT AGT GGA GAT GGG TG R: TTC ATC CCT CTT CCG CCC AC	$(GA)_{14}$	PET	AB286040
Lec10	F: M13-GGT TGG CAA TGC CAG CAA TG R: TGC TTT ACC AAG GTG ACG GC	$(GT)_{7}$	6-FAM	AB286041
Lec11	F: M13-CTG ACA CTG TGT GTG TAG CAG R: GGT TTC ACC TGG TCC ATA CAC	$(GT)_{11}$	NED	AB286042
Lec12	F: M13-GGC ACC AAA GGC AGA TTT TAC R: AGA GTG TGA GAT TAT GGC AGC	$(CT)_{14}CA(CT)_{2}$ $(CA)_{6}$	VIC	AB286043
Lec13	F: M13-GAC GCC ACG ACA AGA CGA AC R: TAT GTG TGG AGG GGG GTG AG	$(CT)_{21}$	NED	AB286044
Lec14	F: M13-ATT AGG AGC ATT ACC CAA CAG C R: CAA AGG AAG CAA AAA CAA GGG C	$(GT)_{7}$	NED	AB286045
Lec15	F: M13-GAG CAA GAG GTG TGT GCT TC R: TGC TGG TTC ACG CTC TAC AC	$(GT)_{11}$	PET	AB286046
Lec16	F: M13-CAC ACT AAC ACT TCT CCA GCG R: CAC AGT GAC CAA AGT CAC CAG	$(CA)_{10}$	6-FAM	AB286047
Lec17	F: M13-GTC CCC ATA AAA CAG GAA ACC C R: GAC TAT TGA GTG AGT GCC ACA C	$(GT)_{7}GCGTGG$ $(GT)_{5}$	VIC	AB286048
Lec18	F: M13-CGA CCA TCT TCT GGG GTT ACG R: CCT CGG ATG GGC TAA ATG ACC	$(GT)_{9}$	NED	AB439725
Lec19	F: M13-CTG TGT GTG GGT GTA TCT GAA C R: AAA GTG GCT CTT CTT CTG CTG G	$(GT)_{6}$	PET	AB439726

[a] Sequence of the M13 tails on forward primers: GCC AGT CAC GAC GTT GTA

Table 1. Characterization of 19 polymorphic microsatellite loci for 32 individuals of the Hotoke loach. Loci with gray color were used in analysis of genetic diversity and population structure in Section 3. (Modified from one of previous study [36])

2.2. Characterization of microsatellite loci

Each microsatellite locus was characterized for polymorphisms among 32 individuals obtained the Koise R., Ibaraki Pref. in 2006. DNA of the individuals was extracted using an automated DNA isolation system (GENE PREP STAR PI-80X, KURABO) following the manufacturer's instructions. PCR amplifications were performed on the 32 DNA extracts across all loci using 10 μl reaction volumes containing approximately 10 ng DNA template, 0.5 U Taq DNA polymerase (BIOTAQ, Bioline), 1×NH_4 buffer (BIOTAQ), 2.5 mM $MgCl_2$, 0.25 mM each dNTP, 0.03 μM M13-tailed forward primer, 0.25 μM reverse primer and 0.25 μM labeled M13 primer (5'-GCC AGT CAC GAC GTT GTA-3') [44]. The M13 primer was labeled at the 5' end with 6-FAM, VIC, NED or PET fluorescent dyes (ABI, Table 1).

Thermal profiles on iCycler and C1000 (both of Bio-Rad) of thermal cyclers were as follows. Initial denaturation at 94°C for 2 min was followed by 40 cycles of denaturation at 94°C for 15 s, annealing at 56°C for 15 s and extension at 72°C for 30 s. A single final extension at 72°C was done for 30 min. PCR products were resolved on a 3130*xl* Genetic Analyser with GeneScan 500 LIZ size standard (ABI). Electropherograms were analyzed with the software GENEMAPPER version 4.0 (ABI).

Measures of genetic diversity, tests for deviations from Hardy-Weinberg equilibrium (HWE) and estimates of linkage disequilibrium (LD) between loci were calculated using the software GENEPOP on the web version 4.0.10 [45]. The possible presence of null alleles was assessed with the software MICRO-CHECKER version 2.2.3 [46].

All the 19 loci were polymorphic (Table 1). The number of observed alleles per locus ranged from 2 to 9. The observed heterozygosity ranged from 0.125 to 0.844, while the expected heterozygosity varied from 0.148 to 0.876. No significant deviations from HWE or signs of LD were observed after sequential Bonferroni correction with the significant level at 0.05 [47] and there was no evidence of null alleles in any of the tested loci. Consequently, the high level of polymorphisms observed in these microsatellite loci may have to support future investigations to improve our knowledge of the genetic differentiation and genetic structure of populations of the Hotoke loach.

3. Analysis of genetic diversity and population structure

3.1. Study sites

In Section 3, genetic diversity and population structure of populations of the Hotoke loach in the upper Kokai R. including 4 adjacent rivers, the southeast part of Tochigi Pref. (Fig. 3) was detailed using the microsatellite loci developed in Section 2 (Table 1). As mentioned in Section 1, populations of the Hotoke loach have been often diminished and isolated by land consolidation projects in rural areas. Therefore it appears difficult to find populations distributed with a certain area. However, rich biota still continues to exist in the upper Kokai R. due to delay of land consolidation. This area sounds attractive for field scientists, and then their some activities were carried out to conserve and recover such a sound rural ecosystem

[48-52]. According to the results of these studies [48, 49], the populations of the Hotoke loach tended to be distributed in the upper zone of hill-bottom valleys in this area and also a negative correlation was observed between the population size and water temperature.

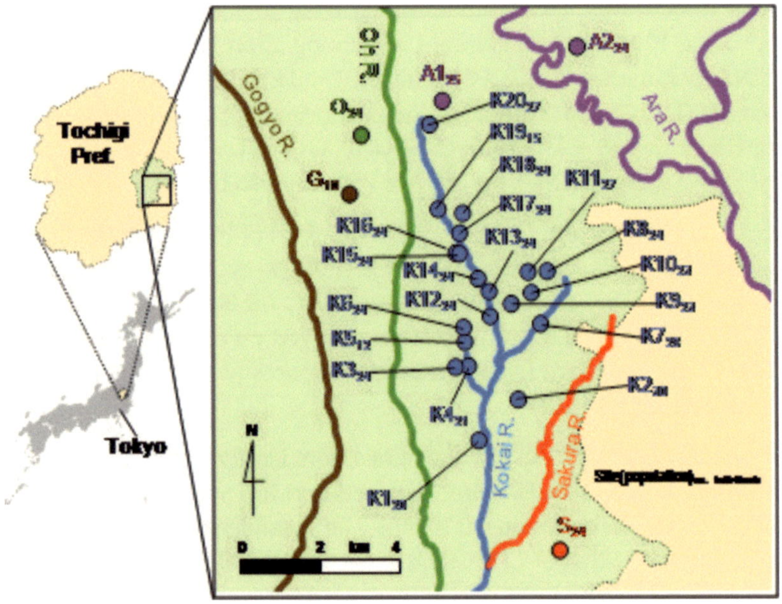

Figure 3. Collection sites for individuals of populations of the Hotoke loach in the upper of Kokai River (K1 to K20) along with adjacent the Oh, Sakura, Gogyo and Ara Rivers (O, S, G and A1, A2, respectively), the southeast part of Tochigi Prefecture (unpublished figure).

Considering such spatial distribution patterns in the previous studies [48, 49] and geographical conditions in this area, a total of 20 sites were established to collect individuals of the populations in the upper Kokai R. (K1 to K20 in Fig. 3). Additionally 5 collection sites of adjacent 4 rivers that are the Oh, Sakura, Gogyo and Ara (O, S, G and A1, A2, respectively in Fig. 3) were decided to compare with the populations of the Kokai R.

3.2. Sample collection

Sample collections in each site (Fig. 3) were performed using hand nets with reticulation at 2 mm, flame width at 30 to 40 cm in August 2007 to June 2008 (Photo 4). 10 to 24 individuals (a total of 573 individuals) of each population were collected in earth canals and ditches with water depth of 2 to 24 cm, water width of 15 to 110 cm, flow velocity of 5 to 25 cm/s and substrates consisting of silts, sands and gravels. There were no rain during the sample collections and a part of the caudal fin (3 mm × 3 mm) of each individual was removed and preserved in 99.5% EtOH at the sites, and then all individuals were immediately released alive. The preserved caudal fins were kept at -30 °C and the mean ± standard deviation in body length for all individuals was 46 ± 11 mm.

http://dx.doi.org/10.5772/53022

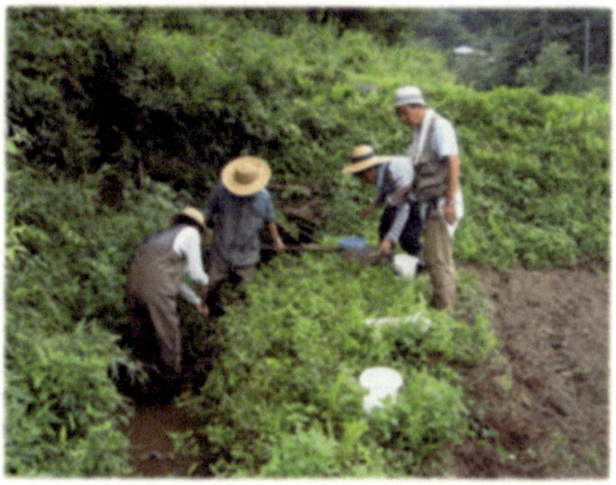

Photo 3. Collection of individuals of the Hotoke loach in an earth ditch at the site K9 in the Kokai River (unpublished photo)

3.3. DNA chemical analysis

Total genomic DNA from the preserved caudal fins of each individual was extracted using an automated DNA isolation system following the manufacturer's instructions, and kept at 4 °C after being diluted to 10 ng/μl.

The microsatellite DNA analysis were performed using the following 11 loci that are *Lec01, Lec05, Lec06, Lec08, Lec12, Lec14, Lec15, Lec16, Lec17, Lec18* and *Lec19* with gray color in Table 1. These loci were confirmed to be appropriate for investigating the populations in the Kokai R. in the preliminary studies [37, 38]. In accordance with the procedure in Section 2, microsatellite amplification with PCR on iCycler and C1000 of thermal cyclers was conducted in 10 μl reaction volumes containing approximately 10 ng DNA templates. PCR products were electrophoresed on a 3130*xl* Genetic Analyzer with GeneScan 500 LIZ of size markers and the electrophoregrams were analyzed with the GENEMAPPER. Consequently genotype data composed of a pair of fragment sizes, which are inherited from both of parents and depends on length of repeat motif, was obtained for each individual in a PCR product of a locus. All genotype data were compiled in the software THE EXCEL MICROSATELLITE TOOLKIT [53].

3.4. DNA data analysis

3.4.1. Genetic diversity within population

The genetic diversity within the populations of the Hotoke loach in each collection site was evaluated with the genotype data of the 11 loci for all individuals. The number of allele (N_A) and allelic richness (A_r) [54], where bias caused by population size (the number of individuals) is removed from N_A, were estimated using the software GENALEX version 6.41 [55] and FSTAT version 2.9.3 [56], respectively. Differences of N_A and A_r among the populations were tested by one-way analysis of variance (ANOVA) using the software EKUSERU-TOUKEI 2010 (Social Survey Research Information Co., Ltd.).

The observed and unbiased expected heterozygosities (H_O and H_E, respectively) [57] were calculated by GENALEX [55]. The software ARLEQUIN version 3.11 [58] was used to test deviations from Hardy-Weinberg equilibrium with Fisher's exact probability test, which was run through 100,000 iterations using the Markov chain Monte Carlo (MCMC). Significance values ($\alpha = 0.05$) of a multiple test were corrected following the sequential Bonferroni procedure [47]. Significant differences of H_O and H_E among the populations were detected by one-way ANOVA using EKUSERU-TOUKEI 2010.

3.4.2. Genetic population structure among populations

Genetic population structure among the populations in the Kokai R. including 4 adjacent rivers was elucidated with three analytical methods based on the assumption that mutation of alleles in each locus confirmed to an infinite allele model [59, 60].

First, genetic differentiation between the populations was evaluated with classical pairwise F_{ST} statistics [61] using ARLEQUIN [58]. Statistical significance ($\alpha = 0.05$) for values of F_{ST} was tested with applying 10,000 permutations, followed by sequential Bonferroni corrections [47] and these values were graded on four classifications for genetic differentiation in the previous study [62]. An analysis of molecular variance (AMOVA) [63] for F_{ST} was performed to estimate hierarchical genetic structure across the populations. In this AMOVA, the populations were divided into 2 to 6 groups according to geographical condition such as rivers and the distances among collection sites. And then variances among groups, among populations within groups, among individuals within populations and within all individuals were computed for 3 cases of genetic structure using GENALEX [55] with 10,000 permutations.

Second, a phylogenetic tree of a genetic distance D_A [64] between the populations was constructed with the neighbor-joining method [65] and the reliability of the obtained phylogenetic tree was evaluated using the aid of 1,000 bootstrap replicates [66]. The software POPULATIONS version 1.2.31 [67] was used to estimate D_A and to construct a phylogenetic tree and an appropriate shape of the phylogenetic tree was edited with the software MEGA version 5.05 [68].

Finally, Bayesian cluster analysis [69-73] that has been recently used as a popular method was implemented in the software STRUCTURE version 2.3.3 [70] to circumstantially investigate the occurrence of genetic structure among the populations without the prior identification of populations. Briefly, this analysis allows the inference of the number of genetically homogeneous clusters (K) that are implicitly genetic populations from individual genotypes at multiple loci and also assignment probability (Q) of individuals to each genetic cluster. The admixture model and correlated allele frequencies model were used along with LOCPRIOR model [74] and the software was run with 20 repetitions of 500,000 iterations of MCMC, following a burn-in of 500,000 iterations at K of 1 to 10.

The most likely number of genetic clusters was evaluated using the rate of change in the log probability between the values of successive K [75]. Distribution of the values of Q across runs for each cluster were organized using the software STRUCTURE HARVESTER web version 0.6.92 [76] and then summarized using the software CLUMPP [77]. When individuals had the values of Q more than 0.7, they were assigned to be members of that particular cluster in this study. And also K usually appears to show the genetic structure at the uppermost hierarchical level [75]. Therefore, when a particular cluster was formed by some populations, additional analysis of each cluster was performed to investigate the detailed genetic structures after the first analysis.

3.5. Results and discussions

3.5.1. *Genetic diversity within populations*

All the 11 microsatellite loci were moderate to highly polymorphic, with the number of alleles (N_A) and observed and unbiased heterozygosities (H_O and H_E, respectively) per locus for all individuals ranging from 2 (*Lec19*) to 40 (*Lec06*) and from 0.147 (*Lec17* and *Lec19*) to 0.846 (*Lec05*) and from 0.155 (*Lec17*) and 0.915 (*Lec08*), respectively. Such a polymorphic level observed in these loci indicated to be beneficial to investigating genetic characteristics of populations in detail.

Means of N_A per locus in the populations varies from 4.5 (Population A2, hereafter Pop A2) to 8.0 (Pop K11). Allele richness (A_r) per locus was standardized by the minimum size of the population (10 individuals of Pop G) and its means per locus varied from 3.7 (Pop A2) to 5.6 (Pop K11) among populations (Fig. 4). The one-way analysis of variance (ANOVA) showed that significant differences of the means of both N_A and A_r were not confirmed among populations ($F_{24, 250}=0.641$, $M_{SE}=11.937$, $p>0.05$ for N_A and $F_{24,250}=0.459$, $M_{SE}=4.803$, $p>0.05$ for A_r).

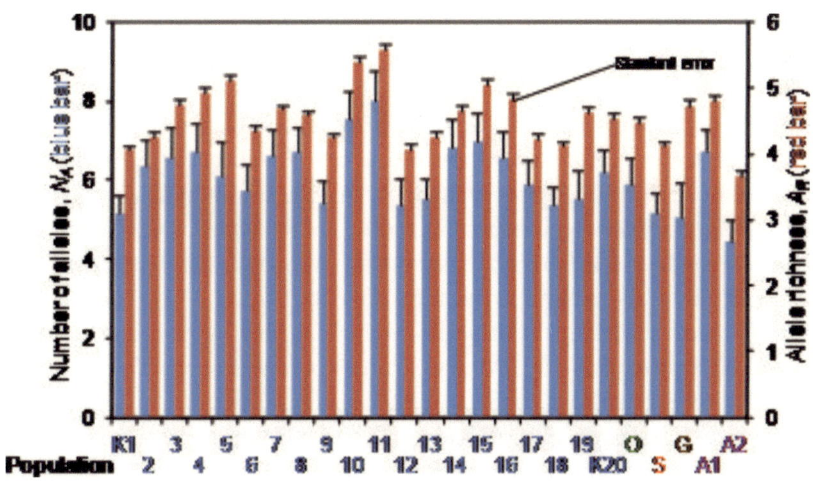

Figure 4. Means and standard errors of the number of alleles (N_A) and allelic richness (A_r) per locus in the populations (unpublished figure). A_r was standardized by the minimum size of the population (10 individuals of Population G) and there were no significant differences among the populations for both N_A and A_R ($p > 0.05$).

Means of the observed and unbiased expected heterozygosities (H_O and H_E, respectively) per locus across all population ranged from 0.418 (Pop A2) to 0.669 (Pop K11) and from 0.507 (Pop A2) to 0.674 (Pop K11), respectively (Fig. 5). Significant departures from the Hardy-Weinberg equilibrium (HWE) were not observed in all the populations. This result indicated that the populations could be applied to the following analyses of genetic population structure, because most analyses are often performed under the assumption that population conforms to HWE. The results of one-way ANOVA showed that there were no significant of the differences among the populations for both H_O and H_E ($F_{24, 250} = 0.377$, $M_{SE} = 0.090$, $p > 0.05$ for H_O and $F_{24, 250} = 0.207$, $M_{SE} = 0.079$, $p > 0.05$ for H_E).

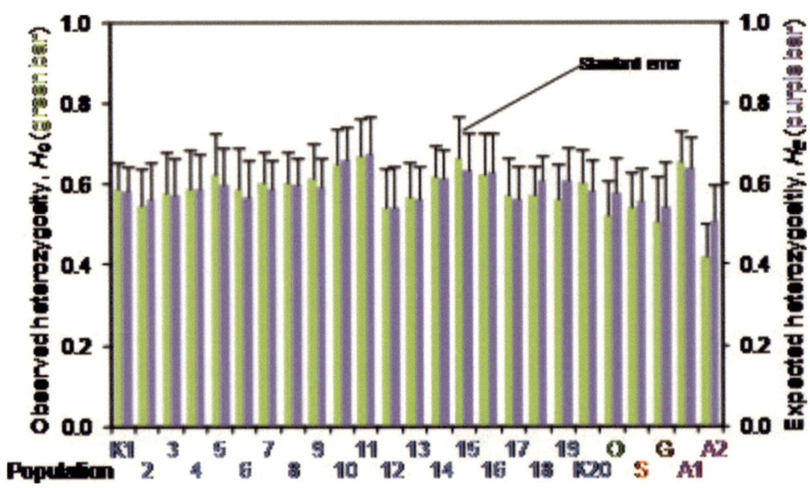

Figure 5. Means and standard errors of the observed and unbiased expected heterozygosities (H_O and H_E, respectively) per locus in the populations (unpublished figure). There were no significant differences among the populations for both H_O and H_E ($p > 0.05$).

Genetic diversity of the populations appeared not to degrade. Generally, when population size is small, inbreeding among individuals appears to progressively occur in a population [30-33] as mentioned in Section 1. It has been observed that such populations had low values of N_A, H_O and H_E [33]. For instance, means of N_A per locus for the Ethiopian wolf, *Canis simensis*, the Mauritius kestrel, *Falco punctatus* and the Northern hairy-nosed wombat, *Lasiorhinus krefftii* which are designated as worldwide endangered species, were only 2.4, 1.4 and 2.1, respectively. Means of H_E for the Ethiopian wolf, the Mauritius kestrel and the Northern hairy-nosed wombat were also 0.21, 0.10 and 0.32, respectively [78]. But then, values of representatively common freshwater fish species inhabiting agricultural canals and ditches in rural area, Japan such as the Dojo loach, the Field gudgeon, *Gnathopogon elongates elongatus* and the Amur goby (orange type), *Rhinogobius* sp. OR ranged from 3.3 to 17.7 (both of the Amur goby) for means of N_A per locus and from 0.463 (the Dojo loach) to 0.905 (the Field gudgeon) for means of H_E per locus [79-81].

Comparing with these values for the endangered and common species, the means of N_A and H_E per locus (4.5 to 8.0 and 0.507 to 0.674, respectively) observed in the populations indicated to be in relatively moderate level. Hence, a serious concern for genetic diversity could not occur in the populations at present. However, there are no confident that such a level of genetic diversity would be sustaining in the future. Monitoring genetic diversity may need including ordinary biological investigation such as an estimation of size and age composition of populations.

3.5.2. Genetic population structure inferred from F_{ST}

The lowest and highest values of F_{ST} were observed between Pops K15 & K16 and between Pops K18 & A2 (F_{ST} = 0.008 and 0.246, respectively, Fig. 6). The permutation test showed that all the F_{ST} were significantly different from zero ($p > 0.05$), except the lowest F_{ST} between Pops K15 & K16 after sequential Bonferroni corrections [47].

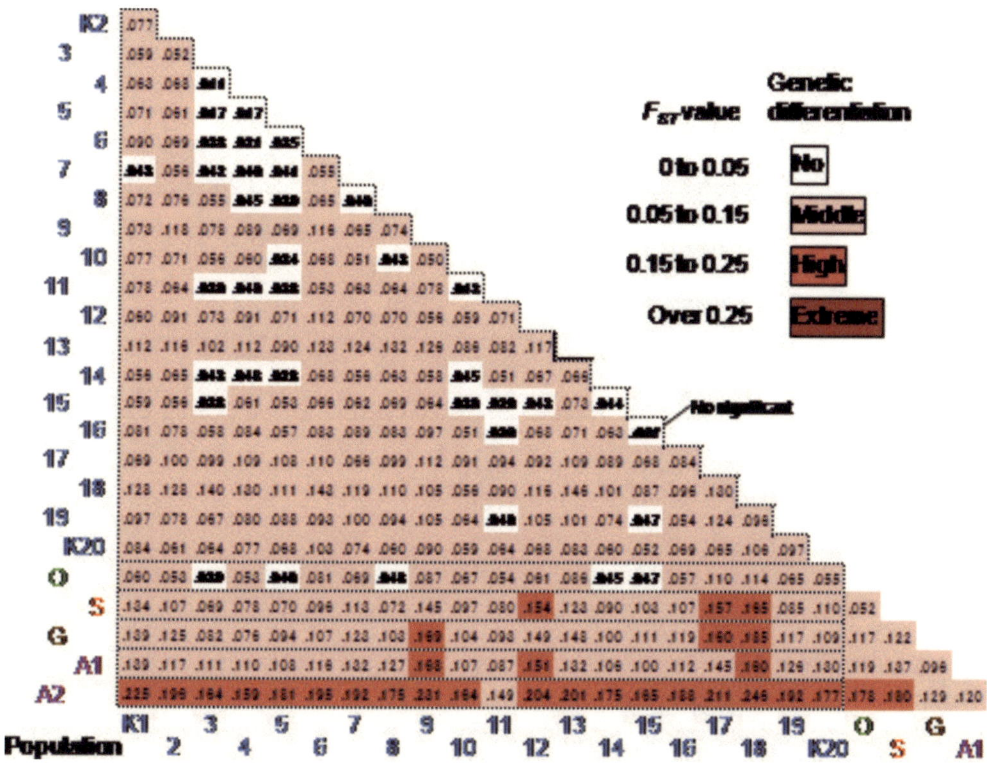

Figure 6. Values of pairwise F_{ST} between the populations and their grades of genetic differentiation composed of four classifications (unpublished figure). All the value of F_{ST} were significantly different from zero ($p > 0.05$), except between Populations K15 & K16 (F_{ST} = 0.008). Four classifications of genetic differentiation derive from the previous study [62].

Values of F_{ST} were graded on four classifications for genetic differentiation based on the previous study [62]. These classifications imply no, middle, high and extreme genetic differentiation when F_{ST} ranges from 0 to 0.05, from 0.05 to 0.15, from 0.15 to 0.25 and over 0.25. Applying this grade, 20.3% of the F_{ST} (32/190) between the populations within the Kokai R. (Pops K1 to K20) were classified into no genetic differentiation and a part of such populations tended to be close located each other (Fig. 6). The remaining F_{ST} within the Kokai R. were classified into middle genetic differentiation. Between the populations in the Kokai R. and adjacent 4 rivers (Pops O to A2), their F_{ST} showed middle to high genetic differentiation, although the F_{ST} between the populations in the Kokai and Oh Rs were partially no differentiation.

The analysis of molecular variance (AMOVA) was implemented for the following Cases I to III, among which the number of groups and composition of the populations in groups differed. In Case I, the populations of the Kokai R. (K1 to K20) and 4 adjacent rivers (Pops O to A2) were divided into $Group_{CaseI}$ 1 and 2, respectively. In Case II, $Group_{CaseII}$ 1 was formed by the populations of the Kokai, Oh and Sakura Rs (Pops K1 to S) and $Group_{caseII}$ 2, 3 and 4 were formed by 3 remaining populations of 2 rivers (Pops G, A1 and A2). There were groups $Group_{CaseIII}$ 1 to 6 composed of the populations of the Kokai (Pops K1 to K20), Oh (Pop O), Sakura (Pop S), Gogyo (Pop G), one Ara (Pop A1) and another Ara (Pop A2) R. in Case III.

Significant genetic differentiations were observed at all hierarchical levels in all cases ($p <$ 0.01, Table 2). The largest genetic variance in all variances was found at the level of within individuals in each case (from 82.5 % in Case II to 86.0 % in Case I). The genetic variances at the levels of among groups and among populations within groups accounted for 2.8% in Case I to 7.3 % in Case II and 6.9 % in Case II and III to 7.9 % in Case I, respectively (Table 2).

Case (no. groups)	Statistic	Hierarchy				
		Among groups (A)	Among pops within groups (B)	Among inds within pops (C)	Within inds (D)	Total (E)
I (2)	d.f.	1	23	548	573	1145
	MS	52.5	16.8	3.4	3.2	
	Var comp	0.102	0.291	0.124	3.184	3.702
	% of var	2.76	7.87	3.35	86.01	100.00
	F	0.028[a]	0.081[b]	0.106[c]	0.038[d]	0.140[e]
II (4)	d.f.	3	21	548	573	1145
	MS	34.6	15.9	3.4	3.2	
	Var comp	0.282	0.267	0.124	3.184	3.858
	% of var	7.32	6.93	3.22	82.53	100.00
	F	0.073	0.075	0.142	0.038	0.175
III (6)	d.f.	5	19	548	573	1145
	MS	28.5	15.6	3.4	3.2	
	Var comp	0.183	0.260	0.124	3.184	3.752
	% of var	4.88	6.94	3.31	84.86	100.00
	F	0.049	0.073	0.118	0.038	0.151

[a]$F_{A/E}$, [b]$F_{B/(B+C+D)}$, [c]$F_{(A+B)/E}$, [d]$F_{C/(C+E)}$, [e]$F_{(A+B+C)/E}$

Table 2. Results of analysis of molecular variance (AMOVA) for three Cases I, II and III (unpublished table). Compositions of the populations in groups for Case I to III are referred in the text. Genetic differentiations were significant at all hierarchical levels for each case ($p < 0.01$).

Genetic differentiation between the populations was significantly inferred from the analysis of F_{ST} and its relevant AMOVA. Geographical condition such as river and the distances among locations appeared to relate to degree of the genetic differentiation as illustrated in the previous studies [37, 38, 82-84]. However, only a part of genetic population structure could be indicated in this analysis, because the proportions of the genetic variances at the level of among groups were relatively low (2.8 to 7.3 % of among groups in Table 2). Investigating schematically and visually genetic structure may have to be implemented as further analysis as commented in the previous study [74].

3.5.3. Genetic population structure inferred from phylogentic tree

The calculated genetic distance D_A between the populations ranged from 0.073 (between Pops K15 & K16) to 0.99 (between Pops K6 & A2). In this phylogenetic tree of D_A using the neighbor-joining method [65] (Fig. 7), there was a few of highly significant divergences of population with the bootstrap probabilities over 90 % (e.g. 98 % between Pops K15 & K16, 93 % between Pops K10 & K11); while the probabilities left were less than 50 % on most divergences. But, the topology of the phylogenetic tree displayed that there were 4 distinct groups, $\text{Group}_{\text{Tree}}$ 1 to 4 despite weak condition of the statistical support. Both $\text{Group}_{\text{Tree}}$ 1 and 2 consisted of 3 populations of the Gogyo and Ara Rs (Pops G, A1 and A2) and of the Kokai, Oh and Sakura Rs (Pops K8, O and S), respectively. $\text{Group}_{\text{Tree}}$ 3 consisted of 7 populations collected in the lower part of the Kokai R. (Pops K1 to K7), while $\text{Group}_{\text{Tree}}$ 4 were formed by the 12 remaining populations coming from the middle and upper part of the Kokai R. (Pops K9 to K20).

The schematic genetic structure of the populations was showed by constructing the phylogenetic tree (Fig. 7). Including the results of the above F_{ST} analysis and AMOVA, the existence of 2 genetic populations that related to $\text{Group}_{\text{Tree}}$ 3 and 4 was indicated in the populations within the Kokai R., but these groups were statistically cryptic. It could be expected that characterization of admixture of gene flow and migrants among the populations was displayed by detailing structures of such cryptic genetic populations.

3.5.4. Genetic structure among populations inferred from Bayesian cluster analysis

The Bayesian clustering analysis supported the occurrence of two defined genetic clusters, Clusters A and B in the uppermost hierarchical level (Fig. 8). By accounting for the number of individuals with more than 70 % of assignment probability (Q) to each cluster, 98.6 6% of all individuals (507/514 individuals) in the populations from the Kokai, Oh and Sakura Rs (Pops K1 to S) were assigned to Cluster A. And also, 91.5 % of the remaining individuals (54/59 individuals) in the populations from the Gogyo and Ara Rs (Pops G to A2) were assigned to Cluster B (Fig. 8).

Further clustering analysis were performed to assign the populations in Clusters A and B to genetic clusters in the second hierarchical level. Applying the same procedure in the first analysis, the appropriate K were 2 in both analyses. According to the values of Q of the individuals, they were assigned to one of Clusters I, II or admixture of Cluster I & II in the analysis of Cluster A and Clusters III or IV in the analyses of Cluster B.

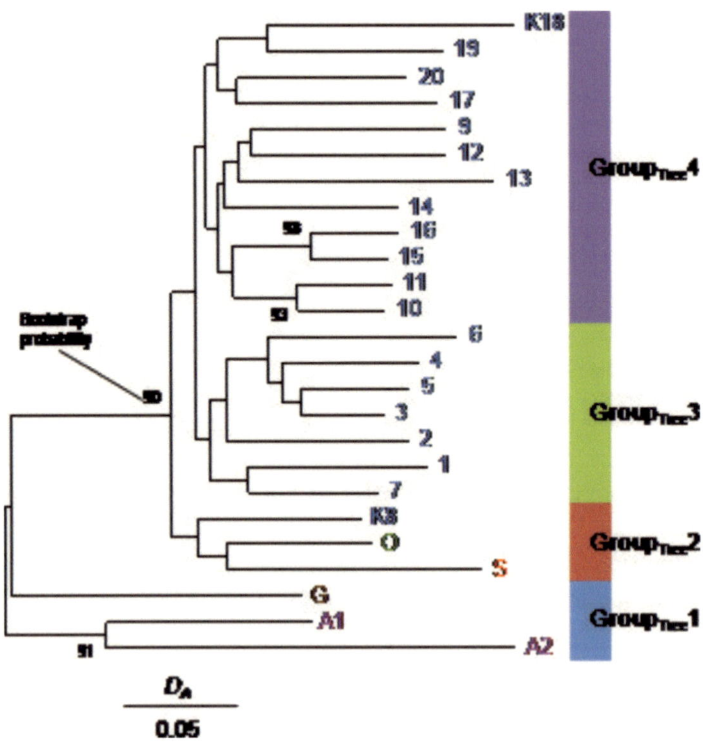

Figure 7. Phylogenetic tree of D_A for the populations with neighbour-joining method (unpublished figure)

http://dx.doi.org/10.5772/53022

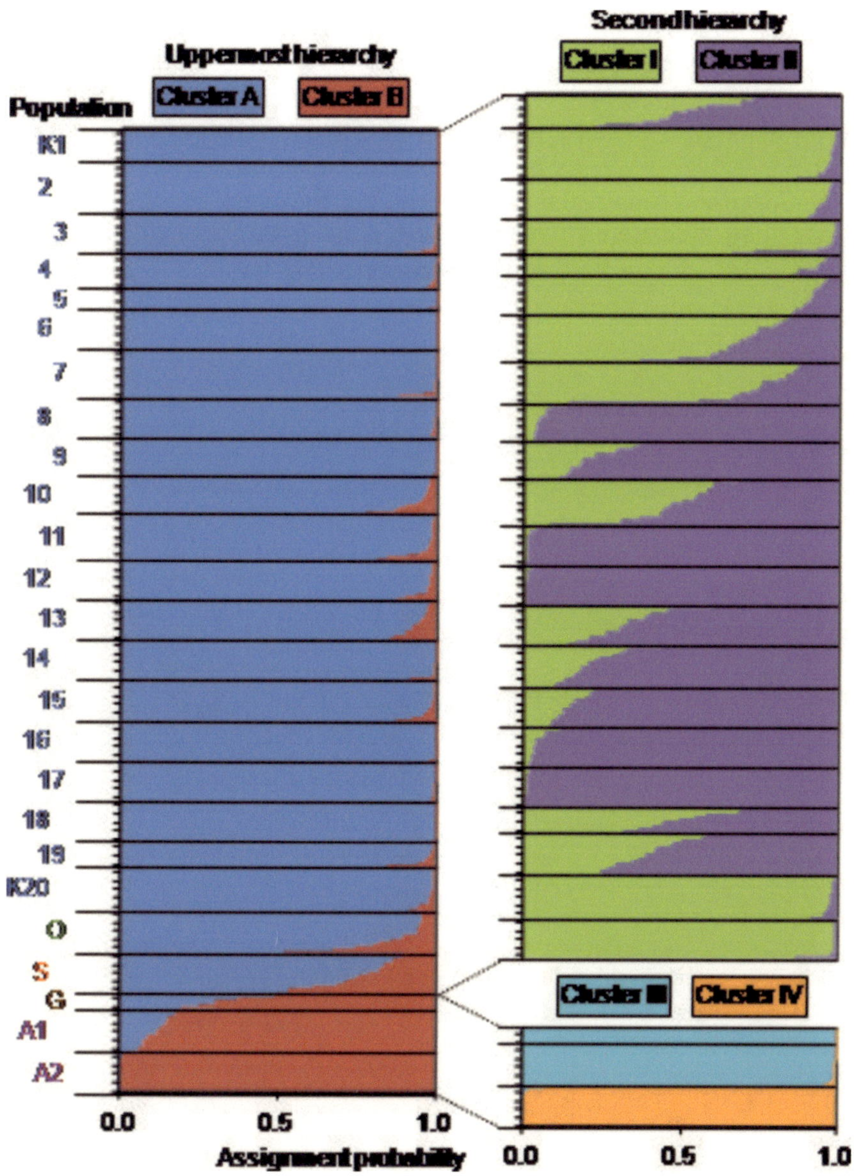

Figure 8. Structures of genetic clusters in the populations inferred by the Bayesian analysis (unpublished figure). Clusters A & B and I to IV imply the genetic populations at uppermost and second hierarchical levels, respectively. Each individual is represented by a horizontal line fragmented by assignment probabilities to the genetic clusters.

In the analysis of Cluster A, 77.0 to 98.6 % of individuals of Pops K2 to K6, K8, O and S (a total of 8 populations) in the Kokai, Oh and Sakura Rs were assigned to members of Cluster I (Fig. 8). Considering the geographical locations of the populations as performed in the previous studies [85-88], Cluster I mainly indicated to be the genetic population of the lower part of the Kokai including the Oh and Sakura Rs (Fig. 9). 77.4 to 99.0 % of individuals of Pops K9, 10, 12, 13, 15 to 18 (a total of 8 populations) in the Kokai occupied members of Cluster II. Cluster II also implied to be the genetic population of the middle and upper parts of the Kokai R. The remaining individuals of Pops K1, K7, K11, K14, K19 and K20 (a total of 6 populations) in the Kokai R. were mainly classified into members of admixtures of Clusters I & II. In the analysis of Cluster B, almost all individuals (more than 99.1 %) of Pops G and A1 in the Gogyo and Ara Rs. and Pop A2 in the Ara R. were assigned to Clusters III and IV, respectively (Fig. 8). Cluster III and IV reflected the genetic populations of the Gogyo and one of Ara R. and another of the Ara R., respectively (Fig. 9).

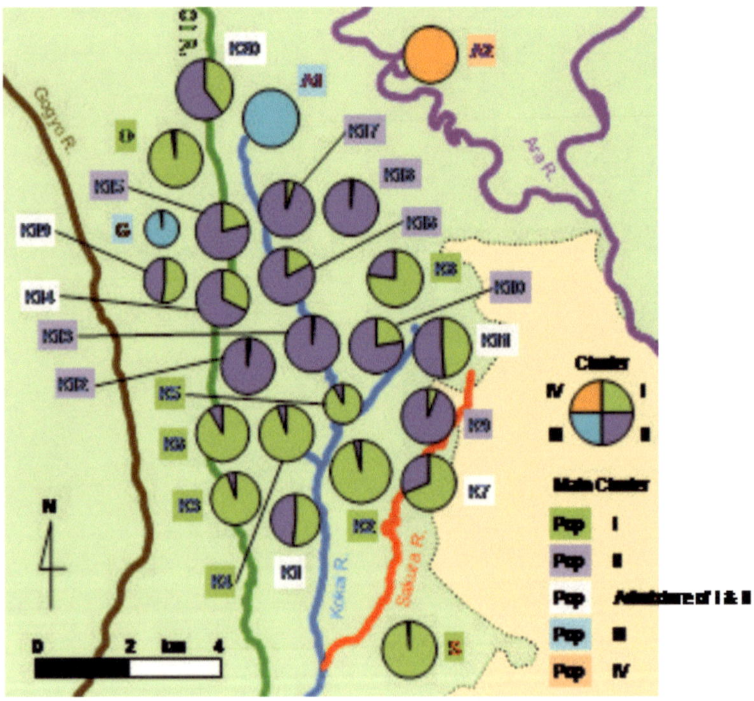

Figure 9. Spatial distribution and composition of genetic clusters in populations (unpublished figure). Size of circle reflects that of population.

Consequently the four genetic populations (Clusters I to IV) and a mixed genetic population (admixture of Cluster I & II) were confirmed in the populations using this clustering analysis. Clusters I, II and a pair of Clusters III & IV nearly coincided with a pair of $\mathrm{Group}_{\mathrm{Tree}}$ 2 & 3, $\mathrm{Group}_{\mathrm{Tree}}$ 4 and $\mathrm{Group}_{\mathrm{Tree}}$ 1 in the phylogenetic tree, respectively (Fig. 7). Moreover, the presence of the mixed genetic population, which could not be usually detected in a phylogenetic tree, was founded by the cluster analysis. As discussed in the previous studies [69-71, 73], this admixture of Cluster I & II may be established through gene flow caused by migrant; thus, events relative to individual movement and breeding could have occurred among some populations in the past.

4. Conclusions

A series of the exhaustive genetic analysis in this chapter demonstrated that the populations of the Hotoke loach indicated to have moderate genetic diversity and to be supported with 4 genetic populations, of which distributions depended on the populations and the geographical locations. These 2 genetic characteristics showed that there could not be serious genetic concerns at present and the populations might be available as valuable biological resources such as bird food. To fulfill the effective utilization of this loach in near future, both biomedical and nutritional investigations for component contained in the body may also have to be practiced in the next research subjects along with proposing an optimal management plan for conserving the populations.

Further, the following 2 suggestions based on the results of this analysis should be realized in conduct of the next research. First, to sustain the present genetic features, habitats of the populations have to be maintained with monitoring the population size. As it is repeatedly described in the above, but reduction of the population size often appears to cause degradation of the genetic diversity and the lost genetic diversity could never be regained in the populations [30-33]. Avoiding such a decrease in the genetic diversity, habitat conservation might be important for a population management. It was also investigated that this species had relatively strict water temperature resistance compared with other common freshwater fish [48, 49]; hence the control of the water quality, especially water temperature could be one of essential factors for conserving habitats of the populations.

Second, spatial distribution and composition of the genetic populations should be taken account in the population management. In this area the genetic populations could be established by only geographical factors such as river and ground conditions (Fig. 9) and related to no human activities. The foregoing genetic populations often appear a kind of genetic heritages and it is recommended that their distributions do not have to be disturbed artificially [30-33, 35]. If perchance size diminishment of a specific population is observed and there is only individual translocation as a method to recover the population, selections of translated individuals and populations should be advisedly carried out based on the distribution of the genetic populations. Finally there still may be various and many biological resources left in the rural ecosystem in Japan. Genetic analyses performed in this chapter would have to contribute substantially to exploration and beneficial utilization of these resources.

Acknowledgement

Our thanks go to Drs Wataru Kakino and Shin-ichi Matsuzawa, Mr. Masumi Matsuzaki and Ms. Zhenli Gao for their aggressive supports in the research field and Mses. Chikusa Suzuki, Ponthip Goto and Kyoko Yamanoi for their assistance in DNA chemical analyses, including valuable discussions with Dr. Hiroshi Aiki. The first author would like to kindly appreciate Dr. Gandhi Rádis Baptista for his invitation to this book and Mses. Adriana Pecar, Ivana Zec and Masa Vidovic and Mr. Dejan Grgur for their thoughtful helps in the publishing process for this manuscript. This study was supported in part by a Grant-in-Aid for Scientific Research (C-18580250, C-20580270, C-23580340, B-18380139 and B-22380133) from the Japan Society for the Promotion of Science.

Author details

Noriyuki Koizumi[1], Masakazu Mizutani[2], Keiji Watabe[1], Atsushi Mori[1], Kazuya Nishida[1] and Takeshi Takemura[1]

1 Institute for Rural Engineering, National Agriculture and Food Research Organization, Ibaraki, Japan

2 Faculty of Agriculture, Utsunomiya University, Utsunomioya, Japan

References

[1] Honda Y (2009) How do the local people think about the release of Toki (*Nipponia nippon*) just before the release?: from the questionnaire survey in whole Sado-city. *Bulletin of the Tokyo University Forests*, 121, 149-172. (in Japanese with English abstract)

[2] Naito K, Kikuchi N, Ikeda H (2011) Reintroduction of oriental white storks: ecological restoration and preparation for release into the wild based on the guidelines of IUCN. *Japanese Journal of Conservation Ecology*, 16, 181-193. (in Japanese with English abstract)

[3] National Institute for Agro-Environmental Sciences (1998) *Biodiversity of Paddy Field Ecosystem*. Yokendo Co., Ltd., Tokyo. (in Japanese)

[4] Makino H (1996) *Dojo Loach*. Rural Culture Association Japan, Tokyo. (in Japanese)

[5] Suzuki R (1983) *Latest Technology of the Dojo Loach Culture*. Soubunkan, Tokyo. (in Japanese)

[6] Ezaki Y, Tanaka T (1998) *Conservation of Waterfront Environment*. Asakura Publishing Co., Ltd., Tokyo. (in Japanese)

[7] Nakagawa S (2000) *Biotope in Rural Area*. Shinzansha Publisher Co., Ltd., Tokyo. (in Japanese)

[8] Mizutani M (2007) *An Introduction to Paddy Field Eco-engineering for Sustaining and Restoring Biodiversity in Rural Areas*. Rural Culture Association Japan, Tokyo. (in Japanese)

[9] Mizutani M, Mori A (2009) *Conserving Habitat of Freshwater Fishes Inhabiting Haruno-ogawa, Irrigation/Drainage Ditches, in Rice Paddies*. Gakuhosya, Tokyo. (in Japanese)

[10] Japan Ministry of the Environment (2003) *Threatened Wildlife of Japan, Red Data Book*. Japan Wildlife Research Center, Tokyo. (in Japanese)

[11] Mitsuo Y, Nishida K, Senga Y (2007) A research on habitat condition of Hotoke loach in "Yatu" waters: case study of the upper stream of the Okuri River. *Irrigation, Drainage and Rural Engineering Journal*, 75, 445-451. (in Japanese with English abstract)

[12] Moriyama T, Mizutani M, Goto A (2007) Seasonal migration of Hotoke-dojo loach *Lefua echigonia* in a spring-derived stream, Nishikinugawa district, Tochigi Prefecture, Japan. *Japanese Journal of Ichthyology*, 54, 161-171. (in Japanese with English abstract)

[13] Fujita H, Okawa K (1975) A preliminary survey of geographic variations of cobitid fish, *Lefua echigonia*, in Japan. *Japanese Journal of Ichthyology*, 22, 179-182. (in Japanese with English abstract)

[14] Hosoya K (2000) Cobitidae. In Nakabo T (ed.) *Fishes of Japan with Pictorial Keys to the Species*, Tokai University Press, Tokyo, p272-277. (in Japanese)

[15] Mochida M, Kuramoto N (2007) Study on native habitat of Hotoke loach, *Lefua echigonia* to live on Yato after farmlad consolidation. *Papers on Environmental Information Science*, 21, 117-122. (in Japanese with English abstract)

[16] Kitano S, Yamagata T, Yagyu M (2008) Distribution, habitat characteristics, and mitochondrial DNA haplotypes of *Lefua echigonia* in Nagano Pref., central Japan. *Bulletin of Nagano Environmental Conservation Research Institute*, 4, 45-50. (in Japanese with English abstract)

[17] Aiki H, Mano N, Sasada K, Shimada M, Hirose H (2008) Distribution and present status of Japanese eight-barbel loach *Lefua echigonia* (Jordan et Richardson, 1907) in Fukushima Prefecture, Japan. *Bulletin of the Bio-geographical Society of Japan*, 63, 5-11. (in Japanese with English abstract)

[18] Moriyama T, Kakino W, Mizutani M (2010) Winter distribution pattern of Japanese eight-barbel loach in a conservation pond supplied with pumped groundwater. *Japanese Journal of Ichthyology*, 57, 161-166. (in Japanese with English abstract)

[19] Suguro N, Suzuki M, Mizutani M (2008) Study of a fish way suitable for Hotoke loach (*Lefua echigonia*). *Bulletin of the Kanagawa Prefectural Fisheries Technology Center*, 3, 87-95. (in Japanese with English abstract)

[20] Mitsuo Y, Nishida K, Senga Y (2010) Utilization of paddy field by Hotoke loach: Case study of Yatsu paddy field in the upper stream of the Okuri River. *Wildlife Conservation Japan*, 12, 1-9. (in Japanese with English abstract)

[21] Suguro N (2002) Early rearing conditions of Hotoke loach, *Lefua echigonia*. *Aquaculture Science*, 50, 55-62. (in Japanese with English abstract)

[22] Suguro N (2005) Numbers of parental fish and artificial spawning beds that result in maximum seed production in *Lefua echigonia*. *Aquaculture Science*, 53, 83-90. (in Japanese with English abstract)

[23] Miyamoto R, Suguro N, Hosoya K (2009) Artificial propagation of an endangered freshwater fish, the Hotoke loach *Lefua echigonia* Jordan et Richardson. *Memoirs of the Faculty of Agriculture of Kinki University*, 42, 119-126. (in Japanese with English abstract)

[24] Sakai T, Mihara M, Shitara H, Yonekawa H, Hosoya K, Miyazaki J (2003) Phylogenetic relationships and intraspecific variations of loaches of the genus *Lefua* (Balitoridae, Cypriniformes). *Zoological Science*, 20, 501-514.

[25] Saka R, Takehana Y, Suguro N, Sakaizumi M (2003) Genetic population structure of *Lefua echigonia* inferred from allozymic and mitochondrial cytochrome *b* variations. *Ichthyological Research*, 50, 301-309.

[26] Mihara M, Sakai T, Nakano K, Martins OL, Hosoya K, Miyazaki J (2005) Phylogeography of loaches of the genus *Lefua* (Balitoridae, Cypriniformes) inferred from mitochondrial DNA sequences. *Zoological Science*, 22, 157-168.

[27] Aiki H, Takayama K, Tamaru T, Mano N, Shimada M, Komaki H, Hirose H (2009) Phylogeography of the Japanese eight-barbel loach *Lefua echigonia* from the Yamagata area of the Tohoku district, Japan. *Fisheries Science*, 75, 903-908.

[28] Koizumi N, Watabe K, Gao Z, Mizutani M, Takemura T, Mori A (2010) Haplotype of mitochondrial DNA for the Japanese eight-barbel loach in the southeast of Tochigi Prefecture. *Irrigation, Drainage and Rural Engineering Journal*, 78, 61-62. (in Japanese)

[29] Nishida K, Koizumi N, Takemura T, Watabe K, Mori A (2012) Mitochondrial DNA D-loop sequence-based analysis of the influence of river basin connectivity and fragmentation on the genetic structure and diversity of the Japanese eight-barbel loach *Lefua echigonia*. *Technical Report of National Institute for Rural Engineering*, 212, 177-188. (in Japanese with English abstract)

[30] Loeschcke V, Tomiuk J, Jain SK (1994) *Conservation Genetics*. Birkhäuser Verlag, Boston.

[31] Avise JC, Hamric JL (1996) *Conservation Genetics*. Chapman and Hall, New York.

[32] Smith TB, Wayne RK (1996) *Molecular Genetic Approaches in Conservation*. Oxford University Press, New York.

[33] Frankham R, Ballou JD, Briscoe DA (2002) *Introduction to Conservation Genetics*. Cambridge University Press, Cambridge.

[34] The Society for the Study of Species Biology (2001) *Molecular Ecology of Woody Species*. Bun-ichi Sogo Shuppan Co., Tokyo. (in Japanese)

[35] Koike Y, Matsui M (2003) *Conservation Genetics*. University of Tokyo Press, Tokyo. (in Japanese)

[36] Koizumi N, Takahashi H, Minezawa M, Takemura T, Okushima S, Mori A (2007). Isolation and characterization of polymorphic microsatellite DNA markers in the Japanese eight-barbel loach, *Lefua echigonia*. *Molecular Ecology Notes*, 7, 836-838.

[37] Koizumi N, Watabe K, Gao Z, Mizutani M, Mori A, Takemura T (2008) Preliminary study on genetic population of the Japanese eight-barbel loach in the upper Kokai River basin, Tochigi Prefecture using microsatellite DNA. *Irrigation, Drainage and Rural Engineering Journal*, 76, 397-403. (in Japanese with English abstract)

[38] Koizumi N (2009) Conservation of freshwater fishes using information obtained by DNA analysis. In Mizutani M, Mori A (ed.) *Conserving Habitat of Freshwater Fishes Inhabiting Haruno-ogawa, Irrigation/Drainage Ditches, in Rice Paddies*, Gakuhosya, Tokyo, p121-148. (in Japanese)

[39] Koizumi N, Hanamura Y, Quinn TW, Nishida K, Takemura T, Watabe K, Mori A, Man A (2012) Thirty-two polymorphic microsatellite loci of the mysid crustacean *Mesopodopsis tenuipes*. *Conservation Genetic Resources*, 4, 55-58.

[40] Koizumi N, Quinn TW, Jinguji H, Nishida K, Watabe K, Takemura T, Mori A (2012) Development and characterization of 23 polymorphic microsatellite markers for *Sympetrum frequens*. *Conservation Genetic Resources*, 4, 67-70.

[41] Asahida T, Kobayashi T, Saitoh K, Nakayama I (1996) Tissue preservation and total DNA extraction from fish stored at ambient temperature using buffer containing high concentration of urea. *Fisheries Science*, 62, 727-730.

[42] Glenn TC, Schable NA (2005) Isolating microsatellite DNA loci. *Methods in Enzymology*, 395, 202-222.

[43] St. John J, Quinn TW (2008) Rapid capture of DNA targets. *BioTechniques*, 44, 259-264.

[44] Lorenz E, Frees KL, Schwartz DA (2001) M13-tailed primers improve the readability and usability of microsatellite analyses performed with two different allele-sizing methods. *BioTechniques*, 31, 24-27.

[45] Rousset F (2008) Genepop'007: a complete reimplementation of the Genepop software for Windows and Linux. *Molecular Ecology Resources*, 8, 103-106.

[46] van Oosterhout C, Hutchinson WF, Wills DPM, Shipley P (2004) Micro-Checker: software for identifying and correcting genotyping errors in microsatellite data. *Molecular Ecology Notes*, 4,535-538.

[47] Rice WR (1989) Analyzing tables of statistical tests. *Evolution*, 43, 223-225.

[48] Kakino W, Mizutani M, Fujisaku M, Goto A (2006) Influence of environmental factors on fish fauna distribution in hill-bottom valleys: case study of the upper stream of the Kokai River. *Irrigation, Drainage and Rural Engineering Journal*, 74, 809-816. (in Japanese with English abstract)

[49] Kakino W, Mizutani M, Fujisaku M, Goto A (2007) Seasonal changes of environmental factors influencing on fish population density in ditches of hill-bottom valleys lo-

cated in the upper stream of the Kokai River, the Tone River basin. *Irrigation, Drainage and Rural Engineering Journal*, 75, 19-29. (in Japanese with English abstract)

[50] Mori A, Mizutani M, Matsuzawa S (2007) Origin estimation of carbon of spiders (Arachnida) by carbon stable isotope ratio. *Irrigation, Drainage and Rural Engineering Journal*, 75, 565-571. (in Japanese with English abstract)

[51] Matsuzawa S, Mizutani M, Mori A, Goto A (2008) Stable isotope ratio of organisms in small ditches used for irrigation and drainage in hill-bottom paddy fields. *Irrigation, Drainage and Rural Engineering Journal*, 76, 95-105. (in Japanese with English abstract)

[52] Kakino W, Mizutani M, Goto A (2009) Proposal of a fish habitat environmental model at hill-bottom valleys waters in Tochgi Prefecture. *Irrigation, Drainage and Rural Engineering Journal*, 77, 567-575. (in Japanese with English abstract)

[53] Park, SDE (2001) *Trypanotolerance in West African Cattle and the Population Genetic Effects of Selection*. PhD thesis, University of Dublin.

[54] El Mousadik A, Petit RJ (1996) High level of genetic differentiation for allelic richness among populations of the argan tree [*Argania spinosa* (L.) Skeels] endemic to Morocco. *Theoretical and Applied Genetics*, 92, 832-839.

[55] Peakall R, Smouse PE (2006) GENALEX 6: genetic analysis in Excel. Population genetic software for teaching and research. *Molecular Ecology Notes*, 6, 288-295.

[56] Goudet J (1999) *FSTAT, a program to estimate and test gene diversities and fixation indices (version 2.9.3)*. University of Lausanne, Lausanne.

[57] Nei M (1987) *Molecular Evolutionary Genetics*. Columbia University Press, New York.

[58] Excoffier L, Laval G, Schneider S (2005) Arlequin ver. 3.0: An integrated software package for population genetics data analysis. *Evolutionary Bioinformatics Online*, 1, 47-50.

[59] Write S (1939) The distribution of self-sterility alleles in populations. *Genetics*, 24, 538-552.

[60] Kimura M, Crow J (1964) The number of alleles that can be maintained in a finite population. *Genetics*, 49, 725-738.

[61] Weir BS, Cockerham CC (1984) Estimating F-statistics for the analysis of population structure. *Evolution*, 38, 1358-1370.

[62] Hartl DL (1981) *A Primer of Population Genetics*. Sinauer Associates Inc., Massachusetts.

[63] Excoffier L, Smouse PE, Quattro JM (1992) Analysis of molecular variance inferred from metric distances among DNA haplotypes: application to human mitochondrial DNA restriction data. *Genetics*, 131, 479-491.

[64] Nei M, Tajima F, Tateno Y (1983) Accuracy of estimated phylogenetic trees from molecular data. *Journal of Molecular Evolution*, 19, 153-170.

[65] Saitou N, Nei M (1987) The neighbor-joining method: a new method for reconstructing phylogenetic trees. *Molecular Biology and Evolution*, 4, 406-425.

[66] Felsenstein J (1985) Confidence limits on phylogenies: an approach using the bootstrap. *Evolution*, 39, 783-791.

[67] Langella O (2007) *Populations 1.2.31*. http://bioinformatics.org/~tryphon/populations/ (accessed 12 June 2012).

[68] Tamura K, Peterson D, Peterson N, Stecher G, Nei M, Kumar S (2011) MEGA5: molecular evolutionary genetics analysis using maximum likelihood, evolutionary distance, and maximum parsimony methods. *Molecular Biology and Evolution*, 28, 2731-2739.

[69] Pritchard JK, Rosenberg NA (1999) Use of unlinked genetic markers to detect population stratification in association studies. *The American Journal of Human Genetics*, 65, 220-228.

[70] Pritchard JK, Stephens M, Donnelly P (2000) Inference of population structure using multilocus genotype data. *Genetics*, 155, 945-959.

[71] Falush D, Stephens M, Pritchard JK (2003) Inference of population structure using multilocus genotype data: linked loci and correlated allele frequencies. *Genetics*, 164, 1567-1587.

[72] Manel S, Gaggiotti OE, Waples RS (2005) Assignment methods: matching biological questions with appropriate techniques. *Trends in Ecology and Evolution*, 20, 136-142.

[73] Falush D, Stephens M, Pritchard JK (2007) Inference of population structure using multilocus genotype data: dominant markers and null alleles. *Molecular Ecology Notes*, 7, 574-578.

[74] Hubisz M, Falush D, Stephens M, Pritchard J (2009) Inferring weak population structure with the assistance of sample group information. *Molecular Ecology Resources*, 9, 1322-1332.

[75] Evanno G, Regnaut S, Goudet J (2005) Detecting the number of clusters of individuals using the software STRUCTURE: a simulation study. *Molecular Ecology*, 14, 2611-2620.

[76] Earl DA, vonHoldt BM (2012) STRUCTURE HARVESTER: a website and program for visualizing STRUCTURE output and implementing the Evanno method. *Conservation Genetics Resources*, 4, 359-361.

[77] Jakobsson M, Rosenberg NA (2007) CLUMPP: a cluster matching and permutation program for dealing with label switching and multimodality in analysis of population structure. *Bioinformatics*, 23, 1801-1806.

[78] Frankham R (2000) Modeling problems in conservation genetics using laboratory animals. In Ferson S, Burgman M (ed.) *Quantitative Methods in Conservation Biology*, Springer-Verlag, New York, p259-273.

[79] Koizumi N, Takemura T, Mori A, Okushima S (2009) Genetic structure of loach population in Yatsu paddy field. *Irrigation, Drainage and Rural Engineering Journal*, 77, 253-261. (in Japanese with English abstract)

[80] Koizumi N, Takahashi H, Minezawa M, Takemura T, Okushima S (2007) Fourteen polymorphic microsatellite loci in the field gudgeon, *Gnathopogon elongatus elongates. Molecular Ecology Notes*, 7, 240-242.

[81] Ohara K, Hotta M, Takahashi D, Asahida T, Ida H, Umino T (2009) Use of microsatellite DNA and otolith Sr:Ca ratios to infer genetic relationships and migration history of four morphotypes of *Rhinogobius* sp. OR. *Ichthyological Research*, 56, 373-379.

[82] Randall1 DA, Pollinger JP, Argaw K, Macdonald DW, Wayne RK (2010) Fine-scale genetic structure in Ethiopian wolves imposed by sociality, migration, and population bottlenecks. *Conservation Genetics*, 11, 89-101.

[83] Brown VA, Brooke A, Fordyce JA, McCracken GF (2011) Genetic analysis of populations of the threatened bat *Pteropus mariannus. Conservation Genetics*, 12, 933-941.

[84] Docker MF, Heath DD (2003) Genetic comparison between sympatric anadromous steelhead and freshwater resident rainbow trout in British Columbia, Canada. *Conservation Genetics*, 2, 227-231.

[85] Massa-Gallucci A, Coscia I, O'Grady M, Kelly-Quinn M, Mariani S (2010) Patterns of genetic structuring in a brown trout (*Salmo trutta* L.) metapopulation. *Conservation Genetics*, 11, 1689-1699.

[86] Lloyd MW, Burnett RK, Engelhardt KAM, Neel MC (2011) The structure of population genetic diversity in *Vallisneriaamericana* in the Chesapeake Bay: implications for restoration. *Conservation Genetics*, 12, 1269-1285.

[87] Junker J, Peter A, Wagner CE, Mwaiko S, Germann B, Seehausen O, Keller, I (2012) River fragmentation increases localized population genetic structure and enhances asymmetry of dispersal in bullhead (*Cottus gobio*). *Conservation Genetics*, 13, 545-556.

[88] Rodriguez D, Forstner MRJ, McBride DL, Densmore LD, Dixon JR (2012) Low genetic diversity and evidence of population structure among subspecies of *Nerodia harteri*, a threatened water snake endemic to Texas. *Conservation Genetics*, 13, 977-986.

Section 3

Molecular Recognition

Chapter 15

The HIV-1 Integrase: Modeling and Beyond

Rohit Arora and Luba Tchertanov

Additional information is available at the end of the chapter

http://dx.doi.org/10.5772/52344

1. Introduction

Molecular recognition is a fundamental phenomenon observed in all biological systems organisation – proteins, nucleic acids and their complexes, cells and tissues. Molecular recognition is governed by specific attractive interactions between two or more partner molecules through non-covalent bonding such as hydrogen bonds, metal coordination, electrostatic effects, hydrophobic and van der Waals interactions. The partners – receptor(s) and substrate(s) or ligands – involved in molecular recognition, exhibit molecular complementarity that can be adjusted over the recognition process. Competition and co-operation, the two opposite natural effects contributing to selective and specific recognition between participating partners, are the basic principles of substrate/ligand/inhibitor or protein binding to its targets.

The tertiary structures of biological objects (proteins and nucleic acids) are formed mainly by hydrogen bonds (enthalpic contributions) and by hydrophobic contacts (mostly entropic contributions). With a few exceptions, (e.g. ligand binding to the Ah receptor), the organisation of ligand-protein complexes depends primarily on hydrogen bonding.

In the process of a ligand binding to its target the hydrogen bonds contribute to (i) the orientation of the substrates/ligands/inhibitors by a receptor, frequently associated with a conformational/structural adjustment of the interacting agents; (ii) the specific recognition of substrates/ligands/inhibitors and selectivity between sterically or structurally similar but biochemically different species; (iii) the affinity of ligands/inhibitors – the most decisive factor in drug design.

To describe the pharmacological properties of a given ligand or inhibitor, the knowledge of the site where the inhibitor is to bind with the target and of which interaction(s) control the specific recognition of the inhibitor by its target(s), represents a corner stone factor. Only a limited number of target-ligand molecular complexes have been characterized experimentally at the atomic level (X-ray or NMR analysis) [1]. Part of them describes the binding mode of therapeutically relevant ligands to biologically non-relevant and non-pertinent targets (e.g., the HIV-1 integrase specific inhibitor RAL was published as a ligand fixed to the PFV intasome [2,3]). Consequently, a large quantity of reliable information on target-ligand binding is based on molecular docking methods which generate insights into the interactions of ligands with the amino acid residues in the binding pockets of the targets, and also predict the corresponding binding affinities of ligands [4]. The first step of a docking calculation consists of the choice or generation/construction of the therapeutically appropriate target. Frequently the target modeling is a hard computational task which requires the application of sophisticated theoretical methods and constitutes a fascinating creative process.

Therefore, theoretical studies contribute first, to establish biologically valid models of the targets; second, through the use of these models, to the understanding of the protein functional properties; and finally to apply this data to rational drug design.

Here we compile and review the data on the molecular structure, properties and interactions of the HIV-1 integrase representing from one side, a characteristic example of a polyfunctional and complex biological object interacting with different viral and cellular partners and from another side, an attractive therapeutical target. We attempt to extract key messages of practical value and complement references with our own research of this viral enzyme. We characterized the structural and conformational features of Raltegravir (RAL), the first integrase specific inhibitor approved for the treatment of HIV/AIDS, and we analyzed the factors contributing to RAL recognition by the viral targets.

2. The HIV-1 integrase and integrase-viral DNA pre-integration complex

2.1. Activities

The HIV-1 integrase (IN) is a key enzyme in the replication mechanism of retroviruses, catalyzing the covalent insertion of the reverse-transcribed DNA into the chromosomes of the infected cells [5]. Once integrated, the provirus persists in the host cell and serves as a template for the transcription of viral genes and replication of the viral genome, leading to production of new viruses (Figure 1a). A two-step reaction is required for covalent integration of viral DNA (vDNA) into host DNA (hDNA). First, IN binds to a short sequence located at either end of the long terminal repeat (LTR) of the viral DNA and catalyzes an endo-nucleotide cleavage. This process is known as 3′-processing reaction (3′-P), resulting in the removal of two nucleotides from each of the 3′-ends of the LTR and the delivery of hydroxyl groups for nucleophilic attacks (Figure 1 b).

The cleaved (pre-processed) DNA is then used as a substrate for the strand transfer (ST) reaction, leading to the covalent insertion of the vDNA into genome of the infected cell [5,7]. The ST reaction occurs at both ends of the vDNA simultaneously, with an offset of precisely five base pairs between the two distant points of insertion. The integration process is accomplished by the removal of unpaired dinucleotides from the 5′-ends of the vDNA, the filling

http://dx.doi.org/10.5772/52344

in of the single-strand gaps between viral and target DNA molecules and ligation of the 3′-ends of the vDNA to the 5′-ends of the hDNA (Figure 1 b). These two reactions are spatially and temporally separated and energetically independent: the 3′-processing takes place in the cytoplasm of the infected cells, whereas strand transfer occurs in the nuclei. They are catalyzed by the enzyme in different conformational and oligomerisation states: dimerization is required for the 3′-processing step [8,9], while tetrameric IN is believed to be required for strand transfer [10-12].

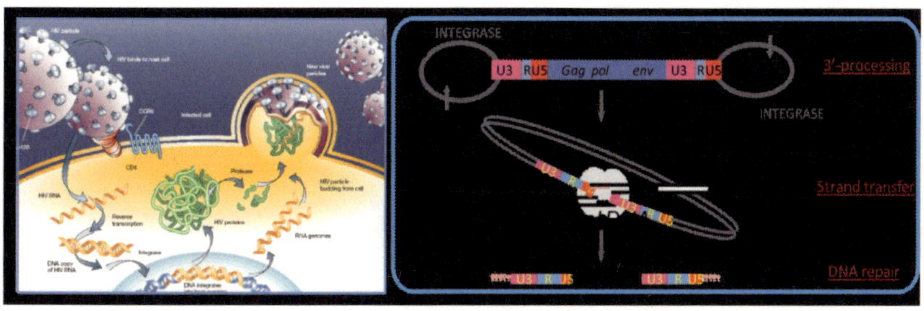

(a) (b)

Figure 1. The HIV-1 replication cycle (a) and catalytic steps involved in the insertion of viral DNA into the human genome (b) [6].

2.2. Structural data

The HIV-1 IN is a 288 amino acids enzyme (32 kDa) that consists in three structurally distinct domains: (i) the N-terminal domain (NTD, $IN^{1–49}$) with a non-conventional HHCC zinc-finger motif, promoting protein multimerization; (ii) the central core domain (CCD, $IN^{50–212}$) containing a canonical D,D,E motif performing catalysis and involved in DNA substrate recognition [35]; (iii) the C-terminal domain (CTD, $IN^{213–288}$), which non-specifically binds DNA and helps to stabilize the IN•vDNA complex [13]. Both integration steps, 3′-P and ST, involve the active site and the active site flexible loop formed by ten residues, $IN^{140-149}$.

Neither the structure of isolated full-length IN from HIV-1 nor that of IN complex with its DNA substrate has been determined. Nevertheless, the structures of the isolated HIV-1 domains or two domains were characterized by X-ray crystallography (34 structures) and NMR analysis (9 structures) [1]. NTD presented by 6 NMR structure solutions (1WJA, 1WJB, 1WJC, 1WJE, and 1WGF) [14-16] was classified by SCOP as the 'all alpha helix' structure and consists of four helices stabilized by a Zn^{2+}cation coordinated with the HHCC motif (His12, His16, Cys40 and Cys43); the sequence from 43 to 49 residue are disordered (Figure 2). Structure of CTD was also characterised by NMR (3 deposited solutions (1IHV, 1IHW and 1QMC) [17,18]. According to the SCOP classification it presents the 'all beta strand' structure and consists of five anti-parallel β-strands forming a β-barrel and adopting an SH3-like fold (Figure 2).

The human IN CCD characterized by X-ray analysis has been reported as 14 different crystal structures (1HYV, 1HYZ, 1EXQ, 1QS4, 1B92, 1B9D, 1BHL, 1BI4, 1BIS, 1BIU, 1BIZ, 1BL3, 1ITG and 2ITG). The wild-type IN was resolved with a poor precision (1ITG) [19], the other structures represent engineered mutants, either single (F185K/H) [20-23], double (W131E and F185K; G149A and F185K or C56S and F185K) [24-26] or multiple (C56S, W131D, F139D and F185K) [27] mutants which were designed to overcome the poor solubility of the protein. The core domain has a mixed α/β structure, with five β-sheets and six α–helices (Figure 2).

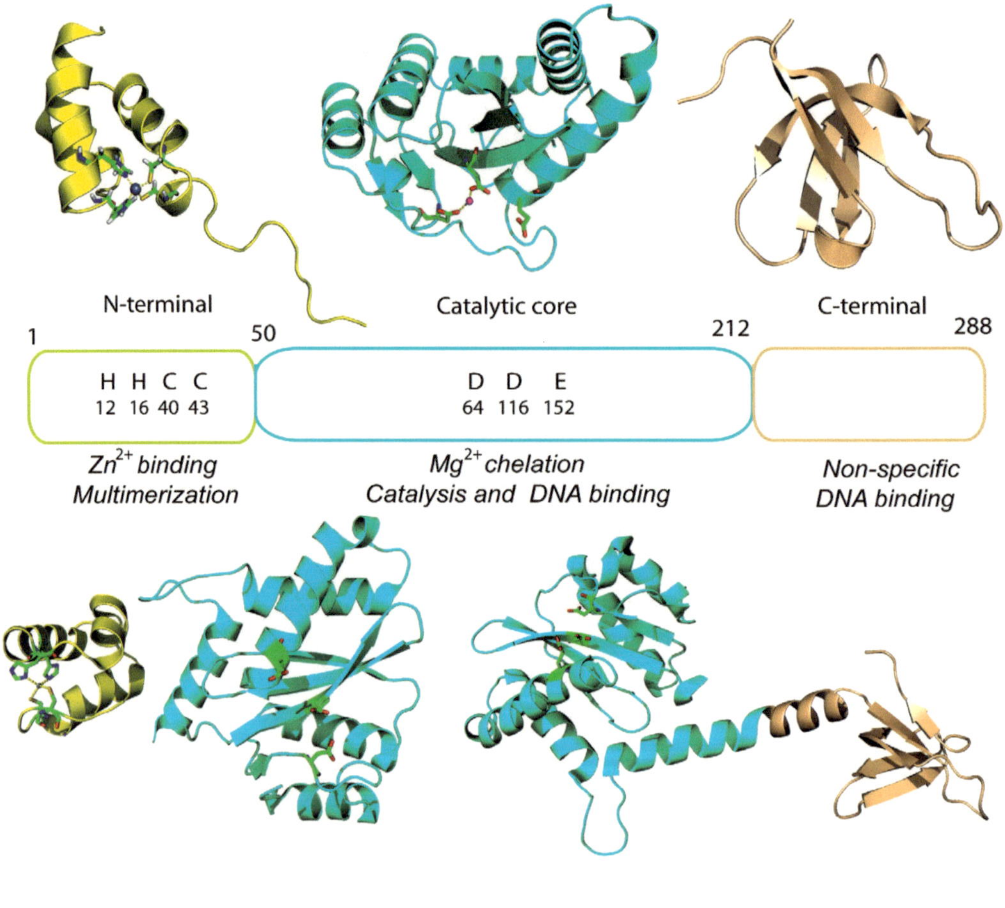

Figure 2. Structural domains of the HIV-1 integrase. (Top) N-terminal (IN^{1-49}, left), catalytic core (IN^{50-212}, middle) and C-terminal ($IN^{219-270}$, right) domains; (bottom) N-terminal with catalytic core domain (IN^{1-212}, left) and catalytic core with C-terminal fragment (IN^{52-288}, right). The structures are shown as cartoon with the side chains of the HHCC and DDE motifs in the N-terminal and catalytic core domains rendered in stick and the Zn^{2+} and Mg^{2+} cations as balls; dashed lines indicate ion coordination [28,29].

The active site residues D64, D116 and E152 are located in different structural elements: β-sheet (β1), coil and helix (α4), respectively. The catalytic core domain also encompasses a flexible loop comprising residues 140–149, in which conformational changes are required for 3′-P and ST reactions. These activities require the presence of a metallic cofactor(s), the Mg^{2+} ion(s), which binds to the catalytic residues D64, D116 and E152. The number of Mg^{2+} cations is different for the distinct enzymatic reactions and consequently, for the different IN states: a single Mg^{2+} cation in non-processed IN, and two in processed IN. The structures of avian sarcoma virus (ASV) IN [21] and the Tn5 transposase[30] have provided evidence of a two-metal active site structure, which has been used to build metal-containing IN models [31-33].

Crystallographic structures of IN^{1-212} and IN^{50-288} two-domain constructs have also been obtained for W131D/F139D/F185K and C56S/W131D/F139D/F185K/C180S mutants, respectively (Figure 2) [34,35]. In the first of these structures, there is an asymmetric unit containing four molecules forming pairs of dimers connected by a non-crystallographic two fold axis, in which the catalytic core and N-terminal domains are well resolved, their structures closely matching those found with isolated IN^{1-45} and IN^{50-212} domains, and connected by a highly disordered linking region (47–55 amino acids). The X-ray structure of the other two-domain construct, IN^{50-288}, showed there was a two-fold symmetric dimer in the crystal. The catalytic core and C-terminal domains were connected by a perfect helix formed by residues 195–221. The local structure of each domain was similar to the structure of the isolated domains. The dimer core domain interface was found to be similar to the isolated core domain, whereas the dimer C-terminal interface differed from that obtained by NMR.

2.3. Theoretical models

All these structural data characterising the HIV-1 IN single or two-domains allow the generation of biologically relevant models, representing either the unbound dimeric enzyme or IN complexed with the viral or/and host DNA [29].

IN acts as a multimer [36]. Dimerization is required for the 3′-processing step, with tetrameric IN catalyzing the ST reaction [37,38]. Dimeric models were built to reproduce the specific contacts between IN and the LTR terminal CA/TG nucleotides identified *in vitro* [39,40]. However, most models include a tetrameric IN alone or IN complex with either vDNA alone or vDNA/hDNA, recapitulating the simultaneous binding of IN to both DNAs required for strand transfer (Figure 3 b–d).

These models were either based on the partial crystal structure of IN [32,44] or constructed by analogy with a synaptic Tn5 transposase complex described in previous studies [42,45,46].

Most models include an Mg^{2+} cationic cofactor and take into account both structural data and biologically significant constraints (Figure 2 b–d). In particular, HIV-1 IN synaptic complexes (IN•vDNA•hDNA) have been constructed taken into account the different enzymatic states occurring during the integration process (Figure 3 d) [41,42]. Such complexes have also been characterized by electron microscopy (EM) and single-particle imaging at a resolution of 27 Å [47]. Recently the X-ray complete structure of the Primate Foamy Virus (PFV) integrase in complex with the substrate DNA and Raltegravir or Elvitegravir has also recently been reported (Figure 3 e) [2].

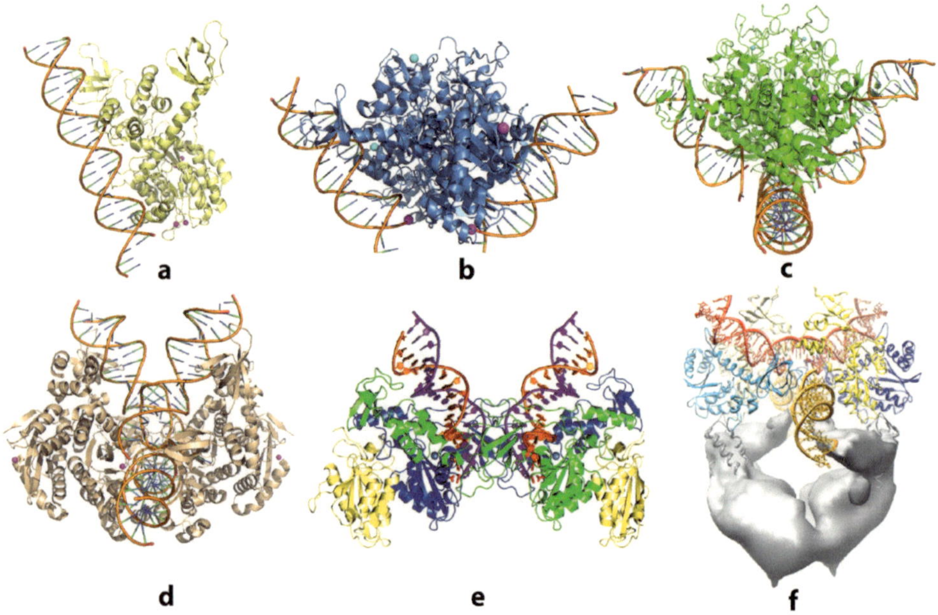

Figure 3. Integrase architecture and organization. Theoretical models: (a) dimeric model of the full-length IN•vDNA-complex [39]; (b) tetramer models of the IN•vDNA [27]; (c and d) synaptic complexes IN4•vDNA•hDNA [41,42]; (e) X-ray structure of the PFV IN•vDNAintasome [2]; and (f) EM maps reconstitution of IN•vDNA•hDNA complex with LEGDF [43]. Protein and DNA structures are presented as cartoon with colour coded nucleotides and Zn^{2+} and Mg^{2+}cations shown as balls. The active site contains two Mg^{2+} cations in (a) and one in (b–d).

In this complex, the retroviral intasome consists of an IN tetramer tightly associated with a pair of viral DNA ends. The overall shape of the complex is consistent with a low-resolution structure obtained by electron microscopy and single-particle reconstruction for HIV-1 IN complex with its cellular cofactor, the lens epithelium-derived growth factor (LEDGF) (Figure 3 d) [43].

2.5. Targets models representing the HIV-1 integrase before and after 3′-processing

Recently new HIV-1 IN models were generated by homology modeling. They represent with a certain level of reliability two different enzymatic states of the HIV-1 IN that can be explored as the biological relevant targets for design of the HIV-1 integrase inhibitors (Figure 4). The generated models are based on the experimental data characterising either the partial structures of IN from HIV-1 or full-length IN from PFV. The models of the separated full-length HIV-1 integrase represent the unbound homodimers of IN (IN1-270) containing either one or two Mg^{2+} cations in the active site – a plausible enzymatic state before the 3′

processing. The catalytic site loop encompassing ten residues forms the boundary of the active site. This loop shows either a coiled structure [20,22,24] or contains an Ω-shaped hairpin [28,48].

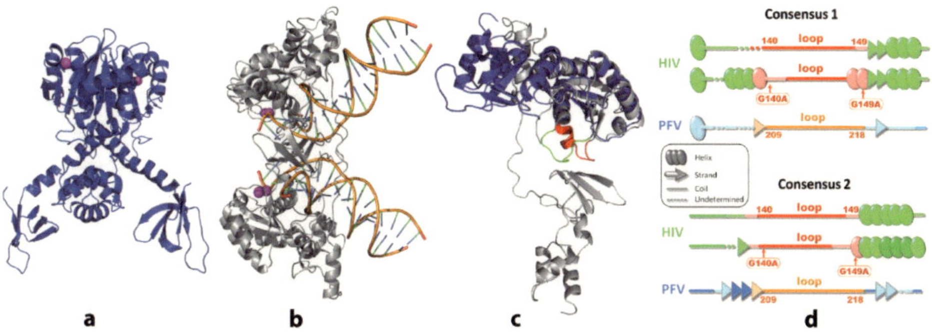

Figure 4. Structural models of the HIV-1 integrase. (a) Model of unbound IN representing the homodimeric enzyme before the 3'-processing; (b) Model of the simplified (dimeric form) IN•DNA pre-integration complex; (c) Superimposition of monomeric subunits from two models in which catalytic site loop residues 140-149 are shown by colours (red and green).The proteins are shown as cartoons, Mg^{2+} ions as spheres (in magenta). (d) Schematic representation of the HIV and PVF active site loop secondary structure prediction, according to consensus 1 and consensus 2.

It will be useful to note that we evidenced a high flexibility of the functional domains in unbound IN by using the Normal Modes Analysis (NMA) [49,50]. Particularly, CTD is characterized by a large scissors-like movement (Figure 5 a). We established that the catalytic site loop in unbound IN with two Mg^{2+}cations in the active site is more rigid due to the stabilising role of the coordination of the Mg^{2+}cations by three active site residues, D64, D116 and E152, whereas the catalytic site loop flexibility increases significantly (Figure 5 b, c).

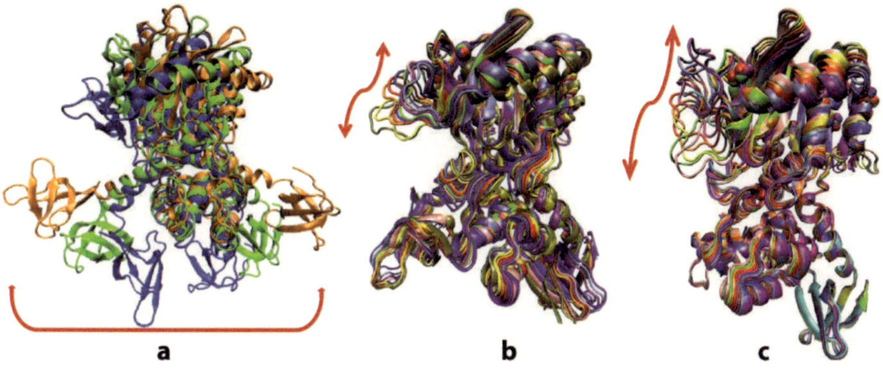

Figure 5. Normal modes illustrating fragments movement in unbound IN. A scissors-like movement in CTD (a); the catalytic site loop displacement in unbound IN with one and two Mg^{2+}cation(s) in the active site (b) and (c) respectively (S. Abdel-Azeim, personal communication).

The simplified model of the HIV-1 IN•vDNA pre-integration complex represents the homodimer of integrase non-covalently attached to the two double strains of the viral DNA with two removed nucleotides GT at each 3′-end (Figure 4 b), and likely depicts the biologically active unit of the IN•vDNA strand transfer intasome. The IN•vDNA model was generated from the X-ray structure of the PFV intasome [2]. Despite the very low sequence identity (22%) between the HIV-1 and PFV INs, the structure-based alignment of the two proteins demonstrates high conservation of key secondary structural elements and the three PFV IN domains shared with HIV-1 IN have essentially the same structure as the isolated IN domains from HIV-1 [51]. Moreover, the structure of the PFV intasome displays a distance between the reactive 3′ ends of vDNA that corresponds to the expected distance between the integration sites of HIV-1 IN target DNA (4 base pairs). Consequently, we suggested that the PFV IN X-ray structure represents an acceptable template for the HIV-1 IN model generation [52].

Two models of different states of the HIV-1 IN show a strong dissimilarity of their structure evidenced by divergent relative spatial positions of their structural domains, NTD, CCD and CTD (Figure 4 c). These tertiary structural modifications altered the contacts between IN domains and the structure and conformation of the linker regions. Particularly, the NTD-CCD interface exhibits substantial changes: in the unbound form the NTD-CCD interface belongs to the same monomer subunit whereas in the vDNA-bound form the interface is composed of residues from the two different subunits. Moreover, IN undergoes important structural transformation leading to structural re-organisation of the catalytic site loop; the coiled portion of the loop reduces from ten residues in the unbound form to five residues in the vDNA-bound form. Such effect may be induced either by the vDNA binding or it can derive as an artefact produced from the use of structural data of the PFV IN as a template for the model generation. Prediction of $IN^{133\text{-}155}$ sequence secondary structure elements indicates a more significant predisposition of IN from HIV-1 to be folded as two helices linked by a coiled loop than the IN from PFV (Figure 4 d). Prediction results obtained with high reliability (>75%) correlate perfectly with the X-ray data characterising the WT HIV-1 integrase (1B3L) [22] and its double mutant G140A/G149A (1B9F) [26]. The helix elongation accompanied by loop shortening may be easily induced by the enzyme conformational/structural transition between the two integration steps prompted by substrate binding.

This structure can be used to generate reliable HIV-1 IN models for Integrase Strand Transfer Inhibitors (INSTIs) design. However, the active site loop adopts a five-residue coil structure, rather than the ten-residue extended loop observed in HIV-1IN. This difference may be due to a difference in the sequence of the two enzymes or an effect induced by DNA binding, and caution is therefore required in the use of this structure as a template for modelling biologically relevant conformations of HIV-1 IN [2,45].

2.6. Transition pathway between two IN states and the allosteric binding sites

Two different states of the HIV-1 IN represent the enzyme structures before and after 3′-processing. Under integration process, IN as many other proteins undergo large conformational transitions that are essential for its functions (Figure 6) [53-55]. Tertiary structural changes precede and accompany these quaternary transitions in the HIV-1 IN as was evidenced by Targeted Molecular Dynamics (TMD) [56] and Meta Dynamics (MD) [57] (Figure 6 c, d).

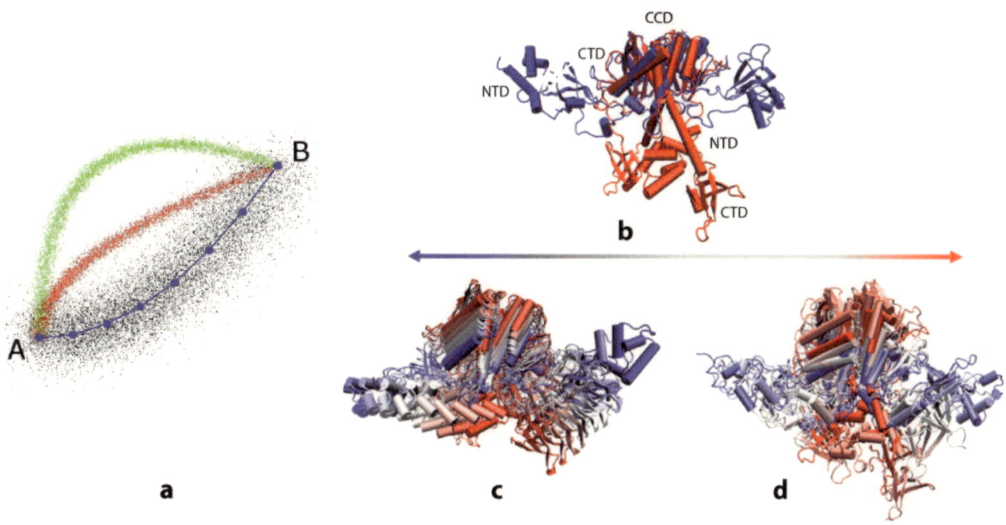

Figure 6. Transition states ensemble between A and B structures (a) (A. Blondel, personal communication). A series of conformations visited by the HIV-1 IN over transition from unbound IN to IN•vDNA complex before (red) and after (blue) 3′-processing (b) obtained by Targeted Molecular Dynamics (TMD) (c) and Meta Dynamics (MD) simulations (d) (S. Abdel-Azeim, personal communication).

Our results, first, provide a description of structure-dynamics-function relationships which in turn supplies a plausible understanding of the IN 3′-processing at the atomic level. Second, the calculated intermediate conformations along the trajectories were scanned for molecular pockets - a means of exploring putative allosteric binding sites, particularly positioned on the IN C-terminal domain (CTD), which is responsible for the vDNA recognition (Figure 7).

3. Raltegravir

The integrase inhibitors were developed to block either the 3′-processing or the strand transfer reaction [58-60]. Raltegravir (RAL), the first IN inhibitor approved for AIDS treatment [61] specifically inhibits the ST activity and was confirmed as an integrase ST inhibitor (INSTI), whereas the 3′-P activity was inhibited only up to a certain concentration [28,62]. The potency of RAL has been described at the level of half-maximal inhibitory concentration (IC50 values) in cellular antiviral and recombinant enzyme assays, kinetic analysis and slow-binding inhibition of IN-catalyzed ST reaction [62-68]. Particularly, it has an IC_{50} of 2 to 7nM for the inhibition of recombinant IN-mediated ST *in vitro* and an IC_{95} of 19 and 31 nM in 10% FBS (fetal bovine serum) and 50 % NHS (normal human serum), respectively. This drug has been reported to be approximately 100-fold less specific for the inhibition of 3'-processing activity compared to strand transfer. The dissociation rate of RAL with IN•vDNA complex was slow, with k_{off} values of $(22 \pm 2) \times 10^{-6}\ s^{-1}$. The dissociative half-life value measured for RAL with the wild type IN•vDNA complex was 7.3 h and 11.0 h obtained at 37°C and at 25°C respectively.

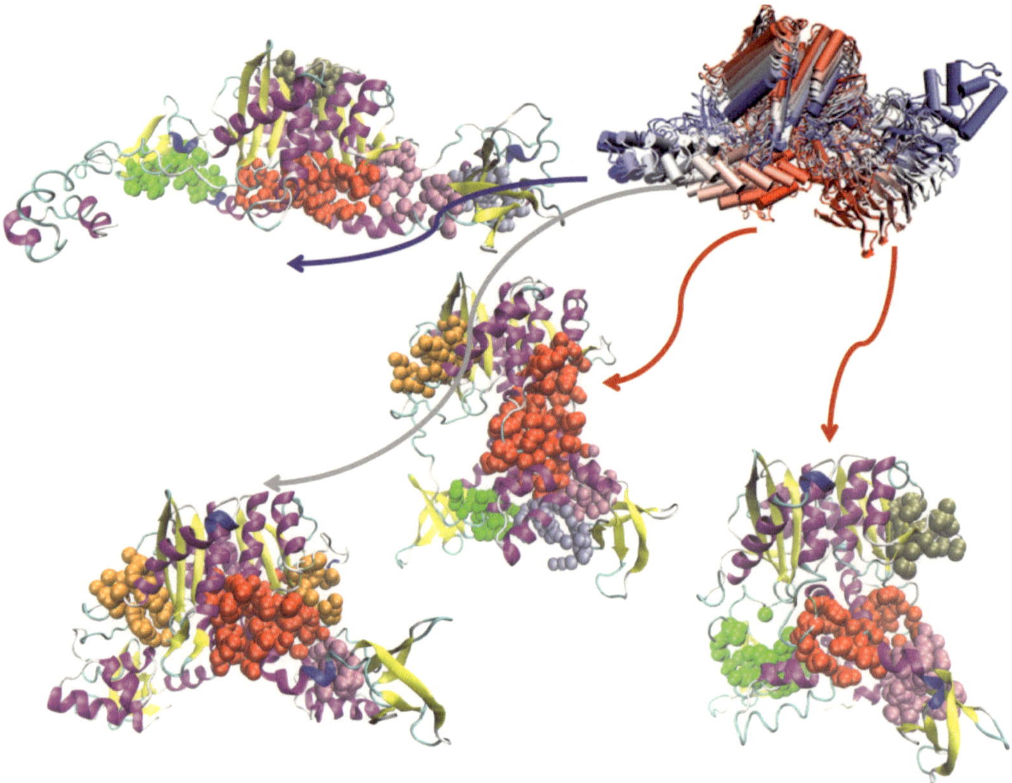

Figure 7. Pockets detected on the surface of the HIV-1 Integrase intermediate conformations obtained by Targeted Molecular Dynamics (TMD) simulations. (S. Abdel-Azeim, personal communication).

Like other antiretroviral inhibitors, RAL develops/induces a resistance effect. Resistance to RAL was associated with amino acids substitutions following three distinct genetic pathways that involve either N155H, either Q148R/K/H or Y143R primary mutation [69,70]. The last mutation was reported as rare [71]. It was supposed that the integrase active site mutation N155H causes resistance to raltegravir primarily by perturbing the arrangement of the active site Mg^{2+} ions and not by affecting the affinity of the metals or the direct contacts of the inhibitor with the enzyme [72].

G140S has been shown to enhance the RAL resistance associated with Q148R/K/H [73]. The kinetic gating and/or induced fit effect have been reported as possible mechanisms for RAL resistance of the G140S/Q148H mutant [74]. A third pathway involving the Y143R/C/H mutation and conferring a large decrease in susceptibility to RAL has been described [75].

3.1. Structure and conformational flexibility

No experimental data characterizing RAL unbound structure or RAL binding mode to the HIV-1 IN has been reported. In this regard, the characterization of RAL conformational preferences and the study of its binding to the HIV-1 IN represent an important task for determining the molecular factors that contribute to the pharmacological action of this drug. Crystallographic data describing the separate domains of the HIV-1 IN and the full-length PFV IN with its cognate DNA deposited in the PDB, provide useful experimental starting guide for the theoretical modeling of the structurally unstudied objects, IN and IN•vDNA complex of HIV-1 as the RAL targets.

RAL, incorporating two pharmacophores, is a multipotent agent capable to hit more than one target in HIV-1, the unbound IN, the viral DNA or IN•vDNA complex. RAL shows the configurational E/Z isomerism and a high conformational flexibility due to eight aliphatic single bonds. Two pharmacophores, (1) 1,3,4-oxadiazole-2-carboxamide and (2) carbonylamino-1-N-alkyl-5-hydroxypyrimidinone, possessing structural versatility through the orientation of carboxamide fragments respective to the aromatic rings, show E-, Z-configuration states characterizing the relative position of the vicinal 1–4 and 1–5 oxygen atoms [48] (Chart 1). The molecule has a set of multiple H-bond donor and acceptor centres. These molecular features together with high structural flexibility provide an abundance of alternative mono- and bi-dentate binding sites in a given RAL conformation.

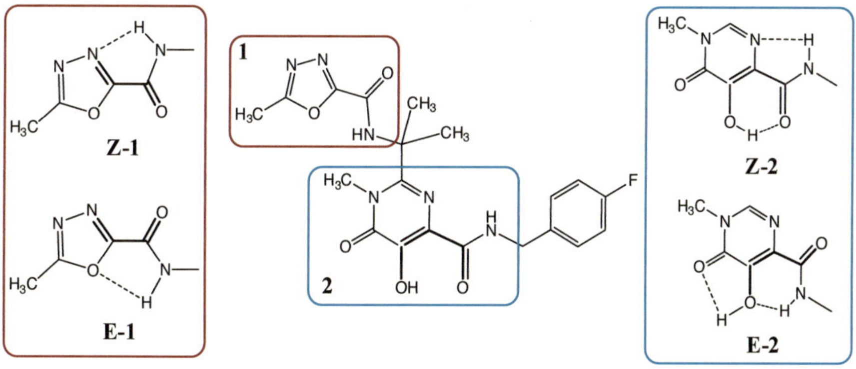

Chart 1. RAL structure. The E- and Z-isomers of 1,3,4-oxadiazole-2-carboxamide (1) and carbonylamino-1-N-alkyl-5-hydroxypyrimidinone (2) pharmacophores are stabilized by intramolecular H-bonds.

The chelating properties of protonated or deprotonated RAL are also determined by the E- or Z- configuration (Chart 2). Consequently, RAL can contribute in the recognition and binding of different partners – H-donor, H-acceptors, charged non-metal atoms and metal cations – in topologically distinct regions of IN by applying the richness of its molecular and structural properties. For instance, RAL as a bioisoster of adenine can block IN interaction with DNA [48] or sequester metal cofactor ions [76].

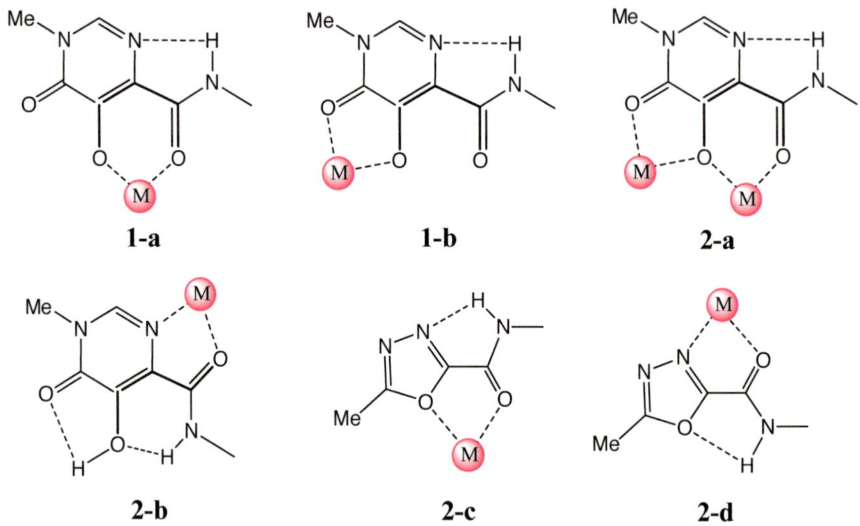

Chart 2. Metal chelating properties of 1, 3, 4-oxadiazole-2-carboxamide (1) and carbonylamino-1-N-alkyl-5-hydroxy-pyrimidinone (2) moieties.

The conformational preferences of RAL were examined in the gas phase (conformational analysis), in water solution (molecular dynamics, MD, in explicit solvent) and in the solid state (the fragment-based analysis using the crystallographic data from Cambridge Structural Database, CSD [77]. Conformational analysis of the different isomeric states of RAL in the gas phase indicates a small difference between the energy profiles of the Z-1/Z-2 and E-1/Z-2 isomers suggesting a relatively low energetical barrier between these two inhibitor states (Figure 8).

A slight preference for the Z-configuration of carbonylamino-hydroxypyrimidinonepharmacophore in the gas phase was observed, in coherence with the established predisposition of β-ketoenols – a principle corner stone of this pharmacophore – to adopt the Z-isomer in the solid state (Figure 9 b) [78-80]. The preference of aliphatic β-ketoenols to form energetically favorable Z-configurartion has been predicted early by *ab initio* studies at the B3LYP/3-G** level of theory [81].

The Cambridge Structural Databank search (CSD) [77] based on molecular fragments mimicking the RAL pharmacophores statistically demonstrates the preferential E-configuration of oxadiazolecarboxamide–like molecules and the Z-configuration of carbonylamino-hydroxypyrimidinone-like molecules in the solid state (Figure 9 a and b respectively). The halogenated aromatic rings, widely used pharmacophores, show a great level of conformational flexibility (Figure 9, c), allowing to contribute to a better inhibitor affinity in the binding site.

http://dx.doi.org/10.5772/52344

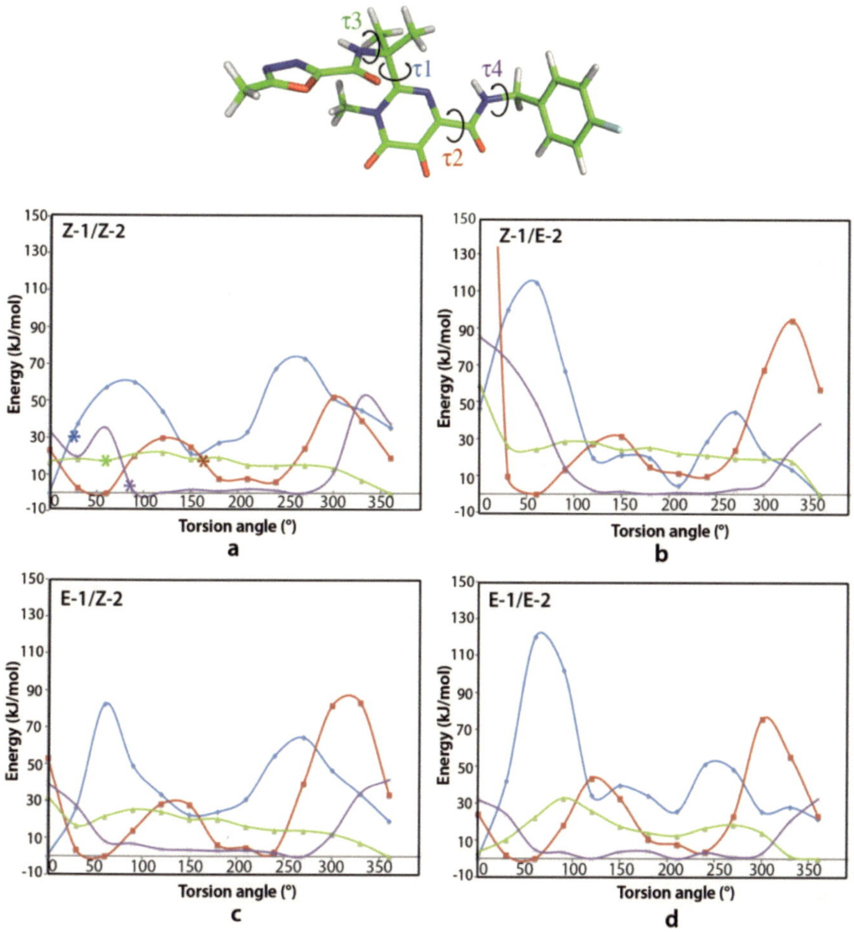

Figure 8. RAL conformations in the gas phase. Free energy profiles obtained by relaxed scans around the single bonds of RAL from 0 to 360º with an increment step of 30º, considering the four RAL isomers: (a) Z-1/Z-2, (b) Z-1/E-2, (c) E-1/Z-2 and (d) E-1/E-2. The curves representing the rotations around torsion angles τ1, τ2, τ3 and τ4 are shown in blue, red, green and violet colours. The values of τ1, τ2, τ3 and τ4 observed in RAL crystal structure 3OYA are indicated by asterisks.

3.2. Raltegravir-metal recognition

Synthesized as a metal cations chelating ligand, RAL can bind the metal by both pharmacophores in different isomerisation states. Probing the RAL chelating features with relevant cations, K, Mg and Mn, we evidenced that in the majority of metal complexes, the carbonylaminohydroxypyrimidinone-like fragments are observed in the Z configuration in the solid state (Figure 10).

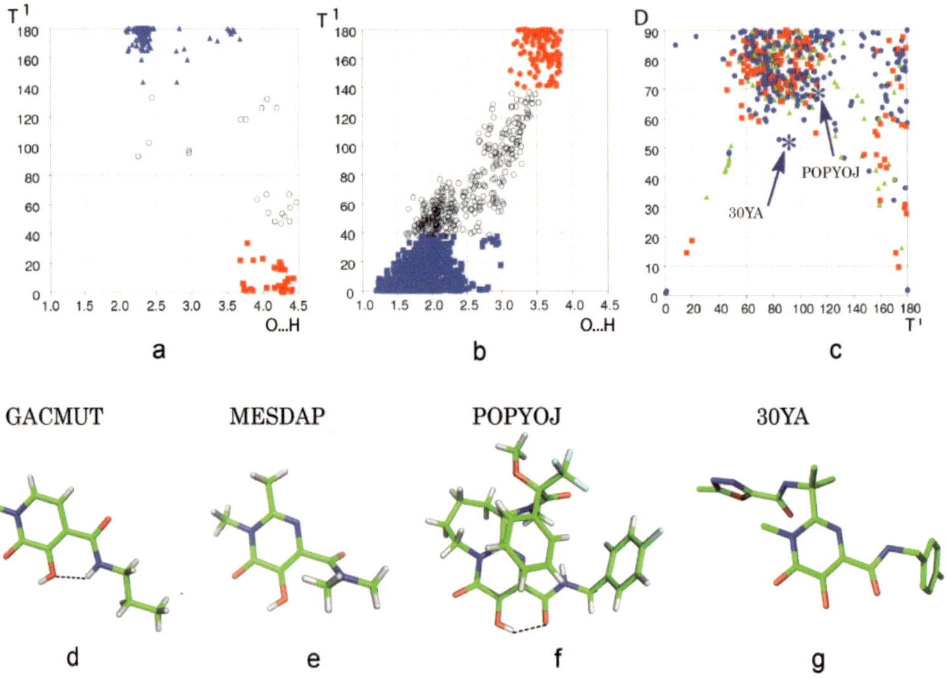

Figure 9. RAL conformations in the solid state. CSD fragment-based analysis of the RAL subunits indicates the E- (blue triangles) and Z- (red squares) conformations of oxadiazolecarboxamide–like molecules (a) and the Z-configuration of carbonylamino-hydroxypyrimidinone-like molecules (b). The halogenated phenyl ring conformation RAL geometry in PFV complex is shown in (c and d respectively). The RAL crystal structure parameters are indicated by asterisks. The alternative configurations of the carbonylamino-hydroxypyrimidinone derivatives are demonstrated by structure of RAL precursor molecules, GACMUT, MEADAP and POPYOJ, and RAL inhibitor (d-g).

The oxadiazolecarboxamide-like pharmacophore is observed in the metal complexes as two isomers and demonstrates a strong selectivity to the metal type: the Z isomer binds K and Mg while the E isomer binds mainly Mn. The higher probability of Mg^{2+}cation coordination by the Z-isomer of both pharmacophores indicates that the presence of two Mg^{2+}cations at the integrase binding site may be a decisive factor for stabilisation of the Z/Z configuration of RAL which is observed in the PFV intasome complex [2,3].

Therapeutically used RAL is in deprotonated state neutralised by K cation. Such drug formula corresponds to the optimal condition allowing efficient cations replacement in cells. The significantly higher affinity of both parmacophores to Mg relatively to K permits a positive competition between these cations, resulting in the change of RAL composition from a pharmaceutically acceptable potassium (K) salt to a biologically relevant Mg complex.

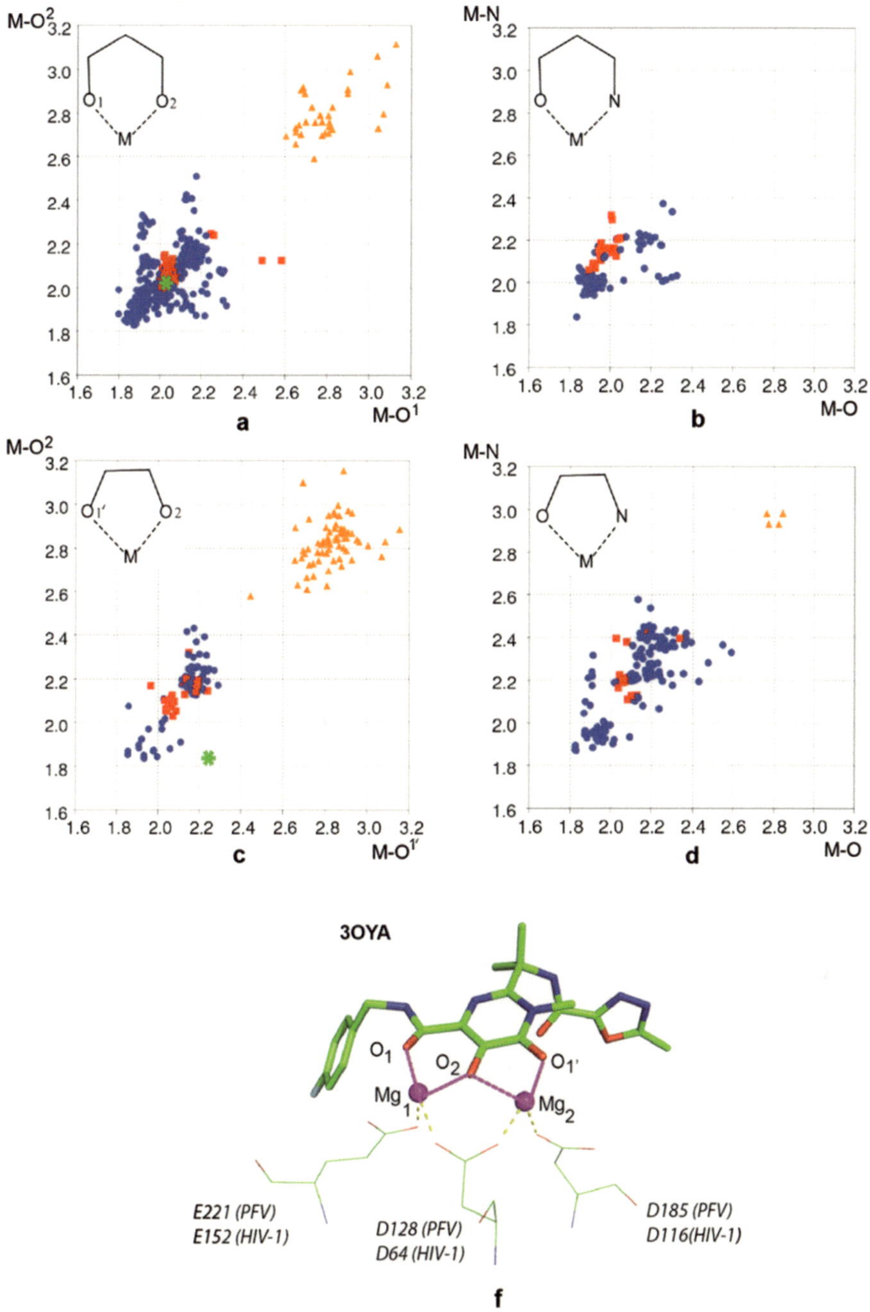

Figure 10. Probing of ligand interactions with Mg, Mn and K by CSD fragment-based search for the metal-ligand complexes (Chart 2, and scatterplots (a-d). Metal complexes are indicated by bull symbols: red squares (Mg), blue circles (Mn) and orange triangles (K). The RAL crystal structure is shown (f) and the RAL parameters are indicated by asterisks in (a and c).

3.3. Raltegravir recognition by the HIV-1 targets

The published docking studies report located within the active site of either unbound IN or IN•vDNA complex. Distinct poses of RAL representing different RAL configuration and modes of Mg^{2+} cations chelation were observed [74,82-84].

Our docking calculations of RAL onto each model evidenced that (i) the large binding pocket delimited by the active site and the extended catalytic site loop in the unbound IN can accommodate RAL in distinct configurational/conformational states showing a lack of interaction specificity between inhibitor and target; (ii) the well defined cavity formed by the active site, vDNA and shortened catalytic site loop provides a more optimised RAL binding site where the inhibitor is stabilised by coordination bonds with Mg^{2+} cations in the Z/Z-configuration (Figure 11).

Additional stabilisation of RAL is provided by non-covalent interactions with the environing residues of IN and the viral DNA bases. Based on our computing data we suggested earlier the stabilizing role of the vDNA in the inhibitors recognition by IN•vDNA pre-integration complex [51]. It was experimentally evidenced that RAL potently binds only when IN is in a binary complex with vDNA [85], possibly binding to a transient intermediate along the integration pathway [86]. Terminal bases of the viral DNA play a role in both catalytic efficiency [87,88] and inhibitor binding [89-91].

It was reported recently that unprocessed viral DNA could be the primary target of RAL [92]. This study is based on the PFV DNA and several oligonucleotides mimicking the HIV-1 DNA probed by experimental and computing techniques.

To explore the role of the HIV-1 viral DNA in RAL recognition we docked RAL onto the non-cleaved and cleaved DNA (the terminal GT nucleotides were removed) [79]. We found that RAL docked onto the non-cleaved vDNA is positioned in the minor groove of the substrate. No stabilising interactions between the partners, RAL and vDNA, were observed. In contrast, in the processed (cleaved) vDNA the Z/Z isomer of RAL takes the place of the remote GT based and is stabilised by strong and specific H-bonds with the unpaired cytosine. These H-bonds characterize the high affinity and specific recognition between RAL and the unpaired cytosine similarly to those observed in the DNA bases pair G-C.

Based on the docking results we suggested that the inhibition process may include as a first step the RAL recognition by the processed viral DNA bound to a transient intermediate IN state. RAL coupled to vDNA shows an outside orientation of all oxygen atoms, excellent putative chelating agents of Mg^{2+}cations, which could facilitate the insertion of RAL into the active site. The conformational flexibility of RAL further allows the accommodation/adaptation of the inhibitor in a relatively large binding pocket of IN•vDNA pre-integration complex thus producing various RAL docked conformation. We believe that such variety of RAL conformations contributing to the alternative enzyme residue recognition may impact the selection of the clinically observed alternative resistance pathways to the drug [29] and references herein.

http://dx.doi.org/10.5772/52344

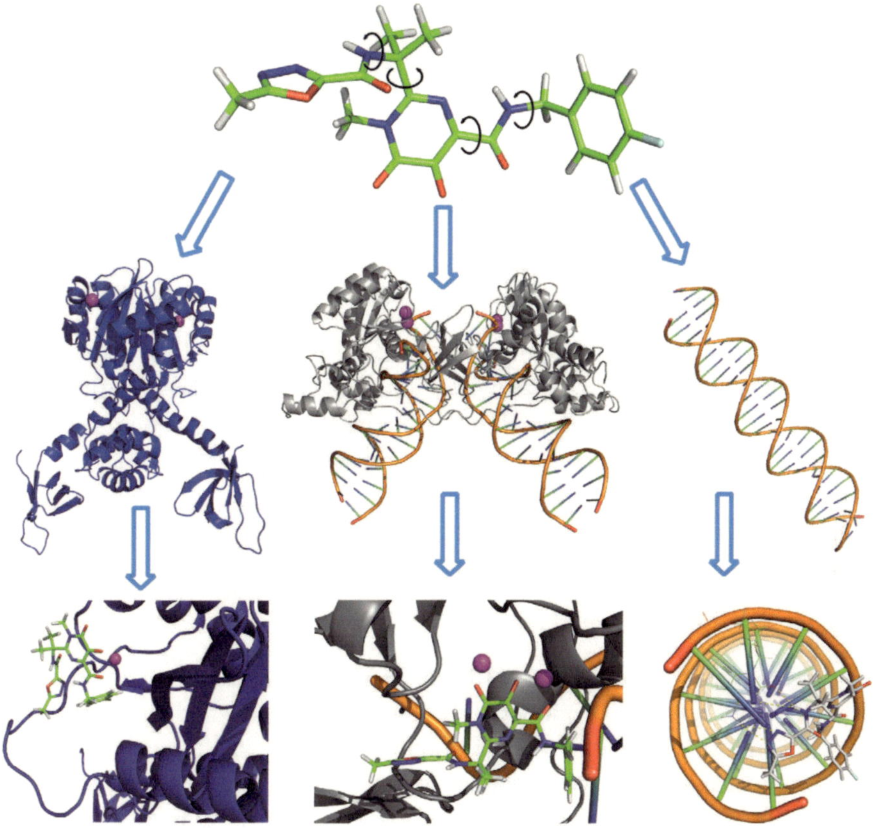

Figure 11. RAL docking onto the active site of unbound IN, IN•vDNA complex and viral DNA. Proteins and DNA are shown as cartoons; inhibitors as sticks and Mg2+ cations as balls.

4. Conclusions and perspectives

The HIV-1 Integrase is an essential retroviral enzyme that covalently binds both ends of linear viral DNA and inserts them into a cellular chromosome. The functions of this enzyme are based on the existence of specific attractive interactions between partner molecules or cofactors – IN, viral DNA and Mg^{2+} cations. Structure-based drug development seeks to identify and use such interactions to design and optimize the competitive and specific modulator of such functional interactions. Drug design and optimisation process require knowledge about interaction geometries and binding affinity contributing to molecular recognition that can be gleaned from crystallographic and modeling data.

We have resumed the available structural information related to the retroviral integrase. We used this data to generate biologically relevant HIV-1 targets – the unbound IN, the viral DNA (vDNA) and the IN•vDNA complex – which represent with a certain level of reliability, two different enzymatic states of the HIV-1 over the retroviral integration process.

We have characterised the RAL binding, a very flexible molecule displaying the E/Z isomerism, to the active site of its HIV-1 targets which mimic the integrase states before and after the 3′-processing. The docked conformations represent a spectrum of possible conformational/configurational states. The best docking scores and poses confirm that the generated model representing the IN•vDNA complex is the biologically relevant target of RAL, the strand transfer inhibitor. This finding is consistent with well-documented and commonly accepted inhibition mechanism of RAL, based on integral biological, biochemical and structural data.

RAL docking onto the IN•vDNA complex systematically generated the RAL chelated to Mg^{2+}cations at the active site by the pharmacophore oxygen atoms. The identification of IN residues specifically interacting with RAL is likely a very difficult task and the exact modes of binding of this inhibitor remain a matter of debate. Most probably the flexible nature of RAL results in different conformations and the mode of binding may differ in terms of the interacting residues of the target, which trigger the alternative resistance phenomenon.

The identified RAL binding to the processed viral DNA shed light on a putative, even plausible, step of the RAL inhibition mechanism.

We have implemented dynamic properties to the HIV-1 targets characterisation, particularly, the internal protein collective motions and the global conformational transition. Such transitions play an essential role in the function of many proteins, but experiments do not provide the atomic details on the path followed in going from one end structure to the other. For the dimeric IN, the transition pathway between the unbound and bound to vDNA is not known, which limits information of the cooperative mechanism in this typical allosteric system, where both tertiary and quaternary changes are involved. Description of the IN intermediate conformations open a way to localise the allosteric pockets, which in turn can be selected as the putative binding sites for small molecules in a virtual screening protocol.

Novel drugs, targeted the HIV-1 Integrase, outcome mainly due to the rapid emergence of RAL analogues (for example, GS-9137 or elvitegravir, MK-2048 and S/GSK 1349572, currently under clinical trials [93]). The clinical trials of several RAL analogues (BMS-707035, GSK-364735) were suspended. All these molecules specifically suppress the IN ST reaction. We conceive that the future HIV-1 integrase drug development will be mainly oriented to design of inhibitors with a mechanism of action that differs from that of RAL and its analogues. Distinct conceptions are potentially conceivable: (i) Design of the allosteric inhibitors, able to recognize specifically the binding sites that differ from the IN active site. Inhibitor V-165, belonging to such type inhibitors, prevents IN binding with the viral DNA such blocking 3′-processing reaction [94]. (ii) Design of the protein-protein inhibitors (PPIs) acting on interaction interface between either viral components (the IN monomers upon multimerization process or sub-units of the IN•vDNA complex) [95,96], or between viral and cellular proteins (IN/LEDGF) [97,98]. These alternative strategies represent rational and prospective directions in the HIV-1 integrase drug developement.

Acknowledgement

The authors thank Dr. E. Laine for valuable discussions and for editorial assistance, I. Chauvot de Beauchêne and S. Abdel-Azeim for providing of illustrative materials. This work is funded by the Centre National de la Recherche Scientifique (CNRS), Ecole Normale Supérieure (ENS) de Cachan and SIDACTION.

Author details

Rohit Arora and Luba Tchertanov

BiMoDyM, LBPA, CNRS -ENS de Cachan, LabEx LERMIT, CEDEX Cachan, France

References

[1] Berman HM, Westbrook J, Feng Z, Gilliland G, Bhat TN, Weissig H, et al. The Protein Data Bank. Nucleic Acids Research 2000 Jan 1;28(1):235-42.

[2] Hare S, Gupta SS, Valkov E, Engelman A, Cherepanov P. Retroviral intasome assembly and inhibition of DNA strand transfer. Nature 2010 Mar 11;464(7286):232-6.

[3] Hare S, Vos AM, Clayton RF, Thuring JW, Cummings MD, Cherepanov P. Molecular mechanisms of retroviral integrase inhibition and the evolution of viral resistance. Proceedings of the National Academy of Sciences of the United States of America 2010 Nov 16;107(46):20057-62.

[4] Krovat EM, Steindl T, Langer T. Recent Advances in Docking and Scoring. Current Computer-Aided Drug Design 2005 Jan;1(1):93-102.

[5] Brown PO. Integration of Retroviral DNA. Current Topics in Microbiology and Immunology 1990;157:19-48.

[6] Weiss RA. Gulliver's travels in HIV land. Nature 2001 Apr 19;410(6831):963-7.

[7] Chiu TK, Davies DR. Structure and function of HIV-1 integrase. Current Topics in Medicinal Chemistry 2004;4(9):965-77.

[8] Hayouka Z, Rosenbluh J, Levin A, Loya S, Lebendiker M, Veprintsev D, et al. Inhibiting HIV-1 integrase by shifting its oligomerization equilibrium. Proceedings of the

National Academy of Sciences of the United States of America 2007 May 15;104(20): 8316-21.

[9] Guiot E, Carayon K, Delelis O, Simon F, Tauc P, Zubin E, et al. Relationship between the oligomeric status of HIV-1 integrase on DNA and enzymatic activity. Journal of Biological Chemistry 2006 Aug 11;281(32):22707-19.

[10] Faure A, Calmels C, Desjobert C, Castroviejo M, Caumont-Sarcos A, Tarrago-Litvak L, et al. HIV-1 integrase crosslinked oligomers are active in vitro. Nucleic Acids Research 2005;33(3):977-86.

[11] Wang Y, Klock H, Yin H, Wolff K, Bieza K, Niswonger K, et al. Homogeneous high-throughput screening assays for HIV-1 integrase 3 '-processing and strand transfer activities. Journal of Biomolecular Screening 2005 Aug;10(5):456-62.

[12] Li M, Mizuuchi M, Burke TR, Craigie R. Retroviral DNA integration: reaction pathway and critical intermediates. Embo Journal 2006 Mar 22;25(6):1295-304.

[13] Asante-Appiah E, Skalka AM. Molecular mechanisms in retrovirus DNA integration. Antiviral Research 1997 Dec;36(3):139-56.

[14] Cai ML, Huang Y, Caffrey M, Zheng RL, Craigie R, Clore GM, et al. Solution structure of the His12 -> Cys mutant of the N-terminal zinc binding domain of HIV-1 integrase complexed to cadmium. Protein Science 1998 Dec;7(12):2669-74.

[15] Cai ML, Zheng RL, Caffrey M, Craigie R, Clore GM, Gronenborn AM. Solution structure of the N-terminal zinc binding domain of HIV-1 integrase. Nature Structural Biology 1997 Jul;4(7):567-77.

[16] Eijkelenboom APAM, vandenEnt FMI, Vos A, Doreleijers JF, Hard K, Tullius TD, et al. The solution structure of the amino-terminal HHCC domain of HIV-2 integrase: a three-helix bundle stabilized by zinc. Current Biology 1997 Oct 1;7(10):739-46.

[17] Eijkelenboom APAM, Sprangers R, Hard K, Lutzke RAP, Plasterk RHA, Boelens R, et al. Refined solution structure of the C-terminal DNA-binding domain of human immunovirus-1 integrase. Proteins-Structure Function and Genetics 1999 Sep 1;36(4): 556-64.

[18] Lodi PJ, Ernst JA, Kuszewski J, Hickman AB, Engelman A, Craigie R, et al. Solution structure of the DNA binding domain of HIV-1 integrase. Biochemistry 1995 Aug 8;34(31):9826-33.

[19] Dyda F, Hickman AB, Jenkins TM, Engelman A, Craigie R, Davies DR. Crystal-Structure of the Catalytic Domain of HIV-1 Integrase - Similarity to Other Polynucleotidyl Transferases. Science 1994 Dec 23;266(5193):1981-6.

[20] Bujacz G, Alexandratos J, ZhouLiu Q, ClementMella C, Wlodawer A. The catalytic domain of human immunodeficiency virus integrase: Ordered active site in the F185H mutant. FEBS Letters 1996 Dec 2;398(2-3):175-8.

[21] Bujacz G, Alexandratos J, Wlodawer A. Binding of different divalent cations to the active site of avian sarcoma virus integrase and their effects on enzymatic activity. Journal of Biological Chemistry 1997 Jul 18;272(29):18161-8.

[22] Maignan S, Guilloteau JP, Zhou-Liu Q, Clement-Mella C, Mikol V. Crystal structures of the catalytic domain of HIV-1 integrase free and complexed with its metal cofactor: High level of similarity of the active site with other viral integrases. Journal of Molecular Biology 1998 Sep 18;282(2):359-68.

[23] Molteni V, Greenwald J, Rhodes D, Hwang Y, Kwiatkowski W, Bushman FD, et al. Identification of a small-molecule binding site at the dimer interface of the HIV integrase catalytic domain. Acta Crystallographica Section D-Biological Crystallography 2001 Apr;57:536-44.

[24] Goldgur Y, Dyda F, Hickman AB, Jenkins TM, Craigie R, Davies DR. Three new structures of the core domain of HIV-1 integrase: An active site that binds magnesium. ProcNatlAcadSci USA 1998 Aug 4;95(16):9150-4.

[25] Goldgur Y, Craigie R, Cohen GH, Fujiwara T, Yoshinaga T, Fujishita T, et al. Structure of the HIV-1 integrase catalytic domain complexed with an inhibitor: A platform for antiviral drug design. Proceedings of the National Academy of Sciences of the United States of America 1999 Nov 9;96(23):13040-3.

[26] Greenwald J, Le V, Butler SL, Bushman FD, Choe S. The mobility of an HIV-1 integrase active site loop is correlated with catalytic activity. Biochemistry 1999 Jul 13;38(28):8892-8.

[27] Chen AP, Weber IT, Harrison RW, Leis J. Identification of amino acids in HIV-1 and avian sarcoma virus integrase subsites required for specific recognition of the long terminal repeat ends. Journal of Biological Chemistry 2006 Feb 17;281(7):4173-82.

[28] Mouscadet JF, Tchertanov L. Raltegravir: molecular basis of its mechanism of action. Eur J Med Res 2009 Nov 24;14 Suppl 3:5-16.

[29] Mouscadet JF, Delelis O, Marcelin AG, Tchertanov L. Resistance to HIV-1 integrase inhibitors: A structural perspective. Drug Resist Updat 2010 Aug;13(4-5):139-50.

[30] Lovell S, Goryshin IY, Reznikoff WR, Rayment I. Two-metal active site binding of a Tn5 transposase synaptic complex. Nature Structural Biology 2002 Apr;9(4):278-81.

[31] Karki R, Tang Y, Nicklaus MC. Model of the HIV-1 integrase-viral DNA complex - A template for structure-based design of HIV in inhibitors. Abstracts of Papers of the American Chemical Society 2002 Aug 18;224:U9-U10.

[32] Karki RG, Tang Y, Burke TR, Nicklaus MC. Model of full-length HIV-1 integrase complexed with viral DNA as template for anti-HIV drug design. Journal of Computer-Aided Molecular Design 2004 Dec;18(12):739-60.

[33] Wang LD, Liu CL, Chen WZ, Wang CX. Constructing HIV-1 integrase tetramer and exploring influences of metal ions on forming integrase-DNA complex. Biochemical and Biophysical Research Communications 2005 Nov 11;337(1):313-9.

[34] Chen ZG, Yan YW, Munshi S, Li Y, Zugay-Murphy J, Xu B, et al. X-ray structure of simian immunodeficiency virus integrase containing the core and C-terminal domain (residues 50-293) - An initial glance of the viral DNA binding platform. Journal of Molecular Biology 2000 Feb 18;296(2):521-33.

[35] Wang JY, Ling H, Yang W, Craigie R. Structure of a two-domain fragment of HIV-1 integrase: implications for domain organization in the intact protein. Embo Journal 2001 Dec 17;20(24):7333-43.

[36] Ellison V, Gerton J, Vincent KA, Brown PO. An Essential Interaction Between Distinct Domains of Hiv-1 Integrase Mediates Assembly of the Active Multimer. Journal of Biological Chemistry 1995 Feb 17;270(7):3320-6.

[37] Faure A, Calmels C, Desjobert C, Castroviejo M, Caumont-Sarcos A, Tarrago-Litvak L, et al. HIV-1 integrase crosslinked oligomers are active in vitro. Nucleic Acids Research 2005;33(3):977-86.

[38] Guiot E, Carayon K, Delelis O, Simon F, Tauc P, Zubin E, et al. Relationship between the oligomeric status of HIV-1 integrase on DNA and enzymatic activity. Journal of Biological Chemistry 2006 Aug 11;281(32):22707-19.

[39] De Luca L, Pedretti A, Vistoli G, Barreca ML, Villa L, Monforte P, et al. Analysis of the full-length integrase - DNA complex by a modified approach for DNA docking. Biochemical and Biophysical Research Communications 2003 Oct 31;310(4):1083-8.

[40] Esposito D, Craigie R. Sequence specificity of viral end DNA binding by HIV-1 integrase reveals critical regions for protein-DNA interaction. EMBO Journal 1998 Oct 1;17(19):5832-43.

[41] Fenollar-Ferrer C, Carnevale V, Raugei S, Carloni P. HIV-1 integrase-DNA interactions investigated by molecular modelling. Computational and Mathematical Methods in Medicine 2008;9(3-4):231-43.

[42] Wielens J, Crosby IT, Chalmers DK. A three-dimensional model of the human immunodeficiency virus type 1 integration complex. Journal of Computer-Aided Molecular Design 2005 May;19(5):301-17.

[43] Michel F, Crucifix C, Granger F, Eiler S, Mouscadet JF, Korolev S, et al. Structural basis for HIV-1 DNA integration in the human genome, role of the LEDGF/P75 cofactor. EMBO J 2009 Apr 8;28(7):980-91.

[44] Gao K, Butler SL, Bushman F. Human immunodeficiency virus type 1 integrase: arrangement of protein domains in active cDNA complexes. Embo Journal 2001 Jul 2;20(13):3565-76.

[45] Davies DR, Goryshin IY, Reznikoff WS, Rayment I. Three-dimensional structure of the Tn5 synaptic complex transposition intermediate. Science 2000 Jul 7;289(5476): 77-85.

[46] Podtelezhnikov AA, Gao K, Bushman FD, McCammon JA. Modeling HIV-1 integrase complexes based on their hydrodynamic properties. Biopolymers 2003 Jan;68(1): 110-20.

[47] Ren G, Gao K, Bushman FD, Yeager M. Single-particle image reconstruction of a tetramer of HIV integrase bound to DNA. Journal of Molecular Biology 2007 Feb 9;366(1):286-94.

[48] Mouscadet JF, Arora R, Andre J, Lambry JC, Delelis O, Malet I, et al. HIV-1 IN alternative molecular recognition of DNA induced by raltegravir resistance mutations. Journal of Molecular Recognition 2009 Nov;22(6):480-94.

[49] Tama F, Gadea FX, Marques O, Sanejouand YH. Building-block approach for determining low-frequency normal modes of macromolecules. Proteins 2000 Oct 1;41(1): 1-7.

[50] Tama F, Sanejouand YH. Conformational change of proteins arising from normal mode calculations. Protein Eng 2001 Jan;14(1):1-6.

[51] Ni X, Abdel-Azeim S, Laine E, Arora R, Osemwota O, Marcelin A-G, et al. In silico and in vitro Comparison of HIV-1 Subtypes B and CRF02_AG Integrases Susceptibility to Integrase Strand Transfer Inhibitors. Advances in Vilology 2012;2012:548657.

[52] Yin ZQ, Craigie R. Modeling the HIV-1 Intasome: A Prototype View of the Target of Integrase Inhibitors. Viruses-Basel 2010 Dec;2(12):2777-81.

[53] Karplus M, Kuriyan J. Molecular dynamics and protein function. Proc Natl Acad Sci U S A 2005 May 10;102(19):6679-85.

[54] Karplus M, Gao YQ, Ma J, van d, V, Yang W. Protein structural transitions and their functional role. Philos Transact A Math Phys Eng Sci 2005 Feb 15;363(1827):331-55.

[55] Gerstein M, Lesk AM, Chothia C. Structural mechanisms for domain movements in proteins. Biochemistry 1994 Jun 7;33(22):6739-49.

[56] Schlitter J, Engels M, Kruger P. Targeted molecular dynamics: a new approach for searching pathways of conformational transitions. J Mol Graph 1994 Jun;12(2):84-9.

[57] Bagley RJ, Farmer JD, Kauffman SA, Packard NH, Perelson AS, Stadnyk IM. Modeling adaptive biological systems. Biosystems 1989;23(2-3):113-37.

[58] Cotelle P. Patented HIV-1 integrase inhibitors (1998-2005). Recent Pat Antiinfect Drug Discov 2006 Jan;1(1):1-15.

[59] Pommier Y, Johnson AA, Marchand C. Integrase inhibitors to treat HIV/AIDS. Nature Reviews Drug Discovery 2005 Mar;4(3):236-48.

[60] Semenova EA, Marchand C, Pommier Y. HIV-1 integrase inhibitors: Update and Perspectives. Adv Pharmacol 2008;56:199-228.

[61] Marchand C, Maddali K, Metifiot M, Pommier Y. HIV-1 IN Inhibitors: 2010 Update and Perspectives. Current Topics in Medicinal Chemistry 2009 Aug;9(11):1016-37.

[62] Hazuda DJ, Felock P, Witmer M, Wolfe A, Stillmock K, Grobler JA, et al. Inhibitors of strand transfer that prevent integration and inhibit HIV-1 replication in cells. Science 2000 Jan 28;287(5453):646-50.

[63] Markowitz M, Morales-Ramirez JO, Nguyen BY, Kovacs CM, Steigbigel RT, Cooper DA, et al. Antiretroviral activity, pharmacokinetics, and tolerability of MK-0518, a novel inhibitor of HIV-1 integrase, dosed as monotherapy for 10 days in treatment-naive HIV-1-infected individuals. J Acquir Immune DeficSyndr. 2006 Dec 15;43(5): 509-15.

[64] Grobler JA, Stillmock K, Hu B, Witmer M, Felock P, Espeseth AS, et al. Diketo acid inhibitor mechanism and HIV-1 integrase: implications for metal binding in the active site of phosphotransferase enzymes.ProcNatlAcadSci USA. 2002 May 14;99(10): 6661-6.

[65] Garvey EP, Schwartz B, Gartland MJ, Lang S, Halsey W, Sathe G, et al. Potent inhibitors of HIV-1 integrase display a two-step, slow-binding inhibition mechanism which is absent in a drug-resistant T66I/M154I mutant.Biochemistry. 2009 Feb 24;48(7):1644-53.

[66] Copeland RA, Pompliano DL, Meek TD. Drug-target residence time and its implications for lead optimization.Nat Rev Drug Discov. 2006 Sep;5(9):730-9.

[67] Dicker IB, Terry B, Lin Z, Li Z, Bollini S, Samanta HK, et al. Biochemical analysis of HIV-1 integrase variants resistant to strand transfer inhibitors. J Biol Chem. 2008 Aug 29;283(35):23599-609.

[68] Hightower KE, Wang R, Deanda F, Johns BA, Weaver K, Shen Y, et al. Dolutegravir (S/GSK1349572) exhibits significantly slower dissociation than raltegravir and elvitegravir from wild-type and integrase inhibitor-resistant HIV-1 integrase-DNA complexes.Antimicrob Agents Chemother. 2011 Oct;55(10):4552-9.

[69] Cooper DA, Steigbigel RT, Gatell JM, Rockstroh JK, Katlama C, Yeni P, et al. Subgroup and resistance analyses of raltegravir for resistant HIV-1 infection. New England Journal of Medicine 2008 Jul 24;359(4):355-65.

[70] Steigbigel RT, Cooper DA, Kumar PN, Eron JE, Schechter M, Markowitz M, et al. Raltegravir with optimized background therapy for resistant HIV-1 infection. New England Journal of Medicine 2008 Jul 24;359(4):339-54.

[71] Sichtig N, Sierra S, Kaiser R, Daumer M, Reuter S, Schulter E, et al. Evolution of raltegravir resistance during therapy. Journal of Antimicrobial Chemotherapy 2009 Jul; 64(1):25-32.

[72] Grobler JA, Stillmock KA, Miller MD, Hazuda DJ. Mechanism by which the HIV integrase active-site mutation N155H confers resistance to raltegravir. Antiviral Therapy 2008;13(4):A41.

[73] Delelis O, Malet I, Na L, Tchertanov L, Calvez V, Marcelin AG, et al. The G140S mutation in HIV integrases from raltegravir-resistant patients rescues catalytic defect due to the resistance Q148H mutation. Nucleic Acids Research 2009 Mar;37(4):1193-201.

[74] Perryman AL, Forli S, Morris GM, Burt C, Cheng YH, Palmer MJ, et al. A Dynamic Model of HIV Integrase Inhibition and Drug Resistance. Journal of Molecular Biology 2010 Mar 26;397(2):600-15.

[75] Delelis O, Thierry S, Subra F, Simon F, Malet I, Alloui C, et al. Impact of Y143 HIV-1 Integrase Mutations on Resistance to Raltegravir In Vitro and In Vivo. Antimicrobial Agents and Chemotherapy 2010 Jan;54(1):491-501.

[76] Kawasuji T, Fuji M, Yoshinaga T, Sato A, Fujiwara T, Kiyama R. A platform for designing HIV integrase inhibitors. Part 2: A two-metal binding model as a potential mechanism of HIV integrase inhibitors. Bioorganic & Medicinal Chemistry 2006 Dec 15;14(24):8420-9.

[77] Allen FH. The Cambridge Structural Database: a quarter of a million crystal structures and rising. Acta Crystallogr B 2002 Jun;58(Pt 3 Pt 1):380-8.

[78] Tchertanov L, Mouscadet JF. Target recognition by catechols and beta-ketoenols: Potential contribution of hydrogen bonding and Mn/Mg chelation to HIV-1 integrase inhibition. Journal of Medicinal Chemistry 2007 Mar 22;50(6):1133-45.

[79] Arora R, Chauvot de Beauchêne I, Abdel-Azeim S, Polanski J, Laine E, Tchertanov L. Raltegravir flexibility and its impact on recognition by the HIV-1 Integrase targets. Journal of Molecular Recognition 2012. Submitted

[80] Arora R, Tchertanov L. Structural determinants of Raltegravir specific recognition by the HIV-1 Integrase. 2012. Les actes: 57-60. http://jobim2012.inria.fr/jobim_actes_2012_online.pdf

[81] Schiavoni MM, Mack HG, Ulic SE, Della Vedova CO. Tautomers and conformers of malonamide, NH2-C(O)-CH2-C(O)-NH2: vibrational analysis, NMR spectra and ab initio calculations. Spectrochim Acta A Mol Biomol Spectrosc 2000 Jul;56A(8):1533-41.

[82] Barreca ML, Iraci N, De Luca L, Chimirri A. Induced-Fit Docking Approach Provides Insight into the Binding Mode and Mechanism of Action of HIV-1 Integrase Inhibitors. Chemmedchem 2009 Sep;4(9):1446-56.

[83] Loizidou EZ, Zeinalipour-Yazdi CD, Christofides T, Kostrikis LG. Analysis of binding parameters of HIV-1 integrase inhibitors: Correlates of drug inhibition and resistance. Bioorganic & Medicinal Chemistry 2009 Jul 1;17(13):4806-18.

[84] Serrao E, Odde S, Ramkumar K, Neamati N. Raltegravir, elvitegravir, and metoogravir: the birth of "me-too" HIV-1 integrase inhibitors. Retrovirology 2009;6:25.

[85] Espeseth AS, Felock P, Wolfe A, Witmer M, Grobler, J, Anthony N., et al.HIV-1 integrase inhibitors that compete with the target DNA substrate define a unique strand transfer conformation for integrase. Proc. Natl. Acad. Sci. U.S.A 2000; 97:11244–49.

[86] Pandey KK., Bera S., Zahm J., Vora A, Stillmock K., Hazuda D, et al. Inhibition of human immunodeficiency virus type 1 concerted integration by strand transfer inhibitors which recognize a transient structural intermediate. J. Virol. 2007; 81: 12189–99.

[87] Sherman PA, Dickson ML. and Fyfe JA. Human immunodeficiency virus type 1 integration protein: DNA sequence requirements for cleaving and joining reactions. J. Virol. 1992; 66: 3593–601.

[88] Johnson AA, Santos W, Pais GCG, Marchand C, Amin, R., Burker, T. R., Jr., Verdine, G., and Pommier, Y. Integration requires a specific interaction of the donor DNA terminal 5′-cytosine with glutamine 148 of the HIV-1 integrase flexible loop. J. Biol. Chem. 2006; 281,:461–7.

[89] Johnson AA, Marchand C, Patil SS, Costi R, DiSanto R, Burke, R. R. Jr. et al. Probing HIV-1 integrase inhibitor binding sites with position-specific integrase-DNA cross-linking assays. Mol. Pharmacol. 2007; 71: 893–901.

[90] Dicker IB, Samanta HK, Li A, Hong Y, Tian Y, Banville J et al. Changes to the HIV long terminal repeat and to HIV integrase differentially impact HIV integrase assembly, activity, and the binding of strand transfer inhibitors. J. Biol. Chem. 2008; 282: 31186–96.

[91] Langley D, Samanta HK, Lin Z, Walker MA, Krystal M, and Dicker IB. The Terminal (Catalytic) Adenosine of the HIV LTR Controls the Kinetics of Binding and Dissociation of HIV Integrase Strand Transfer Inhibitors. Biochemistry 2008; 47: 13481–8.

[92] Ammar FF, Abdel-Azeim S, Zargarian L, Hobaika Z, Maroun RG, Fermandjian S Unprocessed Viral DNA Could Be the Primary Target of the HIV-1 Integrase Inhibitor Raltegravir. PLoS One.oS One. 2012;7(7):e40223.

[93] Korolev S, Agapkina Yu, Gottikh M. Clinical Use of Inhibitors of HIV-1 Integration: Problems and Prospects. Acta Naturae 2011;3;3:12-28.

[94] Pannecouque C, Pluymers W, Van Maele B, Tetz V, Cherepanov P, De Clercq E, et al. New class of HIV integrase inhibitors that block viral replication in cell culture. Curr Biol. 2002 Jul 23;12(14):1169-77.

[95] Mazumder A, Wang S, Neamati N, Nicklaus M, Sunder S, Chen J, et al. Antiretroviral agents as inhibitors of both human immunodeficiency virus type 1 integrase and protease.J Med Chem. 1996 Jun 21;39(13):2472-81.

[96] Tsiang M, Jones GS, Hung M, Samuel D, Novikov N, Mukund S, et al. Dithiothreitol causes HIV-1 integrase dimer dissociation while agents interacting with the integrase dimer interface promote dimer formation. Biochemistry. 2011 Mar 15;50(10):1567-81.

[97] De Luca L, Ferro S, Gitto R, Barreca ML, Agnello S, Christ F, et al. Small molecules targeting the interaction between HIV-1 integrase and LEDGF/p75 cofactor. Bioorg Med Chem. 2010 Nov 1;18(21):7515-21.

[98] Tsiang M, Jones GS, Niedziela-Majka A, Kan E, Lansdon EB, Huang W, Hung M, et al. New Class of HIV-1 Integrase (IN) Inhibitors with a Dual Mode of Action.Biol Chem. 2012 Jun 15;287(25):21189-203.

Chapter 16

Similarities Between the Binding Sites of Monoamine Oxidase (MAO) from Different Species — Is Zebrafish a Useful Model for the Discovery of Novel MAO Inhibitors?

Angelica Fierro, Alejandro Montecinos,
Cristobal Gómez-Molina, Gabriel Núñez,
Milagros Aldeco, Dale E. Edmondson,
Marcelo Vilches-Herrera, Susan Lühr,
Patricio Iturriaga-Vásquez and Miguel Reyes-Parada

Additional information is available at the end of the chapter

http://dx.doi.org/10.5772/35874

1. Introduction

Zebrafish (*Danio rerio*) is an animal model that is attracting increasing interest in pharmacology and toxicology. The relatively ease with which large numbers of individuals can be obtained and their inexpensive maintenance makes zebrafish a particularly suitable tool for drug discovery. Thus, in recent years diverse compounds have been assayed both in larval and adult specimens and changes of behavioral patterns, for instance, have been related to anxiolytic, addictive or cognitive effects. In this context, the molecular characterization of drug targets in zebrafish, comparing them to their mammalian counterparts, arises as a subject of paramount importance.

Monoamine oxidase (MAO) is the main catabolic enzyme of monoamine neurotransmitters and the primary target of several clinically relevant antidepressant and antiparkinsonian drugs. In mammals, it exists in two isoforms termed MAO-A and MAO-B, which share a number of structural and mechanistic features, but differ in genetic origin, tissue localization and inhibitor selectivity. High-resolution structures of MAOs from rat and human have been reported during the last decade, allowing detailed comparison of their overall structures and respective active sites. On the other hand, a few studies have shown that zebrafish contains a single MAO gene and that enzyme activity is due to a single form (zMAO) which resembles, but is distinct from, both mammalian MAO-A and MAO-B. No three-dimensional structural data exist thus far for zMAO. Sequence comparison of the putative substrate binding site of zMAO with those of human MAO isoforms suggests that the fish enzyme resembles mammalian MAO-A more than MAO-B. Nevertheless, biochemical studies have shown that zMAO exhibits such unique behavior toward MAO-A and -B substrates and inhibitors, that the results of studies using zebrafish MAO function, either as a disease model or for drug screening, should be considered with caution.

Functional and evolutionary relationships between proteins can be reliably inferred by comparison of their sequences, structures or binding sites. From a drug-discovery perspective, the study of binding site similarities (and differences) can be particularly insightful since it aids the design of selective or non-selective ligands and the detection of off-targets. In addition, knowledge of ligand-binding site similarity could increase our understanding of divergent and convergent evolution and the origin of proteins, even in those cases where no obvious sequence or structural similarity exists. In recent years, a number of algorithms have been developed for the identification and comparison of ligand-binding sites. Even though each method has its own merits and limitations, the performance of these computational tools is continuously improving. Advances in this field, associated with the increasing availability of structural data and reliable homology models of thousands to millions of protein molecules, provide an unprecedented framework to investigate the mechanisms underlying the molecular interactions between these proteins and their ligands, as well as to evaluate the similarities between the binding sites of related and unrelated proteins

On the basis of the foregoing, the first section of this chapter provides an overview on: a) the relevance of zebrafish as an animal model of increasing interest in pharmacology; b) the impact that MAO crystal structures and molecular simulation approaches have had on the development of novel MAO inhibitors, as well as comparative structural and functional information about zMAO and its mammalian counterparts; c) recent developments in computational methods to evaluate similarities between ligand-binding sites, emphasizing their usefulness for the rational design of multitarget (promiscuous) drugs.

The second part of the chapter describes unpublished results regarding a further characterization of zMAO activity and its comparison with MAOs from mammals. Specific topics in this section include: a) the construction of homology models of zMAO, built using human MAO-A and -B crystal structures as templates; b) a three-dimensional analysis of the binding site similarities between MAOs from different species using a statistical algorithm; c) a functional evaluation of zMAO activity in the presence of a small series of reversible and selective MAO-A and -B inhibitors.

http://dx.doi.org/10.5772/35874

2. Zebrafish as a model in pharmacology, monoamine oxidase and computational methods to evaluate binding site similarities: An overview

2.1. Zebrafish as an animal model in pharmacology and neurobehavioral studies

In order to understand complex behaviors observed in nature, scientists have always tried to develop models that could be used and tested under controlled conditions in the laboratory. In the last 30 years a new animal model, zebrafish (*Danio rerio*), has emerged as a powerful tool mostly for studying developmental biology. The scientific potential of zebrafish was originally assessed by George Streisinger (Streisinger et al., 1981). This work was the starting point for rapid progress in molecular and genetic analysis of zebrafish neurodevelopment, which allowed the construction of many genetic mutants and the identification of several genes that affect different brain functions such as learning and memory (Norton & Bally-Cuif, 2010). During the last decade zebrafish has also become an attractive model for behavioral and drug discovery studies, particularly those related to actions in the central nervous systems (Chakraborty & Hsu, 2009; King, 2009; Rubinstein, 2006; Zon & Peterson, 2005).

Zebrafish develop rapidly and almost all organs are developed at 7 days post-fertilization. Their fecundity makes it easy to obtain large numbers of individuals for experimentation, which are relatively inexpensive to maintain. In addition, they can absorb chemical substances from their tank water, and their genome has been almost fully sequenced, which makes genetic manipulation more accessible. These characteristics have stimulated the use of zebrafish in medicinal chemistry to assay the effects of different compounds in whole animals (Goldsmith, 2004; Kaufman & White, 2009). Another attractive characteristic of zebrafish is its potential for use in *in vivo* high-throughput screening assays. Consequently, a number of studies which take advantage of this possibility have been reported recently (Kokel et al., 2010; Kokel & Peterson, 2011; Rihel et al., 2010; Zon & Peterson, 2005).

Zebrafish exhibit many social characteristics that can be assimilated to those observed in mammals. They recognize each other by sight and odor (Tebbich et al., 2002) and display an interesting social learning (Reader et al., 2003). This teleost also shows a characteristic aggressive behavior (Payne, 1998), a pheromone-mediated danger alarm (Suboski, 1988; Suboski et al., 1990), cognitive and adaptive behaviors such as habituation (Miklosi et al., 1997; Miklosi & Andrew 1999), spatial navigation abilities and Pavlovian conditioning (Hollis, 1999). These features make this species a valuable tool for either the development or the adaptation of behavioral paradigms. Thus, behavioral protocols such as an aquatic version of the T-maze, which is used for studies of discrimination, reinforcement and memory in rodents, had been used to assess color discrimination in zebrafish (Colwill et al., 2005). Another interesting model is the aquatic version of conditioned place preference (CPP), where the fish can be exposed to different stimuli in two separate compartments and is then allowed to freely explore the apparatus without partition (Darland & Dowling, 2001). A further paradigm, the novel tank diving test, has been used by different research groups (Bencan & Levin 2008; Bencan et al., 2009; Egan et al., 2009; Levin et al., 2007) as a model for anxiety. It is conceptually similar to the rodent open field test, because it takes advantage of the instinctive behavior of both zebrafish and rats to seek refuge when exposed to an unfamiliar environment (Levin et al., 2007). In the case of the novel tank diving test, the fish dives to the bottom of the tank and remains there until it presumably feels safe enough to explore the rest of the tank and gradually starts to explore the upper zone (Egan et al., 2009). Similar observations can be made in an open field test for rodents, where initially they spend a lot of time near the walls, which is considered as an indication of an anxious state. The time spent by the zebrafish in the lower or upper part of the tank, as well as erratic movements, have been established as anxiety indices (Egan et al., 2009). It is considered that the zebrafish is anxious when it shows a longer latency to enter the upper part of the tank, or when the time spent at the top is reduced. Conversely, when an anxiolytic drug is administered, animals spend much more time in the upper portion of the tank. Figure 1 illustrates this response by showing the typical traces of motor activity observed for control animals (left) and for animals exposed to nicotine (right), which has been reported to have anxiolytic properties in this paradigm (Levin et al., 2007).

Based on these findings, the potential of zebrafish for neurobehavioral studies is increasingly recognized (Bencan & Levin, 2008; Eddins et al., 2010). Thus, this animal has been used as a model in studies of memory (Levin & Chen, 2006), anxiety (Bencan et al., 2009; Levin et al., 2007), reinforcement properties of drugs of abuse (Ninkovic & Bally-Cuif, 2006), neuroprotection of dopaminergic neurons (McKinley et al., 2005), and movement disorders (Flinn et al., 2008).

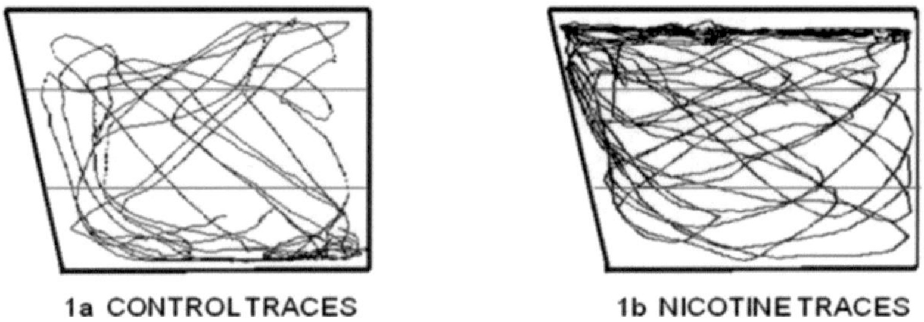

Figure 1. Representative traces of characteristic behavior of control-saline- (left) and nicotine- (right) treated zebra fish. Traces were recorded during 5 min in a glass trapezoidal test tank (22.9 cm long at the bottom, 27.9 cm long at the top, 15.2 cm high, 6.4 cm wide), filled with 1.5 L of artificial sea water. Nicotine was administered 5 min before the test. All other experimental conditions were as previously published (Levin et al., 2007).

A final word of caution should be said regarding the apparent usefulness of zebrafish as a research tool. One critical aspect to be considered when using animal models to understand a specific behavior is its validity. Mammals such as rats and mice have been widely used as models to study several functions since, among other characteristics, many brain regions and their neurotransmitter systems are well characterized. Thus, even though genome and the genetic pathways controlling signal transduction and development appear to be highly conserved between zebrafish and humans (Postlethwait et al., 2000), further validation of this model is needed, particularly if human systems or conditions are the final aims to be addressed.

2.1.1. Monoamine oxidase: general characteristics and the impact of crystal structures on the understanding of enzyme function and inhibition

Monoamine oxidase (monoamine oxygen oxidoreductase (deaminating) (flavin-containing); EC 1.4.3.4; MAO) is a key enzyme in the inactivation of neurotransmitters such as serotonin, dopamine and noradrenaline. In mammals it exists in two isoforms termed MAO-A and MAO-B which have molecular weights of ~60 kDa. Both proteins are outer mitochondrial membrane-bound flavoproteins, with the FAD cofactor covalently bound to the enzyme. MAO-A and MAO-B are encoded by separate genes (Kochersperger et al., 1986; Lan et al., 1989) and the isoforms from the same species show about 70% sequence identity, whereas 85-88% identity is observed between the same isoforms from human and rat (Nagatsu, 2004). Both neurological and psychiatric diseases have been related to MAO dysfunction. Consequently, the search for inhibitors of each isoform has lasted decades. Currently, selective inhibitors of MAO-A are used clinically as antidepressants and anxiolytics, while MAO-B inhibitors are used to reduce the progression of Parkinson's disease and of symptoms associated with Alzheimer's disease (Youdim et al., 2006).

In 2002, Binda and colleagues (Binda et al., 2002) published a groundbreaking article showing the high-resolution structure of human MAO-B in complex with the irreversible inhibitor pargyline. Subsequent structures of this enzyme (Binda et al., 2003, 2004), as well as that of rat MAO-A (Ma et al., 2004), and more recently human MAO-A (De Colibus et al., 2005; Son et al., 2008), have allowed a detailed comparison of the overall structures of both isoforms, and new insights regarding their active sites (Edmondson et al., 2007, 2009; Reyes-Parada et al., 2005). Based on these findings, the substrate/inhibitor binding site of both isozymes can be described as a pocket lined by the isoalloxazine ring of the flavin cofactor and several aliphatic and aromatic residues (in the second part, close ups of this binding site are depicted in Figures 5 and 8). In particular, two conserved tyrosine residues (Y407, Y444 and Y398, Y435 in MAO-A and -B, respectively), whose aromatic rings face each other, are located almost perpendicularly to the isoalloxazine ring defining an "aromatic cage". This conformational arrangement provides a path to guide the substrate amine towards the reactive positions on the flavin ring and therefore seems to be essential for catalytic activity. In addition, a critical role of residues G215 and I180 of MAO-A (G206 and L171 being the corresponding residues in MAO-B) in the orientation and stabilization of the substrate/inhibitor binding can be inferred from the X-ray diffraction data. In MAO-B, the substrate/inhibitor binding site is a cavity (~400 $Å^3$, termed the "substrate cavity") which can be distinguished, in some cases, from another hydrophobic pocket (~300 $Å^3$, termed the "entrance cavity") located closer to the protein surface. It has been demonstrated that the I199 side-chain can act as a "gate" opening or closing the connection between the two cavities by modifying its conformation (Binda et al., 2003). In contrast, the MAO-A binding site consists of a single cavity (De Colibus et al., 2005; Ma et al., 2004). It should be noted that, although residues lining the binding site of human and rat MAO-A are identical, the human MAO-A cavity is larger

(~550 Å^3) than that in rat MAO-A (~450 Å^3). Remarkably, an exchanged location of aromatic and aliphatic nonconserved residues in the active sites of MAO-A and MAO-B (F208/I199 and I335/Y326, respectively) has been implicated in the affinity and selective recognition of substrates and inhibitors, and provides a molecular basis for the development of specific reversible inhibitors of each isoform (Edmondson et al., 2009).

The availability of the aforementioned crystal structures has made an enormous impact on our knowledge about the function and regulation of the enzyme and has also allowed a quicker pace in the rational design of novel MAO inhibitors. Different theoretical approaches and computational methods have been used since, to explore **how**, **where** and **why** some interactions are central in MAO-ligand complexes. For instance, quantum mechanics calculations have been used to obtain insights about the mechanism by which amines are oxidized by MAO (Erdem & Büyükmenekşe, 2011), whereas molecular dynamics simulations have been recently employed to study specific interactions involved in the access of reversible MAO inhibitors to their binding site (Allen & Bevan 2011). In addition, a number of studies describing potent and selective inhibitors have been reported during the last decade and in most of them molecular simulation approaches have been used to rationalize and/or to predict the functional interactions between the proteins and their inhibitors. Figure 2 illustrates this situation by showing the progression of published articles about MAO in which computational methodologies were used.

It should be pointed out however, that crystal structures only provide a snapshot of one of the many conformations available to proteins. Therefore theoretical (and experimental) approaches, adequately considering dynamic aspects, will grow in importance in order to better understand the physiological functioning of these enzymes.

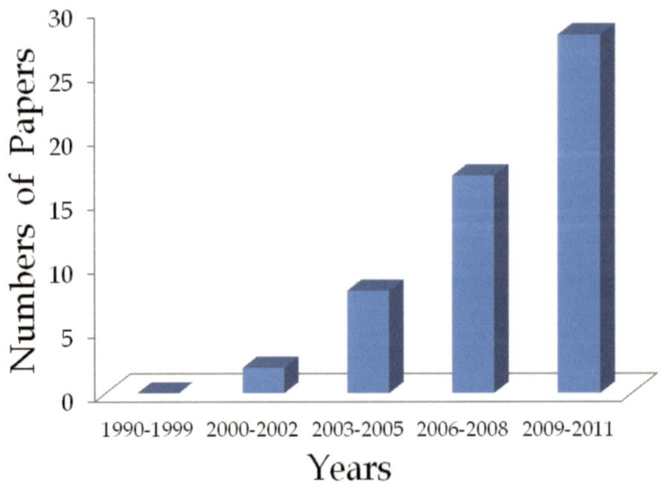

Figure 2. Progression of research articles involving docking studies on MAO before and after (2002) the first three-dimensional structure of MAO was deposited in the Protein Data Bank. Data from PubMed. "MAO" and "docking" were used as keywords.

2.1.2. Comparative functional and structural information about zebrafish MAO and its mammalian counterparts

Unlike mammals, zebrafish have only one MAO gene (Anichtchik et al., 2006; Setini et al., 2005). This gene is located in chromosome 9 and exhibits an identical intron-exon organization as compared to mammals, which suggests a common ancestral gene (Anichtchik et al., 2006; Panula et al., 2010). Sequencing studies have shown that zebrafish MAO (zMAO) contains 522 amino acids and has a molecular weight of about 59 kDa (Setini et al., 2005), which is very similar to that found in mammalian MAO-A and MAO-B. zMAO displays about 70% identity with human MAO-A or -B, and its predicted secondary structure indicates that the flavin-binding-, the substrate- and the membrane-binding- domains, which are typical in other MAOs, should also be present in the fish enzyme. Indeed, a recent study (Arslan & Edmondson, 2010) has demonstrated that (like the mammalian isoforms), zMAO is also a mitochondrial enzyme, presumably bound to the outer membrane, and that the flavin cofactor is covalently bound to the protein via an 8α-thioether linkage likely established with C406. Beyond its overall identity, the amino acid sequence of the presumed zMAO binding domain shows ~67% and ~83% identity with the corresponding binding sites of human MAO-B and MAO-A respectively (Panula et al., 2010). Interestingly, some residues that have been shown to be critical for inhibitor and substrate selectivity in human MAOs such as the pairs F208/I335 (in MAO-A) and I199/Y326 (in MAO-B), are identical or conservatively replaced in zMAO (F200/L327) as compared with MAO-A.

Regarding functional studies, recent data obtained using *para*-substituted benzylamine analogs as substrates suggest that, as in mammalian MAOs, α-C-H bond cleavage is the rate-limiting step in zMAO catalysis (Aldeco et al., 2011). Furthermore, a variety of substrates and inhibitors have been tested against zMAO. Preferential substrates of both MAO-A (e.g. serotonin) and MAO-B (e.g. phenethylamine, benzylamine, MPTP) as well as non-selective substrates such as tyramine, dopamine or kynuramine, have been shown to be deaminated, although with different catalytic efficiency, by zMAO (Aldeco et al., 2011; Anichtchik et al., 2006; Arslan & Edmondson, 2010; Sallinen et al., 2009; Setini et al., 2005). In addition, irreversible selective inhibitors such as clorgyline (MAO-A) or deprenyl (MAO-B) exhibit similar inhibitory profiles toward zMAO (Anichtchik et al., 2006; Arslan & Edmondson, 2010; Setini et al., 2005). Interestingly, the *in vivo* administration of deprenyl to zebrafish increases serotonin levels about 10-fold while levels of dopamine remain unchanged (Sallinen et al., 2009). These data indicate that zMAO is essential for serotonin metabolism in zebrafish, but also underline the distinctive character of this enzyme since in rodents dopamine concentrations are increased after deprenyl treatment, whereas serotonin levels remain unchanged. Structurally diverse reversible MAO inhibitors such as harmane, tetrindole, methylene blue, amphetamine, 8-(3-chlorostyryl)-caffeine, 1,4-diphenyl-1,3-butadiene, farnesol, safinamide or zonisamide display a wide range of inhibitory potencies, from nM to μM to no effect, against zMAO (Aldeco et al., 2011; Binda et al., 2011). Remarkably, methylene blue is the most potent zMAO inhibitor tested thus far, exhibiting a K_i value of 4 nM.

Based on sequence similarity, substrate preference and inhibitor sensitivity, it has been consistently suggested that the functional properties of zMAO resemble more strongly those of

MAO-A than those of MAO-B. Nevertheless, virtually all articles published so far recognize that, although some overlapping properties can be detected, zMAO also shows characteristics of its own that distinguish it from its mammalian counterparts.

2.2. Recent developments in computational methods to evaluate similarities between ligand-binding sites

The concept of protein binding-site similarity and the development of methods to evaluate it are receiving much attention. This is viewed as a step forward in protein classification, as compared with classical sequence-based approaches, since it should allow proteins with low sequence similarity but high similarity at their binding sites to be related (Milletti & Vulpetti, 2010). On the contrary, as will be analyzed below, this approach can also detect subtle differences between highly homologous proteins, and therefore be useful to determine the suitability of non-human proteins as models for drug design aimed to the treatment of human conditions.

One of the newest applications of the study of binding site similarities is polypharmacology. Thus, the classical idea that selective drugs acting on a single target related to one disease will have maximal efficacy has been challenged by increasing evidence showing that most clinically effective drugs bind to several targets, even if these targets are not originally related to the disease (Keiser et al., 2009; Schrattenholz & Soskić 2008). Even though this pharmacological promiscuity may be seen as a negative property, primarily related with the incidence of side effects, recent observations increasingly indicate that multitarget compounds might have better profiles regarding both efficacy and side effects, since they would be acting on a pharmacological network, where several nodes underlie the physiopathology of the disease (Apsel et al., 2008; Hopkins 2008). Thus, the concept of polypharmacology has motivated several groups to find new drug-target associations, based on the idea that a given compound can interact simultaneously with two or more relevant targets if they have similar binding sites. It should be stressed that these associations are pursued considering that two proteins could share a ligand even if they are structurally or functionally very different (Kahraman et al., 2007).

One aspect that has critically fueled this field is the increasing availability of 3D protein structures in public databases (almost 75.000), which allows us to explore the complexity of protein-ligand interactions. This exploration has yielded important insights in order to obtain a good characterization of the binding sites and has confirmed the notion that protein-ligand binding depends not only on shape complementarity but also on complementary physicochemical features (Henrich et al., 2010).

Several algorithms have been developed to compare binding sites of different proteins. In most of them, two main steps are present: the creation of a database that requires the calculation of fingerprints describing each binding site and a pocket screening that requires multiple similarity alignments between the query pocket and the database. These applications are used as a strategy to assess specific issues, such as off-target identification for drug repurposing (Cleves & Jain, 2006; Keiser et al., 2009; Moriaud et al., 2011), functional classification of unknown proteins (Kinnings & Jackson, 2009; Russell et al., 1998), drug discovery by sequence analysis (Xie et al., 2009), detection of evolutionary relationships (Xie & Bourne, 2008) and polypharmacology predictions (Milleti & Vulpetti, 2010; Pérez-Nueno & Ritchie, 2011). The main step before finding similarity between two or more binding sites is their characterization. Several methodologies have been proposed with this purpose: geometrics approaches, which mainly analyze cavities through the exploration of the solvent-accessible protein surface (Weisel et al., 2007); energetics approaches, which use van der Waals and electrostatic energies to define cavities (Laurie & Jackson, 2005); structure and sequence comparison approaches, which use the information of known binding sites to compare and define unknown cavities through the analysis of sequence and structural similarity (Brylinski & Skolnick, 2009); and approaches involving the dynamics of protein structures, which use dynamics simulations to include the natural flexibility of proteins and possible allosteric modifications of binding sites (Landon et al., 2008). Although the determination of similarities between binding sites could seem a simple mathematical method, several approaches have been developed using different characteristics. For example, the Isocleft algorithm measures the similarity by initially defining a cleft in any protein to be compared. These clefts are determined by a set of overlapping spheres that are represented by the van der Waals radii of atoms in the binding sites. Finally each cleft is viewed like a graph and the similarity is measured by finding the largest common subgraph (Najmanovich et al., 2008). The SitesBase algorithm uses a triangular geometric determination of binding sites establishing the cutoff at 5 Å. Similarity is measured by an atom–atom score which finds the largest possible matching constellation (similar atom types with a similar spatial orientation) (Gold & Jackson, 2006). The ProFunc server uses sequence and structural information to find similarities between binding sites. This process includes a phylogenetic component that is used for the identification of homologous proteins (Laskowski et al., 2005). The Sumo algorithm flags each functional group as a node in a graph. Then the similarity is measured through a strategy that does not necessarily find the maximal common subgraph between a pair of binding sites (Jambon et al., 2003). The FLAP algorithm utilizes GRID methodology to calculate the energy of interaction between a molecular probe and the binding sites. These interactions, which include van der Waals and electrostatic terms, are then compared through a geometric approach (Baroni et al., 2007). In another recently developed algorithm (Hoffmann et al., 2010) the binding sites are represented as a set of atoms in the 3D space described by 3D vectors. Initially the algorithm calculates the similarity between two binding sites comparing vectors that only consider the atom coordinates, although different additional parameters such as atom type and charges could be included in the algorithm. The PocketMatch algorithm involves three basic steps: a) each binding site is represented as a sort list of distances between three selected points in every amino acid present at one specific distance from the ligand, b) the two sets of sorted distances are aligned and c) finally the similarity percentage is calculated (Yeturu & Chandra, 2008).

Although most algorithms used to measure the similarities between binding sites have shown high performance when the comparison involves related proteins, doubtful results are obtained when the proteins are not related. In these cases it is very important to select the best algorithm taking into account some critical issues: a ligand may change its orientation in different binding sites; some protein-ligand conformations may have a favorable binding energy, but natural allosteric regulations (not always considered) might not favor such conformations; protein structures from databases could have been determined in different conformational states (active, inactive, closed, open, etc.); finally, it is also very important to consider the solvent and ion concentrations in every system.

Beyond these considerations, the continuous increase in both the number of protein structures and computational power, augurs the development of ever more accurate similarity searching tools, which likely will allow not only better results in virtual screening programs but also a novel view on the evolution of structure and function of proteins.

3. MAO from different species: a biochemical evaluation and a theoretical analysis using molecular simulation and a biostatistical algorithm

As mentioned, even though amino acids lining the zMAO binding site exhibit a high level of identity with those of rat and human MAOs, a few studies have shown that the fish's enzyme shows unexpected sensitivities for known specific substrates and inhibitors. Since zebrafish has been proposed as a model that could be useful for the identification of novel MAO inhibitors (Kokel et al., 2010), we further characterized zMAO using three different approaches. First, we determined the inhibitory potency of a small series of compounds which have been previously evaluated against rat and human MAOs. Then, we built homology models of zMAO based on the crystal structures of human MAO-A or MAO-B and performed docking experiments with a drug selected from the biochemical evaluations. Finally, we used the recently described algorithm PocketMatch (Yeturu & Chandra, 2008) to explore similarities and differences between MAO isoforms from human, rat and zebrafish.

3.1. Biochemical evaluation

3.1.1. Methods

4-Methylthioamphetamine (MTA), 2-naphthylisopropylamine (NIPA), (6-methoxy-2-naphthy)lisopropylamine (MeONIPA), all as hydrochloride salts, 2-(4′-butoxyphenyl)thiomorpholine (BTI), 2-(4′-benzyloxyphenyl)thiomorpholine (ZTI), both as oxalate salts, as well as 2-(4′-butoxyphenyl)thiomorpholin-5-one (BTO) and 2-(4′-benzyloxyphenyl)thiomorpholin-5-one (ZTO) were synthesised following published methods (Hurtado-Guzmán et al., 2003; Lühr et al., 2010; Vilches-Herrera et al., 2009). The expression and purification of zMAO in *Pichia pastoris* was performed as previously described (Arslan & Edmondson, 2010). Enzyme kinetic studies were done spectrophotometrically in 50 mM potassium phosphate buffer (pH = 7.4), 0.5% (w/v) reduced Triton X-100 with kynuramine as substrate. The spectrophotometer used was a Perkin-Elmer Lambda-2 UV–Vis at 25 °C.

3.1.2. Results and discussion

Figure 3 shows the chemical structures of the inhibitors evaluated.

http://dx.doi.org/10.5772/35874

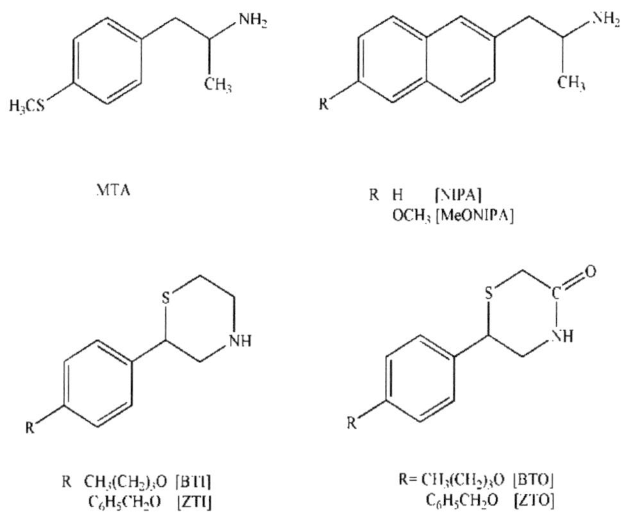

Figure 3. Chemical structures of the compounds used in the biochemical evaluation

Table 1 summarizes the effects of these compounds upon zMAO and also includes, for comparative purposes, the reported values of their inhibitory activities against MAO-A and -B from human and rat (Fierro et al., 2007; Hurtado-Guzmán et al., 2003; Lühr et al., 2010; Vilches-Herrera et al., 2009).

Compound	K_i (μM)				
	zMAO	hMAO-A	rMAO-A	hMAO-B	rMAO-B
MTA [a]	NE	0.13 ± 0.02	0.25 ± 0.02	NE	NE
NIPA [b]	17.7 ± 2.6	0.48 ± 0.31	0.42 ± 0.04	>100	>100
MeONIPA [b]	4.8 ± 0.4	0.24 ± 0.02	0.18 ± 0.05	5.1 ± 0.4	16.3 ± 7.8
BTO [c]	NE	10.0 ± 0.3	50.9 ± 6.1	0.46 ± 0.18	0.16 ± 0.01
ZTO [c]	NE	>100	27.5 ± 4.6	0.048 ± 0.03	0.074 ± 0.003
BTI [c]	30.4 ± 3.8	2.5 ± 0.2	14.1 ± 1.2	0.068 ± 0.05	0.27 ± 0.02
ZTI [c]	NE	>100	19.0 ± 0.4	0.038 ± 0.003	0.13 ±0.01

Table 1. zMAO inhibitory properties of known selective mammalian MAO inhibitors. Comparative data for human and rat MAO inhibition are from: [a]Hurtado-Guzmán et al., 2003; [b]Vilches-Herrera et al 2009; [c]Lühr et al, 2010. NE: No effect

The amphetamine derivative MTA, which is a potent and selective inhibitor of rat and human MAO-A (Fierro et al., 2007; Hurtado-Guzmán et al., 2003), showed no significant effect upon zMAO activity. Similarly, the 2-arylthiomorpholine analogue ZTI, and the 2-arylthiomorpholin-5-one derivatives BTO and ZTO, which are highly selective MAO-B inhibitors

(Lühr et al., 2010), did not inhibit the fish's enzyme. In contrast, naphthylisopropylamine derivatives NIPA and MeONIPA, which are selective inhibitors of MAO-A (Vilches-Herrera et al., 2009), as well as the 2-arylthiomorpholine derivative BTI which selectively inhibits MAO-B (Lühr et al., 2010), exhibited zMAO inhibitory properties with K_i values in the micromolar range. MeONIPA was the most potent compound of the series evaluated, showing a K_i value (4.8 μM) very similar to that found against human MAO-B (5.1 μM). These results agree with a notion that can be inferred from previous data (Aldeco et al., 2011; Anichtchik et al., 2006), indicating that effects on zMAO cannot be straightforwardly used to predict an effect upon either MAO-A or MAO-B. In addition, these data suggest that the zMAO binding site is significantly different from those of both MAO-A and MAO-B from mammals.

3.2. Homology models of zMAO and molecular docking

3.2.1. Modeling methods

Since neither the MAO-A nor MAO-B structure can be chosen *a priori* as a better template for modeling zMAO, we decided to build two different models using each isoform of human MAO as templates. The MAO-A (Protein Data Bank, PDB code: 2BXS) and MAO-B (PDB code: 2BYB) crystal structures at 3.15 Å and 2.2 Å resolution respectively (De Colibus et al., 2005) were employed. The amino acid sequence and crystal structure of each protein were extracted from the National Center for Biotechnology Information (NCBI) and PDB databases. Sequence alignments were prepared separately. Models were built using standard parameters and the outcomes were ranked on the basis of the internal scoring function of the program MODELLER9v6 (Sali & Blundell, 1993). The best model obtained in each case (using MAO-A or MAO-B as template) was submitted to the H++ server (Gordon et al., 2005; http://biophysics.cs.vt.edu/H++) to compute pK_a values of ionizable groups and to add missing hydrogen atoms according to the specified pH of the environment. Each structure selected was inserted into a POPC membrane, TIP3 solvated and ions were added creating an overall neutral system simulating approximately 0.2 M NaCl. The ions were equally distributed in a water box. The final system was subjected to a molecular dynamics (MD) simulation for 5 ns using NAMD 2.6 (Phillips et al., 2005). The NPT ensemble was used to perform MD calculations. Periodic boundary conditions were applied to the system in the three coordinate directions. A pressure of 1 atm was used and temperature was kept at 310 K. The simulation time was sufficient to obtain an equilibrated system (RMSD < 2 Å). Stereochemical and energy quality of the homology models were evaluated using the PROSAII server (Wiederstain & Sippl 2007) and Procheck (Laskowski et al., 1993)

3.2.2. Docking methods

Dockings of (*S*)-MeONIPA in the zMAO models, as well as in the human MAO-A and MAO-B structures were done using the AutoDock 4.0 suite (Morris et al., 1998). MeONIPA was selected for this study since it was the most potent zMAO inhibitor of the series evaluated and because it also inhibited both human MAO-A and MAO-B at low concentrations. The choice of the (*S*)-isomer for MeONIPA docking experiments was done on the basis that

(*S*)-amphetamine derivatives (which are always dextrorotatory) are usually the eutomers at MAO (Hurtado-Guzmán et al., 2003). All other docking conditions were as previously reported (Fierro et al., 2007; Vilches-Herrera et al., 2009). Briefly, the grid maps were calculated using the autogrid4 option and were centered on the putative ligand-binding site. The volumes chosen for the grid maps were made up of 40 × 40 × 40 points, with a grid-point spacing of 0.375 Å. The autotors option was used to define the rotating bond in the ligand. The docked compound complexes were built using the lowest docked-energy binding positions. MeONIPA was built using Gaussian03 (Frisch et al., 2004) and the partial charges were corrected using ESP methodology.

3.2.3. Results and discussion

Figure 4 depicts the global zMAO models obtained using human MAO-A (left) and human MAO-B (right) as templates. As expected, the overall structure of zMAO was similar to those of the human enzymes. The presumed ligand binding site appears lined by a series of hydrophobic residues and the isoalloxazine ring of the flavin cofactor (top inset Fig. 4). Amino acids forming the binding site of zMAO and human MAO-A and -B are shown in insets of Figure 4.

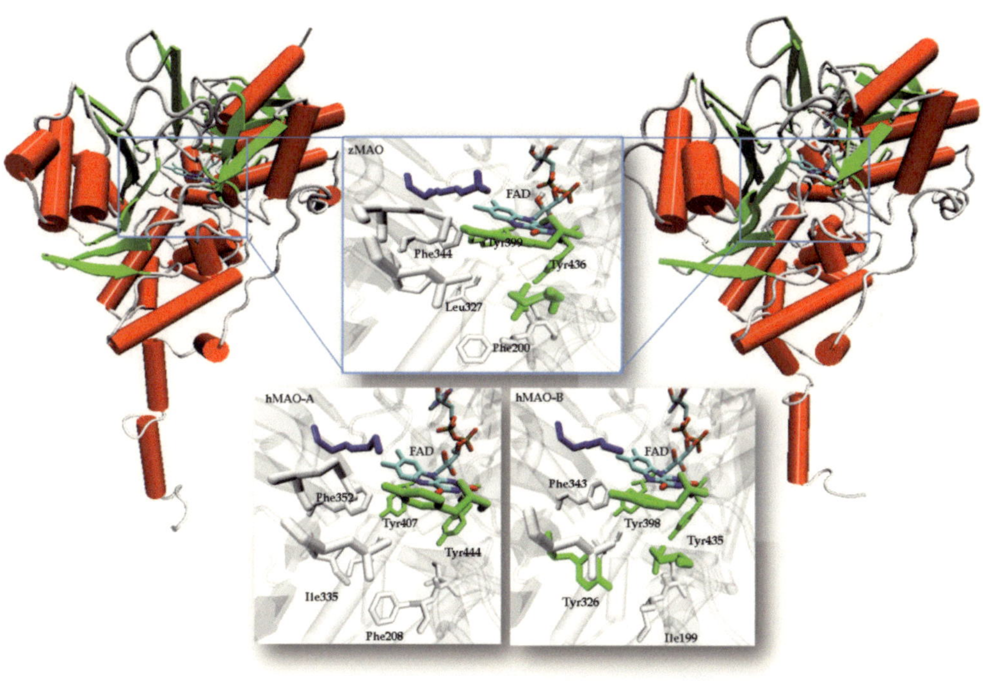

Figure 4. Cartoons of zMAO models obtained using human MAO-A (left) or human MAO-B (right). Insets show the main amino acids of the active sites of zMAO (top), human MAO-A (left) and human MAO-B (right). Amino acids in white, green or blue indicate apolar, polar or positively charged residues respectively.

As shown in Figure 5, docking experiments revealed that in both zMAO models, MeONIPA exhibits a binding mode where the aromatic ring is oriented almost perpendicularly to the isoalloxazine ring of FAD, with the methoxyl group pointing to the binding site entrance, whereas the aminopropyl chain points toward the isoalloxazine ring and appears positioned close to two tyrosine residues which, together with the isoalloxazine ring, form the so-called aromatic cage (Figs. 5 A and 5B). Interestingly, docking of MeONIPA in both human MAO-A and MAO-B, yielded binding modes where the inhibitor molecule adopted an almost opposite orientation to those observed in zMAO models. Thus, the most energetically favorable conformations of MeONIPA were those in which the amino group points away from the flavin ring, whereas the methoxyl group is located between the corresponding tyrosine residues (Figs. 5 C and 5D). These results suggest that the different inhibitory potencies of MeONIPA (and likely other inhibitors) toward zebrafish and human MAOs, might be attributed to the differential binding modes exhibited by the drug. Similar conclusions attempting to explain why MAO inhibitors show differential inhibition properties upon MAO from different species have been reached in previous studies (Fierro et al., 2007; Nandingama et al., 2002). Moreover, our findings suggest that, even in the cases where similar potencies are detected, the mechanism of enzyme inhibition for a given drug might be different in zebrafish and human MAOs.

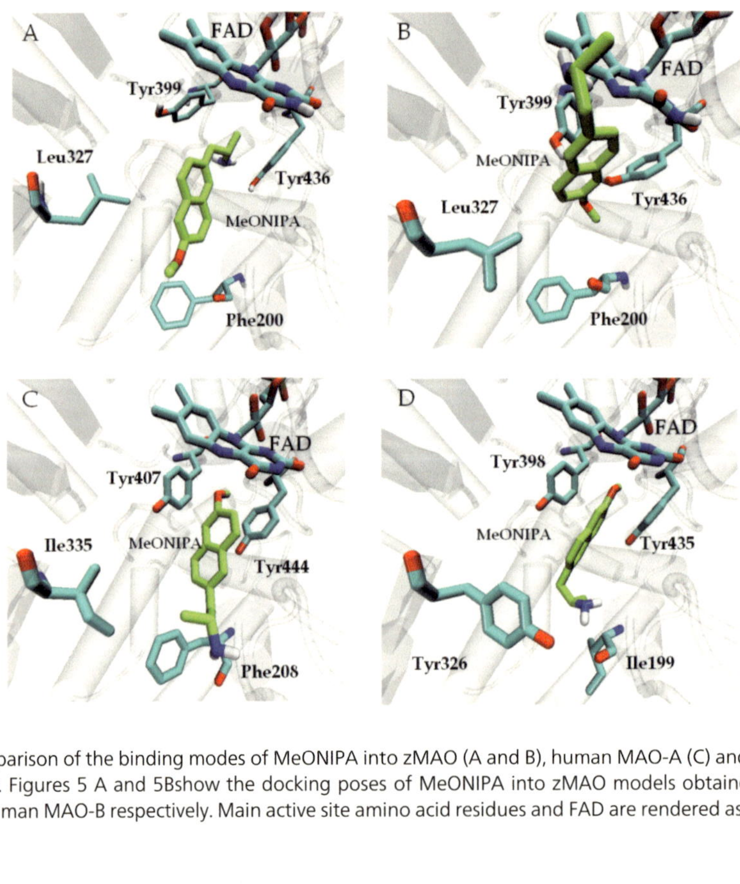

Figure 5. Comparison of the binding modes of MeONIPA into zMAO (A and B), human MAO-A (C) and human MAO-B (D) active sites. Figures 5 A and 5Bshow the docking poses of MeONIPA into zMAO models obtained using human MAO-A and human MAO-B respectively. Main active site amino acid residues and FAD are rendered as stick models.

3.3. Similarities between the binding sites of MAO from different species.

3.3.1. Protein structures employed

The structures of human and rat MAO-A co-crystallized with clorgyline (PDB codes: 2BXS and 1O5W respectively) and human MAO-B co-crystallized with *l*-deprenyl (PDB code: 2BYB) were employed. Furthermore, structures of zMAO models and human MAO-A and MAO-B obtained after docking of MeONIPA (see previous section), were used in additional comparisons.

3.3.2. Binding site comparison methods

The PocketMatch algorithm was selected for this study due to its relatively low computational complexity and high performance. All aspects involved in binding site comparisons followed the procedure published in the original article describing the algorithm (Yeturu & Chandra, 2008). Briefly, each binding site was considered as that determined by the residues for which one or more atoms surround either a crystallographic or a docked ligand at a given distance (4 Å by default; in some cases distances from 3 Å to 10 Å from the ligand were considered; see following section). Each residue was classified into one of 5 groups, taken into account its chemical properties. Then, each residue was represented as a set of three points corresponding to the coordinates of the C-Alpha, the C-Beta and the Centroid Atom of the side chain. Distances between every three points of each residue in the binding sites were measured. All distances computed were sorted in ascending order and stored in sets of distances organized by type of pairs of points and type of pairs of tags. The sorted and organized distances were aligned and compared using a threshold of 0.5 Å, which was established considering the natural dynamics of biological systems. The similarity between sites, referred to as the PMScore, was measured by scoring the alignment of the pair of sites under comparison. Thus, the PMScore represents the percentage of the number of "matches" calculated over the maximal number of distances computed for each binding site. A PMScore of 0.5 (50 %) or higher was considered as indicative of similarity between binding sites.

3.3.3. Results and discussion

Initially, we compared human and rat MAO-A. The amino acid sequence in the active sites of both proteins is identical, and therefore we expected to find a high degree of similarity. Surprisingly, a PMScore value of 0.27 was obtained after comparing the residues located at 4 Å from the ligand (clorgyline in both proteins), which is the PocketMatch default condition. It should be considered that PMScores > 0.5 are indicative of binding site similarity, whereas values below 0.5 indicate lack of similarity. It should also be noted that, as shown in the original report by Yeturu & Chandra (2008), a distance of 4 Å from the ligand was clearly suitable to find similarities between a series of structurally related and unrelated proteins. Therefore, it was rather intriguing that such a low PMScore should be obtained, suggesting the existence of relevant differences between rat and human MAO-A binding sites, most likely in the form in which residues in close proximity to the ligand are arranged. Such a conformational difference has been revealed by the crystal structures of both proteins, which show that the cavity-shaping loop 210–216 and specifically residues Gln215 and Glu216 are differentially oriented in human and rat MAO-A (De Colibus et al., 2005). This differential arrangement determines a larger volume of the active site of human MAO-A (550 Å^3) as compared to that of rat MAO-A (450 Å^3). Thus, our results confirm that rat and human MAOs are not as similar as could be inferred from the analysis of their amino acid sequences, and highlight the sensitivity of PocketMatch to determine subtle differences between highly related proteins.

Despite these considerations, we developed a script that allows the automatic evaluation of PMScores considering distances from 3 Å to 10 Å from the ligand, with the hope that such an analysis could yield further information regarding the similarity of the binding sites of MAOs. Thus, we were able to build "similarity profiles", which graphically show at what distance from the ligand (if any) the binding sites begin to be similar. Figure 6 shows the similarity profile after comparing rat and human MAO-A.

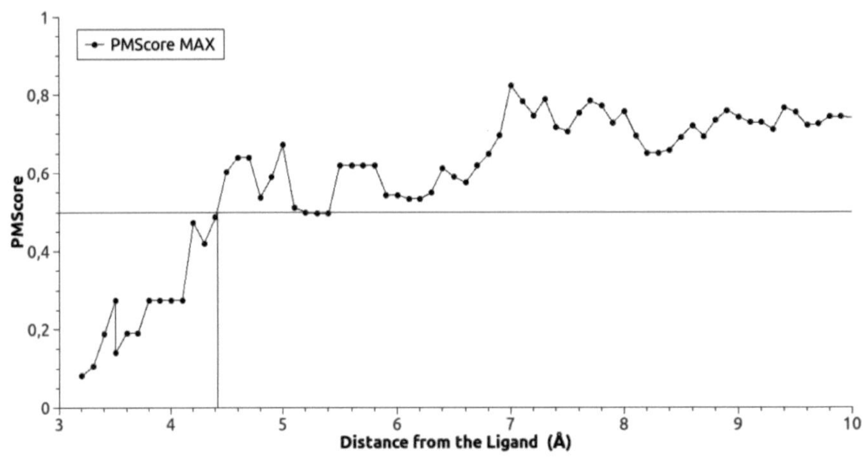

Figure 6. Similarity profile between rat and human MAO-A, both co-crystalized with clorgyline, as calculated using PocketMatch. The horizontal black line indicates PMScore = 0.5. The vertical black line indicates the distance from the ligand where the PMScore begins to be consistently greater than 0.5. Each point corresponds to the PMScore.

As can be seen, PMScores greater than 0.5 appeared at 4.5 Å and were consistently observed at longer distances from the ligand. Since most amino acids located at 4.5 Å from the ligand line the binding site (see Figure 8A and 8B), these results indicate that, beyond the shape differences revealed by crystal structures and detected by PocketMatch, the binding sites of MAO-A from rat and human are quite similar.

In contrast, when binding sites of human MAO-A and MAO-B were compared, PMScores indicating similarity (> 0.5) were only found at distances higher than 6.4 Å from the ligand (Fig. 7).

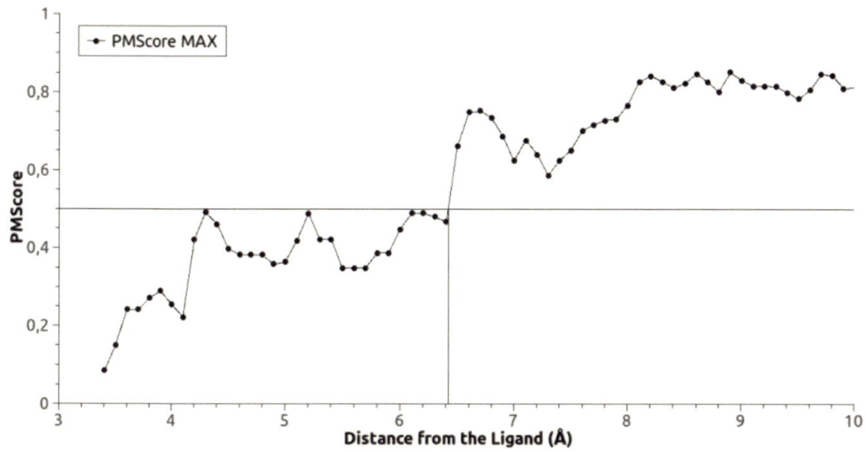

Figure 7. Similarity profile between human MAO-A (co-crystalized with clorgyline) and human MAO-B (co-crystalized with deprenyl), as calculated using PocketMatch. The horizontal black line indicates PMScore = 0.5. The vertical black line indicates the distance from the ligand where the PMScore begins to be consistently greater than 0.5. Each point corresponds to the PMScore.

As shown in Figures 8C and 8D, at a distance of 6.4 Å from the ligand, several amino acids considered in the similarity determination are located outside the binding site.

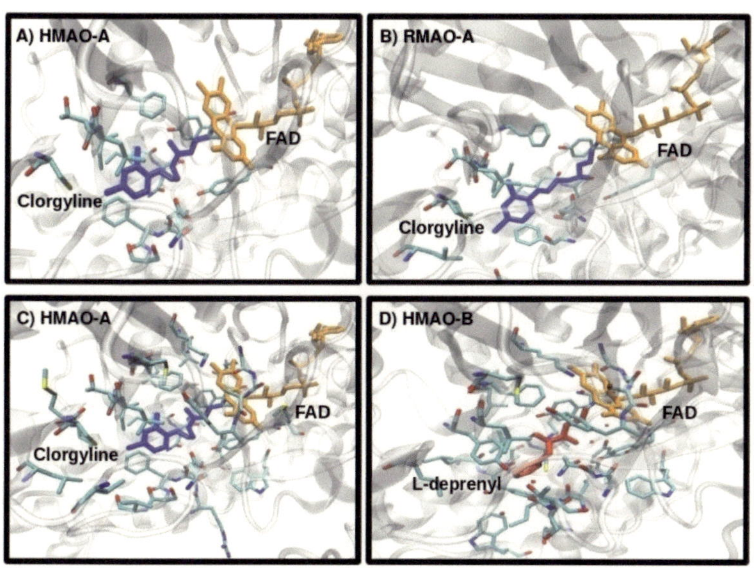

Figure 8. Binding site residues surrounding the inhibitors clorgyline (blue) and deprenyl (pink) bound to human MAO-A (HMAO-A), rat MAO-A (RMAO-A) or human MAO-B (HMAO-B). Figures 8A and 8B show the residues located at 4.5 Å from the ligand, while figures 8C and 8D show the residues located at 6.5 Å from the ligand

Therefore, the similarity profile shown in Figure 7 indicates that human MAO-A and MAO-B binding sites are less similar than those of rat and human MAO-A. It also shows that, although showing differences at their binding sites, human MAO-A and MAO-B exhibit a high degree of global structural similarity (all PMScores obtained at distances longer than 6.5 Å were well over 0.5). Though both findings might be considered obvious from the analysis of each protein sequence and function, they confirm the suitability of PocketMatch to find and predict such characteristics, an aspect that could be particularly useful when comparing proteins from which less functional information is available. In addition, our results suggest that in some cases the determination of similarity profiles can be more informative than point comparisons.

Figures 9 and 10 show the similarity profiles after comparing the homology models of zMAO with those of human MAO-A and MAO-B, respectively. As mentioned, in all cases, MeONIPA docked in each MAO structure was used as ligand.

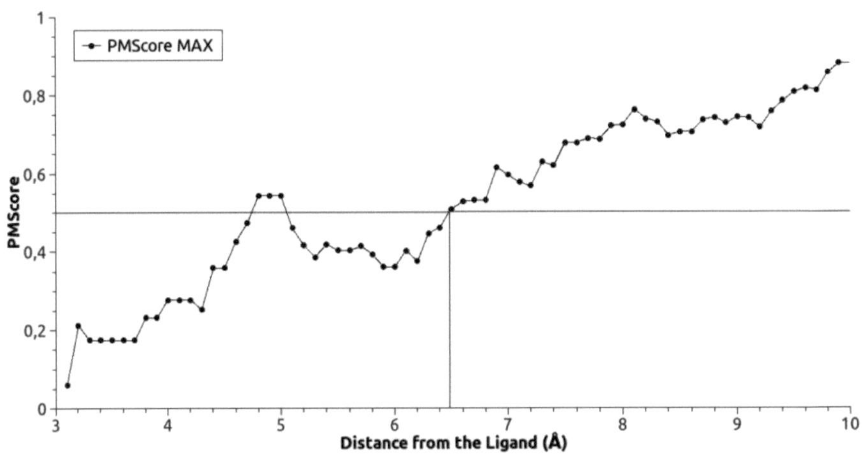

Figure 9. Similarity profile between zMAO (in this case the model corresponds to that based on human MAO-A) and human MAO-A, as calculated using PocketMatch. In both proteins, docked MeONIPA was used as ligand. The horizontal black line indicates PMScore = 0.5. The vertical black line indicates the distance from the ligand where the PMScore begins to be consistently greater than 0.5. Each point corresponds to the PMScore.

As shown in Figures 9 and 10, PMScores indicative of similarity between the binding sites of zMAO and human MAO-A or MAO-B (i.e., PMScore > 0.5) were consistently seen at distances higher than 6 Å from the ligand. It should be noted that comparable values were obtained even though the zMAO model was built using either human MAO-A or MAO-B as templates, and regardless of which human enzyme was used for the comparison. These results suggest that the zMAO binding site is as different from those of both human isoforms as the binding site of MAO-A differs from that of MAO-B. In addition, the similarity profiles of zMAO against both human proteins indicate that global structural similarity is found across these species, while the main differences are found at their binding sites. Since, to perform the similarity determination, PocketMatch considers both the shape and the chemi-

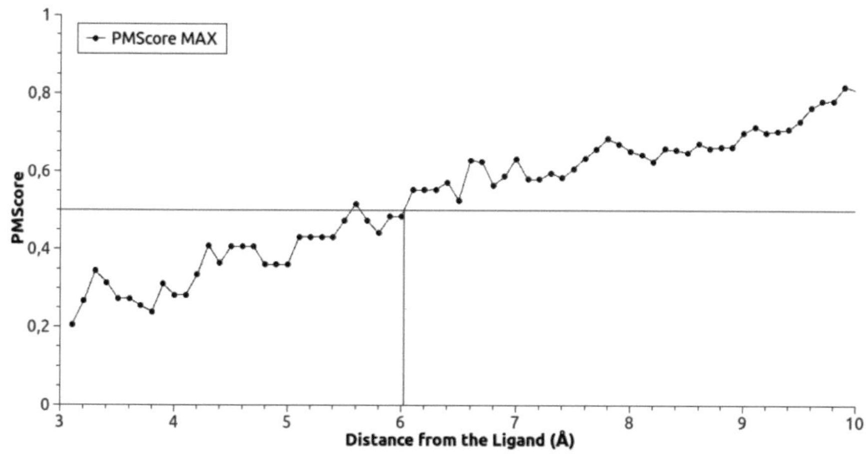

Figure 10. Similarity profile between zMAO (in this case the model corresponds to that based on human MAO-B) and human MAO-B, as calculated using PocketMatch. In both proteins, docked MeONIPA was used as ligand. The horizontal black line indicates PMScore = 0.5. The vertical black line indicates the distance from the ligand where the PMScore begins to be consistently greater than 0.5. Each point corresponds to the PMScore.

cal nature of the residues forming the site (Yeturu & Chandra, 2008), these two factors are likely involved in the differences detected between the MAO isoforms. Considering the sequence identity between zebrafish and human enzymes, one may predict that conformational differences are more important when comparing zMAO and human MAO-A, while the chemical features of the residues are more relevant to the differences between zMAO and human MAO-B. Nevertheless, further analyses are necessary to determine the relative contribution of each aspect to the differences found.

4. Conclusion

In summary, results from biochemical evaluation, molecular simulation and similarity detection studies presented here add novel evidence to the notion that even though zMAO exhibits some functional and structural properties overlapping those of MAO-A and -B, the zebrafish protein behaves quite distinctively from its mammalian counterparts. Therefore, although still an attractive model for drug discovery, in our opinion zebrafish is not a useful model for the identification of novel MAO inhibitors aimed for use in humans.

Acknowledgements

We thank Dr. K. Yeturu and Prof. N. Chandra for their valuable comments regarding Pocket Match results and functioning. We also thank Prof. Bruce K. Cassels for critical reading of the manuscript. This work was funded by MSI Grant P05/001-F, PBCT grant PDA-23 to AF and FONDECYT Grants 110-85002 to AF, 110-0542 to PI-V and 109-0037 to MR-P. D.E.E. acknowledges research support from the National Institutes of Health GM 29433

Author details

Angelica Fierro[1,2], Alejandro Montecinos[1], Cristobal Gómez-Molina[3], Gabriel Núñez[4], Milagros Aldeco[5], Dale E. Edmondson[5], Marcelo Vilches-Herrera[3], Susan Lühr[2,3], Patricio Iturriaga-Vásquez[1] and Miguel Reyes-Parada[2,6*]

*Address all correspondence to: miguel.reyes@usach.cl

1 Faculty of Chemistry and Biology, University of Santiago de Chile, Chile

2 Millennium Institute for Cell Dynamics and Biotechnology, Chile

3 Faculty of Sciences, University of Chile, Chile

4 PhD Program in Biotechnology, University of Santiago de Chile, Chile

5 Department of Biochemistry and Chemistry, Emory University, USA

6 Faculty of Medical Sciences, University of Santiago de Chile, Chile

References

[1] Aldeco, M, Arslan, B. K, & Edmondson, D. E. (2011). Catalytic and inhibitor binding properties of zebrafish monoamine oxidase (zMAO): comparisons with human MAO A and MAO B. *Comparative Biochemistry and Physiology. Part B, Biochemistry & Molecular Biology*, , 159, 78-83.

[2] Allen, W. J, & Bevan, D. R. (2011). Steered molecular dynamics simulations reveal important mechanisms in reversible monoamine oxidase B inhibition. *Biochemistry*, , 50, 6441-6454.

[3] Anichtchik, O, Sallinen, V, Peitsaro, N, & Panula, P. (2006). Distinct structure and activity of monoamine oxidase in the brain of zebrafish (Danio rerio). *Journal of Comparative Neurology*, , 498, 593-610.

[4] Arslan, B. K, & Edmondson, D. E. (2010). Expression of zebrafish (Danio rerio) monoamine oxidase (MAO) in Pichia pastoris: purification and comparison with human MAO A and MAO B. *Protein Expression and Purification*, , 70, 290-297.

[5] Apsel, B, Blair, J. A, González, B, Nazif, T. M, Feldman, M. E, Aizenstein, B, Hoffman, R, Williams, R. L, Shokat, K. M, & Knight, Z. A. (2008). Targeted polypharmacology: discovery of dual inhibitors of tyrosine and phosphoinositide kinases. *Nature Chemical Biology*, , 4, 691-699.

[6] Baroni, M, Cruciani, G, Sciabola, S, Perruccio, F, & Mason, J. S. (2007). A common reference framework for analyzing/comparing proteins and ligands. Fingerprints for Ligands and Proteins (FLAP): theory and application. *Journal of Chemical Information and Modeling*, , 47, 279-294.

[7] Bencan, Z, & Levin, E. D. (2008). The role of $\alpha 7$ and $\alpha 4\beta 2$ nicotinic receptors in the nicotine-induced anxiolyitic effect in Zebrafish. *Physiology & Behavior*, , 95, 408-412.

[8] Bencan, Z, Sledge, D, & Levin, E. D. (2009). Buspirone, chlordiazepoxide and diazepam effects in a zebrafish model of anxiety. *Pharmacology Biochemistry and Behavior*, , 4, 75-80.

[9] Binda, C, Newton-vinson, P, Hubálek, F, Edmondson, D. E, & Mattevi, A. (2002). Structure of human monoamineoxidase B, a drug target for the treatment of neurological disorders. *Nature Structural Biology*, , 9, 22-26.

[10] Binda, C, Li, M, Hubálek, F, Restelli, N, Edmondson, D. E, & Mattevi, A. (2003). Insights into the mode of inhibition of human mitochondrial monoamine oxidase B from high-resolution crystal structures. *Proceedings of the National Academy of Sciences USA.*, , 100, 9759.

[11] Binda, C, Hubálek, F, Li, M, Herzig, Y, Sterling, J, Edmondson, D. E, & Mattevi, A. (2004). Crystal structures of monoamine oxidase B in complex with four inhibitors of the *N*-propargylamino-indan class. *Journal of Medicinal Chemistry*, , 47, 1767-1774.

[12] Binda, C, Aldeco, M, Mattevi, A, & Edmondson, D. E. (2011). Interactions of monoamine oxidases with the antiepileptic drug zonisamide: specificity of inhibition and structure of the human monoamine oxidase B complex. *Journal of Medicinal Chemistry*, , 54, 909-912.

[13] Brylinski, M, & Skolnick, J. (2009). FINDSITE: a threading-based approach to ligand homology modeling. *PLoS Computational Biology*, , 5, e1000405.

[14] Chakraborty, C, & Hsu, C. H. (2009). Zebrafish: a complete animal model for in vivo drug discovery and development. *Current Drug Metabolism*, , 10, 116-124.

[15] Cleves, A. E, & Jain, A. N. Robust ligand-based modeling of the biological targets of known drugs. *Journal of Medicinal Chemistry*, , 49, 2921-2938.

[16] Colwill, R. M, Raymond, M. P, Ferreira, L, & Escudero, H. (2005). Visual discrimination learning in zebrafish (*Danio rerio*). *Behavioral Processes*, , 70, 19-31.

[17] Darland, T, & Dowling, J. E. (2001). Behavioral screening for cocaine sensitivity in mutagenized zebrafish. *Proceedings of the National Academy of Sciences USA.*, , 98, 11691-11696.

[18] De Colibus, L, Li, M, Binda, C, Lustig, A, Edmondson, D. E, & Mattevi, A. (2005). Three-dimensional structure of human monoamine oxidase A (MAO A): Relation to the structures of rat MAO A and human MAO B. *Proceedings of the National Academy of Sciences USA.*, , 102, 12684-12689.

[19] Eddins, D, Cerutti, D, Williams, P, Linney, E, & Levin, E. D. (2010). Zebrafish provide a sensitive model of persisting neurobehavioral effects of developmental chlorpyrifos exposure: Comparison with nicotine and pilocarpine effects and relationship to dopamine deficits. *Neurotoxicology and Teratology*, , 2, 99-108.

[20] Edmondson, D. E, Binda, C, & Mattevi, A. (2007). Structural insights into the mechanism of amine oxidation by monoamine oxidases A and B. *Archives of Biochemistry and Biophysics*, , 464

[21] Edmondson, D. E, Binda, C, Wang, J, Upadhyay, A. K, & Mattevi, A. (2009). Molecular and mechanistic properties of the membrane-bound mitochondrial monoamine oxidases. *Biochemistry*, , 48, 4220-4230.

[22] Egan, R. J, Bergner, C. L, Hart, P. C, Cachat, J. M, Canavello, P. R, Elegante, M. F, El-khayat, S. I, Bartels, B. K, Tien, A. K, Tien, D. H, Mohnot, S, Beeson, E, Glasgow, E, Amri, H, Zukowska, Z, & Kalueff, A. V. (2009). Understanding behavioral and physiological phenotypes of stress and anxiety in zebrafish. *Behavioural Brain Research*, , 205, 38-44.

[23] Erdem, S. S, & Büyükmenekse, B. (2011). Computational investigation on the structure-activity relationship of the biradical mechanism for monoamine oxidase. *Journal of Neural Transmission*, , 118, 1021-1029.

[24] Flinn, L, Bretaud, S, Lo, C, Ingham, P. W, & Bandmann, O. (2008). Zebrafish as a new animal model for movement disorders. *Journal of Neurochemistry*, , 106, 1991-1997.

[25] Fierro, A, Osorio-olivares, M, Cassels, B. K, Edmondson, D. E, Sepúlveda-boza, S, & Reyes-parada, M. (2007). Human and rat monoamine oxidase-A are differentially inhibited by (S)-4-alkylthioamphetamine derivatives: insights from molecular modeling studies. *Bioorganic and Medicinal Chemistry*, , 15, 5198-56206.

[26] Frisch, M. J, Trucks, G. W, Schlegel, H. B, Scuseria, G. E, Robb, M. A, Cheeseman, J. R, et al. (2004). Gaussian 03, Revision C.02, Gaussian, Inc., Wallingford CT.

[27] Gold, N. D, & Jackson, R. M. (2006). SitesBase: a database for structure-based protein-ligand binding site comparisons. *Nucleic Acids Research*, Database issue), , 34, D231-D234.

[28] Goldsmith, P. (2004). Zebrafish as a pharmacological tool: the how, why and when. *Current Opinion in Pharmacology*, , 4, 504-512.

[29] Gordon, J. C, Myers, J. B, Folta, T, Shoja, V, Heath, L. S, & Onufriev, A. (2005). H++: a server for estimating pKas and adding missing hydrogens to macromolecules. *Nucleic Acids Research*, Web Server issue), , 33, W368-W371.

[30] Henrich, S, Salo-ahen, O. M, Huang, B, Rippmann, F. F, Cruciani, G, & Wade, R. C. (2010). Computational approaches to identifying and characterizing protein binding sites for ligand design. *Journal of Molecular Recognition*, , 23, 209-219.

[31] Hollis, K. L. (1999). The role of learning in the aggressive and reproductive behavior of blue gouramis, Trichogaster trichopterus. *Environmental Biology of Fishes*, , 54, 355-369.

[32] Hoffmann, B, Zaslavskiy, M, Vert, J. P, & Stoven, V. (2010). A new protein binding pocket similarity measure based on comparison of clouds of atoms in 3D: application to ligand prediction. *BMC Bioinformatics*, , 11, 99.

[33] Hopkins, A. L. (2008). Network pharmacology: the next paradigm in drug discovery. *Nature Chemical Biology*, , 4, 682-690.

[34] Hurtado-guzmán, C, Fierro, A, Iturriaga-vásquez, P, Sepúlveda-boza, S, Cassels, B. K, & Reyes-parada, M. (2003). Monoamine oxidase inhibitory properties of optical isomers and N-substituted derivatives of 4-methylthioamphetamine. *Journal of Enzyme Inhibition and Medicinal Chemistry*, , 18, 339-347.

[35] Jambon, M, Imberty, A, Deléage, G, & Geourjon, C. (2003). A new bioinformatic approach to detect common 3D sites in protein structures. *Proteins*, , 52, 137-145.

[36] Kahraman, A, Morris, R. J, Laskowski, R. A, & Thornton, J. M. (2007). Shape variation in protein binding pockets and their ligands. *Journal of Molecular Biology*, , 368, 283-301.

[37] Kaufman, C. K, & White, R. M. (2009). Chemical genetic screening in the zebrafish embryo. *Nature Protocols*, , 4, 1422-1432.

[38] Keiser, M. J, Setola, V, Irwin, J. J, Laggner, C, Abbas, A. I, Hufeisen, S. J, Jensen, N. H, Kuijer, M. B, Matos, R. C, Tran, T. B, Whaley, R, Glennon, R. A, Hert, J, Thomas, K. L, Edwards, D. D, Shoichet, B. K, & Roth, B. L. (2009). Predicting new molecular targets for known drugs. *Nature*, , 462, 175-181.

[39] Kinnings, S. L, & Jackson, R. M. (2009). Binding site similarity analysis for the functional classification of the protein kinase family. *Journal of Chemical Information and Modeling*, , 49, 318-329.

[40] King, A. (2009). Researchers find their Nemo. *Cell*, , 139, 843-846.

[41] Kochersperger, L. M, Parker, E. L, Siciliano, M, Darlington, G. J, & Denney, R. M. (1986). Assignment of genes for human monoamine oxidases A and B to the X chromosome. *Journal of Neuroscience Research*, , 16, 601-616.

[42] Kokel, D, Bryan, J, Laggner, C, White, R, Cheung, C. Y, Mateus, R, Healey, D, Kim, S, Werdich, A. A, Haggarty, S. J, Macrae, C. A, Shoichet, B, & Peterson, R. T. (2010).

Rapid behavior-based identification of neuroactive small molecules in the zebrafish. *Nature Chemical Biology*, , 6, 231-237.

[43] Kokel, D, & Peterson, R. T. (2011). Using the zebrafish photomotor response for psychotropic drug screening. *Methods in Cell Biology*, , 105, 517-524.

[44] Lan, N. C, Chen, C. H, & Shih, J. C. (1989). Expression of functional human monoamine oxidase A and B cDNAs in mammalian cells. *Journal of Neurochemistry*, , 52, 1652-1654.

[45] Landon, M. R, Amaro, R. E, Baron, R, Ngan, C. H, Ozonoff, D, Mccammon, J. A, & Vajda, S. (2008). Novel druggable hot spots in avian influenza neuraminidase H5N1 revealed by computational solvent mapping of a reduced and representative receptor ensemble. *Chemical Biology & Drug Design*, , 71, 106-116.

[46] Laskowski, R. A. MacArthur, MW.; Moss, DS. & Thornton, JM. ((1993). PROCHECK: a program to check the stereochemical quality of protein structures. *Journal of Applied Crystallography*, , 26, 283-291.

[47] Laskowski, R. A, Watson, J. D, & Thornton, J. M. (2005). ProFunc: a server for predicting protein function from 3D structure. *Nucleic Acids Research*, Web Server issue), , 33, W89-W93.

[48] Laurie, A. T, & Jackson, R. M. an energy-based method for the prediction of protein-ligand binding sites. *Bioinformatics*, , 21, 1908-1916.

[49] Levin, E. D, & Chen, E. (2006). Nicotinic involvement in memory function in zebrafish. *Neurotoxicology Teratology*, , 6, 731-735.

[50] Levin, E. D, Bencan, Z, & Cerutti, D. T. (2007). Anxiolytic effects of nicotine in zebrafish. *Physiology and Behavior*, , 90, 54-58.

[51] Lühr, S, Vilches-herrera, M, Fierro, A, Ramsay, R. R, Edmondson, D. E, Reyes-parada, M, Cassels, B. K, & Iturriaga-vásquez, P. (2010). Arylthiomorpholine derivatives as potent and selective monoamine oxidase B inhibitors. *Bioorganic & Medicinal Chemistry*, , 18, 1388-1395.

[52] Ma, J, Masato, Y, Yamashita, E, Nakagawa, A, Ito, A, & Tsukihara, T. (2004). Structure of rat monoamine oxidase and its specific recognitions for substrates and inhibitors. *Journal of Molecular Biology*, , 338, 103-114.

[53] Mckinley, E. T, Baranowski, T. C, Blavo, D. O, Cato, C, Doan, T. N, & Rubinstein, A. L. (2005). Neuroprotection of MPTP-induced toxicity in Zebrafish dopaminergic neurons. *Molecular Brain Research*, , 141, 128-137.

[54] Miklosi, A, Andrew, R. J, & Savage, H. (1997). Behavioural lateralisation of the tetrapod type in the zebrafish (Brachydanio rerio). *Physiology & Behavior*, , 63, 127-135.

[55] Miklosi, A, & Andrew, R. J. (1999). Right eye use associated with decision to bite in zebrafish. *Behavioural Brain Research*, , 105, 199-205.

[56] Milletti, F, & Vulpetti, A. (2010). Predicting polypharmacology by binding site similarity: from kinases to the protein universe. *Journal of Chemical Information and Modeling*, , 50, 1418-1431.

[57] Moriaud, F, Richard, S. B, Adcock, S. A, Chanas-martin, L, & Surgand, J. S. Ben Jelloul, M. & Delfaud, F. ((2011). Identify drug repurposing candidates by mining the protein data bank. *Briefings in Bioinformatics*,, 12, 336-240.

[58] Morris, G. M, Goodsell, D. S, Halliday, R. S, Huey, R, Hart, W. E, Belew, R. K, & Olson, A. J. (1998). Automated docking using a Lamarckian genetic algorithm and empirical binding free energy function. *Journal of Computational Chemistry*, , 19, 1639-1662.

[59] Nagatsu, T. (2004). Progress in monoamine oxidase (MAO) research in relation to genetic engineering.*Neurotoxicology*, , 25, 11-20.

[60] Najmanovich, R, Kurbatova, N, & Thornton, J. (2008). Detection of 3D atomic similarities and their use in the discrimination of small molecule protein-binding sites. *Bioinformatics*, , 24, i105-i111.

[61] Nandigama, R. K, Newton-vinson, P, & Edmondson, D. E. (2002). Phentermine inhibition of recombinant human liver monoamine oxidases A and B. *Biochemical Pharmacology*, , 63, 865-869.

[62] Norton, W, & Bally-cuif, L. (2010). Adult zebrafish as a model organism for behavioural genetics. *BMC Neuroscience*, , 11, 90.

[63] Ninkovic, J, & Bally-cuif, L. (2006). The zebrafish as a model system for assessing the reinforcing properties of drug abuse. *Methods*, , 39, 262-274.

[64] Panula, P, Chen, Y. C, Priyadarshini, M, Kudo, H, Semenova, S, Sundvik, M, & Sallinen, V. (2010). The comparative neuroanatomy and neurochemistry of zebrafish CNS systems of relevance to human neuropsychiatric diseases. *Neurobiology of Disease*, , 40, 46-57.

[65] PayneRJH. ((1998). Gradually escalating fights and displays: The cumulative assessment model. *Animal Behavior*, , 56, 651-662.

[66] Pérez-nueno, V. I, & Ritchie, D. W. (2011). Using consensus-shape clustering to identify promiscuous ligands and protein targets and to choose the right query for shape-based virtual screening. *Journal of Chemical Information and Modeling*, , 51, 1233-1248.

[67] Phillips, J. C, Braun, R, Wang, W, Gumbart, J, Tajkhorshid, E, Villa, E, Chipot, C, Skeel, R. D, Kalé, L, & Schulten, K. (2005). Scalable molecular dynamics with NAMD. *Journal of Computational Chemistry*, , 26, 1781-1802.

[68] Postlethwait, J. H, Woods, I. G, Ngo-hazelett, P, Yan, Y. L, Kelly, P. D, Chu, F, Huang, H, Hill-force, A, & Talbot, W. S. (2000). Zebrafish comparative genomics and the origins of vertebrate chromosomes.*Genome Research*, 2000, , 10, 1890-1902.

[69] Reader, S. M, Kendal, J. R, & Laland, K. N. (2003). Social learning of foraging sites and escape routes in wild Trinidadian guppies. *Animal Behavior*, , 66, 729-739.

[70] Reyes-parada, M, Fierro, A, Iturriaga-vásquez, P, & Cassels, B. K. (2005). Monoamine oxidase inhibition in the light of new structural data. *Current Enzyme Inhibition*, , 1

[71] Rihel, J, Prober, D. A, Arvanites, A, Lam, K, Zimmerman, S, Jang, S, Haggarty, S. J, Kokel, D, Rubin, L. L, Peterson, R. T, & Schier, A. F. (2010). Zebrafish behavioral profiling links drugs to biological targets and rest/wake regulation. *Science*, , 327, 348-351.

[72] Rubinstein, A. L. (2006). Zebrafish assays for drug toxicity screening. *Expert Opinion on Drug Metabolism & Toxicology*, , 2, 231-240.

[73] Russell, R. B, Sasieni, P. D, & Sternberg, M. J. (1998). Supersites within superfolds. Binding site similarity in the absence of homology. *Journal of Molecular Biology*, , 282, 903-918.

[74] Sali, A, & Blundell, T. L. (1993). Comparative protein modeling by satisfaction of spatial restraints. *Journal of Molecular Biology*, , 234, 779-815.

[75] Sallinen, V, Sundvik, M, Reenilä, I, Peitsaro, N, Khrustalyov, D, Anichtchik, O, Toleikyte, G, Kaslin, J, & Panula, P. (2009). Hyperserotonergic phenotype after monoamine oxidase inhibition in larval zebrafish. *Journal of Neurochemistry*, , 109

[76] Schrattenholz, A, & Soskic, V. (2008). What does systems biology mean for drug development? *Current Medicinal Chemistry*, , 15, 1520-1528.

[77] Setini, A, Pierucci, F, Senatori, O, & Nicotra, A. (2005). Molecular characterization of monoamine oxidase in zebrafish (Danio rerio). *Comparative Biochemistry and Physiology. Part B, Biochemistry & Molecular Biology*, , 140, 153-161.

[78] Son, S. Y, Ma, J, Kondou, Y, Yoshimura, M, Yamashita, E, & Tsukihara, T. (2008). Structure of human monoamine oxidase A at 2.2-A resolution: the control of opening the entry for substrates/inhibitors. *Proceedings of the National Academy of Sciences USA.*, , 105, 5739-5744.

[79] Streisinger, G, Walker, C, Dower, N, Knauber, D, & Singer, F. (1981). Production of clones of homozygous diploid zebra fish (*Brachydanio rerio*). *Nature.*, , 291, 293-296.

[80] Suboski, M. D. (1988). Acquisition and social communication of stimulus recognition by fish. *Behavioral Processes*, , 16, 213-244.

[81] Suboski, M. D, Bain, S, Carty, A. E, & Mcquoid, L. M. (1990). Alarm reaction in acquisition and social transmission of simulated predator recognition by zebra danio fish. *Journal of Comparative Psychology*, , 104, 101-112.

[82] Tebbich, S, Bshary, R, & Grutter, A. S. (2002). Cleaner fish *Labroides dimidiatus* recognise familiar clients. *Animal Cognition*, , 5, 139-145.

http://dx.doi.org/10.5772/35874

[83] Vilches-herrera, M, Miranda-sepúlveda, J, Rebolledo-fuentes, M, Fierro, A, Lühr, S, Iturriaga-vasquez, P, Cassels, B. K, & Reyes-parada, M. (2009). Naphthylisopropylamine and N-benzylamphetamine derivatives as monoamine oxidase inhibitors. *Bioorganic and Medicinal Chemistry*, , 17, 2452-2460.

[84] Weisel, M, Proschak, E, & Schneider, G. (2007). PocketPicker: analysis of ligand binding-sites with shape descriptors. *Chemistry Central Journal*, , 1, 7.

[85] Wiederstein, M, & Sippl, M. J. (2007). ProSA-web: interactive web service for the recognition of errors in three-dimensional structures of proteins. *Nucleic Acids Research*, Web Server issue), , 35, W407-W410.

[86] Xie, L, & Bourne, P. E. (2008). Detecting evolutionary relationships across existing fold space, using sequence order-independent profile-profile alignments. *Proceedings of the National Academy of Sciences USA.*, , 105, 5441-5446.

[87] Xie, L, Xie, L, & Bourne, P. E. (2009). A unified statistical model to support local sequence order independent similarity searching for ligand-binding sites and its application to genome-based drug discovery. *Bioinformatics*, , 25, i305-i312.

[88] Yeturu, K, & Chandra, N. (2008). PocketMatch: a new algorithm to compare binding sites in protein structures. *BMC Bioinformatics*, , 9, 543.

[89] YoudimMBH.; Edmondson, D. & Tipton, KF. ((2006). The therapeutic potential of monoamine oxidase inhibitors. *Nature Reviews Neuroscience*, , 7, 295.

[90] Zon, L. I, & Peterson, R. T. (2005). In vivo drug discovery in the zebrafish. *Nature Reviews Drug Discovery*, , 4, 35-44.

Chapter 17

Single-Molecule Imaging Measurements of Protein-Protein Interactions in Living Cells

Kayo Hibino, Michio Hiroshima, Yuki Nakamura and Yasushi Sako

Additional information is available at the end of the chapter

http://dx.doi.org/10.5772/52386

1. Introduction

Even though we have several techniques, represented by the electron microscopy, to obtain images of single molecules, in this chapter, we use 'single-molecule imaging' (SMI) for a limited means—that is, imaging of fluorescently labeled biological molecules at work for analyzing their behaviors. To observe biological molecules at work, imaging in aqueous conditions is essential. Therefore, optical microscopy is the main technology in SMI. Fluorescence labeling is good to use for imaging in optical microscopy, because it allows high contrast and selective imaging of molecules that we are interested in. SMI provides information of dynamics and kinetics of molecular reactions. In 1995, two groups firstly and independently realized SMI of biological molecules in aqueous conditions [1,2]. In the early days, SMI was used mainly for the *in vitro* studies of protein motors [1,2] and metabolic enzymes [3]. Detection of enzymatic reaction (reaction kinetics) [1,3] and detection of protein dynamics (lateral and rotational movements) [2] have been the two main usages of SMI since the first development of this technology. After that, the application of SMI has been extended, and in 2000, SMI became to be used in living cells [4,5].

Probably, for the readers, the most familiar usage of SMI is the measurement of molecular dynamics, including conformational changes and lateral and rotational movements. However, kinetic analysis is one of the original applications of SMI as mentioned above, and in many cases, it relates more closely to the higher-order biological functions than does dynamics analysis. This chapter focuses on the kinetic analysis of protein-protein interactions, including molecular recognitions and enzymatic reactions in living cells. As the application of SMI, we introduce a ligand-receptor interaction on the cell surface, and a process of protein activation occurs in a ternary protein complex beneath the plasma membrane. Because the main subject of this chapter is the technical issue, these two examples of applications are chosen to explain how to analyze single-molecule data to understand kinetics of molecular interactions quantitatively in living cells. At the present time, we have several textbooks specialized for the technologies and applications of SMI in a wide field [6-8]. Please refer to these books for information lacking in this chapter.

2. Motivation of Single-molecule Imaging Measurements of Molecular Interactions

2.1. Single-molecule versus ensemble-molecule measurements

Before considering about technological issues, it might be important to discuss why we need SMI measurements of molecular interactions. The operation of biological molecular machines is basically stochastic. Therefore, in ensemble average measurements, in which only the averages over a huge number of reaction events are observed, details of the reaction process are obscured. In SMI measurements, it is possible to virtually synchronize a particular point in the reaction process for kinetic analysis. For example, imagine the observation of an enzyme reaction. The substrate solution is added to the enzyme solution to start the reaction. In ensemble measurements, the time of the two solutions mixing is set to time 0, and the concentration of the product is monitored with time. In the mixture, first, a substrate molecule needs to diffuse and collide with an enzyme molecule to form an enzyme-substrate (ES) complex; then, a chemical reaction starts on the enzyme molecule. The time 0 in ensemble measurements is not the time of ES complex formation. The time of ES complex formation is different for each molecule due to the stochasticity of molecular reactions, and this difference obscures the measurements of chemical reactions. In SMI measurements, the time point of each ES complex formation is detected, and after the observation, all the time points for individual molecules are aligned to time 0. Hence, in SMI measurements, we selectively extract the process of chemical reactions, removing the diffusion and collision for kinetic analysis.

This principle of SMI measurements also allows separation of forward and backward reactions. Here, imagine an association-dissociation reaction between two species of molecules. In the reaction mixture, both association and dissociation occur in parallel (on the different molecules). Even if we monitor the initial process of complex formation soon after the mixing of the two solutions, it is impossible to separate forward and backward reactions completely, and in the equilibrium, it is absolutely impossible to measure reaction kinetics, at least when the numbers of molecules are large. In SMI measurements, each association or dissociation event is detected individually; therefore, after the observations, association (or dissociation) events can be selected for pure kinetic analysis of association (dissociation) reactions. Because of this, kinetic analysis based on SMI, is possible, even in the equilibrium (or steady state) conditions.

Structures of biological macromolecules, especially proteins, often show multiple metastable points (this phenomenon is called polymorphism). Each single molecule is drifting among these metastable points in various timescales. post-translational modifications, such as phosphorylation, may stabilize one or some of the metastable structures, according to each single molecule. SMI measurements are good to detect distributions and fluctuations of reactions and structures caused by static and dynamic polymorphisms of biological macromolecules [3,9-11]. In some cases, non-random reactions of proteins have been detected using SMI [3,9,11].

2.2. Single molecule measurements in living cells

In a cellular context, it is difficult to perform long time-series analyses of the reaction on the same single molecules due to high density and lateral movements of the molecules. However, SMI measurements still have advantages over conventional ensemble average measurements. SMI allows *in situ,* non-destructive quantitative measurements. SMI measurements provide absolute values of the kinetic and dynamic parameters of the molecular reactions and dynamics, including number, density, reaction rate constants, lateral diffusion coefficient, and transport velocity, with the smallest disruption of the living cell systems [8,12,13].

As mentioned above, for the time-series analyses, SMI measurements do not require physical synchronization, which is indispensable in ensemble molecule measurements. Synchronization, like concentration or temperature jumps, generally alters the condition of cell cultures, possibly affecting many cellular reactions in addition to the subject of the experiment. Therefore, it sometimes becomes ambiguous if the changes of the measured value reflect the reaction kinetics itself or the cellular dynamics triggered by the changed culture conditions. SMI measurements allow kinetic analysis in steady state, avoiding changes of culture conditions. For example, Hibino et al. [14] measured dissociation kinetics between two protein species, Ras and RAF, using SMI in quiescent cells in a steady state.

SMI measurements can detect small numbers of reactions in a limited volume inside living cells, because they are based on imaging with spatial resolution and possess the extreme sensitivity to detect single molecules. Using SMI measurement, Ueda et al. [15] measured the numbers and rate constants of the reactions between cAMP and its receptor, comparing the front and rear halves of a single *Dictyostelium* amoeba during chemotaxis. Tani et al. [16] analyzed reaction kinetics at the growth cone of nerve cells. These works have revealed that kinetic parameters of the same reactions diverged according to the positions in single cells. In addition, SMI measurements have directly revealed that cellular responses, such as neurite elongation [16] and calcium response [17], are caused by signaling of tens or hundreds of protein molecules.

The range of application of SMI measurements is broad, covering various fields of biological sciences of cells, including not only basic biochemistry and biophysics but systems biology, pathology of genetic diseases, action points analyses in pharmacology, and toxinology. SMI measurements provide absolute values of reaction parameters, which can be substituted into the reaction models described using mathematical equations. Since these values are determined in live cell conditions, SMI measurements are good to use in combination with mathematical modeling constructed to explain and predict dynamics of complex intracellular reaction networks.

3. Technologies of Single-molecule Imaging in Living Cells

3.1. Microscope and imaging equipment

SMI uses optical microscopy, and since most of the biological molecules are translucent for visible light, some kind of labeling is required. For detection of single molecules, labeling with fluorophore is effective, because it provides high-contrast imaging, which is essential both for detection of small signals from a single molecule and for detection of specific species of molecules in crowded conditions of living cells. Labeling by fluorescent proteins has expanded the application of SMI in living cells.

Fluorescence signal from single fluorophores is small but enough to be imaged individually when recent high-sensitivity video cameras, like EM-CCD or CCD equipped with a multichannel plate image intensifier are used. Standard temporal resolution of SMI in living cells is several tens of ms, and in some cases, under strong illumination, ms sampling has been achieved gathering hundreds of photons from a single fluorophore per single video frame.

For detection of small signals from single molecules, background rejection is essential. Total internal reflection [1] and oblique illumination [18] are useful technologies of wide-field fluorescence microscopy to realize effective background rejection and can be used for SMI in living cells (Figure 1) [19].

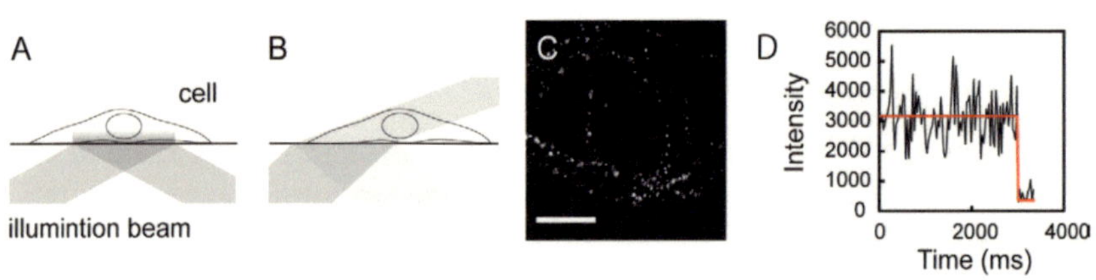

Figure 1. Single-molecule imaging in living cells. Schemes of total internal reflection (A) and oblique illumination (B) microscope and a single-molecule image of tetramethylrhodamine-labeled EGF on the surface of living HeLa cells under an oblique illumination microscope (C) are shown. Bar in C: 10 μm. Detection of singlemolecules can be examined by single-step photobleaching (D).

Figure 2 shows the optical setup of our TIR microscope for SMI, which was home-built based on a commercial inverted fluorescence microscope. Solid-state continuous wave lasers in different emission wavelengths are used for illumination according to the species of fluorophore. Between the lasers and the microscope, a two-dimensional beam scanning system is constructed. This system is composed by a pair of diagonallypositioned Galvanometer-scanning mirrors and a telescope that inserted between the two scanning mirrors. The two scanning mirrors are moved sinusoidally with a π phase difference in a frequency higher than the frame rate of imaging (30 Hz is the typical frame rate). Therefore, the specimen is illuminated from every direction during the acquisition of single frames. Thus, the system achieves pseudo-circular illumination.

http://dx.doi.org/10.5772/52386

Circular illumination is better in TIR-microscopy than the illumination from a fixed single direction that is usually used in commercial TIR system, especially for observations of biological samples having anisotropic structure [19]. It also reduces effects of spatially inhomogeneous illumination pattern often caused by the strong coherence of laser beams. There are several methods to construct circular illumination path using only static optical elements or a rotatory moving mirror with a fixed angle, however, using a pair of Galvanometer, the incident angle of the illumination beam to the specimen is easily adjusted to the best position for each specimen by changing the amplitude of vibration of the scanner mirrors.

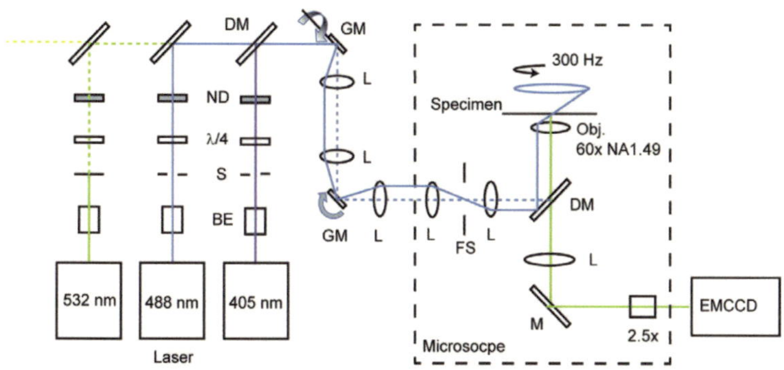

Figure 2. Optical path of a total internal reflection fluorescence microscope for single-molecule imaging.The illumination laser beams are introduced into an inverted fluorescence microscope from the epi-illumination path. Between the microscope and lasers, a two-demensional beam scanning system is inserted to achieve pseudo-circular illumination (see text for details). The violet (405-nm) laser is used for photoconversion of fluorophores. BE: beam expander, DM: dichroic mirror, FS: field stop, GM: Galvanometer scanner mirror, L: lens, λ/4: quarter wave plate, M: mirror, ND: neutral density filter, S: shutter.

3.2. Fluorophores

Both the chemical fluorophores and fluorescent proteins are applicable as the probes of SMI in living cells. To obtain good contrast against autofluorescence of cells and optics, fluorophores with relatively longer wavelength emissions are generally better. As the chemical fluorophores, tetrametylrhodamine (TMR), Cy3, Cy5, Alexa 488, and Alexa 594 are used frequently. Among the fluorescent proteins, as far as we know, eGFP is the best for SMI because of relatively good photostability. As the red fluorescent protein in SMI, tag RFP is applicable. Photoconvertible proteins, Eos and mKikGR, are good in photoactivation localization microscopy (PALM), which is an application of SMI [20]. Protein tags, like HaLo and SNAP, which can be conjugated covalently with chemical fluorophores after expression in living cells, are useful, because chemical fluorophores are generally more photostable than the fluorescent proteins, and colors of fluorescence emission can be changed according to the purpose of the experiment. When an especially strong and stable (long observation time) signal is required, Q-dot or other fluorescent beads will be used. In such cases, steric hindrance and multivalency should be controlled carefully.

3.3. Sample preparation

For SMI, cells are cultured on a coverslip and set on the microscope. Since contamination of small dust on the coverslip prevents SMI, the coverslip must be washed thoroughly before transfer of cells onto it [21]. Usage of glass coverslips (not conventional plastic cell culture dishes) that has the high refractive index was necessary to achieve total internal reflection; however, some cell culture dishes or chambers made of plastic with the refractive index similar to that of glass (1.52) can be purchased recently. One day or more before the observation, the culture medium should be replaced to one that does not contain phenol red to reduce background fluorescence. The culture medium used during observation should also not contain phenol red.

When proteins tagged with fluorescent proteins, like GFP, are expressed and observed in cells, conditions for the transfection of cDNAs should be carefully controlled to avoid overexpression that prevents SMI (see section 3.5). Similarly, when HaLo or SNAP tag is used, staining should be carried out with a much lower concentration of fluorescent regents than that recommended by the manufactures.

3.4. Image processing

The signal-to-noise ratio (S/N) in SMI is usually not good due to small signals and, especially in cells, due to rather large background autofluorescence and scattering. Temporal averaging over successive video frames improves S/N under the sacrifice of temporal resolution. Spatial filtering of the images is also used to improve image quality. But, one must be careful to use any temporal and spatial filtering, because they sometimes do not preserve the linearity of signal intensity. Background subtraction is usually carried out before quantification of single-molecule signals. In cells, because background signals are highly inhomogeneous, the background levels should be determined locally.

After the appropriate pretreatments, the position and signal intensity are determined for individual single-molecule images. For this purpose, fitting with a two-dimensional Gaussian distribution is usually used. Fitting functions can include background signals instead of the pretreatment of background subtraction. We usually use a Gaussian distribution on an inclined background plane as the fitting function [21]. Positions of the molecule can be determined as the centroid of the distribution with sub-pixel spatial resolution. Signal intensity can be calculated by integration of the distribution function. Accuracy of these parameters depends on the measurement system and should be determined statistically from the repeated measurements of the same single molecules.

There are several criteria to judge whether single molecules are really detected or not [4]. Single-step photobleach is the most convenient and used criterion (Figure 1D). To distinguish photobleach from disappearance by the movements of molecules, like release into the solution, illumination intensity should be changed. Photobleaching rate, but not the rate of most of other phenomena, depends on the illumination intensity. Because the size of fluorophores is much smaller than the spatial resolution of the optical microscope, the profile of single-molecule images must be the point spread function of the optics. The intensity distribution of single molecules should be Gaussian, because the photon emission from a fluorophore is a Poisson process; however, when the intensities are small, the distribution becomes binominal or sometimes looks as a log-normal distribution.

3.5. Technical limitations specific for SMI

Photobleach of the fluorophore seems to be the most serious problem in SMI. This brings a trade-off between S/N of the single-molecule measurments and the observation length of each single molecule. By increasing the illumination power, the signals from single molecules increase to improve S/N, which in turn improves the temporal resolution and the accuracy of position determination; however, at the same time, the observation length of each single molecule must be decreased due to increased photobleacing rates. In typical conditions, the emission photon numbers from a single chemical fluorophore, including TMR and Cy3, before photobleach is less than 1 million, and those from fluorescent proteins are several times smaller. Since SMI in typical conditions requires thousands of photon emissions from a fluorophore per frame (due to limited numerical aperture of the objective and tranmittance of the optics, <10% of which reach to the camera), only hundreds of frames can be acquired for each single molecule. If a video rate movie is taken, single molecules could be observed only for about 10 s in average.

Signal intensity (photon flux) of single fluorophores is limited, because the fluorescence emission cycle requires a finite time. The fluorescence lifetime, which is the rate-limiting parameter under strong enough illumination, of typical fluorophores used in SMI is about 1 ns, meaning that the maximum photon flux is about 10^9 s^{-1}. However, strong illuminations that cause such high-rate emission induce higher-order excitation that could be the reason of undesired photochemical reactions. Practical photon emission rate is no more than about 10^6 s^{-1}. This means that because thousands of photons are required to acquire a snapshot of SMI, temporal resolution of SMI is difficult to be improved to more than 1 ms. Accuracy of position detemination depends on the signal intensity. When more than 10,000 photons are obtained on the camera for a single frame, the centroid of a single-molecule image can be determined with 1 nm of accuracy [22]. Such high accuracy cannot be obtained with a temporal resolution better than subseconds.

The special resolution of the optical microscopy is worse than 200 nm. This limits the densities or the concentrations of the molecule to be observed, because in dense conditions, images of molecules overlap to inhibit single-molecule detection. The practical limits of the molecular density and concentration are about 10 μm^{-2} and 10 nM, respectively. Concentrations of most cell signaling proteins are thought to be within these limits, but those of structural proteins could exceed these limits.

4. Applications and DetaAnalysis

4.1. Single-molecule kinetic analysis

4.1.1. Principle

Durations and intervals of molecular interactions contain information about reaction kinetics. Hereafter, we call the durations of the colocalization of two molecules as 'on-times', and the intervals from the dissociation of two molecules to the association of the next molecule with one of the dissociated two molecules as 'off-times'. On-times and off-times can be measured for single events using SMI. Dual-color SMI (Figure 3) is possible to detect on-times, but in practice, due to photobleach, it is difficult to detect successive multiple on-times for a single molecule and not easy to detect even a single off-time.

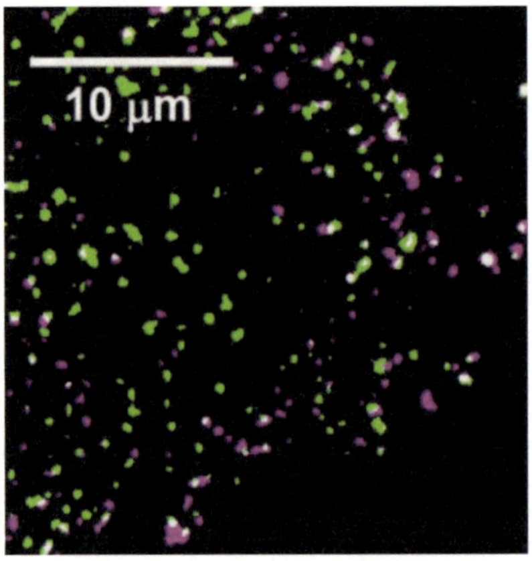

Figure 3. Dual-color single-molecule imaging of TMR-labeled epidermal growth factor (EGF; magenta) and GFP-Sos (green) in a living HeLa cell. Basal cell surface was observed using a dual-colour total internal reflection fluorescence microscope. EGF receptors (EGFR) on the cell surface are activated by EGF binding. Then, Sos molecule,complexed with Grb2, associates to the activated EGFR. White spots represent the EGF-EGFR-Grb2-Sos complexes in the plasma membrane.

More practical single-molecule measurements of on- and off-times are achieved for the interactions between a soluble molecule and a molecule stably attached on stationary structures. Because of the rapid Brownian movements in solution, soluble molecules cannot be observed as clear fluorescent spots and can only be imaged when they associate with fixed or slowly moving molecules. Therefore, *in vitro* SMI measurements, interactions between fluorescently labelled soluble molecules and a (non-labeled) molecule fixed on the substrate are often observed [1, 11]. In such cases, because different soluble molecules interact with a fixed molecule in turn, photobleach has minimal effect. Similar measurements can be achieved in living cells when interactions are observed between a fluorescently labelled soluble molecule (either in the extracellular solution or in the cytoplasm) and molecules in the membrane or cytoskeleton structures. Inside living cells, detection of the successive on-times as well as the single off-time is difficult by this way because of the movements and/or high

http://dx.doi.org/10.5772/52386

density of the non-labeled molecules. However, even in living cells, measurements of the waiting times of the first association after some perturbation and measurements of off-times are usually possible for kinetic analyses.

4.1.2. Estimation of the reaction parameters

Consider a reaction of state change,

$$\mathrm{A}\xrightarrow{k}\phi \tag{1}$$

Here, A and ϕ represent association and dissociation states, respectively, for example, and then k is the dissociation rate constant. The on-time distribution, which is the normalized histogram to show the fraction of on-times observed in each time interval from t to t+Δt, means changes of the nomarlized frequency to observe disappearance of the association state as a function of time. In other words, the on-time distribution represents the reaction rate to produce the dissociation state with time after the formation of the association state. (Disappearance of A state is the appearance of ϕ state in the reaction equation (1).)

Hence, the on-time distribution is the reaction rate equation,

$$\frac{\mathrm{d}\phi(t)}{\mathrm{d}t}=kA(t). \tag{2}$$

Here, the reaction is assumed to proceed according to a simple mass action model. Different from the kinetic analyses in conventional biochemical techniques that deal with the concentration changes, the reaction rate equations in SMI describe state changes of a single molecule with time; i.e., in equation (2), $A(t)$ and $\phi(t)$ do not mean the concentrations but the probabilities with which each of the states is observed. Because every single molecule takes one of the two states in this reaction model, and because at the starting point of each on-time the molecule takes A state, equation (2) has a conservation condition; $A(t) + \phi(t) = 1$, and the initial condition; $A(0) = 1$. Under these conditions, equation (2) is solved as $A(t)=\exp(-kt)$. Then,

$$\frac{\mathrm{d}\phi(t)}{\mathrm{d}t}=kA(t)=k\ \exp(-kt). \tag{3}$$

By fitting the on-time distribution with equation (3), the best-fit value for k is obtained.

This procedure is similar to that used in a conventional biochemical analysis based on ensemble-molecule measurements. However, there are two major different points between SMI and ensemble-molecule analyses. First, the initial condition $A(0) = 1$ is not always applicable in ensemble-molecule analysis. Second, and more importantly, in SMI analysis, the forward and backward reactions can be analyzed completely separately. In the presence of many molecules in the reactant, the association and dissociation reactions take place in parallel; therefore, in ensemble molecules, the reaction equation should be

$$A \underset{k_- L}{\overset{k_+}{\rightleftarrows}} \phi. \tag{4}$$

Then, the rate equation is

$$\frac{d\phi(t)}{dt} = k_+ A(t) - k_- L\ \phi(t). \tag{5}$$

Here, L means the concentration of the ligand molecule, which can be thought of as a constant in the presence of excess amount of the ligand. The solution for $A(t)$ under the same conditions, $A(t) + \phi(t) = 1$ and $A(0) = 1$, is

$$A(t) = \frac{k_+}{k_+ + k_- L} \exp\{-(k_+ + k_- L\ )t\} + \frac{k_- L}{k_+ + k_- L}, \tag{6}$$

indicating that the association (k_+) and dissociation (k_-) rate constants are never able to determined independently by fitting to a timecourse describing the concentration change of A state. (In ensemble-molecule measurements, obtaining multiple timecourses by changing the ligand concentration, L, the association and dissociation rate constants can be determined separately. However, in this case, there is an additional assumption that the rate constants are independent of the concentration.)

Reactions are not always as simple as described in equation (1). Multi-component reactions, described by a sum of exponential functions, are usual for proteins [11,15]. Also, reaction intermediates are sometimes involved. Such reaction structures could be noticed from the shape of the on(off)-time distributions. For example, sequential dissociations of two binding sites in a single molecule are described by the tandem reaction model [14],

$$A \xrightarrow{k_1} B \xrightarrow{k_2} \phi \tag{7}$$

Here, ϕ state is the off state again,and the on-time distribution is

$$\frac{d\phi(t)}{dt} = k_2 B(t). \tag{8}$$

At the same time,

$$\frac{dA(t)}{dt} = -k_1 A(t), \tag{9}$$

and

$$\frac{dB(t)}{dt} = k_1 A(t) - k_2 B(t). \tag{10}$$

Solving the coupled differential equations (8-10) under the conditions $A(t) + B(t) + \phi(t) = 1$, $A(0) = 1$, and $B(0) = \phi(0) = 0$,

$$\frac{d\phi(t)}{dt} = k_2 B(t) = -\frac{k_1 k_2}{k_1 - k_2}\{\exp(-k_1 t) - \exp(-k_2 t)\}. \tag{11}$$

This distribution is peaked; conversely, from the peaked distribution of on-times, presence of a reaction intermediate (or multiple intermediates) can be noticed. By fitting the on-time distribution by equation (11), two reaction rate constants can be determined. However, in this case, even two values of the rate constants are obtained, it is impossible to assign which one is the value of each rate constant, because k_1 and k_2 are interchangeable in equation (11). Additional experiments or information is required for the assignment.

4.1.3. spFRET measurements for detection of molecular interactions

In some case, more direct evidence for interactions between two species of single molecules should be required. Although the spatial resolution of optical microscopy is worse than 200 nm, the position (centroid) of each single-molecule image can be determined at nm-level resolution, if sufficient signal is obtained [22]. Dual-color SMI (Figure 3) allows detection of colocalization within several tens of nm in typical conditions. More accurate detection of direct molecular interactions is allowed by detecting single-pair FRET (spFRET) signal [4,23]. spFRET has a power to detect molecular interactions in crowding conditions, because FRET from sparsely distributed donors to dense acceptors yields sparse signal from the acceptors, which can be detected in single molecules [24]. However, usage of spFRET is limited due to its weakness to photobleach and difficulty to tuning labeling conditions to obtain high FRET efficiency.

4.2. Interactions between epidermal growth factor (EGF) and EGF receptor, and receptor dimerization

4.2.1. EGF and its receptor

Ligand-receptor interactions are one of the basic reactions in cell signaling systems. Here, we used SMI for detection of interactions between an extracellular ligand and receptor on the cell surface.

Epidermal growth factor, EGF, is a soluble cell signaling protein in the extracellular medium. EGF associates with its receptor, EGF receptor (EGFR), in the plasma membrane to stimulate cell proliferation [25]. EGFR is a single membrane spanning protein expressed in various types of animal cells. At the extracellular domain, an EGFR molecule associates with a single molecule of EGF; then, the conformational change of EGFR is thought to induce dimerization of two EGF-associated EGFR molecules. In addition to monomers of vacant

EGFR molecules, predimers of EGFR molecules (dimers without association of EGF molecules) are known to present on the cell surface. However, it is widely believed that only after formation of doubly liganded dimers (signaling dimers), EGFR molecules are activated through phosphorylation at the cytoplasmic domain. These phosphorylations are carried out through the mutual phosphorylations in the signaling dimers using the kinase activity in the cytoplasmic side of EGFR molecules (Figure 4). We tried to determine the kinetic process of EGF-EGFR associations and formation of signaling dimers of EGFR using SMI measurements [26,27].

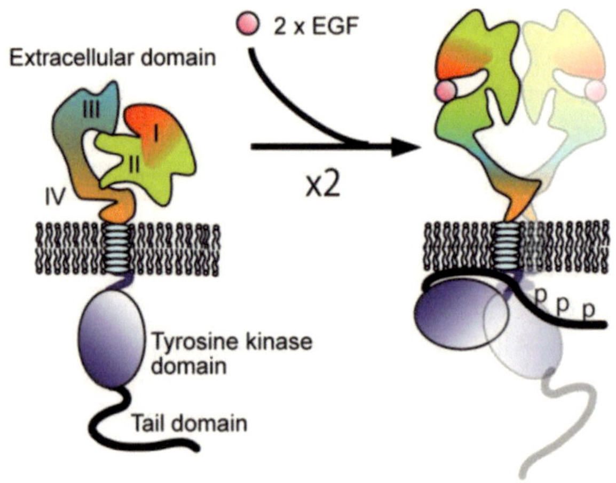

Figure 4. A schematic model of associations between EGF and EGFR and formation of signaling dimers of EGFR.

4.2.2. Single-molecule imaging of EGF association

EGF can be conjugated with chemical fluorophores like TMR at the N-terminus without disruption of its biological activity. After applications of nM orders of TMR-labeled EGF to the culture medium of cells under an oblique illumination fluorescence microscope, associations of single EGF molecules on the apical surface of living cells were observed in real time (Figure 1C). Movies of EGF associations were acquired in 20 frames/s. In this experiment, a human breast cancer cell line, MCF-7, was used. From the single-molecule movies, associations of single EGF molecules were detected individually as the sudden appearance of fluorescent spots on the cell surface (Figure 5A). When the association sites contained more than one EGFR molecule, the second associations were observed at the same positions of the first association sites. Some of the double association sites could be predimers of EGFR, and others could be two EGFR molecules presented in close proximity by accident. In our experimental conditions, no association site showed more than double association.

The association kinetics between EGF and EGFR were analyzed from the distributions of the waiting times for associations of single EGF molecules (Figure 5B,C). The waiting time distribution for the EGF association for the first EGF molecules could be described by a 2-component exponential function with rate constants of k_1 = 1.4 x 10^{-3}nM^{-1}s^{-1} and k_2 = 3.8 x 10^{-2}

http://dx.doi.org/10.5772/52386

$nM^{-1}s^{-1}$. The difference between two types of EGF association sites in the association rate constant of EGF has not been fully known, but it is possible that the latter (k_2) is the association rate constant of the first EGF molecule to the predimers of EGFR, because the association rate constant for the single association sites was the same as k_1 (Figure 5B).

The waiting time distributions for the second associations to the double association sites were peaked (Figure 5C). The distributions were analyzed using the tandem reaction model (equation 7). By changing the concentration of EGF, the rate constants for the intermediate formation (k_3) and for the association of the second EGF molecule (k_4) were assigned: k_3 was independent of the EGF concentration, suggesting that it was the rate constant for a conformational change induced by the first EGF association, while k_4 was proportional to EGF concentration, suggesting they were the association rate constants for the second association of soluble EGF molecules with the singly-liganded EGFR dimers. The values were $k_3 = 4.0\ s^{-1}$ and $k_4/L = 2.4\ nM^{-1}s^{-1}$. The intermediate between the first and the second associations of EGF molecules was first detected using SMI. These results suggest that the association rate constant with EGF is increased by the formation of predimer of EGFR and, after the association of the first EGF molecule to the EGFR dimer, increased further. These properties of EGF-EGFR interactions facilitate the formation of signaling dimers of EGFR. Similar results were observed on HeLa cells [26] and other EGFR family members on MCF-7 cells [27].

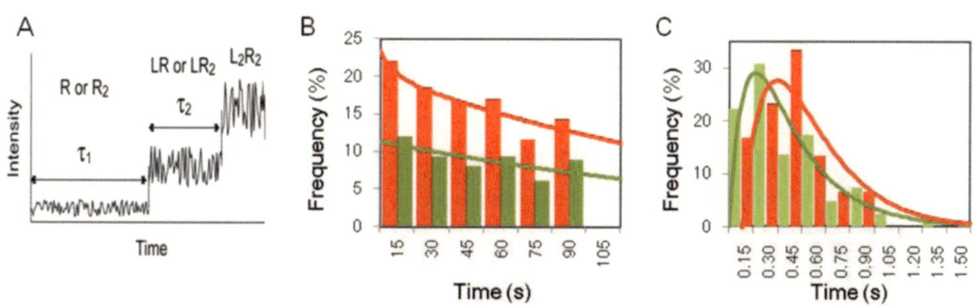

Figure 5. Single-molecule measurement of the associations between EGF and EGFR. (A) Single-molecule detections of the associations of EGF with EGFR are illustrated schematically. Waiting times of the association (appearance) of fluorescent spots on the cell surface (τ_1) were measured individually after the application of TMR-EGF to the cell culture medium. Second associations of TMR-EGF, which could be detected by a step-like increase of the fluorescence intensity, were observed in some association sites. The waiting times of the second association after the first association (τ_2) were also measured. (B) The distributions of τ_1 were measured for all association sites (red bars) and for the single association sites (green bars) in the presence of 4 nM TMR-EGF. The numbers of events were 57 (red) and 31 (green). Lines show the results of fitting with the reaction models. The red histogram was fitted with a two-component exponential function, suggesting the presence of two different association sites. The green histogram was fitted with a single-component exponential function. See text for the values of rate constants. (C) The distributions of τ_2 were measured in the presence of 2 nM (red bars) or 4 nM (green bars) of TMR-EGF. The numbers of events were 30 (red) and 81 (green). The distributions were analyzed by the tandem reaction model. In this model, the first and second steps are the state change and association of the second EGF molecule, respectively. Therefore, the reaction rate of the first step is independent to the EGF concentration, but the second step should be proportional to the EGF concentration. The best-fit values of the first-order reaction rate constants for the second step were 4.7 and 4.7 s^{-1} (2 nM), and 3.4 and 10 s^{-1} (4 nM), suggesting that the rate constant of the first step were 4.7 (2 nM) and 3.4 (4 nM) s^{-1}, and the

second-order rate constants were 4.7/2 (2 nM) and 10/4 (4 nM) $nM^{-1}s^{-1}$. The averages of the rate constants weighted with the event number are 4.0 s^{-1} and 2.4 $nM^{-1}s^{-1}$.

4.3. Interaction between a small GTPaseRaf and a cytoplasmic kinase RAF

4.3.1. Ras and RAF

As the second example of SMI kinetic analysis, intracellular molecular reactions of RAF were analyzed [14,28,29]. As a downstream signaling of EGFR, EGF stimulation induces activation of a small GTPase, Ras, on the cytoplasmic side of the plasma membrane. The active form of Ras is recognized by a cytoplasmic serine/threonine kinase, RAF, which is the MAPKKK of the RAF-MEK-ERK MAPK cascade; thus, RAF translocates from the cytoplasm to the plasma membrane upon activation of Ras (Figure 6A). The active form of Ras induces translocation of RAF but does not activate RAF directory. RAF activation was induced though phosphorylations by still undetermined kinase(s) on the plasma membrane. RAF contains two association sites for Ras (the Ras-binding domain RBD and the cysteine-rich domain CRD). In addition, RAF has at least two conformations, open and closed. In the closed form, due to intramolecular interactions, CRD and the catalytic domain (CAD) of RAF are covered from Ras and the kinase(s), respectively (Figure 6B). Thus, the kinetics of RAF activation in the ternary complex among Ras, RAF, and the kinase(s) should be complicated. Actually, the kinetics of RAF activation has not been known at all. It cannot be studied *in vitro,* since the kinase(s) is(are) not determined. However, in living cells, SMI measurement is applicable.

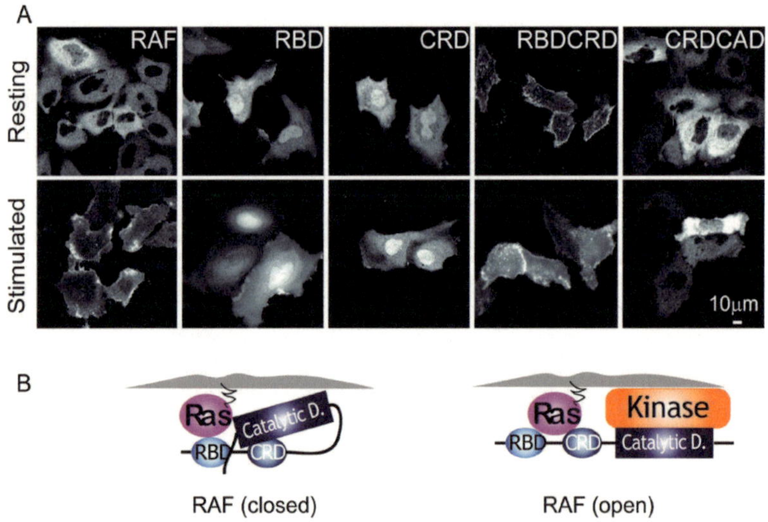

Figure 6. Translocation of RAF.(A) C-RAF1 and its fragments tagged with GFP at the N-terminus was expressed in HeLa cells and observed in ensemble-molecules before (upper panel) and after (lower panel) stimulation of cells with EGF. RAF (whole molecule) translocated from the cytoplasm to the plasma membrane. Translocation was not evident

for RBD, CRD, and CRD-CAD fragments. RBD-CRD fragments accumulated on the membrane independent of EGF stimulation. (B) RAF contains two Ras-association domains (RBD and CRD) and has two conformations (open and closed).

4.3.2. *Single-molecule imaging of RAF translocation*

C-RAF, which is a ubiquitous isoform of RAF, was tagged with GFP (GFP-RAF) and expressed in HeLa cells. GFP-RAF presented in the cytoplasm of quiescent cells and translocated to the plasma membrane upon activation of cells with EGF. The translocation of whole molecules of RAF was observed in ensemble-molecule imaging. Only a small amount of the RBD fragment of RAF showed translocation, and the RBD-CRD fragment bound to the plasma membrane independently of cell stimulation (Figure 6A). The RBD-CRD fragment with a mutation to inactive RBD (CRD) and a mutant of RAF in the open form with inactive RBD (CRD-CAD) did not show remarkable translocation to the plasma membrane in ensemble molecules, even after EGF stimulation.

Reducing the expression levels of GFP-tagged molecules, single molecules of RAF and its fragments were observed on the plasma membrane (Figure 7). For all molecules, transient associations with the plasma membrane were observed in single molecules after EGF stimulation, and for the molecules containing RBD (RAF, RBD, and RBD-CRD), associations of a small amount of molecules were observed, even in quiescent cells. The densities of membrane-associated molecules increased with overexpressions of Ras, suggesting Ras-specific membrane interactions of RAF molecules.

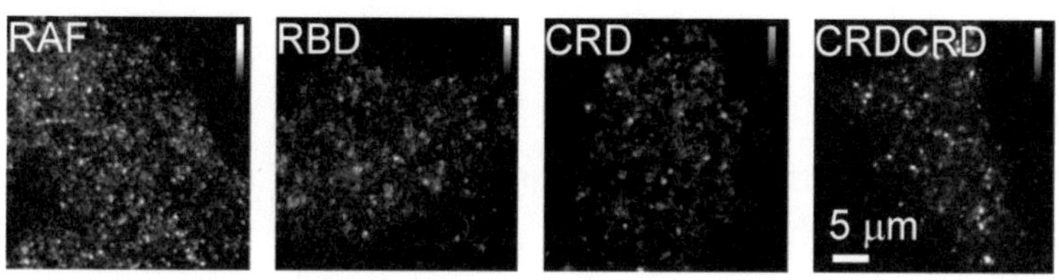

Figure 7. Single-molecule images of RAF and RAF fragments in HeLa cells. These images were observed in a HeLa cells 2-5 min periods after stimulation with EGF.

4.3.3. *Kinetic analysis of RAF activation*

On-time distributions of RAF molecules were obtained in cells after EGF stimulation (Figure 8A). RBD and CRD showed single exponential on-time distributions with the decay rate constants of 3.8 and 2.4 s^{-1}, respectively. Because the decay of on-time distributions is determined by both dissociation and photobleach as the reasons of disappearance of the fluorescent spots, the decay rate constants are the sum of the rate constants for dissociation and photobleach. After the corrections for the photobleaching rate constant, which was determined by SMI in fixed cells, the dissociation rate constants for RBD (k_1) and CRD (k_2) were determined as k_1 = 3.7 and k_2 =2.3 s^{-1}, respectively. Corrections of photobleach were also carried out in the following analyses (see supplement information of [28] for details). The on-time distribution of RBD-CRD was peaked, suggesting sequential dissociation of RBD and

CRD from Ras. Association with Ras using both RBD and CRD could induce firm membrane anchoring of RBD-CRD, even in the quiescent cells. Applying the dissociation rate constants of RBD and CRD, the on-time distributions of RBD-CRD could be described by the following reaction model [29]:

$$RC \underset{k_{1-}}{\overset{k_1}{\rightleftarrows}} C \xrightarrow{k_2} \phi. \tag{12}$$

In this scheme, RC or C represents the state in which the molecule associates with Ras using both RBD and CRD, or only CRD, respectively. Since it is known that CRD of Ras molecules associates with Ras very rapidly after the association of RBD to Ras [14], R state (in which the molecule associates with Ras only with RBD) was neglected in this reaction scheme. Using this scheme, k_{1-} (the association rate constant between RBD and Ras from the C state) was determined to be 1.0 s^{-1}.

RAF and CRD-CAD interact with the kinase(s) on the plasma membrane as the substrate. In addition, RAF contains open-close dynamics. Our previous study using spFRET [14] indicated that the initial association form of RAF with the activated Ras (in our time resolution of ~0.1 s) is an open conformation. The reaction model (equation 12) was extended to include the phosphorylation by the kinase.

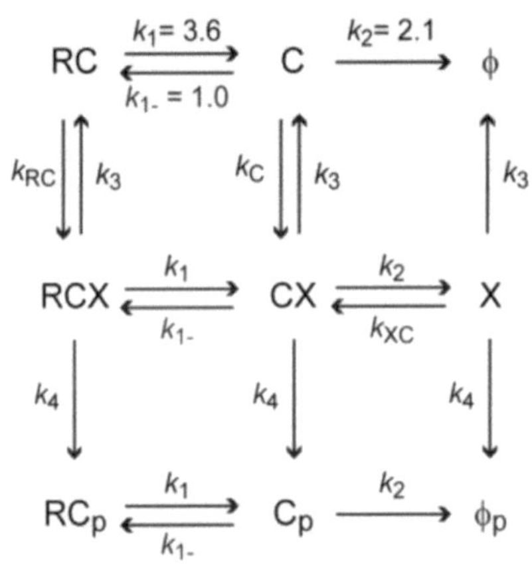

(13)

Here, for simplification, phosphorylation of RAF was assumed to be a single Michaelis-Menten type reaction. Suffixes X and p mean that each state forms complexes with the kinase(s) and is phospholylated, respectively. For the CRD-CAD fragment, RC, RCX, and RCp are not applicable.

Numerically solving the coupled differential equations for the time-dependent probability changes of the molecular states, functions to describe the on-time distributions of RAF and CRD-CAD were calculated and fitted simultaneously to the results of experiments to find the best-fit values of the rate constants. The results are shown in Figure 8B. The deformation of the RAF-kinese complex without enzymatic reaction was slow ($k_3 < 10^{-4}$ s^{-1}) and negligible, and the complex formation mostly took place from the RCX state, not from the C state. The large difference between the rates of complex formation with the kinase from the RC (47 s^{-1}) and C (0.6 s^{-1}) states suggests that interactions with Ras at the RBD and CRD coordinately work for effective presentation of RAF to the kinase. The very rapid association between RAF in the RC state and the kinase to form the RCX complex suggests a preexisting complex between Ras and the kinase. Simulation using the parameters determined by this analysis predicted that once associated with Ras, 95% of RAF molecules are released to the cytoplasm in the phosphorylated (active) form. Thus, efficiency of phosphorylation on the plasma membrane is high, and the overall activation level of RAF in cells should be regulated by the translocation from the cytoplasm to the membrane and/or dephosphorylation in the cytoplasm.

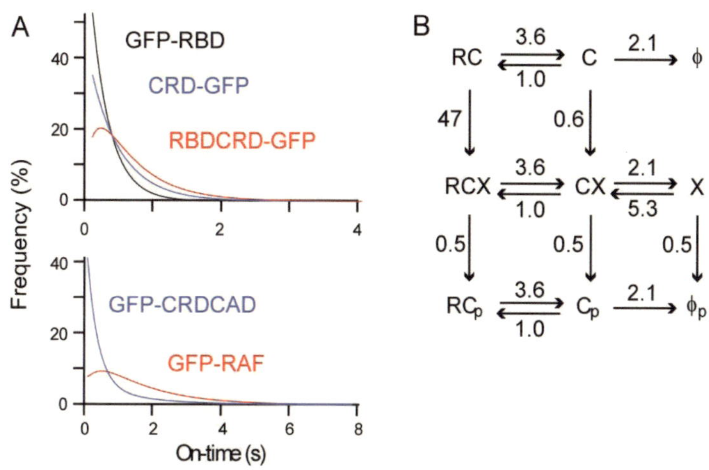

Figure 8. Single-molecule analysis of RAF activation. On-time distributions of RAF and fragments of RAF were analyzed. Results of fittings with the kinetic models are shown (A). The best-fit values of the reaction rate constants (s^{-1}) were determined (B).

4.4. Applications in toxinology

Kinetic analysis of the protein-protein interactions using SMI is a general technology, and there have already been several examples in toxinology. *Staphylococcus aureus* leukocidin fast fraction (LukF) and γ-hemolysin second component (HS) assemble into hetro-oligomeric pores of γ-hemolysin on the cell surface to induce cell lysis. Detecting spFRET between LukF and HS, Nugyen et al. [24] have succeeded in determining equilibrium dissociation constants between the molecules in the intermediate complexes during the pore formation.

A hydrophobic environmental sensitive fluorophore, badan, labeling LukF, has also been used to detect complex formation with HS in single molecules [30].

Groulx et al. [31] measured the stoichiometry of oligomerization of another pore-forming toxin using SMI. Monomers of *Bacillus thuringiensis* toxin Cry1Aa were labeled with a fluorophore at a cysteine residue. After the complex formation, molecules were attached on a coverslip to observe the photobleaching process. Counting the step number during the photobleach, it was concluded that the toxin forms a tetramer.

Nabika et al. [32] used SMI for observation of lateral diffusion of cholera toxin B subunit (CTX) on the artificial lipid bilayer containing GM1, which is the receptor of CTX. The diffusion coefficient was one order smaller than that of lipid molecules in the membrane, and there were higher (0.4 $\mu m^2/s$) and lower (< 0.1 $\mu m^2/s$) diffusive fractions. This observation was explained by assuming multivalent binding between CTX and GM1 molecules.

On the contrary, toxin has been used for single-molecule measurement. Since direct fixation of molecules to a substrate possibly induces artifacts in the measurements, single molecules are sometimes entrapped into fixed tiny liposomes in which the molecules can move more freely. In this case, however, the solution around the molecules cannot be changed during the experiment, limiting experimental conditions. Okumus et al. [33] used liposomes, reconstituting pore-forming toxin, to allow exchange of inside solutions.

5. Conclusions

As shown in this chapter, SMI can be used to detect molecular interactions between proteins and other biological molecules. In addition to detections of static oligomerization states, SMI allows characterization and analysis of dynamic reaction processes, including association-dissociation kinetics and enzymatic reactions.

Kinetic analyses based on SMI measurements have several advantages over analyses using conventional biochemical and ensemble-molecule imaging measurements: SMI allows quantitative measurements with minimal disruption of the system integrity. Actually, SMI is applicable to complex systems, like living cells, and avoids perturbations for synchronization. Measurements in complex systems are useful in analyses of the reaction kinetics between unknown elements, as shown in the case of RAF and the undetermined kinase(s). SMI measurements have often found novel reaction intermediates. This is because virtual synchronization at the reaction steps and complete separation between the forward and backward reactions are allowed.

These advantages of SMI measurements make them effective in quantitative analysis of biological reaction kinetics, providing basic information required in system-level analyses in recent molecular cell biology. In the near future, SMI measurements will be expanded to be used in pharmacology to provide novel drug screening methods and analyses of the sites of action for medical drugs, in pathology to detect currently undetermined dysfunctions of

http://dx.doi.org/10.5772/52386

pathological mutant molecules, and in toxinology for the analyses of molecular mechanisms of toxic functions.

Author details

Kayo Hibino[1], Michio Hiroshima[1,2], Yuki Nakamura[2] and Yasushi Sako[2*]

*Address all correspondence to: sako@riken.jp

1 Laboratory for Cell Signaling Dynamics, RIKEN QBiC, Japan

2 Cellular Informatics Laboratory, RIKEN. 2-1 Hirosawa, Japan

References

[1] Funatsu, T., Harada, Y., Tokunaga, M., Saito, K., & Yanagida, T. (1995). Imaging of single fluorescent molecules and individual ATP turnovers by single myosin molecules in aqueous solution. *Nature*, 374, 555-559.

[2] Sase, I., Miyata, H., Corrie, J. E. T., Craik, J. S., & Kinosita, K. Jr. (1995). Real time imaging of single fluorophores on moving actin with an epifluorescence microscope. *Biophys J*, 69, 323-328.

[3] Lu, H. P., Xun, L, & Xie, X. S. (1998). Single-molecule enzymatic dynamics. *Science*, 282, 1877-1882.

[4] Sako, Y., Minoguchi, S., & Yanagida, T. (2000). Single molecule imaging of EGFR signal transduction on the living cell surface. *Nat Cell Biol*, 2, 168-172.

[5] Shütz, G. J., Kada, G., Pastuchenko, V. Ph, & Schindler, H. (2000). Properties of lipid microdomains in a muscle cell membrane visualized by single molecule microscopy. *EMBO J*, 19, 829-901.

[6] Selvin, P. R., & Ha, T. (2008). Single-molecule techniques. *A laboratory manual. Cold Spring Harbor Laboratory Press New York.*

[7] Yanagida, T., & Ishii, Y. (2009). Single molecule dynamics in life science. *WILEY-VCHWeinhim.*

[8] Sako, Y., & Ueda, M. (2010). Cell Signaling Reactions: Single-molecule Kinetic Analyses. *Springer London.*

[9] Edman, L., & Rigler, R. (2000). Memory landscapes of single-enzyme molecules. *Proc Natl Acad Sci USA*, 97, 8266-8271.

[10] Kozuka, J., Yokota, H., Arai, Y., Ishii, Y., & Yanagida, T. (2006). Dynamic polymorphism of single actin molecules in the actin filament. *Nat Chem Biol*, 2, 83-86.

[11] Morimatsu, M., Takagi, H., Ota, K. G., Iwamoto, R., Yanagida, T., & Sako, Y. (2007). Multiple-state reactions between the epidermal growth factor receptor and Grb2 as observed using single-molecule analysis. *Proc Natl Acad Sci USA*, 104, 18013-18018.

[12] Sako, Y., & Yanagida, T. (2003). Single-molecule visualization in cell biology. *Nature Rev Mol Cell Biol*, 4, SS1-5.

[13] Sako, Y., Hiroshima, M., Park, G. C., Okamoto, K., Hibino, K., & Yamamoto, A. (2011). Live Cell Single-molecule Detection in Systems Biology. *WIREs Systems Biology and Medicine*, 4, 183-192.

[14] Hibino, K., Shibata, T., Yanagida, T., & Sako, Y. (2009). A RasGTP-induced conformational change in C-RAF is essential for accurate molecular recognition. *Biophys J*, 97, 1277-1287.

[15] Ueda, M., Sako, Y., Tanaka, T., Devreotes, P. N., & Yanagida, T. (2001). Single molecule anlaysis of chemotactic signaling in Dictyostelium cells. *Science*, 294, 864-867.

[16] Tani, T, Miyamoto, Y, Fujimori, E.K, Taguchi, T, Yanagida, T, Sako, Y, & Harada, Y. (2005). Trafficking of a ligand-receptor complex on the growth cones as an essential step for the uptake of nerve growth factor at the distal end of axon: a single-molecule analysis. *J Neurosci*, 25, 2181-2191.

[17] Uyemura, T., Takagi, H., Yanagida, T., & Sako, Y. (2005). Single-molecule analysis of epidermal growth factor signaling that leads to ultrasensitive calcium response. *Biophys J*, 88, 3720-3730.

[18] Tokunaga, M., Imamoto, N., & Sakata-Sogawa, K. (2008). Highly inclined thin illumination enables clear single-molecule imaging in cells. *Nat Meth*, 5, 159-161.

[19] Sako, Y. (2006). Imaging single molecules for systems biology. *Mol Syst Biol*, 10.1038/msb4100100.

[20] Betzig, E., Patterson, G. H., Sougrat, R., Lindwasser, O. W., Olenych, S., Bonifacino, J. S., Davidson, M. W., Lippincott-Schwartz, J., & Hess, H. F. (2006). Imaging intracellular fluorescent proteins at nanometer resolution. *Science*, 313, 1642-1645.

[21] Hibino, K., Hiroshima, M., Takahashi, M., & Sako, Y. (2009). Single-molecule imaging of fluorescent proteins expressed in living cells. *Methods MolBiol*, 48, 451-460.

[22] Yildiz, A., Forkey, J. N., McKinny, S. A., Ha, T., Goldman, Y. E., & Selvin, P. R. (2003). Myosin V walks hand-over-hand: single fluorophore imaging with 1.5-nm localization. *Science*, 300, 2061-2065.

[23] Murakoshi, H., Iino, R., Kobayashi, T., Fujiwara, T., Ohshima, C., Yoshimura, A., & Kusumi, A. (2004). Single-molecule imaging analysis of Ras activation in living cells. *Proc Natl Acad Sci USA*, 101, 7317-7322.

[24] Nguyen, V. T., Kamio, Y., & Higuchi, H. (2003). Single-molecule imaging of cooperative assembly of γ-hemolysis on erythrocyte membranes. *EMBO J*, 19, 4968-4979.

[25] Lemmon, M. A. (2009). Ligand-induced ErbB receptor dimerization. *Exp Cell Res*, 315, 638-648.

[26] Teramura, Y., Ichinose, J., Takagi, H., Nishida, K., Yanagida, T., & Sako, Y. (2006). Single-molecule analysis of epidermal growth factor binding on the surface of living cells. *EMBO J*, 25, 4215-4222.

[27] Hiroshima, M., Saeki, Y., Okada-Hatakeyama, M., & Sako, Y. (2012). Dynamically varying interactions between heregulin and ErbB proteins detected by single-molecule analysis in living cells. *Proc Natl Acad Sci USA*, 109, 13984-13989.

[28] Hibino, K., Watanabe, T., Kozuka, J., Iwane, A. H., Okada, T., Kataoka, T., Yanagida, T., & Sako, Y. (2003). Single- and multiple-molecule dynamics of the signaling from H-Ras to c-Raf1 visualized on the plasma membrane of living cells. *Chem Phys Chem*, 4, 748-753.

[29] Hibino, K., Shibata, T., Yanagida, T., & Sako, Y. (2011). Single-molecule kinetic analysis of RAF activation in the ternary complex among RAF, RasGTP, and the kinases on the plasma membrane of living cells. *J Biol Chem*, 286, 36460-36468.

[30] Nguyen, A. H., Nguyen, V. T., Kamio, Y., & Higuchi, H. (2006). Single-molecule visualization of environment-sensitive fluorophores inserted into cell membranes by Staphylococcal γ-hemolysin. *Biochemistry*, 45, 2570-2576.

[31] Groulx, N., Mc Guire, H., Laprade, R., Schwartz-L, J., & Blunck, R. (2011). Single molecule fluorescence study of the Bacillus thuringiensis toxin Cry1Aa reveals tetramerization. *J Biol Chem*, 286, 42274-42282.

[32] Nabika, H., Motegi, T., & Murakoshi, K. (2009). Single molecule tracking of cholera-toxin subunit B on GM1-ganglioside containing lipid bilayer. *e-J Surf Sci Nanotech*, 7, 74-77.

[33] Okumus, B., Arsian, S., Fengler, S. M., Myong, S., & Ha, T. (2009). Single molecule nanocontainers made porous using a bacterial toxin. *J Am ChemSoc*, 131, 14844-14849.

Chapter 18

Molecular Recognition of Glycopolymer Interface

Yoshiko Miura, Hirokazu Seto and
Tomohiro Fukuda

Additional information is available at the end of the chapter

http://dx.doi.org/10.5772/54156

1. Introduction

Saccharides on the cell surfaces play important roles in the living systems. For example, it mediate the cell-cell adhesion, fertilization, protein transportation, infection of pathogens and cancer metastasis etc [1, 2]. The saccharide-protein interactions also involve the various biological events (Table 1). Actualy, the saccharides are the model compounds of some of the medicines like oseltamivir [3]. The interaction between galactose and asialoglycoprotein receptor is a possible mechanism for the hepatocyte-specific drug delivery systems [4]. Therefore, it has been pointed out that the saccharide-protein interaction can be utilized for the novel bio-functional mateials such as cell cultivation, medicine target, and drug delivery systems.

	Target	Saccharide structure
Lectin	Concanavalin A (ConA)	α-Man/α-Glc
	Wheat germ agglutinin (WGA)	GlcNAc, Neu5Ac
Cell	Hepatocyte	β-Gal/β-GalNAc
Pathogen	Shiga toxin (from E. coli O-157etc)	Gb3: Gal1α-4Galβ1-4GlcCer
	Cholera toxin	GM1:Galβ1-3(NeuAcα2-3)GalNAcβ1-4Galβ1-4GlcCer
	Influenza Type A for human	Neu5Acα2-6Galβ1-4(3)GlcNAcβ1-, Neu5Acα2-6Galβ1-3GalNAcβ1

Table 1. The saccharide recognition of proteins, cells and pathogens.

The saccharide-protein interactions are also important in terms of protein analyses (proteome), because the interaction is important to clarify the biological function of proteins. [5] The saccharide immobilized substrates are investigated for the saccharide-microarray. In addition, the saccharide-protein interactions is a potential markar of various diseases like infection of pathogens (e.g. viruses, bacteria, Cholera, and Shiga toxin) and cancer. Therefore, the saccharide-protein interactions are also utilized for the biosensor of diseases.

In this chapter, we describe the materials with molecular recognition ability of sugars. Section 2 reviews the multivalent interaction between sugar and proteins. Section 3 presents the phisycal chemical properties of glycopolymers. Section 4 presents the graft of glycopolymers and the biomaterial fabrication. Section 5 presents the glycopolymer interface with dendrimer.

2. Multivalent interaction

The saccharide-protein interaction plays important roles in the living system, and the novel biomaterial fabriction is expected using the interaction. However, the saccharide-protein interaction is basically weak, and it is difficult to utilize and detect the interactions. It has been reported that the saccharide-protein interaction can be amplified by the multivalency [6, 7, 8]. Actually, saccharides on the cell-surfaces are displayed in a multivalent manner. The glycolipids form densely saccharide structures of lipid-rafts [9], and glycoproteins usually have multivalent saccharide structures, which provies the multivalent saccharide-protein interactions.

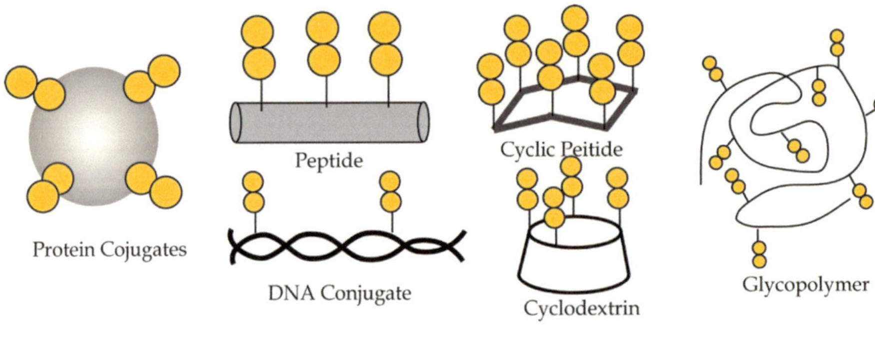

Figure 1. Schematic illustration of multivalent saccharide compounds.

The artificial multivalent saccharide displays also enables the multivalent interaction between saccharide and protein. Various artificial compounds with multivalent saccharides have been reported (Figure 1). Proteis are commonly used as carries for the multivalent presentation of antigens, and bovine serum albumin (BSA) is the representative [10]. Peptides are used as a scaffold of saccharide display [11]. Saccharide conjugates with DNA [12], cyclodextrin [13] and polymers have been also reported to exhibit multivalent interactions.

Saccharide conjugtes with peptides and proteins are appropriate structure for phamaceutical substances because of the biocompatibility and the fine structures. The glycopeptides toward shiga toxins (toxins from *E.coli* O-157 and enterohemorrhagic *E.coli*), influenza virus [14] and lectins [15] were reported.

2.1. Glycopolymer

There have been various multivalent saccharide derivatives as we described in the above section. Glycopolymers have been reported to exhibit larger multivalent effect comparing to other multivalent saccharides, because glycopolymers form large multivalent cluster [16]. The glycopolymers are the interesting compounds with large molecular weights and diverse structures. The glycopolymers are prepared by saccharide addition to polymer via polymer reaction, or by polymerization of saccharide monomers. The technique of synthetic polymer enables the preparation of versatile biomaterials. Especially, living radical polymerization is applicable to various saccharide monomers and provides the facile strategy for functional material preparation [17].

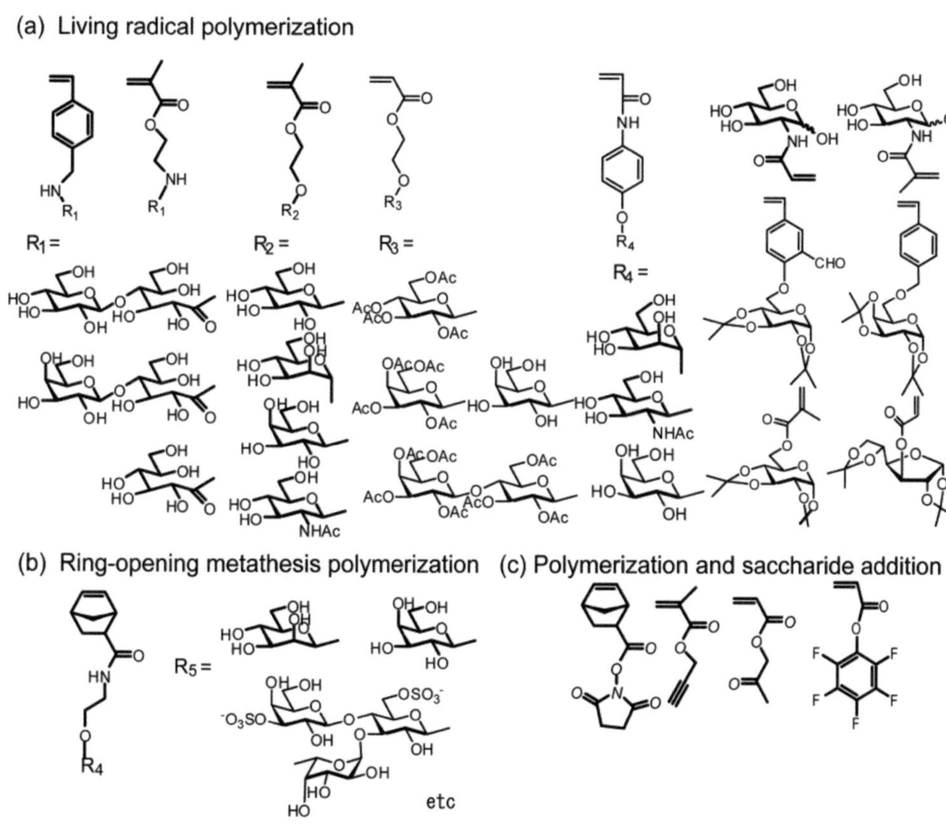

Figure 2. Chemical structure of monomers for glycopolymer preparation for (a) living radical polymerization, (b) ring-opening metathesis polymerization and (c) polymerization with saccharide addition.

The various saccharide monomers have been reported, which were shown in Figure 2. There are various saccahride vinyl compounds. Styrene [18, 19], methacrylate [20], acrylate [21], acrylamide [22] and methacryl amide [23] with saccharide were reported. Living radical polymerizations were reported with them. Norbornene saccharide derivatives were also reported, which provides the fine-tuned polymers via ring opening metastasis polymerization (ROMP) [24]. Reactive functional monomers were also utilized for glycopolymer synthesis. Monomers with acetylene [25] and active ester [26] were reported, where glycopolymers were obtained by polymerization and successive sugar addition.

Saccharide recognition proteins are called lectin, which basically have multiple domain structures [27]. The multivalent saccharides gain in enthalpy due to multiple binding to sugar recognition sites, and gain in entropy due to the various binding modes. The glycopolymers are large sugar cluster to gain the Gibbs free energy in both enthalpy and entropy, and lectins have multiple and valuable structure, which is advantage for binding. The distance of sugar binding sites is different with each lectin, which is easily tuned by copolymerization. The density, distance, and the size of multivalent compounds can be easily adjusted by copolymerization, which can be applied to variable lectins.

The glycopolymers are water soluble polymers, which can be utilized as artificial polymeric ligands or polymer drugs. Choi et al reported polyacrylic acid with sialic acid, and the polymer efficiently inhibited the sialidase of Influenza virus [6] Kobayashi et al reported the various glycopolymers. The lactose substituted polystyrene (poly(*N*-vinylbenzyl-O-β-D-galactopyranosyl-(1-4)-D-gluconamide (PVLA)) strongly interacted with lectin, and it was applied for hepatocyte culture [18]. Polystyrene with sialyl lactose showed the strong binding to influenza virus A [28]. Gestwicki et al prepared various glycopolymers via metastasis reaction, and reported the glycopolymers to bind lectin and *E. coli* [29]. Nishimura reported the glycopolymers interacting with glycosyl transferases to synthesize oligosaccharides, and they developed the oligosaccharide synthesizer with glycopolymers [30].

2.2. Amphiphilic property of glycopolymer

We defined glycopolymers as polymers with pendant saccharides. As we described above, the glycopolymers showed the strong multivalent effect based on the multivalency, with lectins, cells, viruses and bacteria. Another interesting property of glycopolymer is amphiphilicity. Glycopolymers via addition polymerization have hydrophobic backbones with C-C bond, and are amphiphilic due to the hydrophilic side chain. The side chain of glycopolymer is bulky structure, and so the glycopolymer easily form the self-assembling structure. The structure of PVLA in aqueous solution was analyzed by small angle X-ray scattering [31], and it was found that PVLA formed rod-like structure, where the rod had the structure with long axis 10 nm and shot axis 5 nm.The rod-structure was similar to some polysaccharides of amylose and sizofiran.

It has been known that amylose is a host of hydrophobic compound as it is known starch-amylose complex. PVLA also became a host compound of hydrophobic substances. We investigated the supramolecular polymer complex of PVLA. PVLA formed su-

http://dx.doi.org/10.5772/54156

pramolecular complex with various hydrophobic fluorophore and π-conjugate poymer of polythiophen [32].

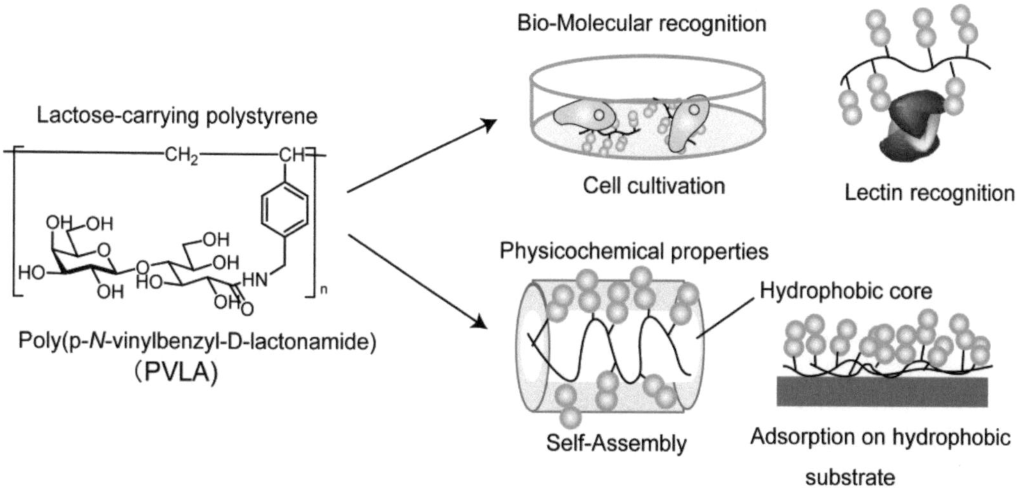

Figure 3. Chemical structure and properties of lactose-carrying polystyrene.

Self-assembling properties of amphiphilic polymers were used in order to organize the glycopolymer interface. The glycopolymer, PVLA, had amphiphilic structure and adsorbed to the hydrophobic interface [33]. PVLA adsorbed the hydrophobic polystyrene culture dish, and the culture dish was used as hepatocyte culture [34]. The adsorption of PVLA was investigated with hydrophobic self-assembled monolayer (SAM) of octadecyltrimethoxysilane [35]. PVLA selectively adsorbed onto the hydrophobic substrate, exhibiting the lectin and hepatocyte affinity. We utilized the adsorption process to fabricate the micropatterned cell cultivation system and protein display.

On the other hand, the self-assembling properties were expanded to the complex and micropatterned cell cultivation systems. We fabricated the micropatterned substrate with hydrophobic and cationic SAM The micropatterned substrates were fabricated by the formation of SAM and micropatterning with photolithography. The orthogonal self-assembly was performed with PVLA and anionic polysaccharide of heparin. PVLA and heparin bound to hydrophobic and cationic part, respectively. PVLA showed affinity to hepatocyte, and heparin binds to bFGF that has affinity to fibroblast cell. The multiple cell cultivation was accomplished with PVLA/hepatocyte and heparin/bFGF/fibroblast in a self-assembling manner [36].

3. Grafted glycopolymers

Glycopolymer-coated substrates were facilely prepared by self-assembly of hydrophobic interaction. However, it is difficult to control the density of glycopolymer by self-assembling process. In addition, the physical adsorbed polymers were fragile in a specific solvent condition. The coatings with spin-coat and Langmuir-Blodgett (LB) technique also provide the well-defined coating, but they are also fragile.

On the other hand, the surface-attached polymers are robust and practical to various purposes. In order to attach the polymer to the substrate, the covalent bond formation between polymers and substrates was necessary. The polymers with functional groups on the side chain and the polymer terminal were subjected to covalent bond formation with substrate. Those method is called "grafting-to" process. The grafting of the polymer was also reported via surface-initiated polymerization, which is called "grafting-from" method. The polymerization was possible to start from the substrate by surface activation with γ-beam, VUV and plasma irradiation, and by the radical initiator immobilization. The properties of the substrates depend on the polymer density, thickness and flatness. The grafting polymers are categorized as "pancake", "mushroom", and "brush". Generally, the grafting to method provides the non-dense grafting substrate like "pancake" or "mushroom" and the grafting from method enables "polymer brush" structure [37].

3.1. Glycopolymer-grafted nanoparticle via RAFT polymerization

In order to prepare the polymer-grafted materials, the living radical polymerizations are actively utilized by many groups. Living radical polymerization provides the uniform polymer, and polymer terminals can be modified. Atom-transfer-radical-polymerization (ATRP) enabled the dense-polymer brush. Since living radical polymer has active terminal end, the polymer terminal is possible to be modified. Specially, the polymers via RAFT process have the active terminal end with dithio- or trithioester. The polymer terminal with reversible-addition-fragmentation chain-transfer polymerization (RAFT) is converted to thiol by reduction or hydrolysis. Thiol is highly reactive and relates to various reaction like thiol-ene reaction, thiol-maleimide coupling, and Au-S interaction [38].

The glycopolymer conjugates have been synthesized via RAFT polymerization. Mancini et al reported a protein with glycopolymer via RAFT polymerization and disulfide bond formation [39]. Narain et al reported the prepration of particle by RAFT polymerization and subsequent Au-S bond formation [40].

We prepared the glycopolymer with *p*-amidophenyl glycosides (α-Man, β-Gal and β-GlcNAc) and acrylamide via RAFT process with (thiobenzoyl)thioglycolic acid [41]. The polydispersities were below 1.5 in spite of random copolymer. The obtained glycopolymers had dithioester terminal, which was reduced thiol by addition of $NaBH_4$. The thiol-terminated glycopolymers were mixed with gold nanoparticle solution. The gold nanoparticle (40 nm) was successfully modified by glycopolymer, which was confirmed by TEM observation and zeta-potential measurement. The glycopolymer modified gold nanoparticle was water soluble and stably dispersed for more than half a year.

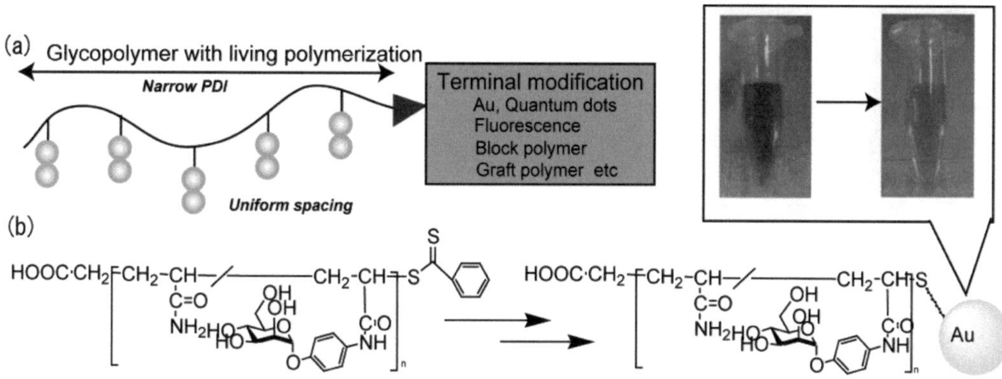

Figure 4. Prepration of a glycopolymer modified nanoparticle via RAFT living radical polymerization. (a) Properties and (b) a synthetic scheme of particle with a color change image of nanoparticle.

A glycopolymer modified gold nanoparticle stained pink color with peak top at 520 nm. ConA (α-Man recognition protein) was added to the α-Man-moidified nanoparticle solution, and the glycopolymer-gold nanoparticle showed the lectin recognition property. The color of the particle solution changed to blue, and the spectra showed the red-shift (Figure 4). The color changed occured based on the aggregation of nanoparticle by α-Man-lectin binding. The nanoparticle showed the affinity to a sugar recognition protein, and bacterium. The sugar recognition *E.coli* (ORN 178) was also added to the solution with glycopolymer-modified gold nanoparticle. The nanoparticle was adsorbed onto the periphery of *E.coli*, which was observed by TEM observation. On the other hand, *E.coli* without sugar recognition property (ORN 258) didn't show the change. The color change slowly occurred in 8 hours, while the color change with protein occurred quickly for 1-3 min. The color change occurred specifically with the corresponding lectin and glycopolymer.

Sugar modified gold nanoparticles were reported by other groups. Otsuka et al reported lactose substituted gold nanoparticles with PEG linker [42]. The gold nanoparticle also showed red-shift by addition of lactose-recognition lectin. Narain et al reported nanoparticle of glycopolymer having biocompatibility [43].

Advantage of the glycopolymer-modified materials is the specific recognition and bioinert property. The detailed protein affinity was investigated with surface plasmon resonance of glyco-polymer-modified gold substrate. The glycopolymer-modified gold substrate had affinity constants of 10^7 (M^{-1}) order, which was much stronger than the monovalent sugar of 10^3 (M^{-1}) order. At the same time, the glycopolymer-modified substrate showed the highly specificity to proteins. The amount of specific protein bounds (α-Man-ConA) was more than 15 times larger than that of non-specific binding (BSA, fibrinogen, and lysozyme) [44]. Interestingly, the glycopolymer-interface showed much better protein specificity than the artificial glycoplipid monolayers of self-assembled monolayer (SAM) and LB membrane. The hydrophilicity of the glycopolymer-modified gold substrate contributed the bioinert property.

3.2. Biosensing with glycopolymer-modified nanoparticles

We investigated the biosensing of the glycopolymer-modified gold nanoparticles.

First, the gold nanoparticles have been applied for biotechnology as a marker. We applied the glycopolymer-modified gold nanoparticle for lateral flow assay (immune-chromatography), where we tested the properties of particle with target analyte of lectin (ConA) [45]. Anti-ConA antigen was immobilized on the nitrocellulose strip, and the detection of target ConA was investigated with glycopolymer-modified gold nanoparticle.

Target protein of ConA was detected by the pink color of gold nanoparticle. We tested the glycopolymer with varying sugar ratio of 0, 6, 12 and 50 %. In terms of red-shift, the glycopolymer with higher sugar ratio (50 %) exhibited more red-shift. However, the nanoparticle with higher sugar ratio (50 %) was not appropriate for lateral flow assay. The gold nanoparticle with higher sugar ratio aggregated at the bottom line with addition of ConA. The glycopolymer with modest sugar content (6 %) exhibited the best indicator of ConA. The glycopolymer with modest sugar content was more flexible than that with higher sugar content, which improves the sensitivity in lateral flow assay. What is interesting about lateral flow assay is the biosensing with naked eye, using a simple device. The detection of ConA was possible from 1 nM level with naked eye.

Electrochemical biosensing was also conducted with glycopolymer-modified gold nanoparticle [46]. The gold nanoparticle was assembled on anti-ConA antigen immobilized electrode. The amount of protein bound was estimated by the electrohemical signal of gold nanoparticle, where the gold nanoparticle was electrochemically reduced in differential pulse voltammetry. The amount of ConA bounds were more sensitively monitored than that with lateral flow assay. The detection limit was around 0.1 nM.

These experiments were conducted using the model target of ConA. Since the protein-saccharide interactions are involved in various infection diseases, the detection of serious disease like influena and cancer will be realizable with the corresponding saccharide modified particle.

3.3. Protein separation with glycopolymer materials

The glycopolymer-modified interface showed specific affinity biomolecules, which can be applied not only for biosensing but also for protein purification devices. We modified the porous filter membrane with glycopolymer grafting, and prepared protein purification device. Basically, the purification and removal of specific biomacromolecules are mainly conducted by the size-exclusion process. For example, bacteria are able to be removed by filtration, which are called "sterile filtration". The size of bacteria was μm order, and so the porous materials with μm order pore are applied for sterilization. However, the size of proteins and viruses are nm level, which is difficult to apply the size-exclusion way. In addition, the filtration speed is strongly dependent on the radius of porous materials, and the flux speed of nano-level porous materials were too slow to use it practically. Therefore, it is almost impossible to attain the protein purification by nm porous membrane, and the affinity purification is appropriate to the purification and removal of protein and viruses [47].

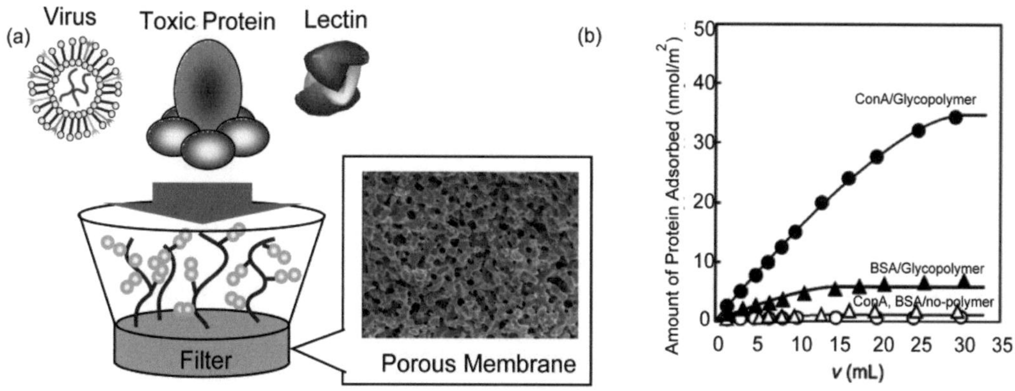

Figure 5. (a) Schematic Illustration of glycopolymer brush for protein and pathogen removal. (b) The amount of protein adsorbed on the glycopolymer brush.

We synthesized the glycopolymer with α-Man and trimethoxysilane units, and the glycopolymer was immobilized onto the porous siliceous materials via Si-O-Si bond [48] (Figure 5). The radius of the porous materials was 2 μm, which was much larger than the size of proteins and viruses. The porous membrane was connected to flow channel, and the protein solutions (ConA and BSA) was injected to the flow. ConA was selectively adsorbed onto the porous membrane, but BSA passed through the membrane due to α-Man-ConA interaction. On the other hand, the porous membrane adsorbed proteins by non-specific interaction. The amount of ConA bound was 34 nmol/m^2, and that of BSA was 4.2nmol/m^2. The modification of glycopolymer provides the affinity to specific protein and the bioinert properties to other proteins.

Li et al reported the filter preparation with sialyl-lactose modified chitosan [49]. The modified chitosan took up the influenza virus. The solution containing influenza virus A was passed through the filter, and the amount of virus was reduced about 1/200. The chitosan filter without sialyl –lactose didn't remove influenza virus. The influenza virus showed the affinity to sialyl-lactose via hemagglutinin. Muschin et al also reported the virus removal by sulfated curdlan modified filter.

Bio-separation with nanomaterials was investigated. Nagatsuka et al reported the protein separation with glycopolymer-modified magnetite. The glycopolymer with lactose modified magnetite was prepared by biotin-streptavidin reaction. The toxic protein of ricin solution was mixed with lactose-substituted nanoparticle [50]. The ricin was separated with maginetic. El-Boubbou et al separated sugar recognition *E.coli* with a similar manner [51].

4. Glyco-interface with precise structure

The affinity between saccharide and protein was strongly affected by multivalency. Therefore, the precise multivalent compound is useful to fabricate the efficient ligand and to clarify the protein function. For example, the precise mulrivalent sugars were reported with a starfish like compound carrying globotriose to exhibit the strong neutralizer of Shiga-toxin [52]. Matsuura et al reported the multivalent sugar with DNA template [12]. The multivalent sugar with precise sugar distance clarified the multivalent interaction based on the sugar distance.

Glycopolymer shows the strong multivalent effect, but generally the structure was not uniform. Dendrimer is regularly branched polymer with precise structure. Glycopolymer with dendrimer is useful to display saccharide in a precise manner [53]. For example, Roy et al reported various glycodendrimers with sialic acid [54]. The efficient ligand fabrication is expected with glycodendrimers.

The precise structure of glycol-dendrimers is applicable to the saccharide microarray, where the multivalent saccharide structure provides the various information. Those saccharide array can reveals the properties of proteins like multivalency, distance of saccharide, and the saccharide binding site.

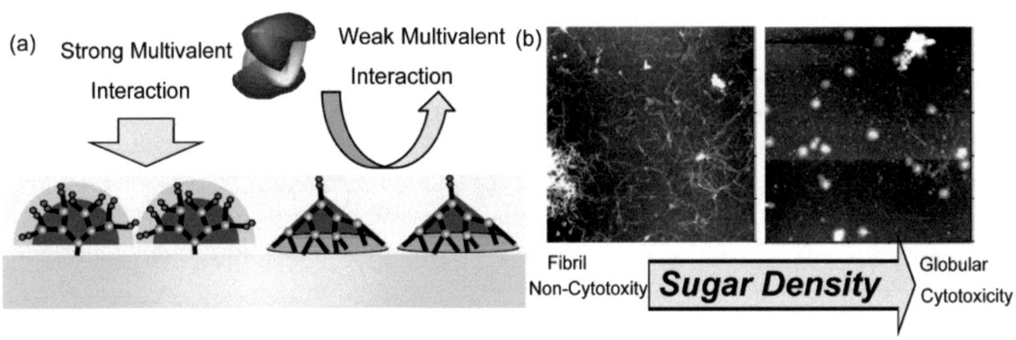

Figure 6. (a) Saccharide microarray with dendrimers. (b) The morphology control of Amyloid beta peptide with sulfonated glyco-dendrimer-interfaces.

The fan-type dendrimers with saccharide terminal was prepared by click chemistry of Huisgen reaction. The saccharide dendrimer with azide-core was immobilized via click reaction onto the acetylene-immobilized SAM. The protein-saccharide interaction of α-Man, β-Gal and β-GlcNAc was measured with surface plasmon resonance. The corresponding lectin showed the remarkable multivalency with higher generation of dendrimer array. Especially, the combination of α-Man and ConA was much affected by dendrimer generation increase [55].

Then, we prepared the glycol-dendrimer interface with 6-sulfo-GlcNAc, which is representative structure in glycosaminoglycans (GAGs) [56] (Figure 6). GAGs have been reported to relate the various biological events. We prepared mono-, di- and tri-valent 6-sulfo-GlcNAc, and the interaction with Alzheimer amyloid β(1-42) (Aβ(1-42)). First, the interaction was measured with SPR, where the divalent and trivalent 6-sulfo-GlcNAc showed the stronger interaction than monovalent one due to the multivalent effect. Interestingly, the morphology of Aβ was strongly affected by the multivalent array. In case of monovalent array, Aβ formed nanofiber with 8-12 nm width and 1-2 mm long. On the other hand, Aβ on the divalent and trivalent induced spherical objects. In the case of trivalent array, Aβ formed spherical objects with 500-600 nm diameter. The cytotoxicity of Aβ was depend on the microarray used, and Aβ showed the strong cytotoxicity on the trivalent 6-sulfo-GlcNAc array, where the cytotoxity of Aβ was related to the morphology of peptide.

Suda et al reported the dendrimer sugar chip with sulfonated trisaccharide of heparin (Suda et al., 2006). They synthesized mono-, tri- and tetravalent sugar chip with as SAM

They investigated the saccharide-protein interaction with hemostatic proteins. They analyzed the affinity of the protein quantitatively. They found the multivalent sugar chip with dendrimer was a useful tool to investigate the protein-saccharide interaction.

5. Conclusion

The molecular recognizable materials were prepared with glycopolymer immobilized substrates. Since the saccharides interact with sugar recognition proteins, cells and viruses, the glycopolymer immobilized substrates exhibited the biomolecules recognition. The substrate were applicable for the biomaterials.

Generally, the saccharide-protein interaction was weak. Therefore, the multivalent saccharide ligands of glycopolymer showed the strong affinity to proteins. Glycopolymers were amphiphilic polymers, and formed self-assembling structure in aqueous solution based on the hydrophobic interaction. The glycopolymer coating by hydrophobic interactionwas also possible in a self-assembling manner, and was used as hepatocyte culture.

The glycopolymers were also prepared via polymer grafting. The glycopolymer grafting was accomplished via both of "grafting to" and "grafting from"methods. The living radical polymerization of glycopolymers was important in both grafting methods. The glycopolymers were immobilized by "grafting to method"via RAFT living radical polymerization. The RAFT polymer terminal was converted to thiol, which modified gold nanoparticle with Au-S bondo formation. The modified gold nanoparticle had both properties of nanoparticles and glycopolymers. The color of the modified gold nanoparticle was basically pink, and the color showed red-shift by addition of the corresponding lectin, and bacterium. The modified gold nanoparticle was applied for the biosensing with lateral flow assay and electrochemistry as a marker. The glycopolymer grafted porous materials were prepared, and the porous materials were selectively filtered the saccharide recognition protein. The glycopolymer-modified materials showed the specific binding properties to the corresponding lectin based on the molecular recognition ability and the bio-inert surface property.

The glycopolymer substrates with glycol-dendrimers were also investigated. The glycol-dendrimers were applied to quantitatively measure the saccharide-protein and the multivalent interaction. These interfaces were useful to measure the detailed interaction and mechanism with pathogens or signal proteins.

Acknowledgements

This work was supported by a Grant-in Aid for Scientific Research on Innovative Areas (20106003).

Author details

Yoshiko Miura[1], Hirokazu Seto[1] and Tomohiro Fukuda[2]

1 Department of Chemical Engineering, Graduate School of Engineering, Kyushu University, Motooka, Nishi-ku, Fukuoka, Japan

2 Department of Applied Chemistry and Chemical Engineering, Toyama National College of Technology, Hongo-machi, Toyoma City, Toyama, Japan

References

[1] Varki A., Biological roles of oligosaccharides: all of the theories are correct. Glycobiology 1993;3(2): 97-130.

[2] Dwek R A., Glycobiology: toward understanding the function of sugars. Chem. Rev. 1996; 96(2): 683-720.

[3] Smith J R., Oseltamivir in human avian influenza infection. J. Antimicrob. Chemother. 2010; 65(2): 25-33.

[4] Hrezenjak A, Frank S, Wo X, Zho Y, Berkel T V, Kostner G M., Galactose-specific asialoglycoprotein receptor is involved in lipoprotein catabolism. Biochem J. 2003; 376(3): 765-771.

[5] Shimaoka H, Kuramoto H, Furukawa J, Miura Y, Kurogochi M, Kita Y, Hinou H, Shinohara Y, Nishimura S I., One-pot solid-phase glycoblotting and probing by transoximization for high-throughput glycomics and glycproteomics. Chemistry. 2007; 13(6): 1664-1673.

[6] Choi S K, Mammen M, Whitesides G M., Generation and in situ evaluation of libraries of poly(acrylic acid) presenting sialosides as side chains as polyvalent inhibitors of influenza-mediated hemagglutination. J. Am. Chem. Soc. 1997; 119(18): 4103-4111.

[7] Lee Y C, Lee R T., Carbohydrate-protein interactions: basis of glycobiology Acc. Chem. Res. 1995; 28(8): 321-327.

[8] Mammen M, Choi S K, Whitesides G M., Polyvalent interactions in biological systems: implications for design and use of multivalent ligands and inhibitors. Angew. Chem. Int. Ed. 1998; 37(20): 2754-2794.

[9] Matsuzaki K, Kato K, Yanagisawa K., A β polymerization through interaction with membrane gangliosides. Biochim. Biophys. Acta. 2010; 1801(8): 868-877.

[10] Amon R, Vangregenmortel M H V., Basis of antigenic specificity and design of new vaccines. FASEB J. 1992; 6(14):3264-3274.

[11] Lundquist J J, Debennham S D, Toone E J., Multivalency effects in protein-carbohydrate interaction: the binding of the Shiga-like toxin 1 binding subunit to multivalent C-linked glycopeptides. J. Org. Chem. 2000; 65(24): 8245-8250.

[12] Matsuura K, Hibino M, Yamada Y, Kobayashi K., Constructions of glycol-clusters by self-organization of site-specifically glycosylated oligonucleotides and their cooperative amplification of lectin-recognition. J. Am. Chem. Soc. 2001; 123(2): 357-358.

[13] Andre S, Kaltner H, Furuike T, Nihsimura S I, Gabius H J., Persubstituted cyclodextrin-based glycoclusters as inhibitors of protein-carbohydrate recognition using purified plant and mammalian lectins and wild-type lectin-gene-transfected tumor cells as targets. Bioconjugate Chem. 2004;15(1):87-98.

[14] Ohta T, Miura N, Fujitani N, Nakajima F, Niikura K, Sadamot R, Guo C T, Suzuki T, Suzuki Y, Monde K, Nishimura S I., Glycotentacles: synthesis of clyclic glycopeptides toward a tailored blocker of influenza virus hemagglutinin. Angew. Chem. Int. Ed. 2003; 42(41): 5186-5189.

[15] Singh Y, Renaudet O, Defrancq E, Dumy P., Preparation of a multitopic glycopeptide-oligonucleotide conjugate. Org. Lett. 2005; 7(7):1359-1362.

[16] Miura Y., Design and synthesis of well-defined glycopolymers for the control of biological functionalities. Polymer J. 2012; 44: 679-689.

[17] Armes M, Narain R., The effect of polymer architecture, composition and molecular weight on the properties of glycopolymer-based non-viral gene delivery systems. Biomaterials 2011; 32(22):5276-5290.

[18] Kobayashi K, Sumitomo H, Inai Y., Synthesis and functions of polystyrene derivatives having pendant oligosaccharides. Polymer J. 1985; 17(4): 565-575.

[19] Narumi A, Matsuda T, Kaga H, Seto T, Kakuchi T., Synthesis of amphiphilic triblock copolymer of polystyrene and poly(4-vinylbenzyl glucoside) via TEMPO mediated livng radical polymerization. Polymer. 2002; 43(17): 4835-4840.

[20] Ting S R S, Min E H, Escale P, Save M, Billon L, Stenzel M H., Lectin recognizable biomaterials synthesized via nitroxide-mediated polymerization of a methacryloyl galactose monomer. 2009; 42(24): 9422-9434.

[21] Fleming C, Maldjian A, Da Costa D, Rullay A K, Haddleton D M, St John J, Penny P, Noble R C, Cameron N R., A carbohydrate-antioxidant hybrid polymer reduces oxi-

dative damage in spermatozoa and enhances fertility. Nat. Chem. Biol. 2005; 1(5): 270-274.

[22] Gotz H, Harth E, Schiller S M, Frank C W, Knoll W, Hawker C J., Synthesis of lipo-glycopolymer amphiphilies by nitroxide-mediated living free-radical polymerization. J. Polym. Sci. PartA; Polym. Chem. 2002; 40(20), 3379-3391.

[23] Deng Z, Ahmed M, Narain R., Novel well-defined glycopolymers synthesized via the reversible addition fragmentation chain transfer process in aqueous media. J. Polym. Sci. PartA, Polym. Chem. 2009; 47(2): 614-627.

[24] Strong L E, Kiessling L L., A general synthetic route to defined biologically active multivalent arrays. J. Am. Chem. Soc. 1999; 121(26): 6193-6196.

[25] Ladmirai V, Mantovani G, Clarkson G J, Cauet S, Irwin J L, Haddleton D M., Synthesis of neoglycopolymers by a combination of "click chemistry" and living radical polymerization. J. Am. Chem. Soc. 2006; 128(14):4823-4830.

[26] Boyer C, Davis T P., One-pot synthesis and biofunctionalization of glycopolymers via RAFT polymerization and thiol-ene reactions. Chem. Cummun. 2009;40:6029-6031.

[27] Rini J M., Lectin structure. Annu. Rev. Biophys. Biomol. Struct. 1995; 24: 551-577.

[28] Tsuchida A, Kobayashi K, Matsubara N, Marumatsu T, Suzuki T, Suzuki Y., Simple synthesis of sialyllacose-carrying polystyrene and its binding with influenza virus. Glycoconjugate J. 1998; 15(11): 1047-1054.

[29] Gestwicki J E, Kiessling L L., Inter-receptor communication through arrays of bacterial chemoreceptors. Nature. 2002; 415:81-84.

[30] Nishimura S I., Toward Automated glycan analysis. Adv. Carbohydr. Chem. Biochem. Adv. Carbohydr. Chem. Biochem. 2011; 65: 219-271.

[31] Wataoka I, Urakawa H, Kobayashi K, Akaike M, Schimidt, M, Kajikawa K., Structural characterization of glycoconjugate postyrene in aqueous solution. Macromolecules 1999; 32(6) 1816-1821.

[32] Fukuda T, Inoue Y, Koga T, Matsuoka M, Miura Y., Encapsulation of polythiophene by glycopolymer for water soluble nano-wire. Chem. Lett. 2011; 40(8): 864-865.

[33] Tsuchida A, Matsuura K, Kobayashi K., A quartz-crystal microbalance study of adsorption behaviors of artificial glycoconjugate polymers with different saccharide chain length and with different backbone structure. Macromol. Chem. Phys. 2000; 201(17): 2245-2250.

[34] Kobayashi A, Goto M, Kobayashi K, Akaike T., Receptor-mediated regulation of differentiation and proliferation of hepatocytes by synthetic polymer model of asaloglycoprotein. J. Biomater. Sci. Polym. Ed. 1994; 6(4): 325-342.

[35] Miura Y, Sato H, Ikeda T, Sugimura H, Takai O, Kobayashi K., Micropatterned carbohydrate display by self-assembly of glycoconjugate polymers on hydrophobic templates on silicon. 2004; 5(5):1708-1713.

[36] Sato H, Miura Y, Nagahiro S, Kobayashi K, Takai O., A micropatterned multifunctional carbohydrate display by an orthogonal self-assembling strategy. Biomacromolecules. 2007; 8(2): 753-756.

[37] Zhao B, Brittain W J., Polymer brushes: surface-immobilized macromolecules. Progress Polym. Sci. 2000; 25(5): 677-710.

[38] Willcock H, O'Reilly R J., End group removal and modification of RAFT polymers. Polym. Chem. 2010; 1(2): 149-157.

[39] Mancini R J, Lee J, Maynard H D., Trehalose glycopolymers for stabilization of protein conjugates to environmental stressors. J. Am. Chem. Soc. 2012; 134(20): 8474-8479.

[40] Housni A, Gai H, Liu S, Pun S H, Narain N., Facile preparation of glyconanoparticles and their bioconjugation to streptavidin. Langmuir. 2007; 23(9):5056-5061.

[41] Toyoshima M, Miura Y., Prepration of glycopolymer-substituted gold nanoparticles and their molecular recognition. J. Polym. Sci. PartA. Polym. Chem. 2009; 47(5): 1412-1421.

[42] Otsuka H, Akiyama Y, Nagasaki Y, Kataoka K., Quantitative and reversible lectin-induced association of gold nanoparticles modified with α-lacotosyl-ω-mercapto-poly(ethylene glycol). J. Am. Chem. Soc. 2001; 123(34): 8226-8230.

[43] Housni A, Ahmaed M, Liu S, Narain R., Monodisperse protein stabilized gold nanoparticles via simpla photochemical process. 2008; 112(32): 12282-12290.

[44] Toyoshima M, Oura T, Fukuda T, Matsumoto E, Miura Y., Biological specific recognition of glycopolymer-modified interfaces by RAFT living radical polymerization. Polymer J. 2010; 42: 172-178.

[45] Ishii J, Toyoshima M, Chikae M, Takamura Y, Miura Y., Preparation of glycopolymer-modified gold nanoparticles and a new approach for a lateral flow assay. Bull Chem. Soc. Jpn. 2011; 84(5): 466-470.

[46] Ishii J, Chikae M, Toyoshima M, Ukita Y, Miura Y, Takamura Y., Electrochemical assay for saccharide-protein interactions using glycopolymer-modified gold nanoparticles. Electrochem. Commun. 2011; 13(8):830-833.

[47] Optiz L, Lenhmann S, Reichi U, Wolff M W., Sulfated membrane adsorbes for economic pseudo-affinity capture of influenza virus particles. Biotechnol. Bioeng. 2009; 103(6) 1144-1154.

[48] Seto H, Ogata Y, Murakami T, Hoshino Y, Miura Y., Selective protein separation using siliceous materials with a trimethoxysilane-containing glycopolymer. ACS Appl. Mater. Interfaces. 2012; 4(1), 411-417.

[49] Li X, Wu P, Gao G F, Cheng S., Carbohydrate-functionalized chitosan fiber for influenza virus capture. Biomacromolecules.2011;12(11): 3962-3969.

[50] Nagatsuka T, Uzawa H, Ohsawa I, Seto Y, Nishida Y., Use of lactose against the deadly biological toxin Ricin. ACS Appl Mater. Interfaces. 2010; 2(4): 1081-1085.

[51] El-Boubbou K, Gruden C, Huang X., Magnetic glycol-nanoparticles: a unique tool of rapid pathogen detection, decontamination, and strain differentiation. J. Am. Chem. Soc. 2007; 129(44): 13392-13393.

[52] Kitov P I, Sadowska J M, Mulvey G, Armstrong G D, Ling H, Pannu N S, Read R J, Bundle D R., Shiga-like toxin are neutralized by tailored multivalent carbohydrate ligands. Nature. 2000; 403: 669-672.

[53] Wolfenden M L, Cloninger M J., Mannose/glucose-functionalizied dendrimers to investigate the predictable tenability of multivalent interactions. J. Am. Chem. Soc. 2005; 127(35): 12168-12169.

[54] Carbre Y M, Roy R., Design and creativity in synthesis of multivalent neoglycoconjugates. Adv. Carbohydr. Chem. Biochem. 2010; 63(10), 165-393.

[55] Fukuda T, Onogi S, Miura Y., Dendritic sugar-microarrays by click chemistry. Thin Solid Films. 2009; 518(2): 880-888.

[56] Fukuda T, Matsumoto E, Onogi S, Miura Y., Aggregation of Alzheimer amyloid β peptide (1-42) on the multivalent sulfonated sugar interface. Bioconjugate Chem. 2010; 21(6):1079-1086.

[57] Suda Y, Arano A, Fukui Y, Koshida S, Wakao M, Nishimura T, Kusumoto S, Sobel M., Immobilization and clustering of structurally defined oligosaccharides for sugar chips: an improved method for surface plasmon resonance analysis of protein-carbohydrate interactions. Bioconjugate Chem. 2006; 17(5): 1125-1135.

Chapter 19

Cyclodextrin Based Spectral Changes

Lida Khalafi and Mohammad Rafiee

Additional information is available at the end of the chapter

http://dx.doi.org/10.5772/52824

1. Introduction

1.1. Cyclodextrins

A cyclodextrin (CyD) is a cyclic oligomer of α-D-glucose formed by the action of certain enzymes, Bacillus amylobacter, on starch. The first reported reference to a cyclodextrin was published by Villiers in 1891 [1]. Three cyclodextrins are readily available: α-CyD, β-CyD and γ-CyD having six, seven and eight glucose units respectively. They are commonly referred to as the native CyDs. For a long time, only the three parent CyDs were known, but during the past decade many covalently modified CyDs have been prepared from the native forms [2].

The glucose units are connected through glycosidic α-1,4 bonds. As a consequence of the $^4C_1$ conformation of the glucopyranose units, all secondary hydroxyl groups are situated on one of the two edges of the ring, whereas all the primary ones are placed on the other edge. The ring, in reality, is a conical cylinder, which is frequently characterized as a doughnut or wreath-shaped truncated cone. It is, of course, the possession of this cavity that makes the CyDs attractive subjects for study. The most notable feature of cyclodextrins is their ability to form inclusion complexes (host–guest complexes) with a very wide range of solid, liquid and gaseous compounds. Complex formation is a dimensional fit between host cavity and guest molecule [3]. This phenomenon bears the name molecular recognition [4].

1.2. Inclusion complex formation

The lipophilic cavity of cyclodextrin molecules provides a microenvironment into which appropriately sized non-polar moieties can enter to form inclusion complexes [5]. No covalent bonds are broken or formed during formation of the inclusion complex [6]. The first driving force of complex formation is release of enthalpy-rich water molecules from the cavity. The second critical factor is the thermodynamic interactions between the different components of the system (cyclodextrin, guest, solvent). The cavity size of the toroidally shaped CyDs and the structural confrmation and size of the guest molecule are the other parameters that mostly affect the formation of a guest-CyD complex [2]. As the results of this inclusion, changes of the chemical or physical properties of both host and guest molecules are generally observed; opening a wide field of applications in many areas and allowing one to monitor the process by several experimental techniques [2,7-9].

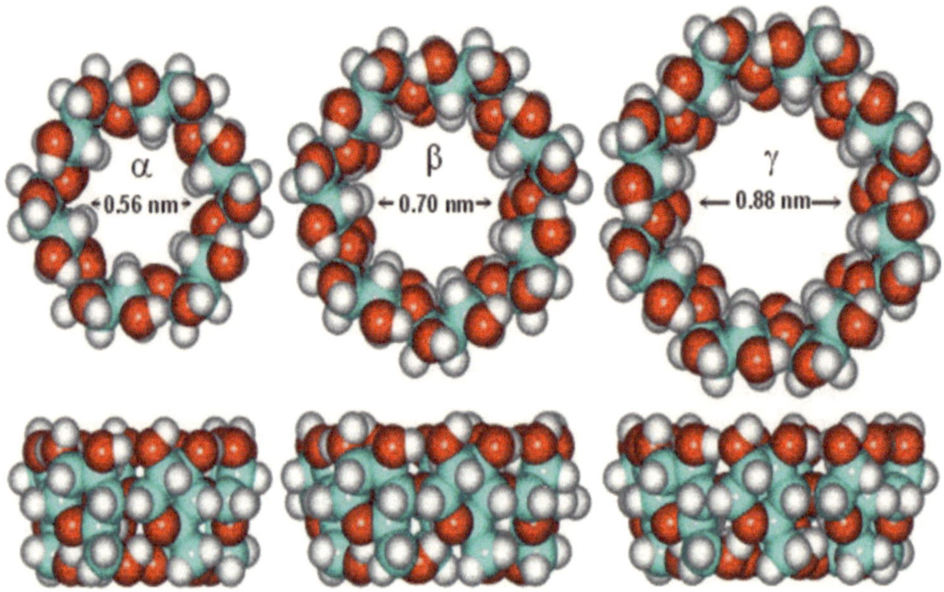

Figure 1. Structure of α-CyD, β-CyD and γ-CyD

2. Results

2.1. Cyclodextrin based spectral changes

As the result of inclusion complexes formation, the guest molecule is surrounded by the hydrophobic microenvironment of the CyD cavity. This environmental changes cause to some considerable changes in chemical properties of guest molecule such as equilibria and kinetic parameters and some changes in physical properties such as absorption coefficient or quantum yield, these changes strongly depend on the difference between CyD cavity and the outer medium.

Spectroscopic techniques are the most frequent ones which have been used for the study of these changes. Although it should be noted that the phase-solubility is one of the simplest techniques which have been used other than spectroscopy [10].

http://dx.doi.org/10.5772/52824

Some of the spectroscopic techniques such as UV-Visible, fluorescence, and NMR spectroscopy are compatible for the spectral study of the complexes that obtained in solution [11]. But the infrared spectroscopy, X-ray diffraction, scanning electron microscopy techniques [12,13] and differential scanning calorimetry [14], are suitable for the inclusion compounds that obtained in the solid state.

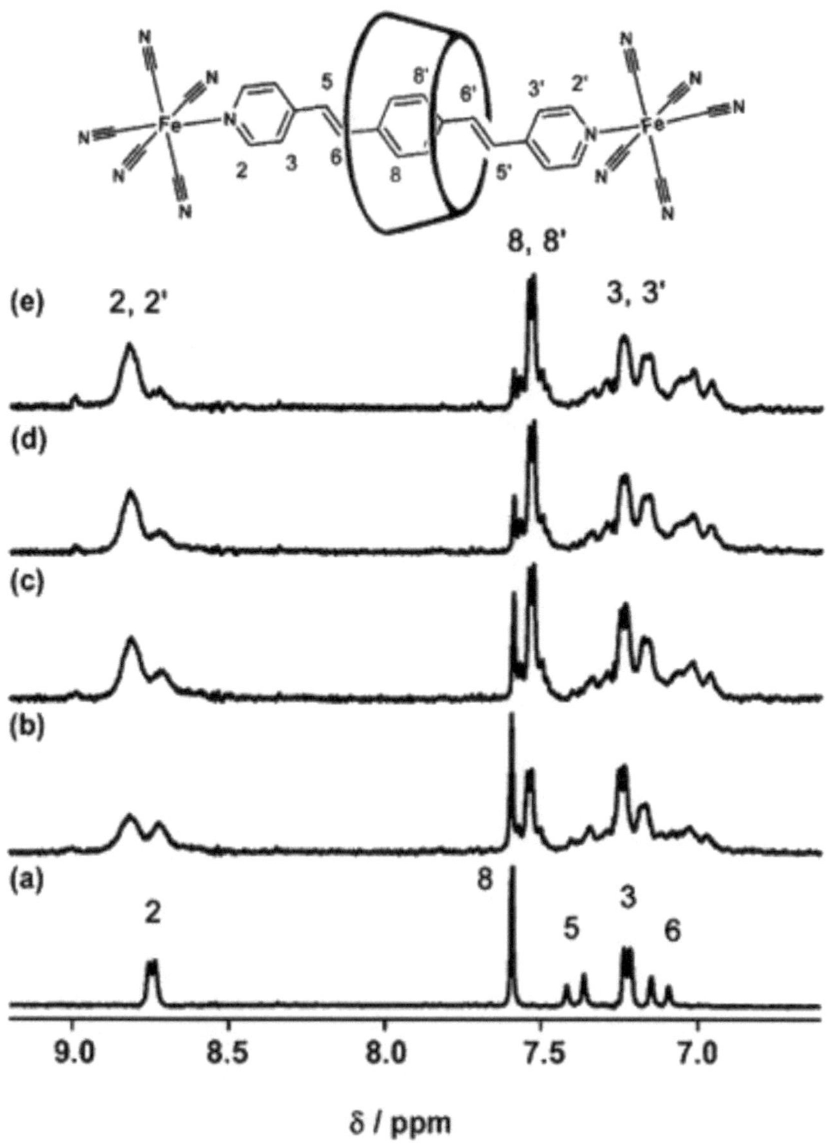

Figure 2. NMR spectra of the trans-1,4-bis[(4-pyridyl)ethenyl]benzene (BPEB) bridged ligand as function of time for the self-assembling $\{[Fe(CN_5)]_2(BPEB.\beta\text{-}CyD)\}^{6-}$ rotaxane, upon addition of 2 equivalents of β-CyD to the dimer in D_2O: (a) 0 min, (b) 5 min, (c) 30 min, (d) 60 min and (e) 24 hours.

Among the above techniques some of them such as X-ray diffraction and NMR are proper for obtaining qualitative information about the inclusion complex. For example ^{1}H NMR spectra can give us some information about the host to guest mole ratios and stability constant and even the orientation of the guest in the host cavity in solution which no other technique can give.

This section provides a condensed overview of the quantitative applications of host-guest interactions and molecular recognition which are well-matched with more quantitative techniques such as UV-Vis absorption and fluorescence.

2.2. UV. Vis. Spectral changes

In spite of the small effects encountered in absorption, peak shifts of the order of a few nm and changes of the absorption coefficients less than ten percent, UV-Vis spectrometry is an easily performed first test of the occurrence of complexation in particular in nonfluorescing systems. Moreover, the power of modern chemometric techniques allows valuable analytical applications of small effects of CyD inclusion on UV-Vis spectra. The emphasis of absorption changes and absorption studies will be on the apparent changes in the chemical properties of guest molecules, such as acid–base equilibrium. The most distinguished work in this field is report by Taguchi [15]. He has demonstrated that upon the binding of phenolphthalein to β-CyD cavity in aqueous solution at pH 10.5, the red-colored dianion form is rapidly transformed into a colorless lactonoid form.

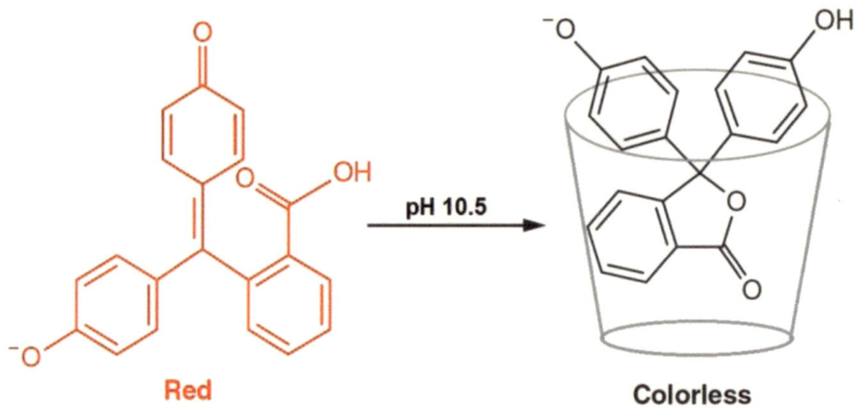

Figure 3. Proposed mechanism for the colour change of phenolphetalein in the presence of β-CyD.

This effect and some other similar spectral changes may reflect the altered polarity of the cavity microenvironment and preferential or specific guest–host interactions and stabilization of the preferred form and suppression of the other form in equilibrium. This is not a comprehensive review but is mainly intended to provide illustrative examples.

The absorption spectrum of mycophenolate mofetil (MMF) at mild acidic solutions shows an absorption band which has an absorption maximum at 302 nm for its acidic form (HMF). With the increasing of pH, the absorption at 302 nm gradually decreased whereas the absorption with the 340 nm maximum, for the basic (MF^-) form, increased, Fig.4. These spectral changes and presence of an isobestic point indicate the presence of acid base equilibrium for this immunosuppressant drug.

The spectra of MMF in the presence of varying amounts of β-CyD at constant pH that both acidic and basic forms are presented in solution are shown in Fig. 5. The spectral change by increasing the β-CyD concentrations at constant pH is similar to the decreasing the pH of aqueous MMF solution. These spectral changes indicate suppression of the basic form and dominance of acidic form in the presence of β-CyD cavity.

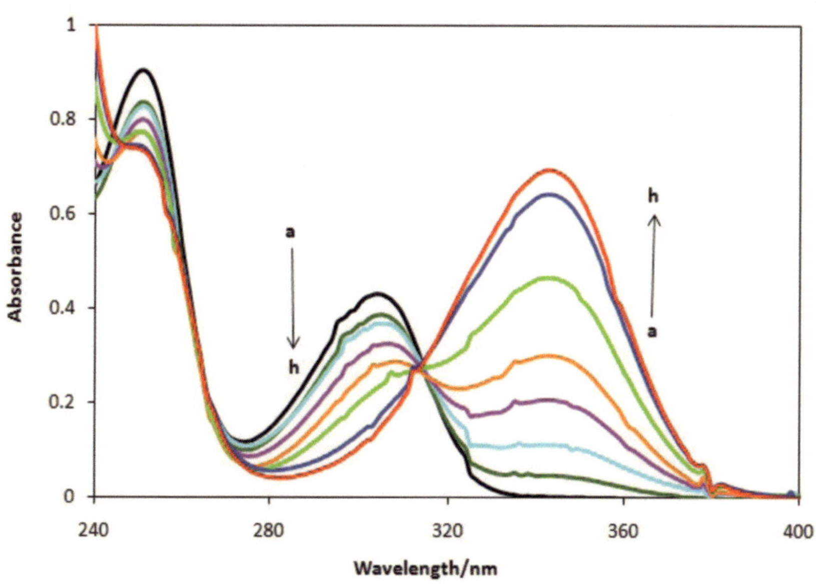

Figure 4. The absorption spectra for 4.0×10^{-4} mol L^{-1}MMF at various pH values. The pH values are (a) 5.0, (b) 6.5, (c) 7.0, (d) 7.5, (e) 8.0, (f) 8.5, (g) 9.0 and (h) 9.5. [Reprinted from Khalafi L, Rafiee M, Mahdiun F, Sedaghat S. / Spectrochim. Acta Part A., 2012; 90 45-49 with permission from Elsevier Science.]

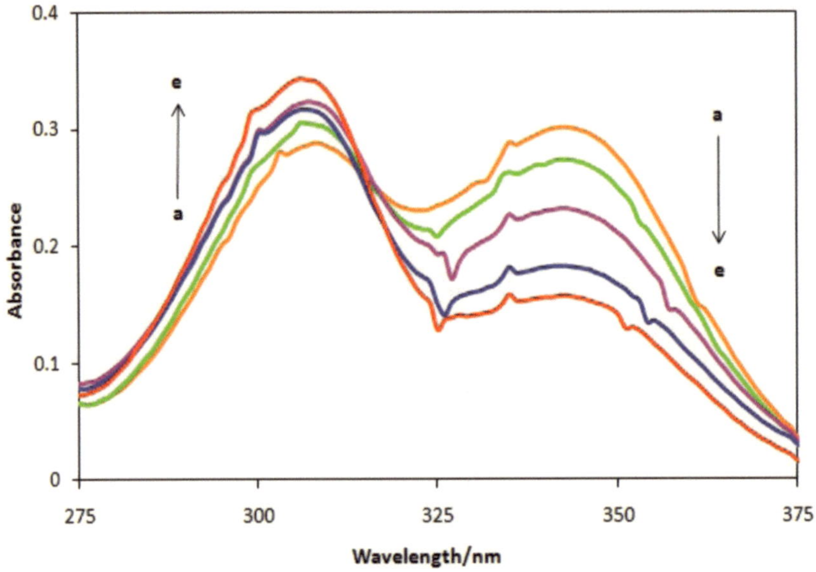

Figure 5. The absorption spectra for 4.0×10^{-4} mol L^{-1}MMF in the presence of different concentrations of β-CyD at pH 8.0. The concentrations of β-CyD are: (a) 0.0, (b) 1.0×10^{-3}, (c) 2.0×10^{-3}, (d) $4.0\times10^{-3}$and (e) 8.0×10^{-3} M. [Reprinted from Khalafi L, Rafiee M, Mahdiun F, Sedaghat S. / Spectrochim. Acta Part A., 2012; 90 45-49 with permission from Elsevier Science.]

Rank Annihilation Factor Analysis (RAFA) is used as an efficient chemometrics algorithm for the analysis of spectrophotometric data and the conditional acidity constant of MMF and the stability constant of its acidic and basic forms were obtained in the absence and presence of β-CyD. Based on these results with increasing β-CyD concentration the acidic form stabilized and the equilibrium of the system driving to produce acidic form. Consequently the conditional acidity constant decrease with increasing the β-CyD concentration [16]. The spectrophotometric study of neutral red and 4-nitrophenol in the presence of β-CyD are the other examples of spectral changes with different preferential complexation.

In the case of neutral red the increase in the acidity constants as a function of β-CyD is indicative of more stabilization of basic (neutral) form rather than positively charged acidic form. Whereas the study of acid-base equilibrium of 4-nitrophenol show that 4-nitrophenolate (the negatively charged basic form) has more affinity than the acidic (neutral) form. It has been claimed that the driving force of more stable inclusion complex of 4-nitrophenolate with β-CyD is the hydrogen bonding [17, 18].

The above results and some other comprehensive studies show the effect of interaction of guest molecules with microenvironment of β-CyD cavity. The CyD nanocavity has the characters similar to an 80% dioxane/water solution and provides a slightly alkaline environment [19]. There are four possible interactions including; hydrophobic, hydrogen binding, Van der Waals forces and donor-acceptor for the cavity that affect the favored interaction, equilibrium shift and spectral changes in the presence of β-CyD [20-22].

http://dx.doi.org/10.5772/52824

2.3. UV. Vis. based Molecular recognition:

The spectral change of an indicator may not be important in molecular recognition itself, but there is an important concept named as "indicator displacement assay" and/or "spectral displacement" which have been developed considering theses spectral changes. Spectral displacement method involves the color changes upon addition of competitive guest molecules; the dye moiety was excluded from the CyD cavity and located in the aqueous media. In that state, by environmental changes around the dye moiety, the dye moiety shows its normal color changes resulting from pH changes [23].

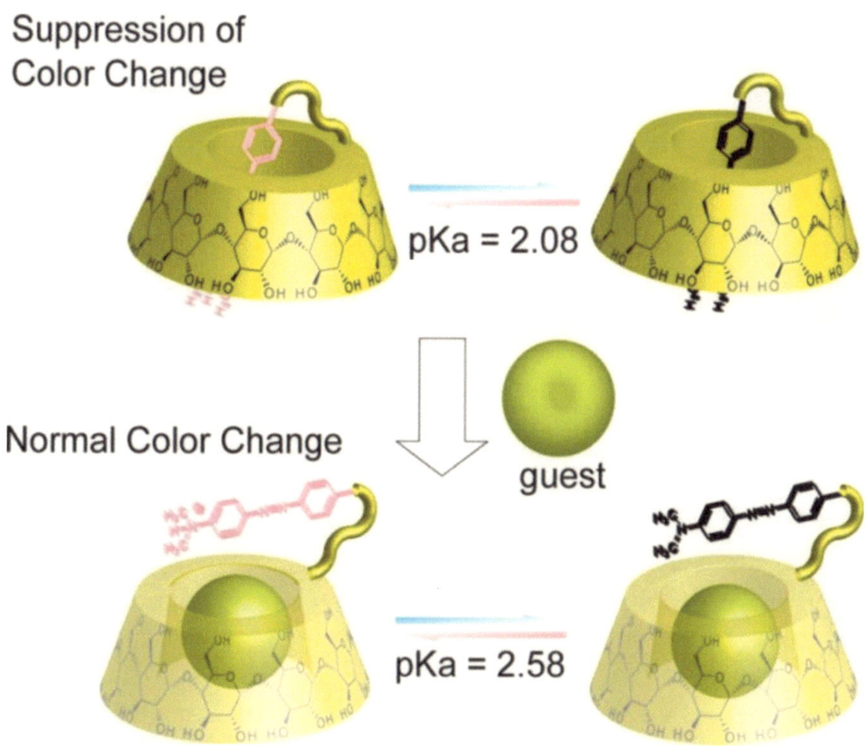

Figure 6. *p*-Methyl red appended β-CyD chemical sensor

A spectroscopic displacement method is used to determine association constants or the concentrations of the compounds that are spectroscopically transparent. Each application may be divided into two classes, the first one is based on competitive inclusion of guest and indicator in the solution, and the second one is the competition of dissolved guest with the CyD bonded indicators.

The success of the visible spectral displacement technique involving methyl red, in bonded form, as the competing reagent applied for the construction of molecular sensor for adamanetanccarboxylic acid, adamantanol, borneol, cyclaxtanol, cyclohexanol and same structures [24,25].

The spectrophotometric technique involving phenolphthalein as the competing reagent appears to be the most promising one. It is based on the fact that in alkaline solutions a colourless 1:1 complex is formed between phenolphthalein and β-CyD that the red phenolphthalein dianion is partially displaced by a competing reagent to an extent depending upon its affinity to form a complex with the CyD host. Phenolphthalein-modified β-CyD was synthesized for the purpose of developing a new type of guest-responsive color change indicator and the guest-induced absorption changes were used for molecule sensing [26, 27].

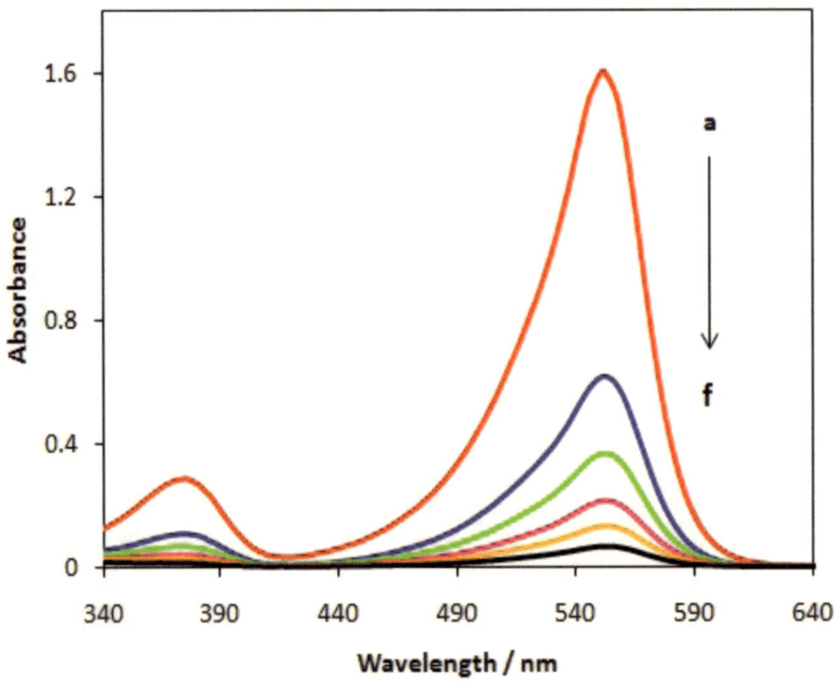

Figure 7. Absorption spectra for 4.8×10^{-5} mol L^{-1} phenolphthalein in the presence (a) 0.0, (b) 1.0×10^{-4}, (c) 2×10^{-4}, (d) 4×10^{-4}, (e) 7×10^{-4}, and (f) 1.0×10^{-3} mol L^{-1} of β -CyD at pH 10.5. [Reprinted from Afkhami A, Madrakian T, Khalafi L. / Anal. Lett, 2007; 40 2317-2328 with permission from Taylor & Francis.]

Several attempts have been also made on color changes based on competitive complexation of some important chemicals with phenolphthalein-CyD inclusion complex. These chemical sensors are relatively inexpensive, rapid and simple for determination of desired compounds, such as pharmaceuticals, surfactants and fatty acids which are transparent in the visible range [28-34]. The sensing abilities of for various guests are roughly parallel to the binding constants. Fig. 8 shows that by addition of ibuprofen to the phenolphthalein-β-CyD complex solution, the absorbance at 554 nm increases. This increase in the absorbance is due to the decomposition of phenolphthalein- β-CyD inclusion complex by displacement of ibuprofen by phenolphthalein. This phenomenon indicates competition of the ibuprofen with phenolphthalein in the formation of inclusion complex with β-CyD. The amount of increase in the absorbance at 554 nm was found to be proportional with the ibuprofen concentration over a certain concentration range.

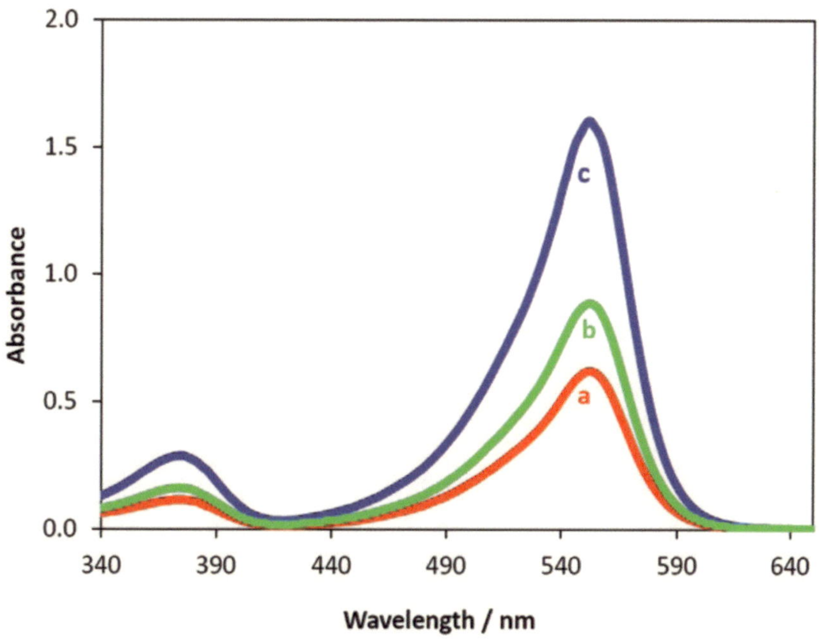

Figure 8. Absorption spectra for 4.8 $\times10^{-5}$ mol L^{-1} phenolphthalein at pH 10.5 in the presence of (a) 1.0×10^{-4} mol L^{-1} β-CyD and 2.0×10^{-4} mol L^{-1}ibuprofen, (b) 1.0×10^{-4} mol L^{-1} β-CyD and (c) in the absence of β-CyD and ibuprofen. [Reprinted from Afkhami A, Madrakian T, Khalafi L. /Anal. Lett, 2007; 40 2317-2328 with permission from Taylor & Francis.]

Color change chemical sensors of CyD derivatives carrying dyes such as nitrophenol [35] and alizarin yellow [36] were reported that relies on direct measurements of some analytes.

Also there is an example of color and spectral change of metal ion-indicators that affected by β-CyD. Recently it has been demonstrated that the addition of β-CyD to the solution containing the complex of calcium and magnesium with Eriochrome Black T (EBT) caused decomposition of the 1:1 metal complex and increase in EBT concentration in solution due to the formation of EBT-β-CyD inclusion complex. At a given pH, the values of metal ion conditional formation constant (K'_f) decreased by increasing β-CyD concentration based due to the formation of an inclusion complex between the desired form of EBT and β-CyD. The amount of decrease in K'_f with increasing β-CyD concentration and the color changes due to complex decomposition depends on the stability of the inclusion complex between EBT and β-CyD [37].

There is a large volume of published studies reporting the affinities and even selective affinity of secondary hydroxyl side of CyDs for metal ion binding and complexation [38]. This complexation ability improves considerably by structural and functional groups modification. The secondary hydroxyl groups are deprotonated and coordinated to bind Pb(II) ions forming a hexadecanuclear lead(II) alkoxide [39]. Two amino groups introduced on the primary hydroxyl side of β-CyD can chelate a platinum ion [40]. 6-amino-glucopyranose analogue of β-CyD had binding affinity for metal ions with Cs^{+} selectivity [41]. In 2010, Pitchumani et al. reported a per-6-amino-β-CyD as a supramolecular host and p-nitrophenol as a spectroscopic probe as a novel colorimetric and ratiometric sensor for transition metal cations, Fe^{3+} and Ru^{3+} in water. Binding of these cations causes an appreciable change in the visible region of the spectrum which can be detected by naked-eye and is insensitive to other metal ions namely Ag^{+}, Cu^{+}, Mn^{2+}, Fe^{2+}, Cu^{2+}, Zn^{2+}, Cd^{2+}, Hg^{2+}, Pb^{2+}, Cr^{3+}, La^{3+} and Eu^{3+}. The color change and consequent sensing ability is significant at equimolar ratio of host and guest and also at very low concentration [42].

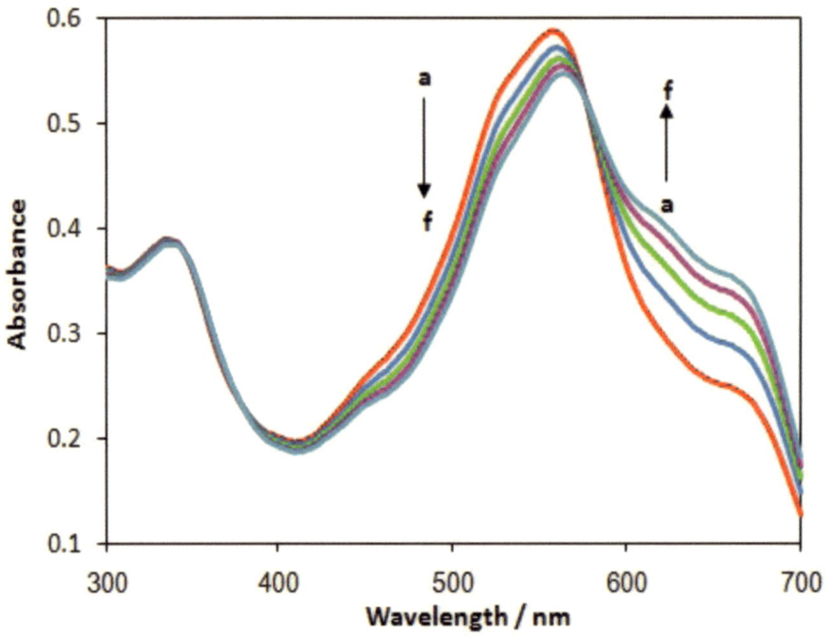

Figure 9. The spectra of Ca-EBT complex (1.0 ×10^{-3} mol L^{-1} Ca^{2+} and 4.0 × 10^{-5} mol L^{-1} EBT) in the presence of (a) 0.0, (b) 3.0 × 10^{-3}, (c) 6.0 × 10^{-3}, (d) 9.0 × 10^{-3}, (e) 1.2 × 10^{-2} and (f) 1.5 × 10^{-2} mol L^{-1} of β-CyD at pH 9.5. [Reprinted from Afkhami A, Khalafi L. / Supramol. Chem., 2008; 19 579-586 with permission from Taylor & Francis.]

http://dx.doi.org/10.5772/52824

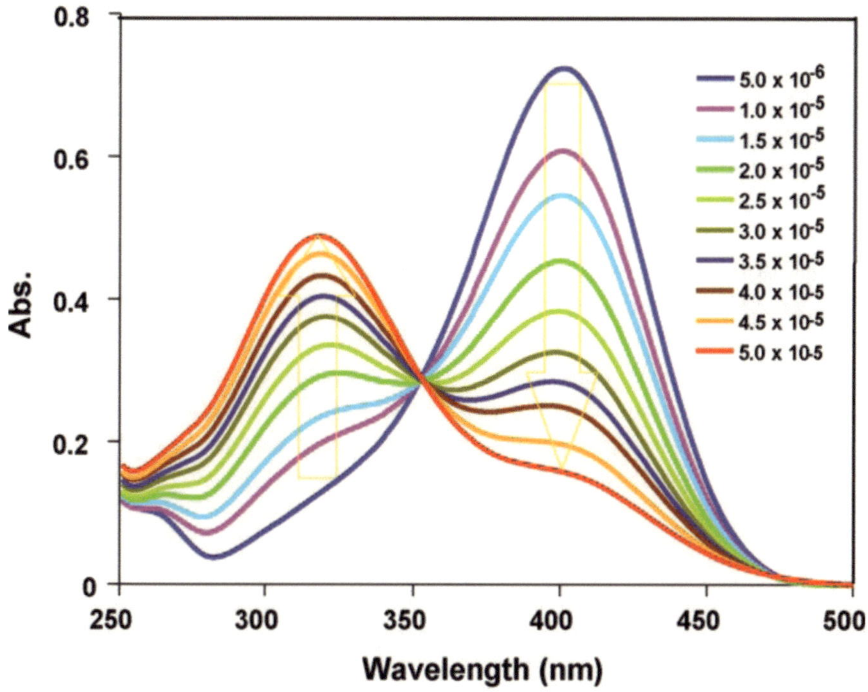

Figure 10. UV–Vis spectra of per-6-amino-β-CyD/p-nitrophenol (5×10^{-5} M) upon addition of Ru^{3+} (5×10^{-6}M to 5×10^{-5} M). [Reprinted from Suresh P. Abulkalam Azath I, Pitchumani K. / Sens. Actuators, B 2010; 146 273-277 with permission from Elsevier Science.]

Numerous studies have attempted to explain the possibility of incorporation of CyDs and modified CyDs in the structures of ternary complexes as ligand. In some of them the whole complex act as a guest and the metal ion has no direct contact with CyD [43]. In some other complexes the CyD appears as a coordinating ligand [44-49]. For example the Imidazole-appended β-CyD forms a ternary complex with a Cu^{2+} ion and l-tryptophanate [50]. The 6-amino and imidazolyl groups of the host molecule and the carboxyl and amino groups of l-tryptophanate are coordinated to the Cu^{2+} ion.

Moreover the cavity microenvironment of CyDs may alter the rate constant of reactions for the guest molecules depend on the reaction, substrate and the differences between cavity and solvent environments [51-53]. The changes in reaction rate cause to spectral time profile of the substrate and may be applicable in selective kinetic measurement of substrates and their recognition [54, 55].

2.4. Luminescence based molecular recognition

CyD inclusion is a means for protection of an excited state luminescent guest from the solvent environment that frequently shows a marked increase of luminescence due to increase in quantum yield and lifetime [56]. It have been mentioned even in some textbook that addition of CyD in solution is an efficient way in attaining the room temperature phosphorescence. This effect is usually much larger than that observed in absorption, and has therefore been used more efficiently and sensitively for luminescencing substrates. 6-bromo-2-naphthol is a good example that exhibited room temperature in the presence of β-CyD owing to protection from O_2 quenching in a nondeoxygenated solution, although nitrogen purging increased the emission intensity 13-fold [57].

For 2-chloronaphthalene solutions containing both d-glucose and α-CyD, the room-temperature phosphorescence of 2-chloronaphthalene has been observed. The 2:1 inclusion complex is responsible for the room-temperature phosphorescence. The quantum yield of the room-temperature phosphorescence from the 2:1 inclusion complex has been determined to be 19% of alcoholic solution at 77 K. When KI is added an enhancement is observed in phosphorescence intensity due to the formation of a ternary inclusion complex with iodide. Also the intensity reduction at higher concentrations of KI seems to be due to the formation of a nonphosphorescent ternary inclusion complex containing two iodides [58]. The notion of "turn-on" fluorescent sensor is used for this molecular recognition mechanism.

For the crown ether fluoroionophore/ β-CyD complex, the dimerization of the fluoroionophore inside the β-CyD is found to be selectively promoted by alkali metal ion binding, thereby resulting in metal-ion-selective pyrene dimer emission in water. This supramolecular function is successfully utilized in the design of a podand fluoroionophore/β-CyD complex for sensing toxic lead ion in water [59, 60].

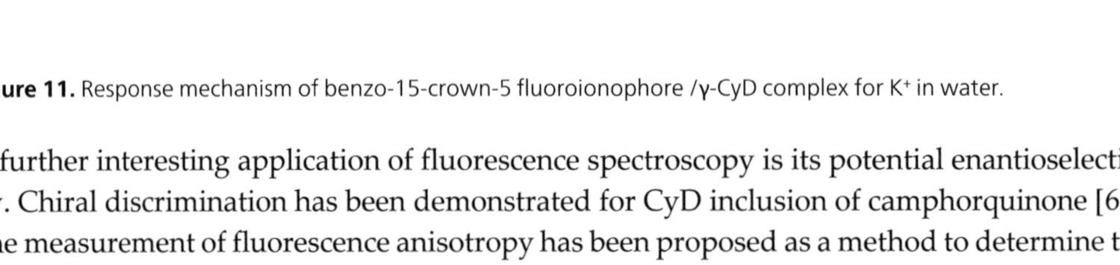

Figure 11. Response mechanism of benzo-15-crown-5 fluoroionophore /γ-CyD complex for K^+ in water.

A further interesting application of fluorescence spectroscopy is its potential enantioselectivity. Chiral discrimination has been demonstrated for CyD inclusion of camphorquinone [61]. The measurement of fluorescence anisotropy has been proposed as a method to determine the enantiomeric composition of samples [62].

As well as UV-Visible spectroscopy; competition of desired analyte with CyD-bonded or dissolved fluorophore yields a significant change in the fluorescence signal that will be useful in molecular recognition. Various "turn-off" fluorescent chemical sensors, in which fluorescence intensity was decreased by complexation with guest molecules, were reported.

http://dx.doi.org/10.5772/52824

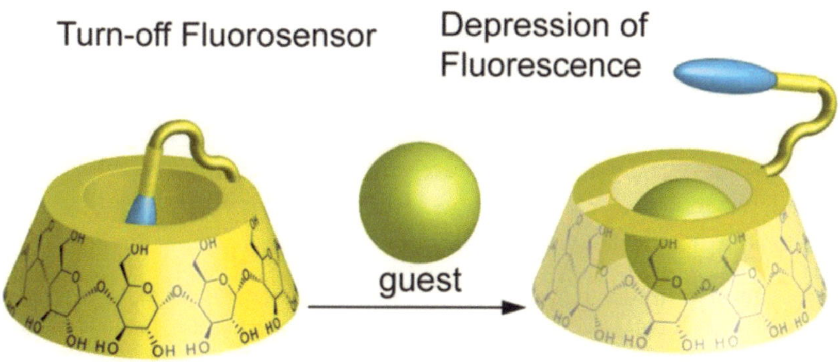

Figure 12. The mechanism of action for a turn-off fluorosensors.

A comprehensive example molecular recognition based on both decrease and increase in fluorescence intensity is the dansyl bonded CyD with diethylenetriamine spacer (CyD-dien-DNS) which have been reported by Corradini et al. In the presence of lipophilic organic molecules, CyD-dien-DNS showed sensing properties due to competitive inclusion of the guest and "in-out" movement of the dansyl group. CyD-dien-DNS was found also to be a fluorescent chemosensor for copper(II) ion, with a linear response and good selectivity, suggesting that a more flexible conformation of the linker and the presence of additional binding sites allow binding of the metal ion by the amino and sulfonamidate groups.

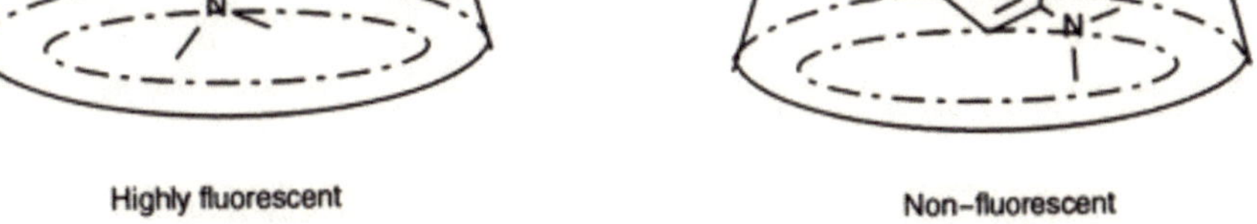

Figure 13. Spectral change of dansyldiethylenetriamine modified cyclodextrin in the presence of copper ion. [Reprinted with permission from Corradini R, Dossena A, Galaverna G, Marchelli R, Panagia A, Sartor G. / J. Org. Chem., 62, 6283 (1997). Copyright 1997, American Chemical Society.]

The CyD-dien-DNS copper(II) complex was shown to behave as a chemosensor for bifunctional molecules, such as amino acids. In fact, upon addition of alanine, tryptophan, and thyroxine, the negligible fluorescence intensity of Cu(CyD-dien-DNS) complex was "switched on", with a response dependent on the amino acid side chain [63]. Fluorescent indolizine modified CyD were studied in aqueous solution to evaluate their potentialities as molecular chemosensors for volatile organic compounds (VOCs) such as adamantanol, benzene, toluene, phenol and p-cresol as guest. The formation constant values measured using a spectral displacement method and also some specific algorithm treatments are reported for their quantitative analysis. [64, 65]. Some phenylseleno derivatives of CyD have been synthesized as chiral molecular sensors. These modified cyclodextrins can recognize both the size and chirality of the guest molecules despite of this fact that their stability constants with aliphatic alcohols are generally smaller than those for native β-CyD [66].

Moreover some chiral amino acid modified CyDs have been synthesized as chiral molecular sensors. N-dansyl-L-Phe-modified β-CyD showed high D-selectivity for norbornane derivatives and N-dansyl-D-Phe-modified β-CyD showed high L-selectivity for menthol [67]. Time-resolved fluorescence studies showed that the fluorescence of the dansyl group was completely quenched in the ternary complexes formed, and that the residual fluorescence was due to uncomplexed ligand. The enantioselectivity in response was found to be due to the formation of diastereomeric ternary complexes [68,69]. Fluorophore-amino acid-CyD were synthesized and characterized as fluorescent indicators of molecular recognition [70]. A novel boronic acid fluorophore 1/β-CyD complex sensor for sugar recognition in water has been designed [71].

2.5. Recognition of toxins based on spectral changes

There are also some successful applications of CyDs based spectral changes which have been used for the recognition of biologically important toxins.

Cyanotoxins are potent toxic compounds produced by cyanobacteria during algal blooms, which threaten drinking water supplies. These compounds can poison and kill animals and humans. The host–guest interactions of CyDs with problematic cyanotoxins were investigated to demonstrate the potential application of CyDs for the removal of these toxins from drinking water or applications related to their separation or purification. The complexation of these cyanotoxins with CyDs was monitored by nuclear magnetic resonance (NMR). The observed changes in chemical shifts for specific protons and competitive binding experiments demonstrate a 1:1 inclusion complex between γ-CyD and microcystins and nodularin, and the results suggest that CyD-type substrates are useful hosts for their complexation [72].

The fluorescence properties of the aflatoxins, as the most important mycotoxins, and the effect of various CyDs on their fluorescence emission were studied. The complex formation constant (K_f) of these compounds with β-CyD was chromatographically determined, and from the results obtained, it has been concluded that K_f cannot be used alone to explain the fluorescence increase [73].

An example of determination of biological toxins is a highly sensitive and rapid strategy for characterizing aflatoxins and the cholera toxin based on capillary electrokinetic chromatography with multiphoton-excited fluorescence. The aflatoxins are a highly mutagenic multiple-ringed heterocycles produced by aspergillus fungi and cholera toxin a-subunit is the catalytic domain of the bacterial protein toxin from Vibrio cholera. The anionic carboxymethyl-β-CyD, used to chromatographically resolve the uncharged aflatoxins, enhances emission from these

http://dx.doi.org/10.5772/52824

compounds without contributing substantially to the background [74]. Also the determination of aflatoxin B1 (AFB1) in wheat has been accomplished by enhanced spectrofluorimetry in the presence of β-CyD. The method is based on the enhanced fluorescence of AFB1 by β-CyD in 10% (w/w) methanol–water solution. The adopted strategy combined the use of parallel factor analysis (PARAFAC) for extraction of the pure analyte signal and the standard addition method, for a determination in the presence of matrix effect caused by wheat matrix [75].

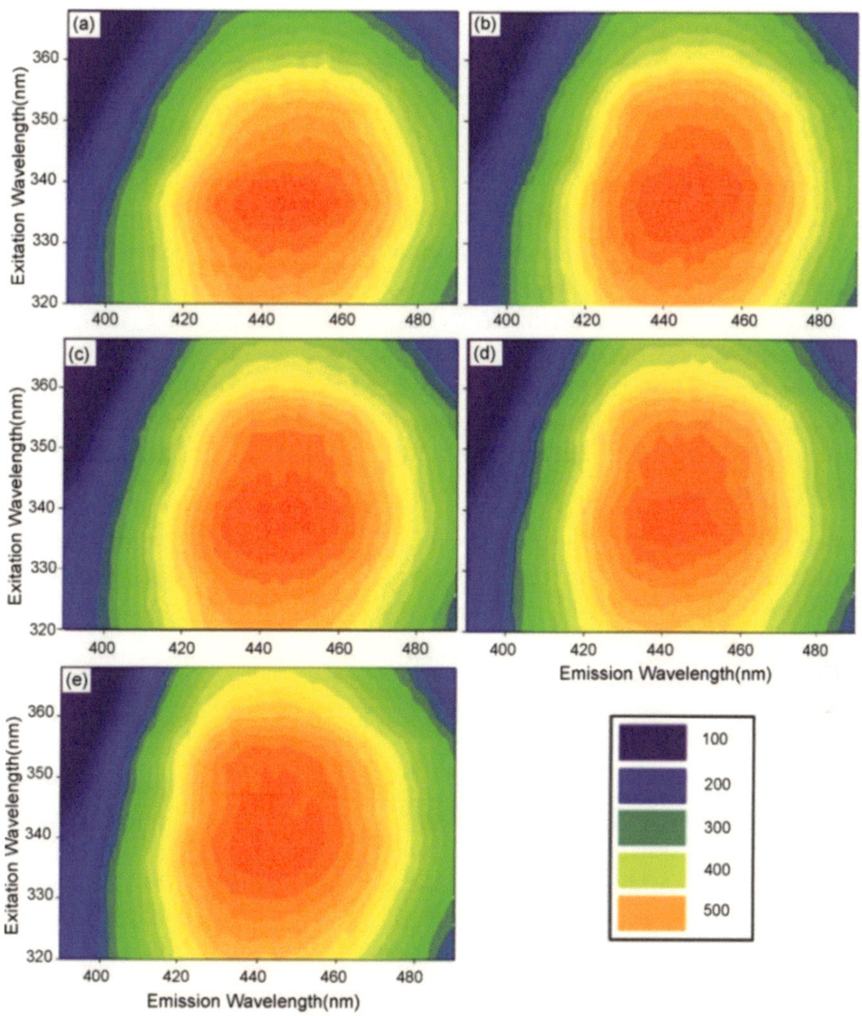

Figure 14. Contour plots (excitation–emission) for an original wheat sample and four AFB1 standard additions; (a) the original sample, (b) plus 2.0 μg kg^{-1}, (c) plus 3.8 μg kg^{-1}, (d) plus 5.7 μg kg^{-1}, (e) plus 7.4 μg kg^{-1}. [Reprinted from Hashemi J, Asadi Kram G, Alizadeh N. / Talanta, 2008; 75 1075-1081 with permission from Elsevier Science.]

2.6. Interaction and recognition of natural compounds

Finally the spectral change and interaction of some natural compounds such as alkaloids and peptides with CyDs is discussed.

Complex formation of the glutathione and some of its derivatives with bridged β-CyD such as 2,2′-diseleno-bridged β-CyD were determined by UV-Vis. absorption and ^{1}H-NMR spectroscopy [76]. Polymerization of the amyloid beta-peptide (Abeta) has been identified as a major feature of the pathogenesis of Alzheimer's disease (AD). Inhibition of the formation of these toxic polymers of Abeta has emerged as an approach for developing therapeutics for AD. NMR and circular dichroism (CD) spectra were used to investigate the interaction between CyD and Abeta. CD spectral analyses show that β-CyD inhibits the aggregation of Abeta. Analysis of the one-dimensional proton NMR spectra of the mixture of Abeta with β-CyD clearly indicates that there are chemical shift changes in the aromatic ring and the methyl groups in the peptide [77].

A series of CyDs –cinchona alkaloid inclusion complexes were prepared from β-CyD and some of its derivaties and four cinchona alkaloids, and their inclusion complexation behavior was investigated by means of fluorescence, UV/Vis and 2D NMR spectroscopy. The results showed that the cinchona alkaloids can be efficiently encapsulated in the CyD cavity in an acidic environment and sufficiently released in a neutral environment, which makes these CyD derivatives the potential carriers for cinchona alkaloids [78,79]. Using colorimetry and ^{1}H-NMR and UV spectroscopy, together with solubility methods,the interaction of natural and hydroxylpropylated CyDs with xanthine, theophylline, theobromine, and caffeine in aqueous solution have been studied [80].

Combination of the spectrophotometric methods and some separation methods such as capillary electrophoresis (CE) and micellar electrokinetic chromatography (MEKC) in the presence of CyDs have been used successfully for the quantitative analysis of natural alkaloids [80,81].

3. Conclusion

CyDs are a versatile tool in the molecular recognition and sensing. Formation of inclusion complex cause to some spectral changes which have been used successfully for the study of host-guest interactions. Additionally the desired spectral changes as the results of complex formation have been used for promote analyte detection and continue to inspire creative applications. The most sensible spectral changes were reported for chemical and fluorescence indicators. These considerable changes have been used for the study and better detection of many absorbing and especially fluorescent species. Moreover many spectrochemically silent organic and some inorganic compounds cause color/fluorescence change in CyD and indicator solutions, because of their competition to form inclusion complex. These changes cause to recognition of the target competitive hosts. On this basis some "indicator modified cyclodextrin" in which indicator is linked to cyclodextrin via a spacer, was synthesized that change color/fluorescence in response to the presence of molecules, ions and many biologically

http://dx.doi.org/10.5772/52824

important compounds. The guest-induced changes that are roughly parallel to its binding constants were used for molecule sensing. These are valuable for qualitative and quantitative chemical analysis. Sensitivity and selectivity improved by appropriate designing of the dye moiety or spacer.

Author details

Lida Khalafi[1] and Mohammad Rafiee[2]

1 Department of Chemistry, Shahr-e-Qods Branch, Islamic Azad University, Tehran, Iran

2 Department of Chemistry, Institute for Advanced Studies in Basic Sciences (IASBS), Zanjan, Iran

References

[1] Villiers A. Sur la fermentation de la fécule par l'action du ferment, Butyriqué Compt. Rend. Fr. Acad. Sci., 1891; 112 435-438.

[2] Szejtli J. Introduction and General Overview of Cyclodextrin Chemistry. Chem. Rev., 1998; 98 1743-1753.

[3] Szente L, Szejtli J, Kis GL. Spontaneous Opalescence of Aqueous γ-Cyclodextrin Solutions: Complex Formation or Self-Aggregation. J. Pharm. Sci., 1998; 87 778-781.

[4] Dodziuk H. Cyclodextrins and Their Complexes Chemistry, Analytical Methods, Applications. Weinheim: WILEY-VCH; 2006.

[5] Loftsson T, Brewster ME. Pharmaceutical Applications of Cyclodextrins: Drug Solubilisation and Stabilization. J. Pharm. Sci., 1996; 85 1017–1025.

[6] Schneiderman E, Stalcup AM. Cyclodextrins: A Versatile Tool in Separation Science. J. Chromatogr. B., 2000; 745 83-102.

[7] Martin Del Valle E.M. Cyclodextrins and Their Uses: A Review. Process Biochem., 2004; 39 1033-1046.

[8] Karathanos VT, Mourtzinos I, Yannakopoulou K, Andrikopoulos, NK. Study of the Solubility, Antioxidant Activity and Structure of Inclusion Complex of Vanillin with β-Cyclodextrin. Food Chem. 2007; 101 652-658.

[9] Buschmann HJ, Schollmeyer E. Applications of Cyclodextrins in Cosmetic Products: A Review. J .Cosmet. Sci. 2002; 53 185-191.

[10] Connors KA. The Stability of Cyclodextrin Complexes in Solution. Chem. Rev., 1997; 97 1325-1357.

[11] Toma SH, Toma HE. Self-Assembled Rotaxane and Pseudo-Rotaxanes based on β-Cyclodextrin Inclusion Compounds with trans-1,4-Bis[(4-pyridyl)ethenyl]benzene-pentacyanoferrate(II) Complexes. J. Braz. Chem. Soc., 2007; 18 279-283.

[12] Perez-Martınez JI, Gines JM, Morillo E, Rodrı´guez ML, Moyano JR. 2,4-Dichlorophenoxyacetic Acid/Partially Methylated-β-Cyclodextrin Inclusion Complexes. Environ. Technol. 2000; 21 209-216.

[13] Saikosin R, Limpaseni T, Pongsawasdi P. Formation of Inclusion Complexes between Cyclodextrins and Carbaryl and Characterization of the Complexes. J. Incl. Phenom. Macro. Chem. 2002; 44 191-196.

[14] Perez-Martinez JI, Arias MJ, Gines JM, Moyano JR, Morillo E, Sanchez-Soto PJ, Novak C. 2,4-D-Alpha-Cyclodextrin Complexes; Preparation and Characterization by Thermal-Analysis. J. Thermal Anal. 1998; 51 965-972.

[15] Taguchi K. Transient Binding Mode of Phenolphthalein- β-Cyclodextrin Complex: An Example of Induced Geometrical Distortion. J. Am. Chem. Soc., 1986; 108 2705-2709.

[16] Khalafi L, Rafiee M, Mahdiun F, Sedaghat S. Investigation of the Inclusion Complex of β-Cyclodextrin with Mycophenolate Mofetil. Spectrochim. Acta Part A, 2012; 90 45-49.

[17] Afkhami A, Khalafi L. Spectrophotometric Determination of Conditional Acidity Constant as a Function of β-Cyclodextrin Concentration for Some Organic Acids Using Rank Annihilation Factor Analysis. Anal. Chim. Acta. 2006; 569 267-274.

[18] Chandra Ghosh B, Deb N, Mukherjee A.K. Determination of Individual Proton Affinities of Ofloxacin from its UV-Vis Absorption, Fluorescence and Charge-Transfer Spectra: Effect of Inclusion in β-Cyclodextrin on the Proton Affinities. J. Phys. Chem. B, 2010; 114 9862-9871.

[19] Bender ML. Cyclodextrin Chemistry. Komiyama M. (Eds.), Berlin: Springer-Verlag; 1978.

[20] Bender ML, Komiyama M. Cyclodextrin Chemistry, Berlin: Springer Verlag; 1978.

[21] Rekharsky MV, Inoue Y. Complexation Thermodynamics of Cyclodextrins. Chem. Rev. 1998; 98 1875-1918.

[22] Khalafi L, Rohani M, Afkhami A. Acidity Constants of Some Organic Acids in the Presence of β-Cyclodextrin in Binary Ethanol–Water Mixtures by Rank Annihilation Factor Analysis. J. Chem. Eng. Data. 2008; 53 2389-2392.

[23] Ogoshi T, Harada A, Chemical Sensors Based on Cyclodextrin Derivatives. Sensors, 2008; 8 4961-4982.

[24] Kuwabara T, Nakamura A, Ueno A, Toda F. Inclusion Complexes and Guest-Induced Color Changes of pH-Indicator-Modified β-Cyclodextrins. J. Phys. Chem. 1994; 98 6297-6303.

[25] Ueno A, Kuwabara T, Nakamura A, Toda F. A Modified Cyclodextrin as a Guest Responsive Color-Change Indicator. Nature, 1992; 356 136-137.

[26] Kuwabara T, Takamura M, Matsushita A, Ikeda H, Nakamura A, Ueno A, Toda F. Phenolphthalein-Modified β-Cyclodextrin as a Molecule-Responsive Colorless-to-Color Change Indicator. J. Org. Chem., 1998; 63 8729-8735.

[27] Kuwabara T, Aoyagi T, Takamura M, Matsushita A, Nakamura A, Ueno A. Heterodimerization of Dye-Modified Cyclodextrins with Native Cyclodextrins. J. Org. Chem., 2002; 67 720-725.

[28] Tutaj B, Kasprzyk A, Czapkiewicz J. The Spectral Displacement Technique for Determining the Binding Constants of β-Cyclodextrin-Alkyltrimethylammonium Inclusion Complexes. J. Incl. Phenom. Macrocyclic Chem. 2003; 47 133-136.

[29] Meier MM, Bordignon Luiz MT, Farmer PJ, Szpoganicz B. The Influence of β- and γ -Cyclodextrin Cavity Size on the Association Constant with Decanoate and Octanoate Anions. J. Incl. Phenom. Macrocyclic Chem. 2001; 40 291-295.

[30] Cadena PG, Oliveira EC, Araujo AN, Montenegro MCBSM, Pimentel MCB, Lima Filho JL, Silva VL. Simple Determination of Deoxycholic and Ursodeoxycholic Acids by Phenolphthalein- β-Cyclodextrin Inclusion Complex. Lipids, 2009; 44 1063-1070.

[31] Skoulika SG, Georgiou CA, Polissiou MG. Interaction of β-Cyclodextrin with Unsaturated and Saturated Straight Chain Fatty Acid Anions Studied by Phenolphthalein Displacement. J. Incl. Phenom. Macrocyclic Chem. 1999; 34 85-96.

[32] Sasaki KJ, Christian SD, Tucker EE. Use of Visible Spectral displacement Method to Determine the Concentration of Surfactants in Aqueous Solution. J. Colloid Interface Sci, 1990; 134 412-416.

[33] Afkhami A, Madrakian T, Khalafi L. Flow Injection and Batch Spectrophotometric Determination of Ibuprofen Based on Its Competitive Complexation Reaction with Phenolphthalein- β-Cyclodextrin Inclusion Complex. Anal. Lett, 2007; 40 2317-2328.

[34] Afkhami A, Madrakian T, Khalafi L. Spectrophotometric Determination of Fluoxetine by Batch and Flow Injection Methods. Chem. Pharm. Bull. 2006; 54 1642-1646.

[35] Kuwabara T, Nakamura A, Ueno A, Toda F. Supramolecular Thermochromism of a Dyeappended β-Cyclodextrin. J. Chem. Soc., Chem. Commun. 1994; 689-690.

[36] Aoyagi T, Nakamura A, Ikeda H, Ikeda T, Mihara H, Ueno A. Alizarin Yellow-Modified β-Cyclodextrin as a Guest-Responsive Absorption Change Sensor. Anal. Chem. 1997; 69 659-663.

[37] Afkhami A, Khalafi L. Investigation of the Effect of Inclusion Erichrome Black T with β-Cyclodextrin on its Complexation Reaction with Ca^{2+} and Mg^{2+} using Rank Annihilation Factor Analysis. Supramol. Chem. 2008; 19 579-586.

[38] Nicolis I, Coleman AW, Selkti M, Villain F, Charpin P, Rango C. Molecular Composites Based on First-Sphere Coordination of Calcium Ions by a Cyclodextrin. J. Phys. Org. Chem., 2001; 14 35-37.

[39] Klufers P, Schuhmacher J. Sixteenfold Deprotonated γ-Cyclodextrin Tori as Anions in a Hexadecanuclear Lead(II) Alkoxide. Angew. Chem. Int. Ed. Engl., 1994; 33 1863-1865.

[40] Cucinotta V, Grasso G, Pedotti S, Rizzarelli E, Vecchio G, Blasio B, Isernia C, Saviano M, Pedone C. A Platinum (II) Diamino-β-cyclodextrin Complex: A Crystallographic and Solution Study. Synthesis and Structural Characterization of a Platinum(II) Complex of 6A,6B-Diamino-6A,6B-dideoxycyclomaltoheptaose. Inorg. Chem., 1996; 35 7535-7540.

[41] Yamamura H, Yotsuya T, Usami S, Iwasa A, Ono S, Tanabe Y, Iida D, Katsuhara T, Kano K, Uchida T, Araki S, Kawai M. Primary hydroxy-modified cyclomaltoheptaose derivatives with two kinds of substituents. Preparation of 6I-(benzyloxycarbonylamino)-, 6I-(tert-butoxycarbonylamino)- and 6I-azido-6I-deoxy-6II,6III,6IV, 6V, 6VI,6VII-hexa-O-tosylcyclomaltoheptaose and their conversion to the hexakis-(3,6-anhydro) derivatives. J. Chem. Soc., Perkin Trans 1 1998; 1299-1304.

[42] Suresh P. Abulkalam Azath I, Pitchumani K. Naked-Eye Detection of Fe^{3+} and Ru^{3+} in Water: Colorimetric and Ratiometric Sensor Based on per-6-amino-β-cyclodextrin/p-nitrophenol. Sens. Actuators, B 2010; 146 273-277.

[43] Alston DR, Slawin AMZ, Stoddart JF, Williams DJ. Cyclodextrins as Second Sphere Ligands for Transition Metal Complexes-The X-Ray Crystal Structure of [Rh(cod) $(NH_3)_2$ α-cyclodextrin][PF_6] $6H_2O$. Angew. Chem. Int. Ed. Engl., 1985; 24 786-787.

[44] Nicolis I, Coleman AW, Charpin P, Rango C. A Molecular Composite Containing Organic and Inorganic Components-A Complex from β-Cyclodextrin and Hydrated Magnesium Chloride. Angew. Chem. Int. Ed. Engl., 1995; 34 2381-2383.

[45] Stoddart JF, Zarzycki R. Cyclodextrins as Second-Sphere Ligands for Transition Metal Complexes. Recl. Trav. Chim. Pays-Bas, 1988; 107 515-528.

[46] Navaza A, Iroulapt MG, Navaza J. A Monomeric Uranyl Hydroxide System Obtained by Inclusion in the β-Cyclodextrin Cavity. J. Coord. Chem., 2000; 51 153-168.

[47] Odagaki Y, Hirotsu K, Higuchi T, Harada A, Takahashi S. X-Ray structure of the α-cyclodextrin–ferrocene (2 : 1) inclusion compound. J. Chem. Soc., Perkin Trans., 1990; 1 1230-1231.

[48] Tabushi I, Shimizu N, Sugimoto T, Shiozuka M, Yamamura K. Cyclodextrin Flexibly Capped with Metal Ion. J. Am. Chem. Soc., 1977; 99 7100-7102.

[49] Klingert B, Rihs G. Molecular encapsulation of transition metal complexes in cyclodextrins. Part 3. Structural consequences of varying the guest geometry in channel-type inclusion compounds. J. Chem. Soc., Dalton Trans1., 1991; 2749-2760.

[50] Bonomo RP, Blasio B, Maccarrone G, Pavone V, Pedone C, Rizzarelli E, Saviano M, Vecchio G. Crystal and Molecular Structure of the [6-Deoxy-6-[(2-(4-imidazolyl)ethyl)amino]- cyclomaltoheptaose]copper(II) Ternary Complex with l-Tryptophanate. Role of Weak Forces in the Chiral Recognition Process Assisted by a Metallocyclodextrin. Inorg. Chem., 1996; 35 4497-4504.

[51] Hoshino T, Ishida K, Irie T, Hirayama F, Uekama K. Reduction of Photohemolytic Activity of Benoxaprofen by β-Cyclodextrin Complexations. J. Incl. Phenom., 1988; 6 415-423.

[52] Hirayama F, Kurihara M, Uekama K. Improvement of Chemical Instability of Prostacyclin in Aqueous Solution by Complexation with Methylated Cyclodextrins. Int. J. Pharmaceut., 1987; 35 193-199.

[53] Gorecka BA, Sanzgiri YD, Bindra DS, Stella VJ. Effect of SBE4-β-CD, a Sulfobutyl Ether β-Cyclodextrin, on the Stability and Solubility of O6-Benzylguanine (NSC-637037) in Aqueous Solutions. Int. J. Pharmaceut., 1995; 125 55-61.

[54] Afkhami A, Khalafi L. Application of Rank Annihilation Factor Analysis to the Determination of the Stability Constant of the Complex XL and Rate Constants for the Reaction of X and XL with the Reagent Z using Kinetic Profiles. Bull. Chem. Soc. Jpn. 2007; 80 1542-1548.

[55] Afkhami A, Khalafi L. Spectrophotometric Investigation of the Effect of β-Cyclodextrin on the Intramolecular Cyclization Reaction of Catecholamines using Rank Annihilation Factor Analysis. Anal. Chim. Acta, 2007; 599 241-248.

[56] Bortolus P, Monti S. Photochemistry in Cyclodextrin Cavities. Adv. Photochem. 1996; 21 1-133.

[57] Munoz de la Pena A, Rodriguez MP, Escandar GM. Optimization of the Room-Temperature Phosphorescence of the 6-Bromo-2-Naphthol–A-Cyclodextrin System in Aqueous Solution. Talanta, 2000; 51 949-955.

[58] Hamai S. Inclusion of 2-Chloronaphthalene by α-Cyclodextrin and Room-Temperature Phosphorescence of 2-Chloronaphthalene in Aqueous d-Glucose Solutions Containing α-Cyclodextrin. J. Phys. Chem. B, 1997; 101 1707-1712.

[59] Hayashita T, Yamauchi A, Tong AJ, Chan Lee J, Smith BD, Teramae N. Design of Supramolecular Cyclodextrin Complex Sensors for Ion and Molecule Recognition in Water. J. Incl. Phenom. Macrocyclic Chem. 2004; 50 87-94.

[60] Suzuki I, Ito M, Osa T, Anzai JI, Molecular Recognition of Deoxycholic Acids by Pyrene-Appended β-Cyclodextrin Connected with a Rigid Azacrown Spacer. Chem. Pharm. Bull. 1999; 47 151-155.

[61] Bortolus P, Marconi G, Monti S, Mayer B. Chiral Discrimination of Camphorquinone Enantiomers by Cyclodextrins: A Spectroscopic and Photophysical Study. J. Phys. Chem. A, 2002; 106 1686-1694.

[62] Xu YF, McCarroll ME. Determination of Enantiomeric Composition by Fluorescence Anisotropy. J. Phys. Chem. A, 2004; 108 6929-6932.

[63] Corradini R, Dossena A, Galaverna G, Marchelli R, Panagia A, Sartor G. Fluorescent Chemosensor for Organic Guests and Copper(II) Ion Based on Dansyldiethylenetriamine-Modified β-Cyclodextrin, J. Org. Chem., 1997; 62 6283-6289.

[64] Fourmentin S, Surpateanu GG, Blach P, Landy D, Decock P, Surpateanu G. Experimental and Theoretical Study on the Inclusion Capability of a Fluorescent Indolizine β-Cyclodextrin Sensor Towards Volatile and Semi-volatile Organic Guest. J. Incl. Phenom. Macrocyclic Chem. 2006; 55 263-269.

[65] Surpateanu GG, Becuwe M, Catalin Lungu N, Dron PI, Fourmentin S, Landy D, Surpateanu G. Photochemical Behaviour Upon the Inclusion for Some Volatile Organic Compounds in New Fluorescent Indolizine β-Cyclodextrin Sensors. J. Photochem. Photobiol. Chem, 2007; 185 312-320.

[66] Liu Y, You CC, Wada T, InoueY. Molecular Recognition Studies on Supramolecular Systems. 22. Size, Shape, and Chiral Recognition of Aliphatic Alcohols by Organoselenium-Modified Cyclodextrins. J. Org. Chem., 1999; 64 3630-3634.

[67] Ikeda H, Li Q, Ueno A. Chiral Recognition by Fluorescent Chemosensors Based on N-Dansyl-Amino Acid-Modified Cyclodextrins. Bioorg. Med. Chem. Lett. 2006; 16 5420-5423.

[68] Pagliari S, Corradini R, Galaverna G, Sforza S, Dossena A, Montalti M, Prodi L, Zaccheroni N, Marchelli R. Enantioselective Fluorescence Sensing of Amino Acids by Modified Cyclodextrins: Role of the Cavity and Sensing Mechanism. Chem. Eur. J., 2004; 10 2749-2758.

[69] Khalafi L. Modified Cyclodextrins as Molecular Sensors. (Mini Review) Res. J. Chem. Environ. 2008; 12 102-103.

[70] Ikeda H, Nakamura M, Ise N, Oguma N, Nakamura A, Ikeda T, Toda F, Ueno A. Fluorescent Cyclodextrins for Molecule Sensing: Fluorescent Properties, NMR Characterization, and Inclusion Phenomena of N-Dansylleucine-Modified Cyclodextrins. J. Am. Chem. Soc., 1996; 118 10980-10988.

[71] Tong AJ, Yamauchi A, Hayashita T, Zhang ZY, Smith BD, Teramae N. Boronic Acid Fluorophore/β-Cyclodextrin Complex Sensors for Selective Sugar Recognition in Water. Anal. Chem., 2001; 73 1530-1536.

[72] Chen L, Dionysiou DD, Oshea K. Complexation of Microcystins and Nodularin by Cyclodextrins in Aqueous Solution, a Potential Removal Strategy. Environ. Sci. Technol., 2011; 45 2293-2300.

[73] Franco CM, Fente CA, Vazquez BI, Cepeda A, Mahuzier G, Prognon P. Interaction between Cyclodextrins and Aflatoxins Q1, M1 and P1: Fluorescence and Chromatographic Studies. J. Chromatogr. A. 1998; 815 21-29.

[74] Wei J, Okerberg E, Dunlap J, Ly C, Shear JB. Determination of Biological Toxins Using Capillary Electrokinetic Chromatography with Multiphoton-Excited Fluorescence. Anal. Chem., 2000; 72 1360-1363.

[75] Hashemi J, Asadi Kram G, Alizadeh N. Enhanced Spectrofluorimetric Determination of Aflatoxin B1 In Wheat by Second-Order Standard Addition Method, Talanta, 2008; 75 1075-1081.

[76] Ya-Qiong H, Xing-Chen L, Jun-Qiu L, Yu-Qing W. Association Mechanism of S-Dinitrophenyl Glutathione with Two Glutathione Peroxidase Mimics: 2, 2′-Ditelluro- and 2, 2′-Diseleno-bridged β-cyclodextrins, Molecules, 2009; 14 904-916.

[77] Qin XR, Abe H, Nakanishi H. NMR and CD Studies on the Interaction of Alzheimer Beta-Amyloid Peptide (12-28) with Beta-Cyclodextrin, Biochem. Biophys. Res. Commun., 2002 ; 297 1011-15.

[78] Yu L, Guo-Song Ch, Yong Ch, Fei D, Jing Ch. Cyclodextrins as Carriers for Cinchona Alkaloids: a pH-Responsive Selective Binding System, Org. Biomol. Chem., 2005; 3 2519-2523.

[79] Liu Y, Li L, Zhang HY, Fan Z, Guan XD. Selective Binding of Chiral Molecules of Cinchona Alkaloid by β- and γ-Cyclodextrins and Organoselenium-Bridged Bis(β-cyclodextrin)s, Bioorg. Chem., 2003; 31 11–23.

[80] Tewari BB, Beaulieu-Houle G, Larsen A, Kengne-Momo R, Auclair K, Butler, IS. An Overview of Molecular Spectroscopic Studies on Theobromine and Related Alkaloids, Appl. Spectrosc. Rev., 2012; 47 163–179.

[81] Sohajda T, Varga E, Ivanyi R, Fejos I, Szente L, Noszal B, Beni S. Separation of Vinca Alkaloid Enantiomers by Capillary Electrophoresis Applying Cyclodextrin Derivatives and Characterization of Cyclodextrin Complexes by Nuclear Magnetic Resonance Spectroscopy, J. Pharmaceut. Biomed. Anal. 2010; 531258–1266.

Chapter 20

Potentiometry for Study of Supramolecular Recognition Processes Between Uncharged Molecules

Jerzy Radecki and Hanna Radecka

Additional information is available at the end of the chapter

http://dx.doi.org/10.5772/52803

1. Introduction

Recently one could observe a continuous increase of scientific interest in host-guest chemistry, and more specifically in the intermolecular recognition processes occurring at liquid-liquid interface [1-3, 7, 8]. The fundamental chemical processes occurring in liquid membrane of potentiometric sensor are guest- induced selective changes in the charge separation across the interface between the liquid membrane and aqueous sample solution. The organic/aqueous interface, often named as "the third phase", possesses unique properties, which are very different from the properties of the bulk phases. In this particular place, many of biological processes of intermolecular recognition occur, demonstrating extremely high selectivity and sensitivity. Numerous instrumental methods were applied for study this phenomenon. Electrochemical one have a significant share in this research.

Potentiometry with using of ion selective electrodes (ISEs) is one of the most popular techniques enable to observe the recognition processes between the ligand and cationic or anionic species occurring in the liquid/liquid interface. The mechanism of potentiometric signal generation relies on the charge separation between two phases, which is the result of a perm selective transfer of analyte ions from the aqueous to the organic phases at the liquid /liquid interface with high sensitivity and selectivity [9, 10]. This type of sensors have some outstanding advantages including simple design and operation, wide linear dynamic range, relatively fast response and rational selectivity and because of these parameters there are particularly interesting from the perspective of the supramolecular chemist. The potentiometric sensors could be applied as a tool for observation of molecular recognition processes at the border of two phases.

In pioneering paper written by Umezawa and co-workers the possibilities of potentiometric signals generation of polymeric membrane modified with permanently charged ligand such as quaternary ammonium salts [4] and lipophilic polyamines [5, 6] after their stimulation with uncharged phenol derivatives were described the first time. According to authors the mechanism of signal generation by membrane modified with quaternary ammonium salts consist of two processes.

First is the complexation of extracted ArOH and Q^+X^- leading to a net movement of anionic species (X^-) from the aqueous to the membrane phase. In second step there is proton dissociation of complexed ArOH and simultaneous ejection of HX to aqueous phase, involving a net movement of cationic species (H^+) from membrane to the aqueous phase [4].

Being inspired by this paper, we have done systematic study on potentiometric signals generated by membranes modified with electrically neutral host molecules and stimulated with uncharged guest molecules [11-25].

As a receptors (host) molecules for recognition of uncharged phenol derivatives, corroles, calix[4]pyrroles, calix[4]phyrins and metalloporphyrines we have applied. Whereas, for recognition of unprotonated aniline derivatives we have used: *p-tert*-butylthiacalix[4]arene (BTC[4]ene), tetrabromodialkoxythiacalix[4]arene (BATC[4]ene), tetra-undecylcalix[4]resorcinarene (UDC[4]Rene), tetra-undecyl-tetra-*p*-nitrophenylazocalix[4]resorcinarene (UDAC[4]Rene), tetra-undecyl-tetra-hydroxycalix[4]resorcinarene (UDHC[4]Rene), tetra-undecyl-tetra-bromocalix[4]resorcinarene (UDBC[4]Rene.

2. Potentiometric response of tetrapyrrolic macrocyclic compounds liquid membrane electrode towards neutral chloro- and nitrophenols

The calix[4]pyrroles, calix[4]phyrins and corroles are tetrapyrrolic macrocyclic compounds. All of them belong to very large group of porphyrin analogs and they are well known as sensitive and selective receptors for anions [26-32].

The main differences between corroles, calix[4]pyrroles and calix[4]phyrins are the following. The corroles are almost planar, aromatic macrocycles. Imine nitrogen atoms from the corrole cavity can be protonated at low pH [33-36].

This is not expected in the case of calix[4]pyrrole and calix[4]phyrins. The calix[4]phyrins (porphodimethenes) demonstrate partly conjugated character similar to porphyrins and partly the non conjugated character of calix[4]pyrroles. Calix[4]pyrroles possess in their structure the relatively dip cavity [26, 32]. Only the individual pyrroles rings have some aromatic character.

Figure 1 illustrates the structures of calix[4]pyrroles, calix[4]phyrins and corroles being applied for this research.

In Table 1 the values of responses of membrane modified with particular host molecules after stimulation with nitrophenols derivatives are collected.

http://dx.doi.org/10.5772/52803

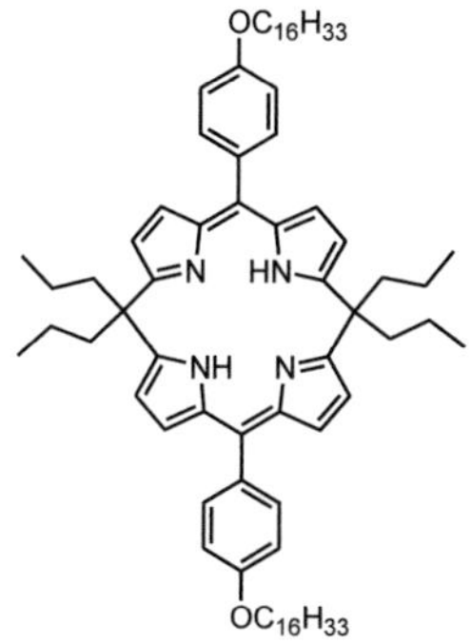

Calix[4]phyrin

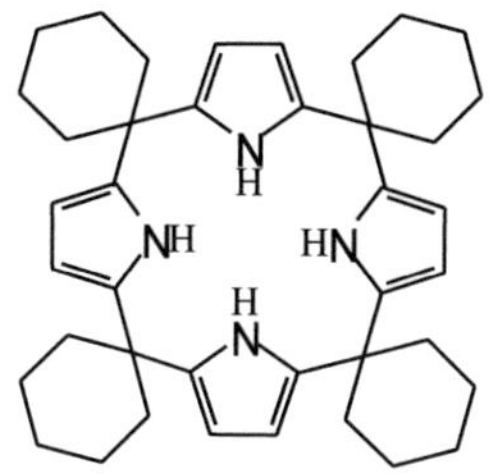

Calix[4]pyrrole

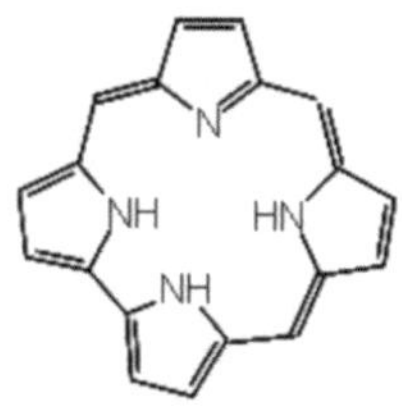

Corrole

Figure 1. The structure of pyrrole hosts.

The results presented indicate that generally, the membrane incorporating calix[4]pyrrole generated the higher potential changes after stimulation with nitrophenols in comparison to calix[4]phyrin and the corrole-containing membrane.

Guests	ΔEMF = EMF_0-EMF_f *					
	Calix[4]pyrrole		Calix[4]phyrin		Corrole	
	pH=4.0	pH=6.0	pH=3.0	pH=6.0	pH=3.0	pH=6.0
ortho-nitrophenol	-3.0	-3.0	-0,7	----	-4.3	-6.0
meta-nitrophenol	-25.9	-24.0	-2,8	----	-9.7	-9.9
para-nitrophenol	-25.9	-35.0	-4,1	----	-14.1	-10.3

*EMF_0 – potential measured in buffer free of analyte

*EMF_f – potential measured in buffer with analyte at final concentration

Table 1. The potentiometric responses of ISE_s incorporating of calix[4]pyrrole, calix[4]phyrin,corrole towards of nitrophenols isomers

The potentiometric signal generated by membranes modified with corrole and calix[4]phyrin and stimulated with nitrophenol derivatives are very week and comparable. In spite of significant differences of signal magnitude for each type of membranes, generally all of them displayed the same signal magnitude sequence:

$para-\text{nitrophenol} \geq meta-\text{nitrophenol} > ortho-\text{nitrophenol}$

This sequence is in good order with the lipophilicity and acidity of the nitrophenolic derivatives (see Table 2)

Guest compound	pKa	Log P_{oct}	Neutral form [%]			
			pH = 2.0	pH = 4.0	pH = 6.0	pH = 8.0
Para-nitrophenol	7.16	1.91	99.99	99.93	93.54	12.63
Meta-nitrophenol	8.39	2.00	99.99	99.99	99.6	71.05
Ortho-nitrophenol	7.21	1.79	99.99	99.94	94.25	13.95
2.4-dinitrophenol	4.11	1.54	99.23	56.31	1.27	0.01
2.5-dinitrophenol	5.22	1.75	99.94	94.32	14.24	0.16
2.6-dinitophenol	4.15	1.25	99.30	58.54	1.39	0.01

Table 2. Acidity and lipophilicity of nitrophenol derivatives. Log $P_{oct/water}$ – logarithm of partition coefficient between n-octanol and water [36,37] pKa – acidity constants [35,36]

The weak response of the membranes studied towards *ortho*-nitrophenol probably is a consequence of formation of an intramolecular hydrogen bond because of adequate closeness of two functional groups – OH and – NO_2 [14,16].

The relationship between the magnitude of the potentiometric response of the polymeric membrane modified with calix[4]pyrrole and the acidity of the undissociated phenolic guests we have although confirmed by the study of isomers of chloro- and fluorophenols [20]. Generally, the sequence of the magnitude of signal generated by discussed phenol derivatives follow their acidity sequence and is as follow:

nitrophenols >> chlorophenols >>fluorophenols

Presented results indicate that the acidity of the guest molecules is one of the most important parameters decisive about quality of potentiometric signal generation by membranes modified with ligands under discussion. An increase of the acidity of guest molecules causes an increase of the potentiometric response. The magnitude sequence of the signal generated by the isomeric chlorophenols was the same as in the case of nitrophenols:

$para-\text{chlorophenol} > meta-\text{chlorophenol} >> ortho-\text{chlorophenol}$

Again, the response of *ortho*-chlorophenol was the weakest, because the intermolecular hydrogen bounds formed between –OH and –Cl groups hamper the recognition process of host (calix[4]pyrrole) molecule and guest (*ortho*-chlorophenol). In consequence this leads to decrease of membrane potential changes [20].

Because the potentiometric signals of calix[4]phyrins and corrole modified membranes were very weak towards nitrophenols, the dinitrophenol isomers as strongest acids were selected as the guest molecules [14].

Guests	Calix[4]phyrin		Corrole	
	pH=3.0	pH=6.0	pH=3.0	pH=6.0
2,4-dinitrophenol	-77.1	-4.7	-36.2	-22.8
2,5-dinitrophenol	-22.2	-14.9	-7.8	-19.6
2,6-dinitrophenol	-54.6	-17.3	-6.1	-13.1

Table 3. The potentiometric responses of ISE_s incorporating of calix[4]phyrin and corrole towards of dinitrophenol isomers.

The responses of both of investigated membranes towards dinitrophenols were stronger than observed for mono – nitrophenols [14].

The sequence of signal magnitude in account of host molecules was as follow:

calix[4]phyrin> corrole

in account of isomer of dinitrophenol (for calix[4]phyrin host) was as follow:

2.4 –dinitrophenol > 2.6- dinitrophenol > 2.5- dinitrophenol

Again the results obtained support our previous hypothesis that the acidity of target phenol derivatives is crucial for the potentiometric signals of liquid membrane incorporated with host molecules such as calix[4]pyrrole [19], calix[4]phyrin or corrole [14]. The lipophilicity of analytes is rather a secondary parameter. Similar results were reported for polyamines [5, 6, 38-40].

The nitrophenol guests might interact with calix[4]phyrin, corrole or calix[4]pyrrole via "sinking" into the host cavity with the phenolic OH pointed towards the NH units of macrocycles. This was confirmed by NMR measurements [14]. Taking into account this mechanism of interaction, we can explain the good correlation between the signal magnitude sequences for all type of membranes and steric hindrance around the OH group present in guest molecule.

3. Elucidation of the mechanism of the potentiometric signal generation of calix[4]pyrrole, calix[4]phyrin and corrole –ISEs upon stimulation by undissociated phenol derivatives

The results we have obtained for calix[4]pyrrole [16, 17, 19, 20], calix[4]phyrin or corrole [14, 15] modified membranes and the results reported for macrocyclic polyamines [5, 6, 38-40] suggest that the intermolecular recognition processes between the ligands investigated and undissociated nitrophenol isomers occurring at the organic/aqueous interface, leading to the potentiometric signal generation, is a general phenomenon.

The results show a higher potentiometric response in all of discussed membranes for the more acidic guest. This fact confirms the influence of the acidity and the lipophilicity of the neutral guest on the signal generation process by membranes incorporating calix[4]phyrin, corrole or calix[4]pyrrole derivatives.

A comparison of the results for investigated host molecules shows that calix[4]pyrrole modified membranes are the considerably more sensitive towards phenolic guests that the calix[4]phyrin or corrole [15, 17, 19]. While calix[4]pyrrole, calix[4]phyrin and corrole modified membranes do not respond towards the dissociated form of phenol derivatives, the polyamine modified membranes do respond [38-40].

Investigated membranes displayed the signal magnitude sequence as follow:

calix[4]pyrrole >calix[4]phyrin > corrole

The generation of membrane potential changes after stimulation with undissociated isomers of phenols derivatives could be explained as follows. In the first step, a supramolecular complex between the host molecules located at the surface of liquid membrane phase, and the neutral phenol guest placed at the surface of the aqueous phase is formed. This interaction relays on the hydrogen bond creation between the OH group of nitrophenol and pyrrole NH groups from the macrocyclic hosts. This was proved by NMR measurements [14].

The formation of such a supramolecular complex, according to mesomeric and inductive effects, causes an increase of acidity of the phenol OH function. This may decrease the pK_a of the phenol derivatives at the surface of the polymeric phase. This leads to the dissociation of OH group and finally to proton ejection from the interface to the aqueous layer adjacent to the organic phase. The energy gained from the proton solvation process is probably the driving force allowing for the dissociation of phenol derivatives at the aqueous/organic membrane interface. This event is responsible for the generation of an anionic response of calix[4]pyrrole, calix[4]phyrin and corrole incorporating membranes after their stimulation with undissociated phenols.

$ArOH_{(aq)} \leftrightarrow ArOH_{(mem)}$ extraction (i)

$Host_{(membrane)} + ArOH_{(mem)} \leftrightarrow Host\text{---}ArOH_{(membrane)}$ complexation (ii)

$Host\text{---}ArOH_{(membrane)} \leftrightarrow Host\text{---}ArO^- + H^+$ dissociation and proton ejection to water surface (iii)

The increase of the proton concentration in the very thin aqueous layer containing 1.0×10^{-2} M *para*-nitrophenol in 1.0×10^{-2} M of KCl (pH 4.0), adjacent to the calix[4]pyrrole or corrole membrane surface, supported this assumption [14, 17]. According to the mechanism proposed, the lack of the potential changes of calix[4]pyrrole, calix[4]phyrin and corrole ISEs observed in the presence of phenolic guests at alkaline pH could be explained as follows.

At this pH the concentration of OH^- in the water phase is high enough to block the cavity of all investigated host molecules by creation of host –OH^- complex [14, 17]. Thus, the formation of a supramolecular complex with phenolic guests is not possible. To confirm that such complex could block the cavity of the calix[4]pyrrole, in our previous investigation we have tested the membrane modified with a calix[4]pyrrole substituted with bromine atoms at the β - carbons. The lack of any response towards nitrophenol isomers of a membrane incorporating bromine derivatives of calix[4]pyrrole, even in strong acid solution supports this assumption [14, 17]. The electron withdrawing bromine atoms increase the affinity of calix[4]pyrrole towards OH^-. Such a complex could be created even in acidic medium. Therefore, in this case the cavity of calix[4]pyrrole is blocked and the supramolecular ligand – phenol complex based on hydrogen bonds can not be created [14, 17].

The lack of any response of the membrane modified with calix[4]phyrin or corrole towards dinitrophenol isomers and very low response towards nitrophenol isomers in alkaline medium (Table 1) could be explained as follow. The consequence of host-OH^- complex creation is the negatively charged surface of polymeric membranes. Dinitrophenols in such circumstances also exist in the anionic forms. Thus, the host-guest electrostatic repulsion force is probably the main reason preventing interaction between them.

The magnitude sequence of the potentiometric signals observed for calix[4]pyrrole, calix[4]phyrin and corrole membranes suggests that the acidity of the target molecules is one of the important factors affecting the process of potentiometric signal generation. A similar relation was observed in the case of macrocyclic polyamine-ISEs [5, 6]. In Table 2 the values of pK_a and $logP_{oct}$ of target molecules investigated were collected.

On the other hand, the recognition of phenol derivatives by calix[4]pyrrole calix[4]phyrin and corrole is such that guests respectively bury themselves into the host cavity or are perpendicular to the macrocycle, with (in both cases) the phenolic OH pointed toward the pyrrole end, where the hydrogen bonds with NH units are formed [14, 17, 42]. Because of this, the sensitivity sequences observed for nitrophenol as well dinitrophenol isomers reflect also the magnitude of the steric obstacle, which is the lowest in the case of *para*-nitrophenol and 2,4-dinitrophenol. Therefore, for these two guests, the strongest potentiometric responses of ISEs studied were observed. A comparison of the results we have obtained for calix[4]pyrrole and [16, 17] calix[4]phyrin and corrole [14, 21, 42] and the results reported for macrocyclic amines [5, 6, 38-40] showed that the potential generation by the membranes modified with nitrogen-containing macrocyclic compounds after stimulation with phenol derivatives is a general phenomenon. The most important parameters governing this phenomenon are the differences between the acidity of the OH group of the target molecules and the ability of the NH group of the macrocyclic ligands to create the hydrogen bonds with OH group of the phenol derivatives.

The signal magnitude sequence based on the host molecules incorporated into the membranes is as follows:

polyamines > calix[4]pyrroles > calix[4]phyrins >corroles

This sequence reflects the sequence of availability of hydrogen atoms coming from NH or NH^+ group of ligand for OH group of phenol derivatives. This availability is crucial for host –guest complex creation.

Calix[4]pyrrole changes its conformation upon complexation of target molecules, and this macrocycle adopts a cone conformation with the four pyrrole NH groups forming hydrogen bonds with OH group of phenol derivatives. The similar reorganization of the calix[4]pyrrole cavity upon complexation with halide anions was reported [26, 27, 29]. In the case of corrole, such conformational change is not possible because of its rigid structure [41]. As a consequence a strong four-center hydrogen bond can not be created. This is probably the explanation of the weaker potential signal generated by the membrane modified with corrole stimulated with nitrophenols in comparison to membranes modified with calix[4]pyrrole. This statement is supported by results obtained for membranes modified with protonated macrocyclic polyamines, which because of their highest flexibility and ionic character are able to create the strongest supramolecular complex based on hydrogen bonds [40]. This leads to the strongest polarization of O-H bond of phenol derivatives. Such membranes generated the strongest signal for nitrophenol derivatives and only these types of membranes are able to recognize dihydroxybenzene isomers, which are very weak acids [6, 40]. The relationship between acid –base properties of guest is in good agreement with the proposed mechanism. The dissociation of the O-H group at the liquid /liquid interface from the phenol – ligand complex is necessary for the generation of membrane potential changes. In the case of macrocyclic polyamines, the hydrogen bond between the N-H and OH phenolic group is the strongest, and as a consequence, this causes the highest increase of the acidity of proton from –OH. In the case of calix[4]pyrrole and corroles, the hydrogen bonds are weaker than macrocyclic polyamines. Therefore, the increase of the acidity of OH group from phenolic guest upon creation of supramolecular complexes with calix[4]pyrrole and corrole are lower in the comparison to this observed for polyamines.

The response properties of ISEs based on ion carriers are strongly influenced by the membrane composition, in particular by the presence of ionic sites in the organic membrane [44-46]. The type of ionic sites depends on the charge of ionophore. In the case of ISEs based on neutral host molecules, ionic sites with the charged sign opposite to that of primary ions are necessary to obtain a Nernstian response, to decrease the membrane resistance, to reduce the ion interference, and to improve the detection limit and selectivity. On the other hand, in ISEs based on electrically charged host, ionic sites with the same charge sign as the primary ions are recommended. In case of potentiometric sensors destined for the detection of neutral compounds there is no general knowledge about the influence of ionic sites on response property.

The calix[4]pyrroles are neutral molecules. On the contrary, the corroles could exist in the three forms: cationic, neutral or anionic [32]. Therefore, two types of ionic sites (anionic and cationic) were used for additional modification of liquid membrane electrodes incorporating both hosts.

The membranes containing corrole and lipophilic cationic salt, tridodecylmethyl -ammonium chloride (T-DDMACl), demonstrated a better sensitivity and a wider dynamic range of potentiometric response towards mono- and dinitrophenol isomers in comparison to membranes containing only corrole [14]. On the other hand, the corrole membranes additionally incorporating an anionic lipophilic salt, potassium tetrakis(p-chlorophenyl)borate (K-TpCPB), gave no response towards phenolic guests.

A similar influence of both type of lipophilic salts were observed for calix[4]pyrrole liquid membrane electrodes [17].

The addition of a lipophilic anion-exchanger into calix[4]pyrrole or corrole-incorporating membranes induces the increase of their pH and phenol response.

This supports the hypothesis, that in the mechanism of their potentiometric response towards pH or phenol derivatives, the reversible hydroxide transport form aqueous to organic phase is involved [17].

4. Potentiometric responses of Mn(III)-porphyrin and dipyrromethene Cu(II) containing sensors toward paracetamol

The potentiometric responses of these sensors toward paracetamol were measured in 0.01 M phosphate buffer at pH = 5.5 [22]. Under these conditions, paracetamol (pKa= 9.5) exists as the undissociated compound in solution. The polymeric liquid membrane and carbon paste based sensor were tested toward paracetamol. Both of the sensors contain Mn(III)-porphyrin as the host molecule.

The generation of membrane potential changes after stimulation with undissociated paracetamol molecules could be explained as follows. In the first step, chloride ligated Mn(III)-porphyrin creates an aqua-complex via simple binding of water as a sixth ligand. The creation of such a complex was described by Meyerhoff *et al.* [47]:

$$\mathrm{Mn(TPP)Cl + H_2O \leftrightarrow Mn(TPP)ClH_2O} \tag{1}$$

$$\begin{gathered}\mathrm{Mn(TPP)ClH_2O + paracetamol \leftrightarrow Mn(TPP)ClH_2O\text{---}paracetamol} \\ \mathrm{Mn(TPP)Cl\text{---}paracetamol\ complexation + H_2O}\end{gathered} \tag{2}$$

$$\begin{gathered}\mathrm{Mn(TPP)Cl\text{---}paracetamol \leftrightarrow Mn(TPP)Cl\text{---}paracetamol^- + H^+} \\ \text{dissociation of paracetamol and ejection of proton to water phases}\end{gathered} \tag{3}$$

In the next step, a second-sphere supramolecular complex of paracetamol molecules with $\mathrm{Mn(TPP)ClH_2O}$ is created. The existence of such a complex at the surface of a polymeric liquid membrane modified with metalloporphyrins was postulated by Kibbey *et al.* [48]. This second-sphere interaction with paracetamol molecules occurs probably at a low sample concentration. When the concentration of paracetamol increases, an exchange of second-sphere coordinated paracetamol for inner-sphere water ligands occurs, and, as a consequence, a complex between the Mn(III) centers and paracetamol, *via* the oxygen atom from the amide group is created.

In the measuring condition (pH = 5.5), paracetamol molecules exists in undissociated form (pK_a =9.5). The formation of the above mentioned complex, according to a combination of mesomeric and inductive effects, causes an increase of the acidity of the phenolic OH function from paracetamol molecule. As a consequence, this leads to a more facile dissociation of the OH group and finally to H^+ ejection from the interface to the aqueous layer adjacent to the organic phase.

This event is responsible for the generation of an anionic response of the polymeric liquid membranes modified with metalloporphyrins after their stimulation with undissociated paracetamol.

The reaction of the metalloporphyrin complex with paracetamol was confirmed by spectroscopic measurements at the border between water and the polymeric membrane. The UV-Vis absorption spectrum of a thin membrane film containing Mn(III)-porphyrin deposited onto glass slides conditioned in 0.01 M phosphate buffer solution (pH = 5.5) exhibited one main band at 470 nm and two weaker bands at 376 and 400 nm. After conditioning in phosphate buffer with an increasing concentration of paracetamol, the absorbance maximum decreased and shifted to shorter wavelength. This blue shift was expected due to the increase in electron density around the Mn(III) centers by the coordinated amide. These data confirm the creation of a complex between the Mn(III)-porphyrin and paracetamol [22].

The electrochemically active Cu(II) dipyrromethene complex immobilized on the surface of gold electrodes previously modified with a dodecanethiol monolayer was successfully applied for voltammetric determination of paracetamol [23]. The interaction of paracetamol with Cu(II) redox centers was a base of analytical signal generation. The presence of human plasma in the measuring solution influence very little on the sensor performance. Its linear dynamic range (0.2-3.2 mM) was sufficient for controlling the toxic level of paracetamol in human plasma [23].

5. Potentiometric response of membranes modified with undecylcalix[4] – resorcinarene derivatives towards of unprotonated diaminobenzene isomers

According to presented mechanism of anionic potentiometric signal generation by membranes modified with nitrogen containing macromolecules as host molecules and stimulated with neutral form of phenol derivatives the crucial phenomenon is transfer of protons from the membrane surface to surface of water phase. From this point of view it was logical and interesting to check if generation of cationic potentiometric signal by membranes modified with macrocycles containing the phenolic group stimulated with unprotonated derivatives of aniline would be possible [25, 52]

There are summarization of systematic research results of the intermolecular recognition processes at the water/polymer membrane border between some derivatives of undecylcalix[4]resorcinarene (Figure 2) and neutral (unprotonated) forms of aniline and its derivatives

http://dx.doi.org/10.5772/52803

such as: aminoaniline, chloroaniline, hydroxyaniline, methylaniline, methoxyaniline and nitroaniline obtained with using potentiometry.

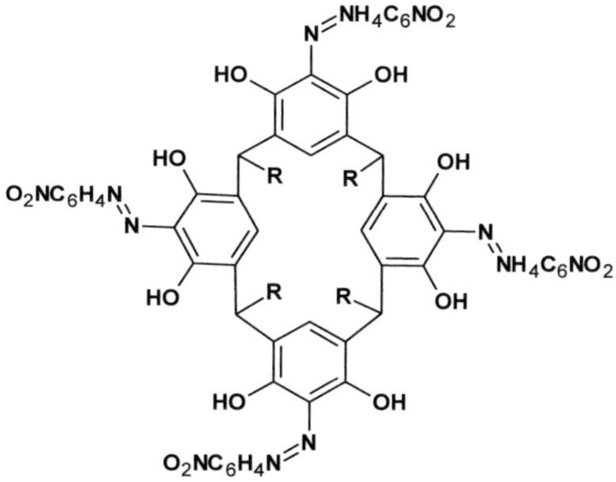

Ligand 1

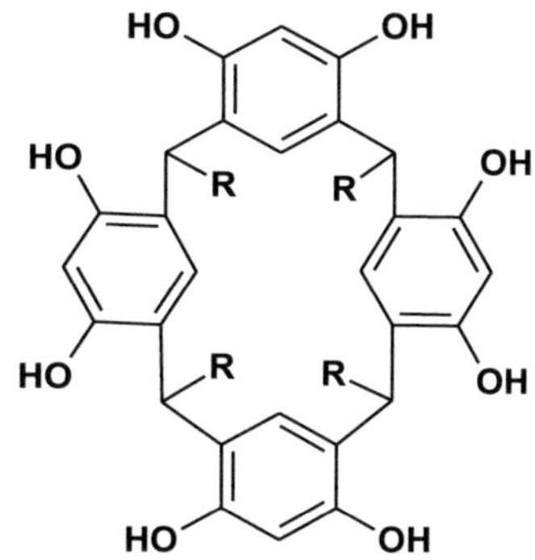

Ligand 2

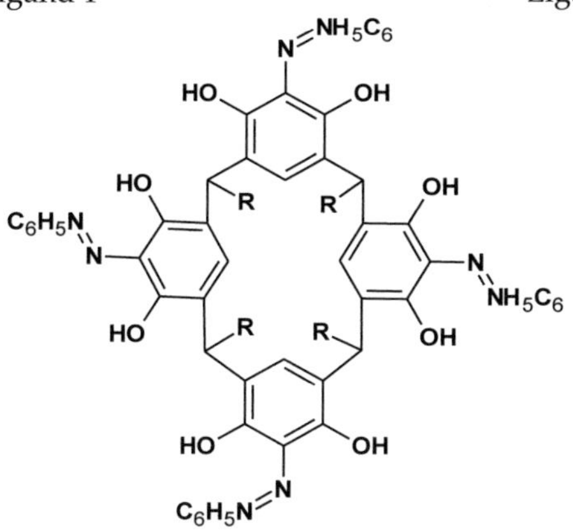

Ligand 3

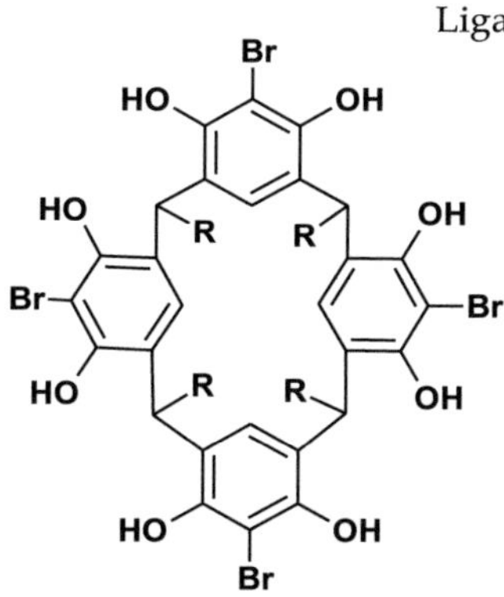

Ligand 4

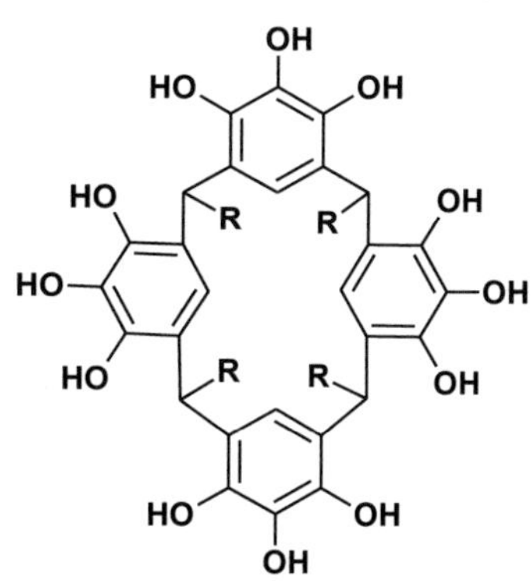

Ligand 5

Figure 2. The structure of host molecules.

In Table 4 the values of potentiometric response of PVC supported liquid membranes incorporated with calixarene host generated in the presence of aniline derivatives are collected. The measurements for all membranes studied were done at pH 7. At this pH investigated aniline derivatives exist in water almost entirely as neutral (unprotonated) compounds (see Table 5).

As it is seen from results introduced from Table 4, all types of membranes generate cationic response towards aniline derivatives

Guests	pK_1	Log $P_{o/w}$	ΔE[mV] Lig 1	ΔE[mV] Lig 2	ΔE[mV] Lig 3	ΔE[mV] Lig 4	ΔE[mV] Lig 5
p-aminoaniline	6.22	-0.26	148.9	138.4	88,4	86.9	41.5
p-anisidine	5.36	1.15	118.6	68.9	53,9	59.4	37.4
m-anisidine	4.20	1.32	92.6	62.2	55,1	20.1	28.4
o-aminoaniline	4.61	0.37	66.8	57.2	64,2	31.0	31.5
m-aminoaniline	5.01	0.03	36.2	42.1	35,8	13.8	7.6
p-toluidine	5.08	1.43	92.3	36.2	44.1	27.0	30.2
p-chloroaniline	3.98	1.81	31.5	24.2	22,8	-0.6	6.2
o-anisidine	4.53	1.65	62.7	20.1	35,7	19.8	7.8
p-hydroxyaniline	5.48	-0.24	27.6	15.5	25,2	-2.1	2.4
aniline	4.87	1.24	57.7	12.8	34,5	10.7	13.1
m-toluidine	4.71	1.59	84.2	9.7	32,9	14.9	22.0
o-toluidine	4.45	1.61	75.8	9.4	20,8	10.7	7.7
p-nitroaniline	1.02	1.19	4.7	3.0	-	-	2.4
m-chloroaniline	3.52	1.88	19.8	0.7	2	-	9.2
o-chloroaniline	2.66	2.02	8.6	-4.5	1,2	-	1.9

ΔE[mV] = E_0 -E_i E_0 – potential recorded in buffer solution, E_i – potential record in the presence of analyte at is final concentration

Table 4. Potentiometric response of PVC supported liquid membranes incorporated with host undodecylcalix[4] resorcinarene derivatives generated in the presence of aniline derivatives. Log $P_{oct/water}$ – logarithm of partition coefficient between n-octanol and water [36, 37] pKa – acidity constants [35, 36]

	Analyte	pK_1	pK_2	pH 7.0	
				RNH_2 (%)	RNH_3^+ (%)
1	*p*-nitroaniline	1.02		100.0	0.0
2	*o*-chloroaniline	2.66		100.0	0.0
3	*m*-chloroaniline	3.52		100.0	0.0
4	*p*-chloroaniline	3.98		99.9	0.1
5	*m*-anisidine	4.20		99.8	0.2
6	*o*-toluidine	4.45		99.7	0.3
7	*o*-anisidine	4.53		99.7	0.3
8	*o*-aminoaniline	4.61	1.81	99.6	0.4
9	*m*-toluidine	4.71		99.5	0.5
10	aniline	4.87		99.3	0.7
11	*m*-aminoaniline	5.01	2.56	99.0	1.0
12	*p*-toluidine	5.08		98.8	1.2
13	*p*-anisidine	5.36		97.8	2.2
14	*p*-hydroxyaniline	5.48		97.1	2.9
15	*p*-aminoaniline	6.22	2.99	85.8	14.2

Table 5. Percentage of protonated and neutral species at pH 7 [25]

The comparison of the results we have got for all of guest molecules showing the following general tendency: with increase of analyte basicity the response increases. This is truth for all of modified membranes. In most of the cases the isomer *para* generate the highest response. For another isomers is difficult to estimate with one generate higher signal. In some cases it is isomer *ortho*, in another meta.

Explanation of weak response of membranes after stimulation with *ortho* isomers is the possibility to form intramolecular hydrogen bonds.

The correlation between the partition coeffiction of guest (Table 4) and value of potentiometric response is very week. And this suggests that this parameter is rather less important for observed phenomena.

The weakest response we have observed for nitro- and chloro- derivatives of aniline. They are the strongest acids between the investigated compounds.

The main differences between the host molecules under study are structure of upper rim. Ligand 1 poses in their upper rim dihydroxybenzene substituents in which the OH groups are in position 1, 3 in relation to each other. Because of this distance the intramolecular hydrogen bounds are very week [43]. Additionally this ligand is substituted in position 2 with azonitrobenzene. The presence of this substituent, because of its inductive and rezonance effect causing the increase of acidity of phenol groups from upper ring. Ligand 2 contains in its structure dihydroxybenzene with OH groups in positions 1 and 3.

Next host, number 3, in its upper rim contains the dihydroksybromobenzene. The OH groups are in position 2, 6 in relation to azabenzene substituent. This substituent, because of its inductive and mesomeric effect, increased the acidity of phenols in relation to previous one.

The upper rim of ligand 4 contains the bromo- 2, 5 hydroksybenzene. The close vicinity of OH groups creates the very good conditions for creation of intramolecular network of hydrogen bonds [43]. The last ligand (no 5) posses in upper rim trihydroksybenzene. Similarly as in previous one this system allows to create the intramolecular hydrogen bound network.

Comparison of value of potentiometric response we have got for each ligand showing the general tendency which is as follow:

Ligand 1 > ligand 2 > ligand 3, ligand 4 > ligand 5

This indicates that increase of the acidity of phenols groups in upper rim causing the increase of response value.

The strongest response we have observed for membrane modified with ligand 1 containing in its structure dihydroxybenzene substituted with azonitrobenzene. Acidity of these OH groups is the highest.

Next in this sequence is ligand 2 substituted with dihydroxybenzene. In this case the acidity of OH groups is lower in relation to the previous one, but the accessibility of them for guest is much easier. As consequence the creation of hydrogen bound (H...O...H...N) between host and guest is relatively easy. The next ligand in the discussed sequence, ligand 3 contained in its structure dihydroxybenzene substituted with azobenzene. This causing the increase the acidity of phenolic group in upper rim, but at the same time presence of rather large substituent makes the hindrance in accessibility of OH groups for guest molecules. The value of generated potentiometric signal is the consequence of these two opposite effects.

Membrane modified with host containing the bromo-derivatives of dihydrobenzene in its structure (no 4) is next in sequence of response value. In this case from one side the inductive effect bromine atom causing increase of acidity of phenolic group and from another one large atom of bromine constitute hindrance in accessibility of phenols groups for guest.

The lowest answer we have got for membrane modified with ligand 5, which poses in its structure trihydroksybenzene. In this ligand the network of intramolecular hydrogen bounds is the strongest. And because of this the formation of supramolecular complex with guest is the most difficult between the ligand under study.

The comparison of lipophilicity of investigated guest molecules showing that there is no direct relation between the lipophilicity of amines and values of signal generated by them.

In order to confirm the supramolecular complex formation between undecylcalix[4]resorcinarene and aniline derivatives at the border of organic/aqueous interface UV-Vis measurements were performed according to procedure reported [52].

http://dx.doi.org/10.5772/52803

Upon complexation of *para*–diaminobenzene, the absorbance decrease at 214 nm, characteristic for UDC[4]Rene was observed. The absorbance at 239 nm characteristic for *para*–diaminobenzene also decrease and shifted towards red. Additionally, new peak was visible at 267 nm. These absorbance changes clearly indicated that a supramolecular complex UDC[4]Rene-*para*-diaminobenzene is formed at the membrane surface.

Therefore, it might be concluded that the cationic potentiometric signals observed in the study presented were generated as a result of the supramolecular recognition phenomenon occurring at the organic/aqueous interface.

Based on obtained results and literature data we have proposed the following mechanism of cationic potential signal generation by membranes modified with derivatives of undecylcalix[4]resorcinarene after stimulation with unprotonated derivatives of aminobenzene. In the first step, which is going during the membrane conditioning some of phenolic groups of derivatives of undecylcalix[4]resorcinarene located at the surface of polymeric membranes dissociated and membranes became minus charged. Such type of dissociation of OH groups of upper rim of undecylcalix[4]resorcinarene was described in [53, 54]. In next step, the network of hydrogen bonds between the derivatives of aminobenzene and phenolic groups is formed. In such situation the amino groups are donors of hydrogen atoms and polarity of them are correlated with acidity of phenol groups. The formation of such network is described in [49-51]. As a result of this, the supramolecular complex of undecylcalix[4]resorcinarene – aminobenzene derivatives located at the interface is formed. As a consequence of above complex formation the density of electrons on nitrogen of aminobenzene increases. The measurements were carried out at pH 7. In this condition all of investigated amines exist in solution mostly as unprotonated compounds (Table 5). The increase of the density of electrons at amine nitrogen atoms causing the increase of their basicity. Because of this, they became protonated in spite of pH condition in bulk solution. This protonation is done by means of transfer of proton from surface of water face to surface of organic one. The transfer of proton leading to the increase of plus charge of membrane and we can observe the generation of potentiometric cationic signal.

Proposed mechanism is based on the three steps:

The first one concerns dissociation of some phenolic groups from upper rim of investigated ligands.

i. $$\mathrm{HostOH_{membrane} + H_2O \leftrightarrow HostO^- + H_3O^+}$$

Next step consist of transfer of analyte from bulk solution to the interface and formation of supramolecular complex ligand –analyte through hydrogen bonds.

ii. $$\mathrm{HostO^-_{interface} + NH_2\text{-}AR \leftrightarrow HostO^-\text{----}H\text{---}NH\text{-}AR_{interface}}$$

The consequence of this is the increase of basicity on nitrogen atom from supramolecular complex and its protonation.

iii. $$\mathrm{HostO^-\text{----}H\text{---}NH\text{-}AR_{interface} + H_3O^+ \leftrightarrow HostO^-\text{----}H\text{---}NH_2\text{-}AR^+_{interface} + H_2O}$$

The formation of such complex at the border we confirmed by means of spectroscopic method. The conformation of first step is based on result we have got for membrane modified with ligand 1 in which the acidity of phenolic groups is the highest.

The results we observed for bromo- and azobenzo- derivatives of investigated undecylcalix[4]resorcinarene showing that the accessibility of phenols groups is very important parameter for intermolecular recognition processes which are going between investigated ligands and analytes.

The weakest response we have observed in case of membranes modified with ligand which has in its structure trihydroxybenzene was explained by possibilities to form the network of intramolecular hydrogen bonds. This is a relatively strong energetic barrier for the described phenomenon.

The second step of proposed mechanism relays on transfer of protons from water phase to organic one. This is supported by fact that independently on the host structure, the strongest signal we have observed for the strongest base between guest compounds under study. The results we have got showed that lipophilicity of analytes it is not crucial parameter.

6. Conclusions

We have presented the systematic research on the potentiometric response of membranes modified with macrocyclic compounds containing in their structures amino groups stimulated by the undissociated phenol derivatives and membranes modified with macrocycles containing the phenolic groups stimulated by unprotonated derivatives of aniline.

The results showed that membranes modified with calix[4]pyrrole, calix[4]phyrin and corrole derivatives are able to generate an anionic potentiometric response after stimulation with undissociated forms of phenols derivatives, whereas the membranes modified with undecylcalix[4]resorcinarene derivatives are able to generate the cationic potentiometric response after stimulation with unprotonated aniline derivatives. Our experimental date indicated that in two types of membranes the movement of protons across the interface is responsible for potentiometric signal generation.

The general mechanism of the potentiometric signal generated by membranes modified with discussed host molecules stimulated by uncharged guest relies on:

- the formation of supramolecular host -guest complex at the liquid membrane/water interface
- the transfer of protons from water surface to organic phase surface generated cationic response, whereas transfer of proton from surface of organic phase to the surface of water generate of anionic response.

In both of cases the acidity of host and basicity of guest are crucial parameters for course of processes under discussion.

http://dx.doi.org/10.5772/52803

- The sensitivity and selectivity of these processes are governed by the acidity of the target molecules studied as well as the ability of host molecules for creation of hydrogen bonds. The lipophilicity of analytes it the secondary parameter.

The described phenomena open the totally new and very promising field of analytical application of potentiometric method.

Author details

Jerzy Radecki* and Hanna Radecka

*Address all correspondence to: j.radecki@pan.olsztyn.pl

Institute of Animal Reproduction and Food Research of Polish Academy of Sciences, Olsztyn, Poland

References

[1] Bakker, E., *Talanta*, 2004 , 63, 21.

[2] Gale, P.A., *Coordination Chemistry Reviews* , 2003, 240, 191.

[3] Umezawa Y., "Ion-Selective Electrodes" , in "Encyclopedia of Supramolecular Chemistry", 2004, Marcel Dekker, New York, p.747.

[4] Ito, T., Radecka, H, Tohda, K., Odashima, K., Umezawa,Y. *J. Am. Chem. Soc.* 1998, 120, 3049.

[5] Odashima , K., Naganava, R., Radecka, H., Kataoka, M., Kiura, E., Koike, T., Tohda, K., Tange, M., Furta, H., Sessler, J. L.,. Yagi, K., Umezawa, Y. *Supramolecular Chemistry* 1994, 4,101.

[6] Ito, T., Radecka, H., Umezawa, K., Kiura, T., Yashiro, A., Lin, X., Kataoka, M., Kiura, E., Sessler, J.L., Yagi, K., Umezawa, Y. *Anal. Sciences*. 1998 14, 89.

[7] M. De Serio H. Mohapatra , R. Zenobi , V. Deckert , Chemical Physics Letters 417 (2006) 452–456

[8] Russell, E., Morris *Nature Chemistry* 2011, 3, 347–348.

[9] Spichiger –Keller U.E., "Chemical Sensors and Biosensors for Medical and Biological Applications" , 1998, Wiley-VCH, Weinheim, Germany.

[10] Pretsch, E., Bühlmann, P., Bakker, E., *Chem Rev.,* 1997, 97, 3083; 1998 , 98, 1593.

[11] L. Bulgariu, H. Radecka, M. Pietraszkiewicz, O. Pietraszkiewicz, Analytical Letters, 2003, 36, 1325-1334.

[12] Radecka, H., Szymańska, I., Pietraszkiewicz, M., Pietraszkiewicz, O., Aoki, H., Umezawa, Y. *Chem. Anal. (Warsaw)*, 2005, 50, 85-102.

[13] Szymańska, I., Radecka, H.,.Radecki, J., Gale, P.A., Warriner, C.N. *Journal of Electroanalytical Chemistry*, 2006, 591, 223-228.

[14] Radecki, J., Stenka, I., Dolusic, E., Dehaen, W., Plavec, J. *Comb. Chem. High. Throughput Screening* 2004, 7,375-381.

[15] Radecki, J. Radecka , H., *Current Topice In Electrochemistry*, 2008, 13, 27-35.

[16] Piotrowski, T., Radecka, H., Radecki, J., Depraetere, S., Dehaen, W. *Electroanalysis* 2001, 13, 342-346.

[17] Radecki, J., Radecka, H., Piotrowski, T., Depraetere, S., Dehaen, W., Plavec, J. *Electroanalysis* 2004, 16, 2073-2081.

[18] Szymańska, I., Orlewska, Cz., Janssen, D., Dehaen, W., Radecka, H. *Electrochimica Acta* 2008, 53, 7932 - 7940.

[19] Piotrowski, T., Radecka, H., Radecki, J., Depraetere, S., Dehaen, W., *Material Science and Engineering* 2001, 18, 223-228.

[20] Piotrowski, T., Radecka, H., Radecki, J., Depraetere, S., Dehaen, W., *Anal. Letters* 2002, 35, 1895-1906.

[21] Radecki, J., Stenka, I., Dolusic, E., Dehaen, W., *Electrochimica Acta* 2006, 51, 2282-2288.

[22] Saraswathyamma, B., Pająk, M., Radecki, J., Maes, W., Dehaen, W., Kumar, K.G., Radecka, H. *Electroanalysis*, 2008, 20, No. 18, 2009 – 2015.

[23] Saraswathyamma, B., Grzybowska, I., Orlewska, Cz., Radecki, J., Dehaen, W., Kumar, K.G., Radecka, H. *Electroanalysis*, 2008, 20, No. 21, 2317-2323.

[24] Ocicka, K., Radecka,H., Radecki, J., Pietraszkiewicz, M., Pietraszkiewicz O. *Sensors and Actuators B*, 2003, 217-224.

[25] Poduval, R.,. Kurzątkowska, K., Stobiecka, M., Dehaen, W.F.A., Dehaen, W., Radecka, H., Radecki, J. *Supramolecular Chemistry*, 2010, 22, No. 7-8, 412 – 418.

[26] Gale, P., A., Anzenbacher Jr, P., Sessler, J., L., *Coordination Chemistry Reviews*, 2001, 222, 57.

[27] Sessler, J. L., Camiolo, S., Gale, P. A., *Coordination Chemistry Reviews*, 2003, 240, 17.

[28] Custelcean, R., Delmau, L.H., Moyer, B.A., Sessler J.L., Cho, W.S., Gross, D., Bates, G.W., Brooks, S.J., Light, M.E., Gale, P.A., *Angew. Chem.*, 2005, 117, 2593.

[29] Gale, P.A., Sessler, J.L., Král, Lynch, V., *J. Am. Chem.Soc.*, 1996, 118, 5140.

[30] Bucher, Ch., Zimmerman, R.S., Lynch, V., Kral, V., Sessler, J. L., *J.Am.Chem Soc* 2001 , 123, 2099-2100.

http://dx.doi.org/10.5772/52803

[31] Camiolo, S., Coles, S.J., , Gale, P.A., Hursthouse, M.B., Sessler, J.L., *Acta Crystallogr. Sect. E*, 2001, 75, 816.

[32] Mahammed, A., Weaver, J.J., Gray, H. B., Abdelas , M., Gross, Z., *Tetrahedron Letters*, 2003, 44, 2077.

[33] Jonson, A., W,. Kay, I.T. *J. Chem. Soc.* 1965, 1620.

[34] Broadhurst, M.J., Grieg, R., Shelton, G., Johson, A.W. *J. Chem.Soc. Perkin Trans I* 1972, 143.

[35] Wroński, M. J., *Chromatogr. A*, 1997 , 772, 19.

[36] Dimitrienko, S.G., Myshak, E. N., Pyatkova, L. N., *Talanta* , 1999, 49, 309.

[37] Leo, A., Hansch, C., Elkins, D., *Chem Rev.* 1971, 71, 525.

[38] Piotrowski, T., Szymańska, I., Radecka, H., Radecki, J., Pietraszkiewicz, M., Pietraszkiewicz, O., Wojciechowski, K., *Electroanalysis* , 2000 , 12, 1397.

[39] Szymańska, I., Radecka, H., Radecki, J., Pietraszkiewicz, M., Pietraszkiewicz, O., *Combinatorial Chemistry & High Throughput Screening* , 2000, 3, 509.

[40] Szymańska, I., Radecka, H., Radecki, J., Pietraszkiewicz, M., Pietraszkiewicz , O. *Electroanalysis* , 2003 , 15, 294-302.

[41] Asokan, C.V., Smeets, S., Dehaen, W., *Tetrahedron Lett.*, 2001, 42, 448.

[42] Stenka, I., Radecka, H., Radecki, J., Dolusic, E., Dehaen, W. *Pol. J. Food Nutr. Sci.*, 2003, 53, 127.

[43] Aakeröy, C.B., Seddon, K.R., *Chem. Soc. Rev.*, 1993, 22,397-407.

[44] Tohda, K., Higuchi, T., Dragoe, D., Umezawa, Y., *Analytical Sciences*, 2001, 17, 833.

[45] Amemiya, S., Bühlmann, P., Pretsch, E., Rusterholz, B., Umezawa, Y., *Anal. Chem.* 2000, 72, 1618

[46] Bühlmann, P., Yajima, S., Tohda, K., Umezawa, K., Nishizawa, S., Umezawa, Y., *Electroanalysis*, 1995, 7, 811

[47] Chaniotakis, N., Chasser, A., Meyerhoff, M.E., Grovers, J. *Anal. Chem.* 1988, 60, 185.

[48] Kibbey, C.E, Park, S.B., DeAdwyler, G., Meyerhoff, M.E., *J Electroanal. Chem.*, 1999, 335 135-194.

[49] Woods, C.J., Camiolo, S., Light, M.E., Coles, S.J., Hursthouse, M.B., King, M.A., Gale, P.A., Essex, J.W., *J. Am. Chem. Soc.*, 2002, 124, 8644.

[50] Beer, P.D., Cadman, J. *Coord. Chem. Rev.* 2003, 240, 131- 155.

[51] Ammico, D.A, Di Natale, C., Polasse, R., Macagnanon, A., Mantini A. *Sens. Actuator B* 2000, 65, 209-215.

[52] Kurzatkowska, K., Radecka, H., Dehaen, W., Wasowicz, M., Grzybowska, I. *J. Comb. Chem. Throughput. Screen.* 2007, 10, 604 – 6010.

[53] Akecylan, E., Bahidir, M., Yilmaz, M.J. *Hazard. Mater*. 2009, 162, 960-966.

[54] Gustasche, C. D., Iqbal, M., Alam, I. *J. Am. Chem. Soc*. 1987, 109, 4314-4320.

Chapter 21

Molecular Recognition of Trans-Chiral Schiff Base Metal Complexes for Induced CD

Takashiro Akitsu and Chigusa Kominato

Additional information is available at the end of the chapter

http://dx.doi.org/10.5772/52226

1. Introduction

Schiff base is one of the most popular ligands in the field of coordination chemistry [1-5]. Conventionally, transition metal complexes having Schiff base ligands have been investigated about stereochemistry and corresponding electronic properties mainly. For example, solution paramagnetism of Ni(II) complexes, structural phase transition of Cu(II) complexes, chiral catalysts, and some types of molecule-based magnets and other interesting facts about correlation between structures and properties are known and these facts are cooperative effect involving intermolecular interactions and molecular recognition. Because of developing importance as functional chiral materials, many researchers have investigated crystal structures (including thermally-induced structural phase transition and polymorphism by solvents) of *trans*-type chiral Schiff base metal complexes and extract important features of chiral molecular recognition in the solid states.

As mentioned in Abstract section, we have tested observation of some novel phenomena associated with chirality or CD spectroscopy based on intermolecular interactions. Induced CD on various nano-scaled (inorganic) materials from chiral Schiff base metal complexes is one of them and not only electronic and magnetic dipole moments but also molecular recognition between chiral compounds and nano-scaled materials are important factors for these phenomena [6, 7]. For example, we have observed induced CD peaks from chiral Schiff base Ni(II) complexes at d-d region for achiral or chiral Schiff base Cu(II) complexes (without exchanging ligands) [8], at d-d and CT regions for Cu(II)-coordinated metallodendrimers (PAMAM), and surface plasmon region for Cu-clusters prepared in PAMAM by irradiation of UV light for the first time [9, 10]. In this way, we have also reported on induced CD peaks of metal complexes (both achiral and chiral ones), organometallics (ferrocene) [11], metallodendrimers, metal nano-clusters, and nano-particles [9, 10] of metal-semiconductors [12]. Additionally, we have successfully observed size-dependence of wavelengths of induced CD peaks from chiral Schiff base Zn(II) complexes involving azo-groups at surface plasmon region on colloidal gold particles [13].

As for the induced CD between chiral Schiff base Ni(II) or Zn(II) complexes and Cu-clusters prepared in PAMAM, we have also investigated the role of chiral ligands for molecular recognition. For example, naphtylgroups are appropriate for induced CD, while more flexible groups are not [14] (Figure 1). Therefore, several examples indicated that supramolecular or molecular recognition must be a key reason for specific intermolecular interactions. In this review article, we have summarized several examples of crystal structures and optimized structures (as a model of them in solutions) of *trans*-type chiral Schiff base Ni(II), Cu(II), and Zn(II) complexes. In order to derive important steric factors for molecular recognition, we will point out characteristic features of molecular shapes or their conformational changes *in silico*.

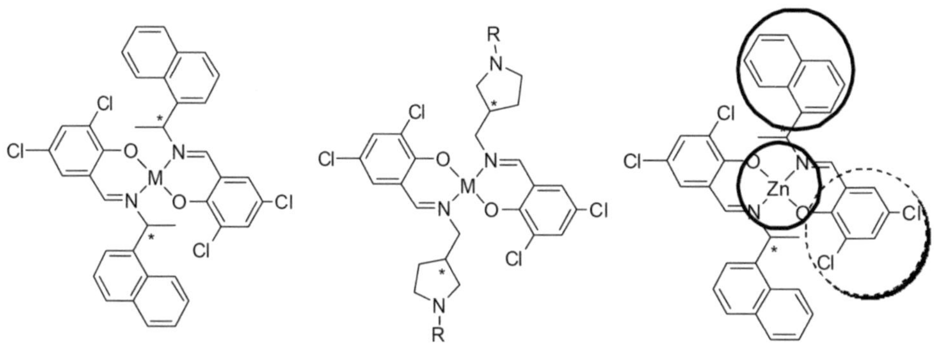

Figure 1. Examples of suitable [left] and unsuitable [center] ligands for induced CD based on experiments [9, 10, 14]. [Right]Important (bold circles) and unimportant (broken circle)moieties of ligands for induced CD.

2. Computation

According to a CCDC database [15], we selected some crystal structures of *trans*-type Schiff base metal complexes. As modeling conformational changes in solutions, we obtain optimized structures and their heat of formation by using MM2. We will search appropriate features of molecular shapesfor induced CD.

3. Results and discussion

12 examples of *trans*-type Schiff base complexes investigated are mentioned below, molecular structures [top], crystal structures [middle], and optimized structures [bottom] as space-filling models with comments.

http://dx.doi.org/10.5772/52226

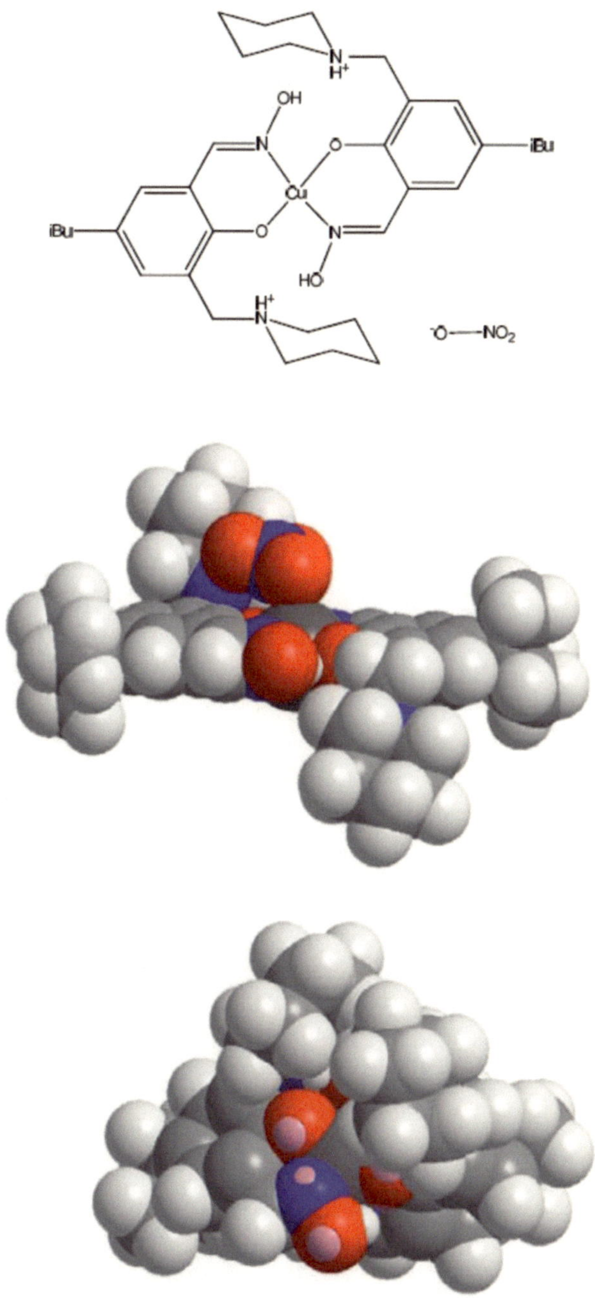

Figure 2. CCDC MIMTOS01 [16].The compound has a formula $C_{34}H_{52}CuN_4O_4^{2+}$, $2(NO_3^-)$. Novel feature mentioned is that attaching dialkylaminomethyl arms to commercial phenolic oxime copper extractants yields reagents which transport base metal salt vary efficiently by forming neutral 1:1 or 1:2 complexes with zwitterionic forms of the ligands. Apparently conformational changes were from a square planar geometry to an umbrella form and twist form (about 45 degree).

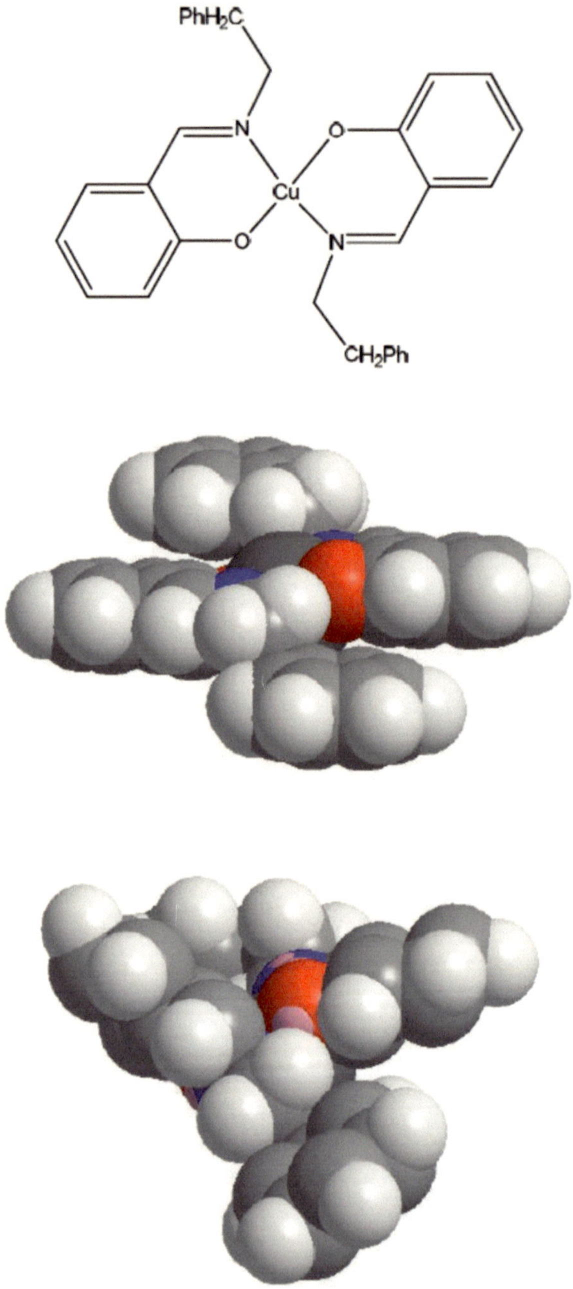

Figure 3. CCDC **MAHYEA** [17].The compound has a formula $C_{30}H_{28}CuN_2O_2$. Novel feature mentioned is that it adopts a stepped conformation and displays a square-planar *trans*-[CuN_2O_2]coordination geometry. The asymmetric unit contains two independent half molecules and each Cu atom is located on acenter of symmetry.

http://dx.doi.org/10.5772/52226

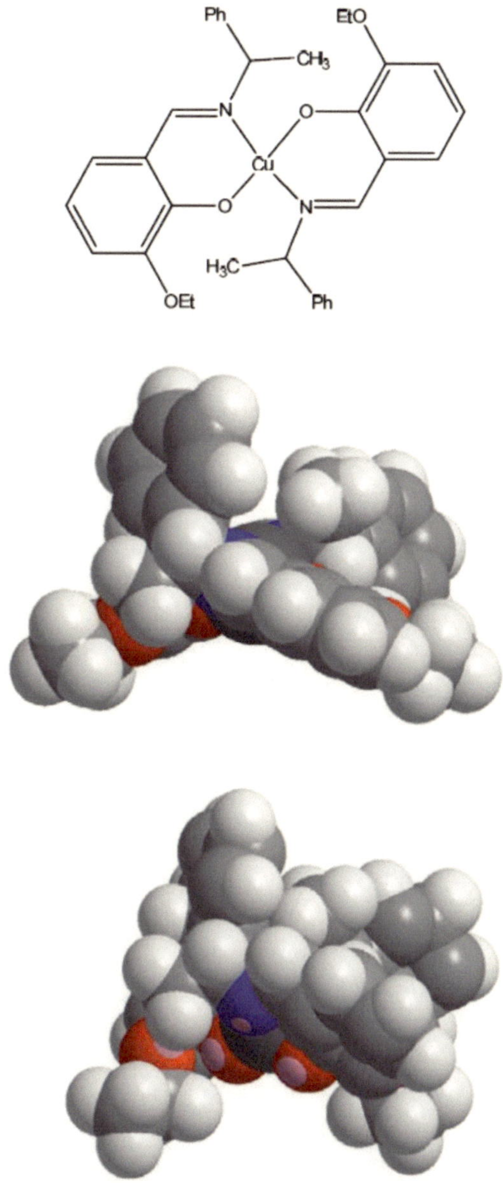

Figure 4. CCDC **MAJNIV** [18].The compound has a formula $C_{34}H_{36}CuN_2O_4$. Novel feature mentioned is that compressed tetrahedral coordination geometry with an *(R,R)*-absolute configuration. These complexes differ from one another with respect to the 1-phenylethylamine moieties, the direction of the benzene rings being inside and outside of the molecules. Apparently conformational changes were from an umbrella and twist (about 45 degree) form to same and twist (about 90 degree) form. The extended conformation of the phenethylimine pendant groups results in crystal packing formed by weakly aggregated planar molecules. Apparently conformational changes were from a relatively flat step form to a significantly sharp step form.

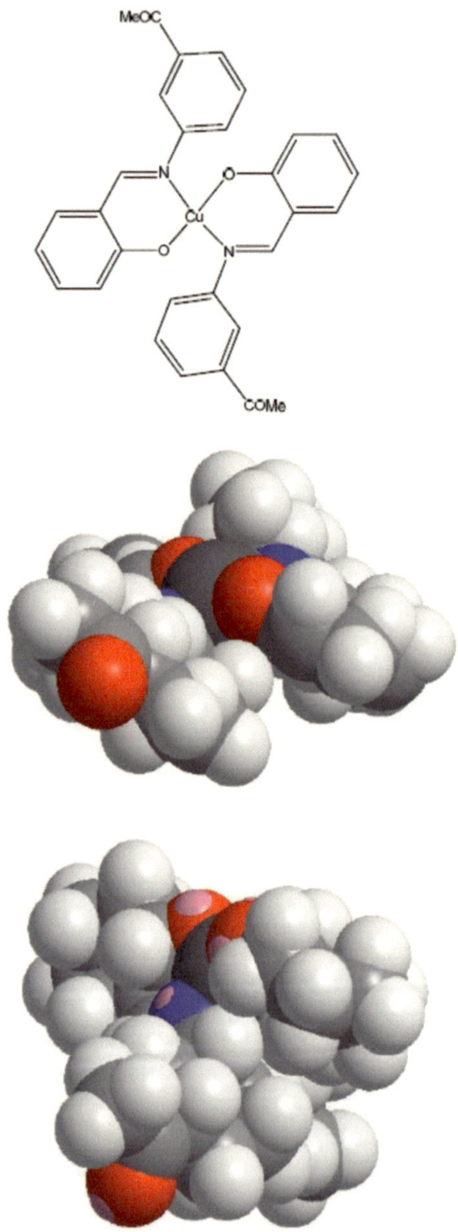

Figure 5. CCDC **MIZGIM** [19].The compound has a formula $C_{30}H_{24}CuN_2O_4$. Novel feature mentioned is that the coordination geometry around the copper atom in the complex is intermediate between square-planar and tetrahedral with two salicylaldimine ligands in trans arrangement. The molecular chains are linked via additional C-H····O hydrogen bonds to form a three-dimensional supramolecular network. Apparently conformational changes were from a moderately umbrella and slightly twist form to a twist (about 90 degree) form.

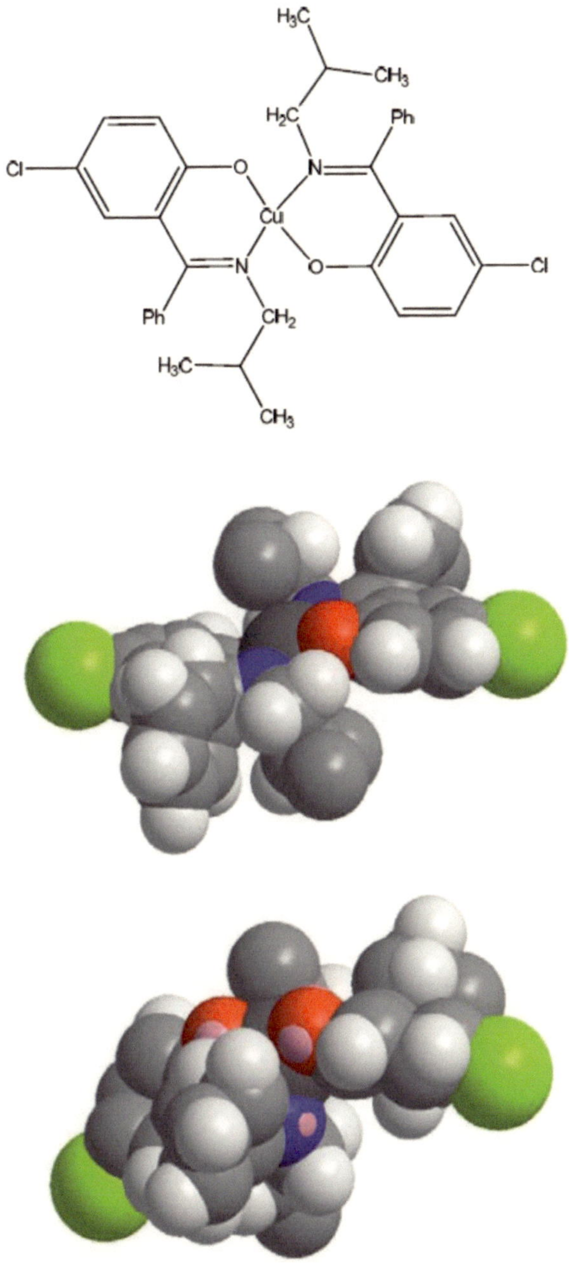

Figure 6. CCDC **IBHBCU01** [20].The compound has a formula$C_{34}H_{34}Cl_2CuN_2O_2$. Novel feature mentioned is that the isobutyl complex exists in two distinct crystalline forms, green and red. The green isomerhas the isobutyl groups pointing to the same side of the approximate [CuO_2N_2] plane. The red isomer of the isobutyl complex contains two crystallographically independent molecules having the isobutyl groups. Apparently conformational changes was from a step form to an umbrella and twist (about 90 degree) form.

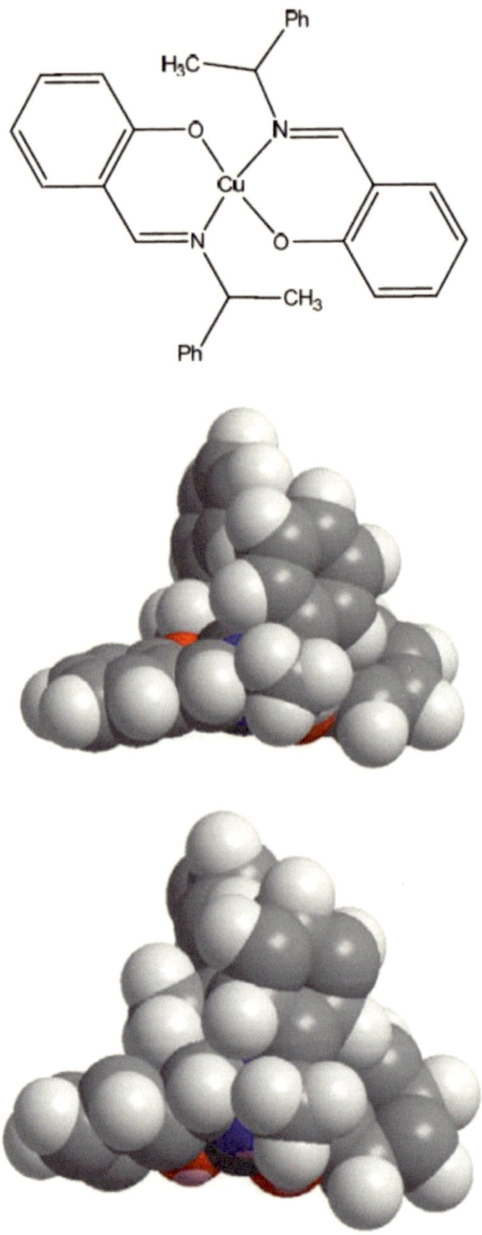

Figure 7. CCDC **DPESCU11** [21].The compound has a formula $C_{30}H_{28}CuN_2O_2$. Novel feature mentioned is that copper(II) complexes of three chiral enantiomeric pairs of o-hydroxy Schiff bases derived from (R)-(+)-1-phenylethylamineand/or (S)-(-)-1-phenylethylamine, were prepared and characterized.The geometry around the metal atom is distorted square planar. Apparently conformational change was from a twist (about 45 degree) form to a twist (about 90 degree) form.

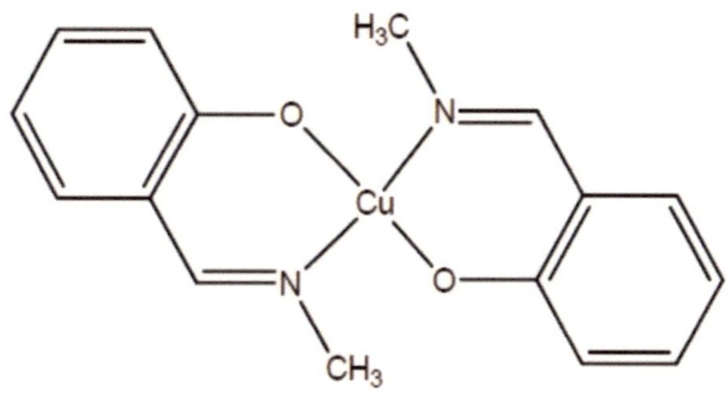

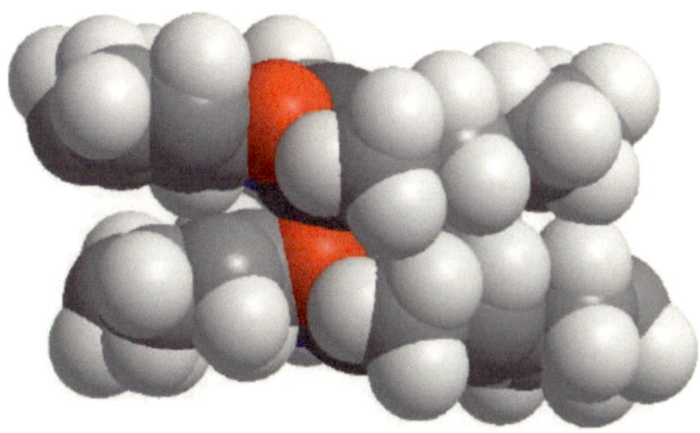

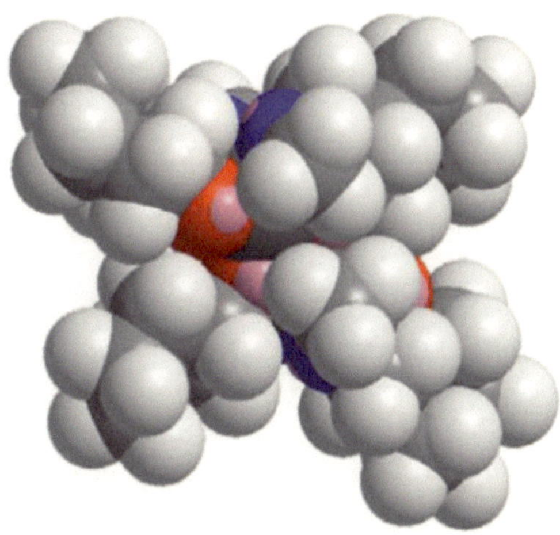

Figure 8. CCDC **MSACOP12** [22].The compound has a formula $C_{16}H_{16}CuN_2O_2$. Novel feature mentioned is that a dimeric molecule in which monomeric halves is joined by two Cu-O bondsto complete a square-pyramidal configuration about each copper atom. Distortions in the molecule are evidentlydue to the close approach of non-bonding regions. It is now seen that this compound displays three differentcoordination arrangements in its three polymorphic forms. Apparently conformational change was from a step form to an umbrella and twist (about 45 degree) form.

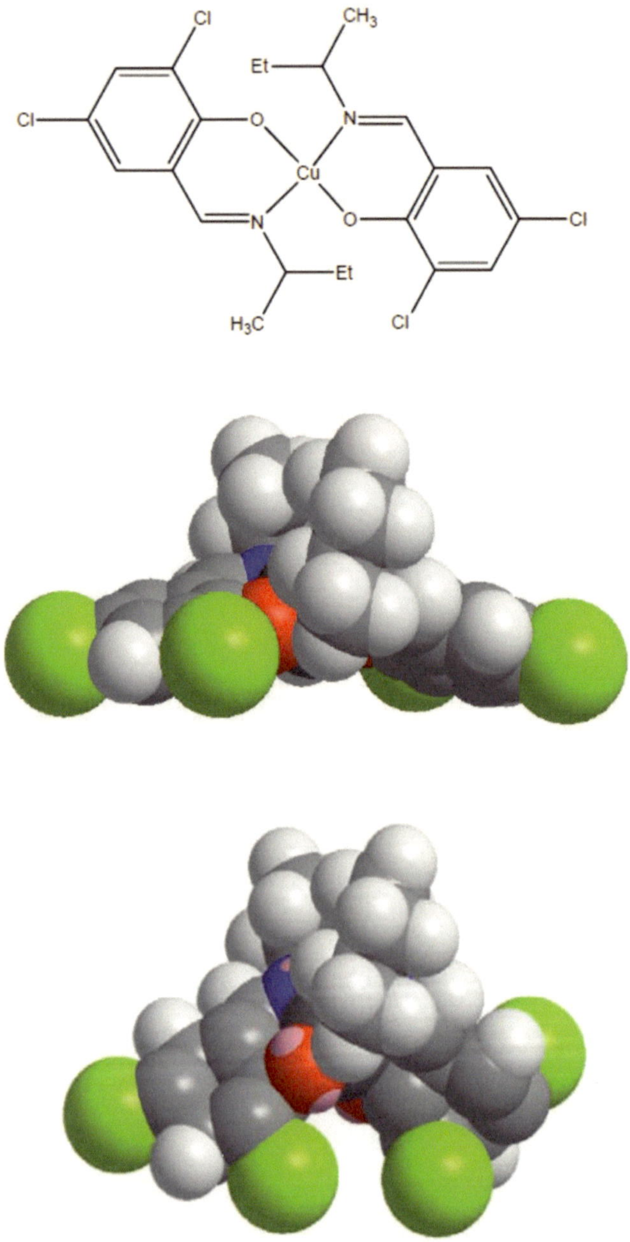

Figure 9. CCDC **MAJCUW** [23].The compound has a formula $C_{22}H_{24}Cl_4CuN_2O_2$. Novel feature mentioned is that it has a compressed tetrahedral *trans*-[CuN_2O_2] coordination environment with an umbrella conformation of the overall molecule.The absolute configuration is found to be *(S,S)* for the crystalexamined.Molecular recognition for the chiral molecules could not be carried out using hydrogen bonding because of no possible hydrogen bonding sites in the crystal packing. Apparently conformational change was from an umbrella and twist form to a twist (about 45 degree) form.

http://dx.doi.org/10.5772/52226

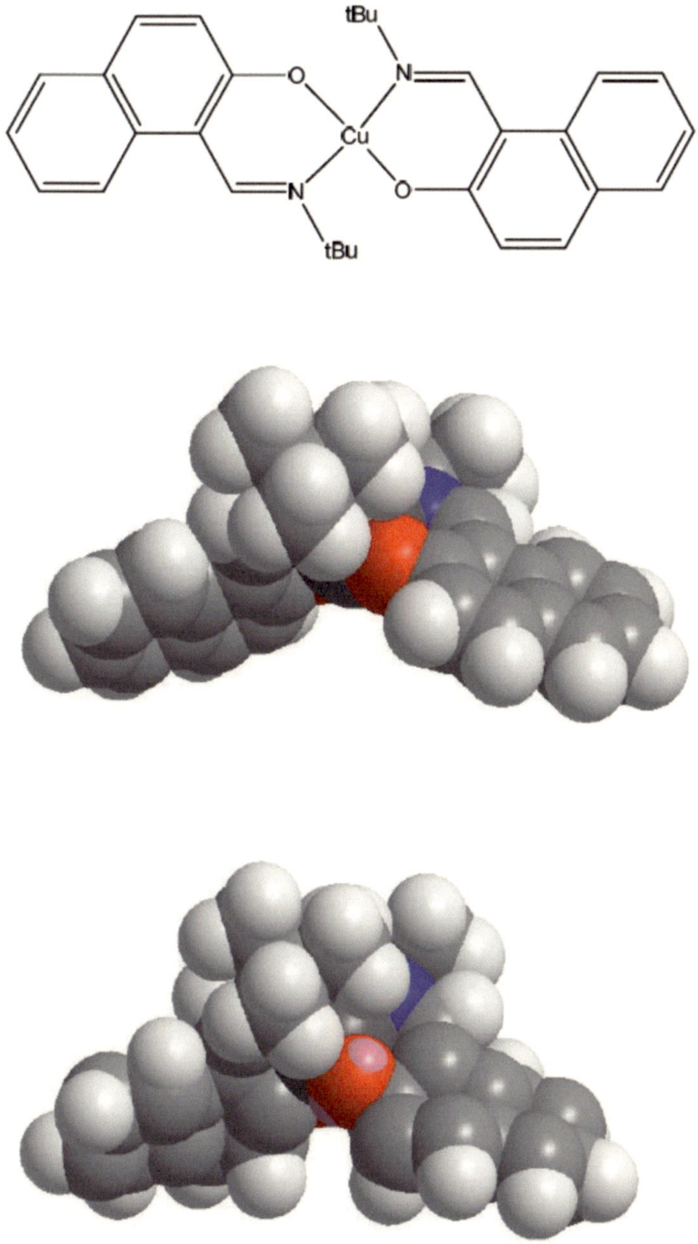

Figure 10. CCDC **KUPBIH** [24].The compound has a formula $C_{30}H_{32}CuN_2O_2$. Novel feature mentioned is that correlation between the bulkiness of the imine nitrogensubstituent, deformation of the copper coordination sphere is important and tBu group in the *N*-tBu derivative prevents such dynamic action. In the crystal, this *N*-tBu complex changes upon DFT geometry optimization to a more tetrahedralconfiguration. Apparently conformational change was from an umbrella and slightly twists form to an umbrella and twist (about 90 degree) form.

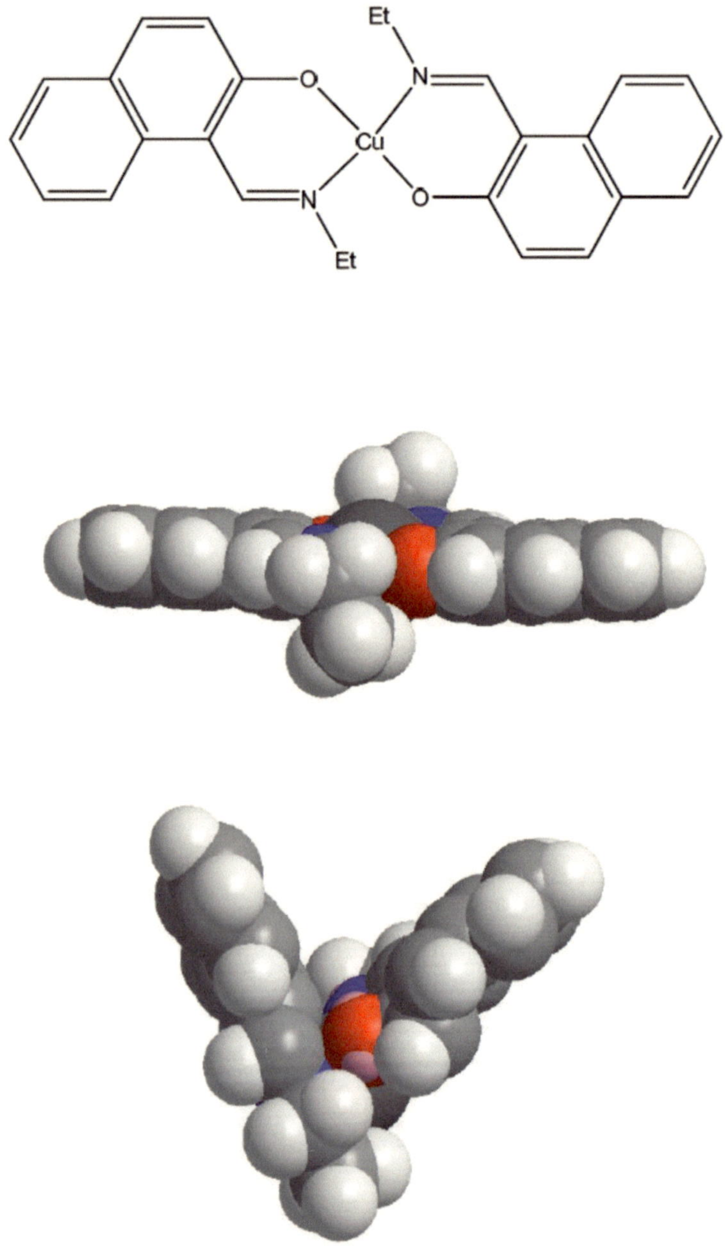

Figure 11. CCDC **KUPBON** [24].The compound has a formula $C_{26}H_{24}CuN_2O_2$. Novel feature mentioned is that the coordination sphere of the N-ethyl derivative has a flat-tetrahedral geometry. TheN–Cu–Nand O–Cu–O angles and the dihedral angle betweenthe planes N–Cu–O and N–Cu–Oin the solid state found by X-ray diffraction in this study are affected by crystalpacking forces according to these DFT calculations. Apparently conformational change was from a flat and square planar form to an umbrella and V-shaped form drastically.

http://dx.doi.org/10.5772/52226

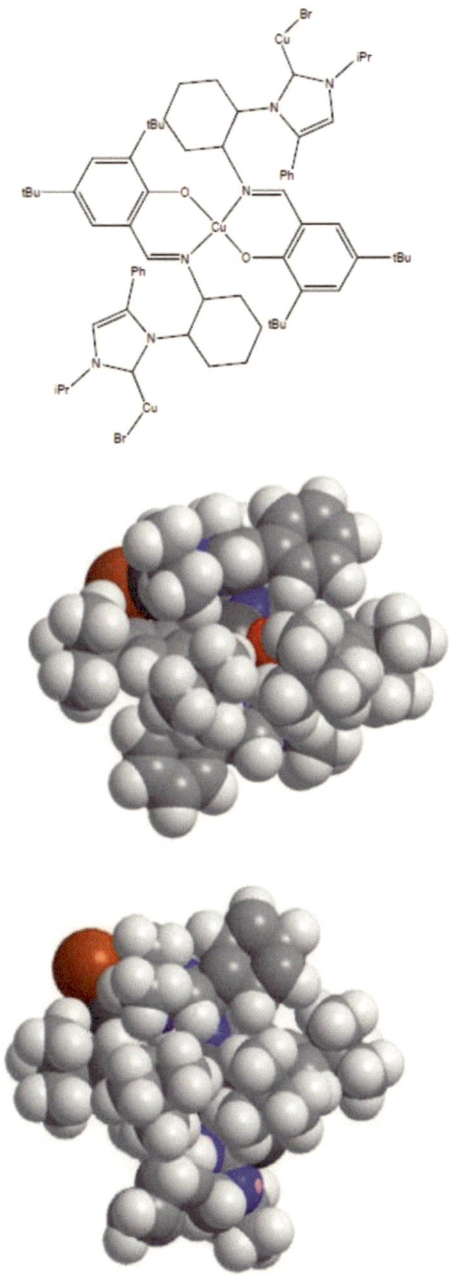

Figure 12. CCDC **YUBLAJ** [23].The compound has a formula $C_{66}H_{88}Br_2Cu_3N_6O_2$. Novel feature mentioned is that it appears that problematic deprotonation of the phenol to give a chelating or bridging ligand is the primary reason for the observed instability based on the stability of related copper NHC–aryl oxide compounds (including mixed valence Cu(I)/Cu(II) centers Cu(I) sites in ligands) Apparently conformational change was from a step and slightly twist form to an umbrella and twist (about 90 degree) form.

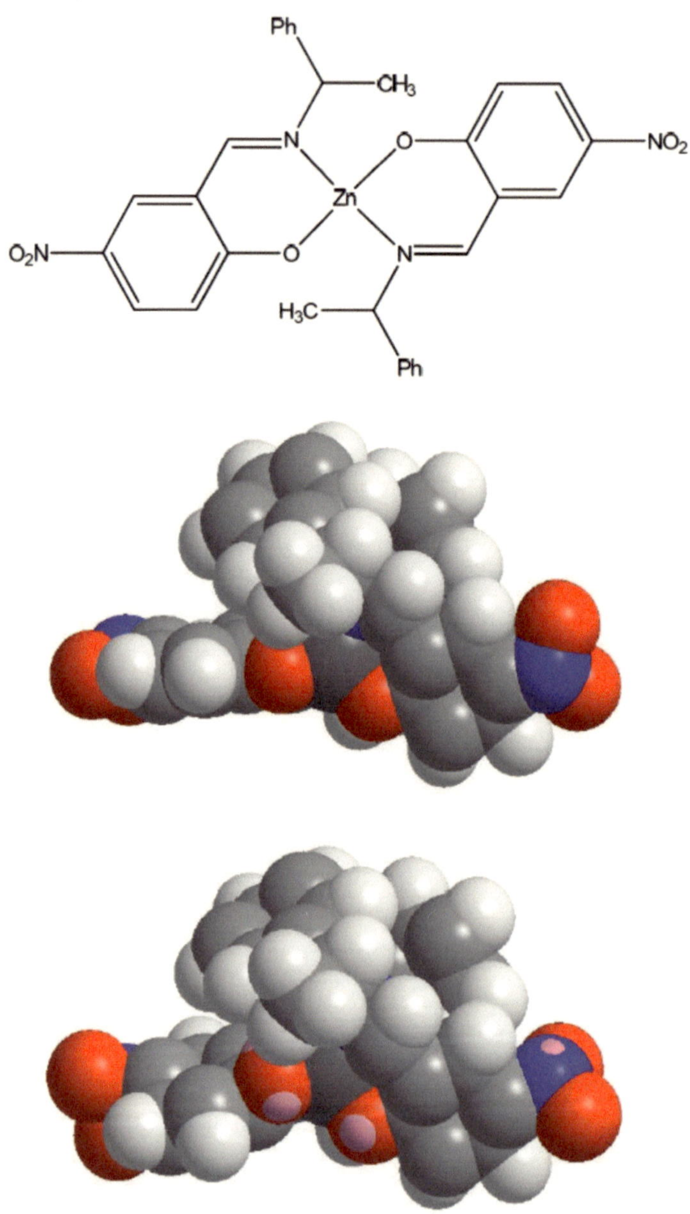

Figure 13. CCDC **METSUZ** [24].The compound has a formula $C_{30}H_{26}N_4O_6Zn$. Novel feature mentioned is that it crystallizes in the noncentrosymmetric space groups. The geometry around the Zn(II) metalcenter is pseudo-tetrahedral with two oxygen and two nitrogen atoms from the ligands and has the Λ absoluteconfiguration. Apparently conformational change was slight, namely it remained a twist (about 90 degree) from.

In principle, induced CD is caused by non-contact interactions between (electric) dipole moments of chiral additives and achiral materials. Because it is an electromagnetic phenomenon essentially, contact intermolecular interactions, in other words molecular recognition, may not be an important factor for it. However, the experimental facts that only complexes with specific ligands or metal ions (which determine their coordination geometries) suggested that induced CD appears under appropriate steric (as well as stereochemical) conditions for metal complexes. One of the important factors of steric factors for metal complexes may be distance between (electric) dipole moments at the surface achiral materials which keep their shapes rigidly. The reason for this assumption is that both metallodendrimers metal and nanoparticles have approximately spherical shapes essentially even surrounded in softmaters.

As for biomolecules such as proteins, however, CD spectra are used for monitoring folding or unfolding of peptide chains after binding small molecules of metal complexes [25]. This different phenomenon is not classified into the induced CD mentioned in this article. By including small molecules into proteins with weakly supramolecular forces, molecules of proteins change their molecular conformation, which attributed to shift of strong π–π^* bands of C=O moieties electronic or CD spectra. This docking mechanism is directly molecular recognition accompanying with conformational changes of proteins as well as small molecules, which is also confirmed by quenching of fluorescence intensity due to energy transfer.

In contrast, non-contact interactions of (electric) dipole moments for CD spectra have complicated problems. Our preliminary results of CD spectra of chiral Schiff base metal complexes in viscous solutions dissolved a certain protein exhibited concentration dependence of so-called artifact peaks of solid-state CD spectra [26]. The artifact CD peaks are attributed to anisotropic molecular orientation and removed in matrix environment which permits molecular rotation isotropically accompanying with (magnetic) dipole moments of chiral molecules [27]. Therefore,not only CD spectra of chiral molecules in anisotropically oriented matrix such as biomolecules but also induced CD bands involving softmaters is still an open question.

4. Conclusion

As summarized in Figure 1[right], according to chemical structures, Zn(II) center and naphtylgroups are suitable factors for induced CD, while 3,5-dichlorosalycilaldehyde moieties are not regardless of common factors. Previous study [11] revealed that in optimized structure, naphtylgroups act as largely spread planar parts outside of a molecular face, which plays an important role in induced CD for this case. In the present study, compounds having identical features were also investigated in view of optimized structures. According to not only3,5-dichlorosalycilaldehyde moieties (**IBHBCU01** and **MAJCUW**) but also tert-Bu-groups (**MIMTOS01** and **YUBLAJ**), EtO- groups (**MAJNIV**), and NO_2- groups (**METSUZ**) gave significantly large steric hindrance resulting in steric repulsion between ligands. However, specific geometry could not be induced by bulky groups. Generally, Zn(II) complexes afford a tetrahedral coordination geometry, which prevents from forming flatten planar molecular shapes in view of ligands. Therefore, these two factors may not be definitive factors solely. On the other hand, besides in amine parts (Figure 1), naphtylgroups in aldehyde parts (**KUPBIH** and **KUPBON**) are also keeping appropriate conditions, namely largely spread planar parts outside of a molecular face. As far as in the sense of molecular recognition, it has advantage for penetrating into inside of dendrimer as well as contacting to the surface of metal nano-particles. Further experimental and/or theoretical investigation including electric factors will be necessary to understand deeply.

Author details

Takashiro Akitsu and Chigusa Kominato

Department of Chemistry, Faculty of Science, Tokyo University of Science, Tokyo, Japan

References

[1] Yamada, S. (1999). Advancement in stereochemical aspects of Schiff base metal complexes. Coord. chem. rev. 190-192:, 537 EOF.

[2] Yamada, S., & Takeuchi, A. (1982). The conformation and interconversion of schiff base complexes of nickel(II) and copper(II). Coord. chem. rev. , 43, 187-204.

[3] Yamada, S., Ohno, E., Kuge, Y., Takeuchi, A., Yamanouchi, K., & Iwasaki, K. (1968). Schiff base nickel(II) complexes with coordination number exceeding four. Coord. chem. rev. , 3, 247-254.

[4] Yamada, S. (1967). The visible and ultraviolet spectra of d6-, d7- and d8-metal ions in trigonalbipyramidal complexes. Coord. chem. rev. , 2, 83-98.

[5] Yamada, S. (1966). Recent aspects of the stereochemistry of Schiff-base-metal complexes.Coord. chem. rev. , 1, 415-437.

[6] Govorov, A. O., Fan, Z., Hernandez, P., Slocik, J. M., & Naik, R. R. (2010). Theory of Circular Dichroism of Nanomaterials Comprising Chiral Molecules and Nanocrystals: Plasmon Enhancement, Dipole Interactions, and Dielectric Effects. Nano lett. , 10, 1374-1382.

[7] Abdulrahman, N. A., Fan, Z., Tonooka, T., Kelly, S. M., Gadegaard, N., Hendry, E., Govorov, A. O., & Kadodwala, M. (2012). Induced Chirality through Electromagnetic Coupling between Chiral Molecular Layers and Plasmonic Nanostructures. Nano lett. , 12, 977-983.

[8] Akitsu, T., Uchida, N., Aritake, Y., Yamaguchi, J., & (200, . (2008). Induced d-d Bands in CD Spectra due to Chiral Transfer from Chiral Nickel(II) Complexes to Achiral Copper(II) Complexes and Application for Structural Estimation. Trend. inorg. chem. , 10, 41-49.

[9] Akitsu, T., Yamaguchi, J., Uchida, N., & Aritake, . Y((2009). The Studies of Conditions for Inducing Chirality to Cu(II) Complexes by Chiral Zn(II) and Ni(II) Complexes with Schiff Base. Res. lett. mater. sci. 484172.

[10] Akitsu, T., Yamaguchi, J., Aritake, Y., Hiratsuka, T., & Uchida, N(201. N((2010). Observation of enhanced CD bands of metal complexes, metallodendrimers, and metal clusters by chiral Schiff base metal complexes. Int. j. curr. chem. , 1, 1-6.

[11] Akitsu, T., & Uchida, N(201. N((2010). Induced d-d bands in CD spectra of solution of chiral Schiff base nickel(II) complex and ferrocene. Asian chem.lett. , 14, 21-28.

[12] Aritake, Y., Nakayama, T., Nishizuru, H., & Akitsu, T. ((2011). Observation of induced CD on CdSenano-particles from chiral Schiff base Ni(II), Cu(II), Zn(II) complexes. Inorg. chem. commun. , 14, 423-425.

[13] Kimura, N., Nishizuru, H., & Akitsu, T. unpublished results.

[14] Yamaguchi, J., & Akitsu, T(201. T((2011). Molecular recognition of chiral Schiff base metal complexes for induced CD bands to metallodendrimers. Int. j. curr. chem. , 2, 165-172.

[15] Cambridge Structural Database System, Cambridge Crystallographic Data Centre, University Chemical Laboratory, Cambridge, UK.

[16] Forgan, R. S., Davidson, J. E., Galbraith, S. G., Henderson, D. K., Parsons, S., Tasker, P. A., & White, F. J. (2008). Transport of metal salts by zwitterionic ligands; simple but highlyefficient salicylaldoximeextractants.Chem.commun. , 4049-4051.

[17] Akitsu, T., Einaga, Y., (200, , Bis, N-2 -phenylethyl-salicydenaminato-k. N., & O)copper, I. (2004). Bis(N-2-phenylethyl-salicydenaminato-k^{2}N,O)copper(II). Acta. crystallogr. E60:m1555-m1557.

[18] Akitsu, T., Einaga, Y., (200, , Bis[-N-(1-phenyl-ethyl)salicylideneaminato-k, R)-3 5 -dichloro., O]copper, N., & , I. (2004). Bis[(R)-3,5-dichloro-N-(1-phenyl-ethyl)salicylideneaminato-k^{2}N,O]copper(II) andbis[(R)-3-ethoxy-N-(1-phenylethyl)salicylideneaminato-k^{2}N,O]copper(II). Acta. crystallogr. E60:m640-m642.

[19] Banerjee, S., Mukherjee, A. K., Banerjee, I., De Neumann, R. L., & Louer, L. (2005). Synthesis, spectroscopic studies and ab-initio structuredetermination from X-ray powder diffraction ofbis-(N-acetophenylsalicylaldiminato)copper(II).Cryst.res.technol. 4815-4821., 3.

[20] Chia, P. C., Freyberg, D. P., Mockler, G. M., & Sinn, E. (1977). Synthesis and Properties ofBis[N-R- (5-chloro- a-phenyl- 2-hydroxybenzylidene) aminatolcopper (11) Complexesand Crystal and Molecular Structures of the Derivatives with R = mButyl and R =Isobutyl (Two Structural Isomers).Inorg.chem., 16, 254-264.

[21] Fernandez-G, J. M., Ausbun-Valdes, C., & Gonzalez-Guerrero, Toscano. R. A. (2007). Characterization and Crystal Structure of some Schiff Base Copper(II)Complexes derived from Enantiomeric Pairs of Chiral Amines. Z.anorg.allg.chem., 633, 1251-1256.

[22] Hall, D., Sheat, S. V., & Waters, T. TN((1968). The Colour Isomerism and Structure of Some Copper Co-ordinationCompounds. Part XV1.l The Crystal Structure of the gama-Form of Bis-(N-methyfsalicylaldiminato)copper(II). J. chem.soc.A , 460-463.

[23] Akitsu, T., & Einaga, Y. (2004). Bis[(S)-N-(2-butyl)-dichlorosalicylideneaminato-k^2N,O]copper(II). Acta. crystallogr. E60:m1605-m1607., 3, 5.

[24] Villagran, M., Caruso, F., Rossi, M., Zagal, J. H., & Costamagna, J. (2010). Substituent Effects on Structural, Electronic, and Redox Properties ofBis(N-alkyl-2 -oxy-1-naphthaldiminato)copper(II) Complexes Revisited-Inequivalence in Solid- and Solution-State Structures by ElectronicSpectroscopy and X-ray Diffraction Explained by DFT. Eu. r. j.inorg.chem. 1373-1380.

[25] Simonovic, A., Whitwood, A. C., Clegg, W., Harrington, R. W., Hursthouse, M. B., Male, L., & Douthwaite, R. E. (2009). Synthesis of Copper(I) Complexes of N-Heterocyclic Carbene-Phenoxyimine/amine Ligands: Structures of Mononuclear Copper(II), Mixed-ValenceCopper(I)/(II), and Copper(II) Cluster Complexes. Eur.j.inorg.chem. , 1786-1795.

[26] Evans, C., & Luneau, D. (2002). New Schiff base zinc(II) complexes exhibiting second harmonicgeneration.J. chem.soc.,daltontrans. , 83-86.

[27] Ray, A., Seth, B. K., Pal, U., & Basu, S. (2012). Nickel(II)-Schiff base complex recognizing domain II of bovine and human serum albumin: Spectroscopic and docking studies. spectrochimicaacta A. , 92, 164-174.

[28] Hayashi, T., & Akitsu, T. Unpublished results ("Environmental effect on CD spectra of chiral Schiff base 3d-4f complexes"presented in the 40th International Conference on Coordination Chemistry, (2012). Spain).

[29] Okamoto, Y., Nidaira, K., & Akitsu, T. (2011). Environmental Dependence of Artifact CD Peaks of Chiral Schiff Base 3d-4f Complexes inSoftmater PMMA Matrix. Int.j.mol. sci. , 12, 6966-6979.